PROFESSIONAL NURSING

*Foundations, Perspectives
and Relationships*

PROFESSIONAL NURSING

Foundations, Perspectives and Relationships

EUGENIA KENNEDY SPALDING, R.N., M.A., D.H.L.

Professor Emeritus, Teacher's College, Columbia University; Formerly Special Consultant International Cooperation Administration, Washington, D.C.; Professor of Nursing Education, Division of Nursing Education, Teacher's College, Columbia University; Director, Division of Nursing Education, Indiana University, Bloomington, Ind.; Associate Professor of Nursing Education, School of Nursing Education, The Catholic University of America, Washington, D.C.; Associate Director (Lt. Colonel), U.S. Cadet Nurse Corps, Public Health Service, Federal Security Agency, Washington, D.C.

LUCILLE E. NOTTER, R.N., M.A., ED.D.

Editor, Nursing Research *and Editor,* International Nursing Index; *Formerly Adjunct Associate Professor, Department of Nursing Education, Hunter College of the City University of New York*

EIGHTH EDITION

J. B. LIPPINCOTT COMPANY
Philadelphia and Toronto

Preface

The eighth edition of this book, like all previous editions, is presented as a guide to an understanding of the major trends and problems affecting nursing—historical, political, social, economic, legal, educational, professional, and personal. It is not intended to offer solutions to all problems. In fact, following each chapter current problems are presented which have been selected to extend the student's thinking on the chapter content. Additional reading from among the references at the end of the chapter will also be helpful in dealing with these problems.

Three new chapters have been written for this edition, 2 of which are an addition to the book and 1 of which replaces a previous chapter. The additions are Chapter 4, *Responsibility for Nursing Practice,* and Chapter 23, *American Nurses' Foundation.* Chapter 6, *Legal Issues in Nursing Practice,* is a new chapter written for this edition by the well-known authority on nursing and the law, Nathan Hershey, Research Professor of Health Law at the University of Pittsburgh and the author of many articles on the various aspects of law and the nurse. This chapter replaces the former one on *Legal Problems, Responsibilities and Relationships.*

The book continues to be organized into 4 parts, but the chapters have been reorganized somewhat in order to present the material, especially the new content, in the most logical sequence. Many new and interesting illustrations have been added.

Besides the addition of the new chapters, extensive revisions have been made in the other chapters. The social setting as it affects and is affected by nursing is presented. Consideration has been given to the current status and responsibilities of the nursing profession. Trends in patterns of nursing service and nursing education are presented together with emerging functions of the various types of personnel in nursing. Throughout the book historical influences are pointed out in order to add this dimension to the thinking about current trends and problems. The problems and references at the end of each chapter also bring into perspective the historical foundations, as well as significant emerging trends. It is recommended that current reference material be constantly added to each phase of the book, especially from periodical literature.

As stated before, the book is divided into 4 parts, with a preview preceeding each part. Students are encouraged to read the previews before proceeding to the chapters because these overall views provide orientation for the reader.

Part One consists of 3 chapters dealing with nursing as a profession, its historical background and its present social setting. Chapter 1, *Historical Foundations of the Profession of Nursing*, discusses the influence of the past on the events of today, thus gives perspective to the consideration of current problems and relationships. This chapter traces the significant major influences on nursing from ancient to present times, using broad strokes to paint the picture of nursing and the relationship of the past to the present. *Chapter 2, Professional Nursing in Its Present Social Setting*, has been revised in the light of current social and political changes in our country and the world and the corresponding changes in the responsibilities and problems facing the health professions. Chapter 3, *Nursing as a Profession*, was also revised considerably in terms of the current status of nursing as a profession. Chapter 4, *Responsibility for Nursing Practice*, a completely new chapter, deals mainly with the individual nurse's responsibility for her practice and the responsibility of other groups, such as employment agencies and society as a whole, to provide adequate nursing services and to strive for improvement of these services. The importance of developing a philosophy of nursing which will insure ethical and technically competent nursing care is stressed. Characteristics of effective modern practice are reviewed and examples given.

Part Two, *Legal, Professional and Personal Problems and Relationships*, includes the new chapter, *Legal Issues in Nursing Practice*, which deals in a very practical way with the legal issues nurses face when they practice their profession. The section on liability as it applies to the various positions in nursing is especially relevant today in view of the accent on the nurse's legal responsibility for her own acts. The other 2 chapters in Part Two, *Problem Solving: A Major Activity of the Professional Nurse* and *Relationships and Personal Growth*, have been considerably revised in light of current concepts and trends.

Part Three, *Choosing, Preparing for, and Succeeding in a Field of Nursing*, has been expanded to include material on additional fields of health work. All chapters in this section have been greatly revised in line with modern changes in the provision of nursing services and in nursing education. Chapter 8, *General Survey of Occupational Opportunities for Nurses*, reflects many of these changes, including those occasioned by the fact that so large a proportion of nursing service is now provided by part-time workers, many of whom are married and carry family responsibilities. Chapter 9, *Fields of Work in Nursing Services*, has undergone many revisions to make the material current. Chapter 10, *Fields of Work in Nursing Education, Consultation, Research and Professional Organizations*, also includes much new material. Chapter 12 has a new and more descriptive title, *Nurses in the Federal Government*. It has been considerably revised and reflects the many changes which have occurred in these services. Because of advances in programs for assistance and care during national disasters. Chapter 13, *Nurses in a National Disaster or Emergency*, was rewritten with the assistance of Jean E. Lazar, Nurse Consultant Training, from the Division of Health Mobilization Services and Mental Health, Public Health Service, U.S. Department of Health, Education, and Welfare. All other chapters, (14, 15 and 16) in this section have been carefully revised to bring them up-to-date.

Part Four, *Organizations and Related Activities,* like the 3 previous parts of the book, reflects many revisions required by the changes that have characterized nursing. Several chapters have been almost completely re-written; these are Chapter 18, *National Student Nurses' Association of the United States of America,* Chapter 20, *American Nurses' Association,* Chapter 21, *National League for Nursing,* Chapter 26, *American National Red Cross,* and Chapter 27, *Legislation Affecting Nursing.* The new Chapter 23, describing the origin and development of the American Nurses' Foundation, is part of this section.

The Appendix continues to include a valuable and up-to-date guide to reference tools for nurses and a suggested form for minutes.

The authors hope that this eighth edition will be as helpful as preceding editions and that it will have the same cordial reception by students and teachers of nursing, members of the nursing profession and of allied profes-sions and by the public.

EUGENIA K. SPALDING

LUCILLE E. NOTTER

Note to Students

The suggested problems following each chapter will require additional reading from among the references listed at the end of the chapter, as well as from current literature. Interviews with experts in various fields of concern could also be most helpful.

Preface to First Edition

In the preparation for a nursing career there are several periods where nursing students need special help in solving professional problems and in learning how to establish fine relationships. There are two stages, however, where it is necessary to provide more definite opportunity for them to raise problems, to consider and solve them, and to have some experience that will aid them in making good personal and professional adjustments. One of these is upon admission to the school of nursing, when the students are first entering upon a new vocation, and the other is just before graduation, when they are preparing to go out into the world to practice as graduate professional nurses. It is with this second stage of the nurse's life in the school of nursing that this book deals.

This edition of *Professional Adjustments in Nursing* is designed to be used by senior students in schools of nursing offering the basic curriculum, under the direction of the instructor who is responsible for coordinating their planned experiences. It is based upon and is an outgrowth of the work which the author did in connection with a publication of the National League of Nursing Education in 1933,[1] and in the preparation of the course of study on "Professional Adjustments II" that is included in *A Curriculum Guide for Schools of Nursing*.[2]

When the author became interested in this subject several years ago she made several studies among graduate and nursing students to determine their problems and needs and what they believed might have helped them to make better personal, professional and social adjustments. A vast amount of enlightening and interesting comments was collected. It is upon the materials collected from this and several other groups that a large part of the content of this book is based.

All of the materials have been tested through actual discussions with nursing students in the classroom, graduate nurses, or experts in the various fields treated in the text.

This book is being presented as a text for senior nursing students and as a reference for graduate nurses, with the idea that it will be used as a nucleus from which to work and as a guide to other helpful sources.

Since one of the principal aims of the course is to keep in touch with contemporary social and professional trends, it is suggested that the reference

[1] F. K. Spalding, *A Suggested Vocational Guidance Program for Schools of Nursing*, New York, National League of Nursing Education, 1935.

[2] National League of Nursing Education, Committee on Curriculum, *A Curriculum Guide for Schools of Nursing*. New York, The League, 1937, pp. 270-292.

lists be added to constantly from the related currently published books, other types of literature, and especially periodicals.

The material has been organized in units, each of which covers an important aspect of the study of professional adjustments in nursing. A list of these units may be found in the table of contents.

It is assumed that students in some schools of nursing, because of their past experience, could omit certain units if they have covered the materials. This applies particularly to the Introduction, the content of which is usually included before the undergraduate nursing student reaches her senior year. It is also assumed that, in addition to the problems raised in this text, other problems, issues, and situations will be brought from the students' own past and present experience for discussion.

A statement of the guiding objectives, as formulated in light of the evident needs of graduate professional nurses and senior nursing students in schools of nursing offering basic curricula, may be helpful to both teachers and students to understand the distinctive purposes of this text. For that reason they are included here.

OBJECTIVES OF THE COURSE

1. "To learn to use intelligently the resources of current literature and other means which will help [you] in continued growth and in successful adjustment [in the profession of nursing]."[3]

2. To get a bird's-eye view of nursing in the present social and economic situation so you will appreciate the social and professional responsibilities of the professional worker.

3. "To [learn] the [vocational] opportunities open to the professional nurse and the qualifications [required] in the main branches of nursing; and to make a vocational plan based upon . . . a careful analysis of [your] own interests and qualifications [and the requirements of the various types of work which you will study in attempting to make a wise vocational choice]."[4]

4. To understand more fully what brings success or failure in any type of work, and to appreciate the important practices in securing and resigning from positions.

5. To understand and appreciate your professional activities and the responsibilities as a graduate professional nurse to yourself, to your own and other professional groups, to society and to your Creator.

6. "[To become acquainted with some of the personal and professional problems with which you might be confronted as a graduate nurse]; to acquire some facility in analyzing and judging situations which [you] are likely to meet in professional life; and to learn some of the principles and

[3] *Ibid.,* p. 274.
[4] *Op. cit.*

[practices that can be used as a guide in dealing with various types of professional problems and situations]."[5]

7. To realize that it is through your own self-directed reasoning and effort, based upon a sound religious and professional philosophy, that you will be able to make fine personal and professional adjustments.

EUGENIA KENNEDY SPALDING.

January, 1939
The Catholic University of America
Washington, D.C.

[5] *Ibid.*

Acknowledgments

Acknowledgments and thanks are given to the following who have given suggestions on content, references and illustrations: Helen H. Augustin, Office Nurse; Anne L. Austin, Nursing Historian; Florence C. Austin, Executive Director, Visiting Nurse Association of Hartford, Inc.; Lois M. Austin, Professor of Nursing Education, University of Pittsburgh School of Nursing; Edward G. Benz, Director of Nursing, Wilmington Medical Center; Elsie T. Berdan, Chief, Nursing Branch, Office of Professional Services, Division of Direct Health Services, Public Health Service, U.S. Department of Health, Education, and Welfare; Mary E. Brackett, Associate Director, Nursing Service, Hartford Hospital; Viola C. Bredenberg, Nursing Service Consultant, The Catholic Hospital Association; Mary Louise Brown, Chief Nurse, Occupational Health Program, National Center for Urban and Industrial Health, Public Health Service, U.S. Department of Health, Education, and Welfare; Elizabeth Cantwell, Director, Economic Security Unit, American Nurses' Association (ANA); Josephine A. Cipolla, Nursing Staff Coordinator, Bell Telephone of New York; Shirley S. Chater, Associate Professor, University of California (San Francisco) School of Nursing; Luther Christman, Dean, Vanderbilt University School of Nursing, and Director of Nursing, Vanderbilt Hospital; Helen V. Connors, Director, Government Relations Department, ANA; Mrs. A. Lionne Conta, Executive Director, California Nurses Association; Laurel A. Copp, Associate Professor, Department of Nursing, College of Human Development, Pennsylvania State University; Helen Creighton, Nursing Consultant, Barnes Hospital, St. Louis; Mrs. Bertha Cunliff, Executive Secretary, Alameda County Nurses Association, California; Elizabeth V. Cunningham, Associate Editor, *Perspectives in Psychiatric Care;* Alice W. Davies, Nurse Specialist, Medical Division, U.S. Department of State; E. Mae Davis, Administrative Assistant, Department of Nursing, St. Anselm's College; Doris DeVincenzo, Director, International Affairs, ANA; Mrs. Madolin M. Dickinson, Director, Nursing Education and Licenses, Colorado State Board of Nursing; Ann E. Donovan, Director, Professional Credentials and Personnel Service (PC&PS), Massachusetts Nurses Association; Margery E. Drake, Executive Secretary, Conference of Catholic Schools of Nursing; Laura C. Dustan, Dean, College of Nursing, University of Iowa; Mrs. Evelyn B. Ferguson, Director, PC&PS, ANA; Martha C. Forejt, Office Nurse, Lavonne M. Frey, Director of Nursing, St. Elizabeths Hospital, Washington, D.C.; Mary Ann Garrigan, Professor of Nursing and Curator,

Nursing Archives, Boston University; Betty Pitt Geiger, Office Nurse; Doris A. Geitgey, Associate Professor and Project Director of Kellogg Foundation Grant for Associate Degree Nursing Programs, University of Washington School of Nursing; Agnes Gelinas, Executive Secretary, Nursing Education Alumni Association, Teachers College, Columbia University; Lucy D. Germain, Associate Administrator, Pennsylvania Hospital; Elizabeth S. Gill, Associate Dean, Department of Nursing, Faculty of Medicine, Columbia University; Mrs. Marjorie B. Glaser, Assistant Educational Director, St. Joseph Infirmary School of Nursing; Stella Goostray, Nursing Historian (Deceased May 8, 1969); A. Welsey Handy, Benedict and Benedict Insurance; Eva E. Hansen, Nurse in Private Practice; Mrs. Ruth W. Harper, Executive Director, District 14, New York State Nurses Association; Evelyn Harrison, Deputy Director, Bureau of Policies and Standards, U.S. Civil Service Commission; Margaret Harty, Director, Division of Nursing Education, National League for Nursing (NLN); Alice Haywood, Writer-Editor, Public Health Service, U.S. Department of Health, Education, and Welfare; Kenneth F. Herrold, Professor of Psychology, Teachers College, Columbia University; Nathan Hershey, Esq., Research Professor of Health Law, Department of Public Health Practice, Graduate School of Public Health, University of Pittsburgh; Elizabeth Hilborn, Chief Nurse Advisor, Office of International Health, Public Health Service, U.S. Department of Health, Education and Welfare; Historical Unit, U.S. Army Medical Service, Walter Reed Army Medical Center; Col. Ethel A. Hoefly, Chief, Air Force Nurse Corps, Office of the Surgeon General, U.S. Air Force; Aileen I. Hogan, Executive Secretary, American College of Nurse-Midwifery; Thelma Ingles, Consultant for Nursing, Rockefeller Foundation; Lucy Johns, National Director, Nursing Programs, American National Red Cross; Clifford H. Jordan, Assistant Professor, Graduate Division, University of Pennsylvania School of Nursing; Angie C. Kammeraad, Institutional Nursing Consultant, Region IV, Public Health Service, U.S. Department of Health, Education, and Welfare; Jane D. Keeler, Executive Director, Visiting Nurse Association of New Haven; Dorothy N. Kelly, Executive Director, National Council of Catholic Nurses; Katherine W. Kendall, Chief, Nursing Section, Children's Bureau, Social and Rehabilitation Service, U.S. Department of Health, Education, and Welfare; Robert E. Kennedy, Associate Editor, Chicago Sun-Times; Virginia Stewart Keyes, Houston, Texas; Marion M. Klappmeier, formerly Executive Director, New York State Nurses Association; Anne Kloiber, Supervising Nurse, Pabst Brewing Company; Mrs. Florence Knowles, Consultant, Division of Training, Rehabilitation Services Administration, Social and Rehabilitation Service, U.S. Department of Health, Education, and Welfare; Col. Ethel R. Kovach, Former Chief, Air Force Nurse Corps, Office of the Surgeon General, U.S. Air Force (retired); William A. Lang, Executive Director, D.C. Nurses Association; Jean E. Lazar, Nurse Consultant, Training, Division of Health Mobilization, Health Services and Mental Health Administration,

Public Health Service, U.S. Department of Health, Education, and Welfare; Barbara J. Lee, Associate Program Director, W. K. Kellogg Foundation; Dolores E. Little, Professor, University of Washington School of Nursing; Mary Jane McCarthy, Director, Nursing Service, Veterans Administration; Audrey M. McCluskey, Associate Director, Visiting Nurse Association of New Haven; Margaret McLaughlin, Assistant Surgeon General, Chief Nurse Officer, Public Health Service, U.S. Department of Health, Education, and Welfare; Florence A. McQuillen, Executive Director, American Association of Nurse Anesthetists; Sandy F. Mannino, Director, Pennsylvania Hospital School of Nursing; Helen F. Marsh, Assistant Professor, School of Nursing, University of Wisconsin-Madison; Eleanor D. Marshall, Assistant Director, Research and Statistics Department, ANA; Mrs. Rose Martin, President, National Association for Practical Nurse Education and Service; R. Maureen Maxwell, Director, Graduate Program in Nursing, Loma Linda University; Robert K. Merton, Giddings Professor of Sociology, Columbia University; Mrs. Lois B. Miller, Librarian, Sophia P. Palmer Library, American Journal of Nursing Company; Mildred L. Montag, Professor, Nursing Education, Teachers College, Columbia University; Charles N. Morris, Associate Professor of Education, Teachers College, Columbia University; M. Ruth Moubray, Executive Director and Counselor, Maryland Nurses Association; Mrs. Edward C. Moynihan, Vice-Chairman, Women's Committee, President's Committee on Employment of Handicapped, and President, Christ Child Society of Washington, D.C.; Helen Nahm, Formerly Dean, University of California, San Francisco (retired); Mrs. Dorothy D. Nayer, Associate Editor, *American Journal of Nursing;* Zelda L. Nelson, Executive Director and Counselor, Nebraska Nurses Association; Mrs. Joan Viehmann Nettleton, Chief Nurse, Medicine, D.C. General Hospital; Richard F. Newcomb, Editor, *RN*; Dorothea E. Orem, Associate Professor of Nursing Education, School of Nursing, The Catholic University of America; Mrs. Daisy Wright Phinney, National President, Guild of St. Barnabas; Helen K. Powers, Chief, Health Occupations Unit, Division of Vocational and Technical Education, Bureau of Adult, Vocational and Library Programs, Office of Education, U.S. Department of Health, Education, and Welfare; Frances Purdy, formerly Dean, Director, and Professor of Nursing, Downstate Medical Center, State University of New York; Sheila Quinn, Executive Director, International Council of Nursing; Dorothy E. Reilly, Associate Professor of Nursing, College of Nursing, Wayne State University; Juliann Ritter, Executive Director and Counselor, West Virginia Nurses Association; Alice M. Robinson, Editor, *Nursing Outlook;* Helen C. Rush, Executive Director, American Association of Industrial Nurses, Inc.; Helen L. Salmon, Public Health Nursing Consultant, Division of Occupational Health, County of Los Angeles Health Department, Mrs. Etta B. Schmidt, Executive Director, National Federation of Licensed Practical Nurses, Inc.; Paul K. Schneider, Publisher, *The Journal of Nursing Education;* Barbara G. Schutt, Editor,

American Journal of Nursing; Doris R. Schwartz, Associate Professor of Public Health Nursing, Cornell University-New York Hospital School of Nursing; Mary D. Shanks, Carolyn Ruppert, Professor of Nursing and Director, School of Nursing, Illinois Wesleyan University; Sister Mary Augustine, Director, Provincial Development, Missionary Sisters of the Society of Mary; Sister Delphine, Director, St. Vincent School of Nursing, Indianapolis; Sister Maria Del Rey, Director of Communications, Maryknoll Sisters; Sister M. Cornile Dulohery, Hospital Administrator, St. Joseph Hospital, Savannah; Sister Jane Gates, Superior General, Medical Mission Sisters; Sister Mary Ruth Owen, General Superior, Sisters of St. Joseph of Wheeling; Sister Mary Regis, Missionary Sisters of the Society of Mary; Sister Xavier Richardson, Provincial Superior, Sisters of Charity of Providence; Mrs. Maurean Skiba, Counselor, PC&PS, California Nurses Association; Myra K. Slavens, Educational Director, Association of Operating Room Nurses; Eleanor J. Smith, Advisor, State Boards of Nursing, ANA; Louise C. Smith, Acting Dean, School of Nursing, University of Wisconsin-Madison; Alphonse C. Sootkoos, Editor-in-chief, *Journal of Psychiatric Nursing and Mental Health Services;* Mrs. D. Ann Sparmacher, Secretary, Committee on Nursing, American Medical Association; Harriet Stambach, former Director, Private Duty Nursing Section, ANA (deceased); Elizabeth C. Stobo, Professor, Nursing Education, Teachers College, Columbia University; Dorothy J. Sutherland, Nurse Advisor, Office of International Health, Public Health Service, U.S. Department of Health, Education, and Welfare; Jean E. Sutherland, Nursing Consultant, New York State Employment Service; Berdine Thompson, Associate Executive Director and Counselor, Minnesota Nurses Association; Esther M. Thompson, former Director of Graduate Studies, Department of Nursing, University of Rochester; Julia C. Thompson, Director, Washington Office, ANA; Frances Thompkins, Executive Director, National Student Nurses' Association; Dorothy C. Tipple, Supervisor of School Nursing, New York State Education Department; Ghislane Van Massenhove, General Secretary, International Committee of Catholic Nurses, CICIAMS; Phyllis J. Verhonick, Professor of Nursing, University of Virginia School of Nursing; Janet F. Walker, Professor of Nursing, Arizona State University; Lucille Wall, Executive Director, Indiana State Nurses Association; Grace Wallace, Director, Nurses Christian Fellowship; Patricia Walsh, Director, Nursing Service, Washtenaw County Health Department and Affiliated Agencies, Michigan; Mrs. Anne R. Warner, Director, Public Relations, ANA; Ernestine Wiedenbach, Associate Professor Emeritus of Maternal and Newborn Health Nursing, Yale University; Sidney H. Willig, Professor of Law of the Health Sciences, Temple University and author of *Legal Aspects of Nursing*, McGraw-Hill; Margaret B. Woodruff, Program Coordinator, Division of Community Health Nursing Practice, ANA; Edward O. Wray, Director of Nursing, New York State Psychiatric Institute and Assistant Professor of Nursing, Department of Nursing, Faculty of Medicine, Columbia University; Mrs. Dora H. C. Yang, Senior Social Worker, Veterans Administration Hospital, Washington, D.C.; Mrs. Mary Jane Zusy and Anne Zusy, Kensington, Maryland.

We wish to thank the publishers and the organizations that have granted permission for the use of quotations, figures, charts, tables and other materials, for which special acknowledgment has been made in the text.

We wish especially to thank Elizabeth V. Cunningham, Ernestine Wiedenbach, Dorothy D. Nayer, Joan Viehmann Nettleton and Dorothea E. Orem who made suggestions on the new chapter, "Responsibility for Nursing Practice"; to Helen Creighton and Sidney H. Willig who reviewed and made suggestions on the chapter on "Legal Issues in Nursing Practice," written by Nathan Hershey; to Jean Lazar who assisted in rewriting the chapter on *Nurses in a National Disaster or Emergency;* and to Mrs. Lois Miller for assistance with the section in the appendix on *Reference Tools for Nurses.*

EUGENIA K. SPALDING

LUCILLE E. NOTTER

Contents

PART TWO

Legal, Professional, and Personal Problems and Relationships

PART THREE *SR*.

Choosing, Preparing for and Succeeding in a Field of Nursing

PART FOUR

Organizations and Related Activities

PART I

The Profession of Nursing and Its Social Setting: Past and Present

PREVIEW

This, the opening part of *Professional Nursing: Foundations, Perspectives, and Relationships,* sets the stage for the parts that will follow. The chapters in it are designed to help you think about the problems that confront nurses because our society is what it is and because of the historical foundations of nursing, and about those problems which stem from the professional status of nursing within our society. This part also points up some major trends, relationships and responsibilities of the professional nurse and others concerned with nursing, which may provide some perspective for your study of remaining chapters.

Later chapters of this book will delineate in more detail the problems of your profession and your responsibility for assisting in their solution. It is hoped that as you study these specific problems you will think back on this part and see them in the context of their social setting.

CHAPTER

1

Historical Foundations
of the Profession
# of Nursing[1]

Throughout the ages and in the world today, you will find men and women who have consistently struggled to improve their personal and occupational way of life. Some have succeeded, and others have failed. Four influences have deeply affected their chances for success: religion, war, self-determination and education.

Religion, in one form or another, has influenced men's work, attitudes and relationships by winning allegiance to a cause greater than self. Military strife has created havoc and horror, but it has released men from tyranny. Self-assertive, democratic trends have moved man from the status quo to a status in which individual rights and abilities could be developed most effectively. Self-improvement through education began with man's earliest attempts to learn through experience and so to develop better practices and clearer vision.

You may trace these same 4 influences in the development of nursing. Men and women as individuals with a high sense of personal commitment and responsibility, and men and women as organized groups with a common goal have brought about the events that are woven together to form the background of nursing.

In this chapter the strands making up this tapestry will be followed through the centuries, without adhering to strict chronologic sequence. Only

[1] The original of this chapter was prepared by Mildred E. Newton, R.N., Ed.D., former Director, School of Nursing, The Ohio State University, Columbus, Ohio.

3

the strands which were most important in creating today's picture of nursing will be included. Because of the brevity of this chapter, many interesting and significant facts and people will, perforce, be omitted; but perhaps the spirit and the direction of their efforts will remain.

RELIGIOUS INFLUENCE

In ancient times the medicine man, the priest-physician and the temple attendant ministered to the sick as part of their religious duties. However, you will find no groups of women who were assigned to visit and care for the sick as part of their religious obligations, prior to those of the early Christian period. There were, in fact, no nurses except women who served as children's or wet nurses and men nurses in Indian hospitals whose primary function was nursing of the sick.

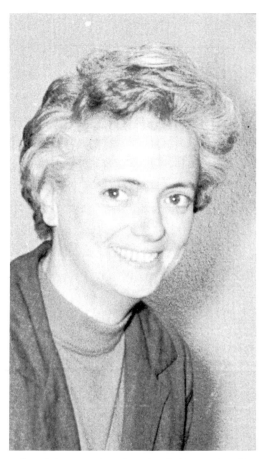

Fig. 1-1. A modern Maryknoll Sister who, like many other members of religious orders, wears civilian clothes today.

Early Christian Period

The "Acts of Charity" of the early Christian church included such admonitions as "Give food to the hungry," "Clothe the naked" and "Visit the sick." These admonitions did not originate with the church but came from the Hebrew tradition. Fortunately, this visitation of the sick was expanded to include the actual care of the sick at home. Women's groups — widows, virgins and deaconesses — acted on the principle that service to man was the equivalent of service to God. They served joyously as an expression of their newly found faith. In reality, they were imbued with the concept that "Inasmuch as ye have done it unto one of the least of these my brethren, ye have done it unto me."[2] At first, these women lived at home, and their early dress was not distinctive; but later religious habits were adopted. Many religious orders today are discarding the religious habit and returning to the early Christian practice of dressing in accord with the current fashion (see Figure 1-1).

Throughout these early centuries, the care which the Christians gave the sick made a great impression on their adversaries. Emperor Julian said that the brotherly love that they showed toward the sick was one of the factors which made them such powerful enemies of the Roman gods. Dionysius of Alexandria also commented that, during a 3rd-century plague, the Christians visited the sick without fear and gave them the best of care.

Monastic Orders

These first Christian groups were forerunners of the monastic orders. Again, nursing was likely to be one of a number of activities carried on by the monks and the nuns; purely nursing orders developed later. The great monastic movement that began in the 4th and the 5th centuries A.D. set a pattern, some traces of which may be found in later nursing practices. The dedication, or setting apart of the worker, began with the nun's novitiate and was followed by the taking of the veil. You will in some instances still find its counterpart in today's preclinical educational period in nursing and in the various capping and banding ceremonies.

While some women entered monastic life to escape from home or to avoid an undesirable marriage, undoubtedly the strongest motivation came from the women's idealism and desire to serve God. Perhaps these ideals were supported by other factors. Economic security was assured. St. Benedict's emphasis on the importance and the value of manual work and his command, "Work and pray!" helped to dignify the work done with one's hands.

The influence of the Roman matrons, early converts to Christianity, in monastic life was great. These highborn women had gained considerable social liberty; they were characterized by great intellectual powers and force of character. Many probably entered the monastic life in order to lead lives independent of their families and to find freedom to pursue activities which could not be carried out in their homes.

[2] Matthew 25:40.

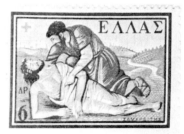

Fig. 1-2. The Good Samaritan, typi-
fying Christian concern for the sick.
(Greece)[3]

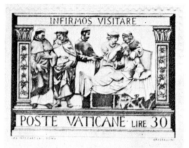

Fig. 1-3. Visiting the sick—one of
the acts of charity of the early
church. (Poste Vaticane)

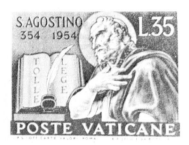

Fig. 1-4. St. Augustine. The first
purely nursing order followed the
rule of St. Augustine. (Poste Vaticane)

The willingness and the ability of nurses to "do everything" possibly became too well established in the first purely nursing order, the Augustinian Sisters. They did the nursing, the housekeeping, the cooking and the laundry and ran the hospitals as well. During the Middle Ages, the two extremes of nursing may be found. On the one hand, you see the Augustinian Sisters breaking the ice of the Seine River and wading into its freezing waters to do the "great wash" for the famous hospital in Paris staffed by them, the Hotel Dieu. On the other hand, you see women rising to the heights of power and prestige as Lady Abbesses in charge of convents, hospitals and, at times, Twin Communities. Such an Abbess, Hildegarde of Germany, was a prophetess, a political expert, a medical author and a nurse.

These few Abbesses were not typical of the hundreds of nuns and monks, serving the poorest of the poor sick with the crude medieval nursing appliances, often at variance with the doctors. They were imbued with the spirit that the more menial and humiliating the work, the greater its value as a means of penance. Thus, nursing became associated with backbreaking, ser-

[3] Illustrations in this chapter are copies of stamps from the history of nursing collection begun by June A. Ramsey and continued by Mildred E. Newton.

vile labor, and as Lavinia Dock says, its practitioners were without the light of knowledge and understanding which makes the hardest toil bearable.[4]

The Protestant Reformation

Until the time of the Protestant Reformation in the 16th century, the Catholic Church had provided most of the hospital facilities, and its nursing Brothers and Sisters had given most of the care afforded the sick (although some, but not many, civil hospitals had developed after the 12th century where the Church's facilities were inadequate or where cities recognized that the care of the sick was one of their responsibilities). Hence, after the Protestant Reformation, countries that became predominantly Protestant were in a serious predicament. Monasteries, convents and hospitals were closed, and the personnel driven out. The cities had no staff prepared to direct and to give care to the sick, the orphans and the aged. As civil institutions sprang up, staffed by crude and ignorant women, nursing plunged deeper into its own Dark Age.

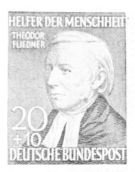

Fig. 1-5. Pastor Theodor Fliedner, the founder of the Kaiserswerth Deaconess Order. (Deutsche Bundespost)

Nursing in the New World

The contrast between the provision for nursing under Catholic and under Protestant auspices in North America is clearly marked. The explorers from Catholic countries, such as France, brought their nursing Brothers with them and sent for their nursing Sisters in the early stages of colonization. Cortez established the Immaculate Conception Hospital in Mexico City in 1524 — some say to assuage his conscience for his perfidy to the natives.

Three Augustinian Sisters arrived in Sillery, Canada, in 1639 with the early settlers. Shortly after the Sisters' arrival, a smallpox epidemic broke out and, as patients flocked to them for this and other ailments, the Sisters were forced to train Indian women to help them. Thus the first nurse-aide training courses in this country were organized. Later the Augustinian Sisters, an enclosed order, built the Hotel Dieu in Quebec. The priests claimed that hospitals like this did more to convert the savages than did

[4] M. A. Nutting and L. L. Dock. *A History of Nursing*, vol. 1. New York, Putnam, 1907, p. 296.

their sermons. The persuasive and competent Mlle. Jeanne Mance, a lay woman, has sometimes been called the "Florence Nightingale of Canada." Against all advice of the Governor of Quebec, Jeanne took her party on to Montreal to establish a hospital there in 1644. They brought equipment, supplies and nursing nuns of the Order of St. Joseph, but had no doctor. This did not deter them, and with such help as they could get from "circuit riding" doctors, they carried on under Jeanne Mance's guidance.

The Ursuline nuns, also an enclosed order, came with the French missionaries and built their famous Old Charity Hospital in New Orleans in 1727. Mother Elizabeth Seton (canonization 1969) founded her Daughters of Charity of St. Joseph at Emmitsburg, Maryland, in 1809. Many orders were either transplanted to North America or were founded here during the 18th and the 19th centuries, and they flourished in the soil of the New World, on both coasts.

Colonists and explorers from Protestant countries brought no such nursing groups with them, because almost none existed. True, the Pilgrims had a deaconess nurse in Holland, but whether she came to this country or not is uncertain.

Revival of the Deaconess Movement

During the centuries following the early Christian era, the deaconesses had continued their work, although with diminished activity as the monasteries became more powerful. However, little is heard of this. At the time of the Protestant Reformation in the 16th century, feeble attempts were made to revive the early church deaconess order. In 1836, Pastor Theodor Fliedner of Kaiserswerth, Germany, met Mrs. Elizabeth Fry of England during a fund-raising trip and was deeply impressed by the reforms that she had brought about at the infamous Newgate Prison in England. In his travels he also had seen some deaconesses at work in Holland. When his enthusiasm for prison reform did not meet with support in Kaiserswerth, he and his first wife, Friederike, decided in 1836 to establish a training institute for deaconesses at Kaiserswerth. Among other activities, such as caring for discharged prisoners and training teachers, they very early began to prepare nursing deaconesses.

Their hospital was established to provide nursing experience for the students, rather than training students in order to staff the hospital. Some very sound practices were developed by Theodor and Friederike Fliedner, and later by his second wife, Caroline. You still find some of these practices in the nursing education systems of today – such as careful selection of students using letters of reference, a preliminary period of study, a uniform, formal instruction and assignments to clinical services. Probably the first syllabus in nursing was Friederike's journal.

The influence of the Kaiserswerth plan was far-reaching. First, nursing became a respectable vocation for young German women. Secondly, this movement soon spread to 4 continents, including establishment of the first Motherhouse in Pittsburgh, Pa., in 1849. Thirdly, the Kaiserswerth Institution gave Florence Nightingale her only formal nurse's training. She spent 2 weeks in Kaiserswerth in 1850 and 3 months in 1851. She wrote that she believed that the strength of the Institution lay in its spirit rather than its practices. One of Miss Nightingale's strongest convictions was that, regardless of the auspices under which it was practiced, nursing must always be carried on in a deeply religious spirit.

Protestant Religious Orders in England

With the dissolution of monasteries in England, the sad conditions of the sick were evident. Elizabeth Fry organized her nursing Sisters in 1840 to meet their needs. Her Sisters were women of good character. They had a short experience in Guy's Hospital in London and then began their care of the sick at home. After this, several Anglican sisterhoods developed which included friendly visiting and sometimes hospital nursing among their activities. These Anglican and other Protestant sisterhoods soon began to organize branches in the United States in such cities as Pittsburgh, Chicago, Milwaukee, New York, Baltimore and Boston.

Schools of Nursing

After schools of nursing were opened in the United States under secular organizations, churches began founding training schools in the hospitals under their control. The religious influence was evident in many aspects of the training school pattern — such as reference letters from pastors, chapel exercises, religious organizations for students like the Sodalities in Catholic schools of nursing and in the St. Barnabas Guild for nurses, as well as courses in religion and ethics in church schools. Today, in many of the schools under church jurisdiction, you will find such phrases as this in their philosophy and objectives: "... diligent preparation for professional competence and purposeful living in the service of God and humanity."

At present, you will find secular groups and the state taking more and more responsibility for education and health care. Some hospitals and schools of nursing that began under religious auspices are now under secular control. This is a rapidly growing trend. Although the numbers of church-related schools and hospitals are diminishing, still the church will always carry on the Lord's command to "Heal the sick"; and young people of today and tomorrow may still wish to serve God through nursing the sick.

MILITARY INFLUENCE

Every war has had special nursing problems because of geographic location and the diseases or the methods of destruction associated with it. The first well-organized military nursing groups were established primarily to serve the Crusaders. The motives of these groups were as much religious as they were military.

The Crusades

For almost 200 years after 1096, seven Crusades were launched in an effort to wrest the Holy Land from the Moslems. In the end, the Crusaders lost ground and were driven out of the Holy Land; but they had gained many new experiences, and military nursing orders were well established. These orders brought prestige and recognition to nursing. Fine hospitals were built by them, principles and practices of hospital administration developed and good care was provided the soldier and in fact all who participated in the Crusades and other pilgrimages.

Three of the orders were the Knights of St. Lazarus for the care of lepers; the Teutonic Knights Hospitallers, largely from Germany; and the Knights Hospitallers of St. John of Jerusalem. Less important companion women's orders were formed for each. The Teutonic Rule indicated that women were to be admitted because services to cattle and hospitalized sick were better performed by females. The Knights of St. John was the largest, wealthiest and most influential of the orders. Nursing was done by the serving Brothers or half-knights, who fought during periods of conflict and nursed between engagements.

When Pope Urban II sent the first Crusaders on their way, he urged them to wear the cross on their heads and breasts. Various forms of the cross were used by different orders, each with its special significance. The Knights of St. John adopted the Maltese Cross, with its 8 points, each representing one of the 8 Beatitudes. The badge designed for the Nightingale School used this same cross. When the USA Cadet Nurse Corps was formed during World War II, it fittingly chose the Maltese Cross as its insignia. The first lines of the Cadet Hymn read, "The Maltese Cross is marching again, To answer the call—a new Crusade."[5] If you will examine nurses' school and organization pins or badges you will find this same symbolism in many of their designs. The former St. Luke's Hospital School of Nursing pin of Chicago carried the Lorraine Cross of relief; the Johns Hopkins pin incorporates the Pattee Cross of protection; and the Red Cross nurse's pin has the St. George's Cross of unselfish service, with its 4 arms, representing faith, hope, love and service.

Other traditions that you can trace from the Crusades to modern times are as follows: military orders and etiquette, rounds with doctors, instruction of medical students, and the physical pattern of nursing units. These included a large ward for convalescents, smaller subwards for sicker patients, and cubicles for those who were critical.

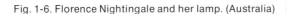

Fig. 1-6. Florence Nightingale and her lamp. (Australia)

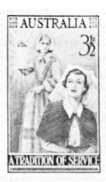

Florence Nightingale's Military Influence

Time and circumstances often provide the opportunity for action that climaxes a lifetime's experience and preparation. The Crimean War, 1854-1856, did this for Florence Nightingale, and, more than that, it engendered an interest in the British soldier which dominated her activities for the next 20 years. For years she had sought some type of work that would benefit mankind and also draw on every resource and ability that she possessed. She was strongly attracted to nursing but had to battle against her family's opposition, society's disapproval and her own lack of adequate preparation. During her years of bitter frustration, she sensed an estrangement from her family and friends that brought a terrible loneliness. Only her intense religious commitment and belief that in all she did she was acting directly under God's commands and in harmony with his purpose, kept her struggling toward her own self-fulfillment.

For 2 brief years of her 90-year life span she organized, maneuvered, commanded, threatened and nursed her way through the Crimean War. Working with a heterogeneous group of Catholic nuns, Anglican Sisters and lay nurses: struggling against medical opposition; and constantly tearing through miles of red tape, she accomplished the impossible. Quite typically as in all her activities, she had comparative facts and figures on which to base her dramatic Blue Book Reports. She could show her results in statistical tables and in the lives of men.

Only Miss Nightingale's major military nursing accomplishments can be listed here. Through her work she:

1. Improved the nursing care of the sick by introducing female nurses, serving proper diets, training orderlies and by her personal example of tender concern for the individual.

2. Lowered death rates, by sanitary reforms coupled with better care, until the death rate on cases treated had dropped from 315 per 1,000 to 22 per 1,000 in 6 months.

3. Established the principle of unified command of nursing in a military situation.

4. Established exacting standards of proficiency and conduct for military nurses.

In the years that followed, Miss Nightingale was driven, and in turn drove others, by her fear of her own imminent death. Action must be taken today — tomorrow might be too late! She fought the cause of the British soldier from her own bedchamber. Her invalid condition made it necessary for people to come to her, and she worked through her "Nightingale Cabinet."

The creation of one Royal Commission after another was demanded by this "drivin' woman," secured, and instructed by her in its duties. Some of these Commissions were formed to remodel military hospitals and barracks, to reorganize military statistics, to institute an Army Medical School, to reorganize the Army Medical Department and to introduce female nursing into military hospitals. In all of these ventures, partial or full success was achieved.

Because the British soldier was assigned to India, Florence Nightingale's interest and concern followed him there. She prescribed what he should eat, what he should wear, and means for controlling the epidemics to which he was exposed. Death rates for the soldiers, which were 69 per 1,000, dropped to 5 per 1,000 after the first year of her reforms. Similar saving of soldier lives was demonstrated in peacetime England after the recommendations she made were implemented by her strongest supporter, Sidney Herbert.

To Miss Nightingale, statistics were sacred. Because of her statistical ability she was made a Fellow of the Royal Statistical Society and an honorary member of the American Statistical Society. For over 20 years she used sanitation and statistics to help her decrease the illnesses and the deaths of her British soldiers.

Henri Dunant and Clara Barton

An interrupted journey, a nightmare following a battle, and a dream that would not let him rest, were the events in Jean Henri Dunant's life which culminated in the birth of the Red Cross Societies.[6] This Swiss businessman literally stumbled onto the Solferino battlefield in northern Italy in 1859, the day after the rout of 2 armies following a disorganized engagement. After heroic efforts by Dunant to bring order out of chaos and to organize the terrified villagers so that the sketchiest of care could be given the wounded, he concluded that only volunteer nurses, previously trained and officially recognized by both armies, could prevent the repetition of the senseless suffering and death that he had just seen.

The nightmare in which he lived during the next months and years haunted him until, as an act of mental catharsis, he wrote *Un Souvenir de Solferino* in 1862. He had it translated and distributed throughout Europe at his own expense. In it he posed a plan that involved international agreements and cooperation. At his instigation, the Geneva Society of Public Utility called a conference in 1863 to discuss plans for the relief of suffering in war. Delegates from 14 nations attended and returned the next year,

[6] See also Chapter 26 for the story of the development of Red Cross Societies.

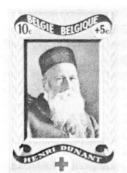

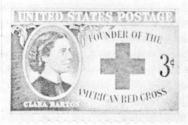

Fig. 1-8. Clara Barton, the founder of the American Red Cross. (USA)

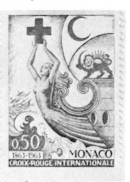

Fig. 1-7. Henri Dunant, the originator of principles followed by the Red Cross Societies. (Belgie Belgique)

Fig. 1-9. Red Crescent and Red Lion and Sun — official variations of Red Cross Insignia. (Monaco)

when 12 powers signed the Treaty. Out of courtesy to their host, the reverse of the Swiss flag was adopted as their emblem, and the organization was called the International Committee of the Red Cross.

Five of the principles agreed on were preparedness of personnel and supplies; centralization of authority; neutrality of personnel, supplies, conveyances and shelters for the wounded; impartiality between friend and foe in the care given; and solidarity, which permitted neutral nations to give aid. Details of organization were wisely left up to each country. Though the use of the Red Cross Symbol had been intended to be universal, yet in countries where the cross is not an acceptable symbol you will see a substitute, e.g., a Red Crescent in Turkey, and a Red Lion and Sun in Iran. No further adaptation of the insignia is now permitted.

Few meetings have ever had such far-reaching results as the 1863 Geneva Convention. Red Cross Societies injected a patriotic motive into nursing and stimulated the organization of Red Cross Schools. They put into action the greatest humanitarian movement, outside of the church, that the world has ever known.

The USA, involved as it was in the Civil War (1861-1865) and steeped in the Monroe Doctrine, did not sign the Treaty. Clara Barton, who served as a volunteer nurse during the Civil War, happened to see the Red Cross in action at the Franco-Prussian front in 1871. From then on, every day of her life was committed to the cause of the Red Cross as interpreter, organizer and later as president of the American Association of the Red Cross. She worked with influential people in Washington without avail in her attempt to persuade the President, the Congress and the people of the United States informing them that if they were diligent they might be 32nd on the roll of civilized nations, but at the moment were standing with the heathens and the barbarians. President Garfield finally agreed to sign but was assassinated before doing so. Despairing, but not defeated, Clara Barton organized the

American Association in 1881, demonstrated its effectiveness in a terrible Michigan forest fire, and secured President Arthur's signature the next year.

The "American Amendment" of 1886, drawn up by Miss Barton and accepted by the International Society, greatly expanded the usefulness of the International Red Cross. Its provisions covered relief of suffering not only in time of war but also when pestilence, famine, fire, floods and other calamities struck a community.

Wars Involving the United States of America

During the early wars—the Revolutionary War, the War of 1812, and even as late as the Civil War—enlisted men or volunteers, including wives, mothers and paid practical nurses, did the nursing in military hospitals. Since 1861, the USA has been involved in serious war 6 times. In this brief sketch of the influences of 3 of those wars, only the type of nursing personnel used, the major nursing problems and the more lasting effects will be outlined.

During the *Civil War*, the only women with any nurses' training were Catholic and Protestant Sisters. Someone commented that they were particularly effective because they were trained, disciplined and not hunting husbands. Their contribution was immeasurable. The largest group of nurses was made up of volunteer, untrained women who patriotically gave of their very best. Familiar names on this list are Dorothea Lynde Dix, Katharine Wormeley, Sister Anthony O'Connell, Louisa May Alcott, the Woolsey sisters and Mother Bickerdyke. A small number were sent to Bellevue Hospital and the New York Hospital in New York to be trained. All of these women cared for soldiers at the front, in the makeshift Army hospitals and on the hospital ships. They even organized rowboat brigades, searched the sloughs and the river banks after a battle to find the wounded and rowed them to points where they could receive care. Men, equally untrained, also served as nurses. In time a hospital corps of men, with an official manual to guide them, was established.

When Dorothea Dix was appointed Superintendent of Female Nurses in the United States Sanitary Commission, under whose auspices the nurses were sent to the hospitals, she was 60 years old and worn out from her years of insane-asylum reform. But she knew hospital organization, typified humanity itself, was most considerate of her nurses and was utterly devoted to duty. She set the first standards for Army Nurses, which required that they be 35 to 50 years old and plain in dress and appearance. Our attractive military nurses of today never would have qualified! The Confederacy had many outstanding nurses but no official agency similar to the USA Sanitary Commission.

The chief nursing problems confronting these nurses were those arising from deficiency diseases and gastrointestinal conditions caused by poor sanitation. Infections spread rapidly through surgical wards where the wounds of all men were washed with the same sea sponge. Anesthesia was known but not used routinely; morphine was administered by sprinkling a few crystals of the drug on the surgeon's pen knife and then jabbing it under the skin.

Aside from the first standards set for military nurses, the most important outcome of the Civil War was the impetus it gave to the development of schools of nursing.

The Spanish-American War (1898) brought nurses closer to a military nurse corps. Graduate nurses were now available and also a national nursing organization, the Nurses' Associated Alumnae, which could have acted as a recruiting agent but offered too late. Dr. Anita Newcomb McGee, sponsored by the Daughters of the American Revolution, took charge. Her standards were 2-fold—a girl must be a graduate nurse and have a certificate of character. Later Dr. McGee was appointed Acting Assistant Surgeon General of the USA Department of the Army in charge of the Army Nurse Division.

In this war, as in the Crimean War, the Civil War, and even World War I, far more men died of disease than wounds. Typhoid fever and yellow fever led the causes of death. One outcome of this period was far better knowledge of the spread and the control of both diseases.

The most important result for nursing was the formation of the Army Nurse Corps in 1901. The Navy Nurse Corps followed in 1908.

In *World War I* (1914-1918) the nurses of this country were prepared and ready to serve. Through the Red Cross Nursing Service, 8,000 were available in 1917. The standards adopted assured the military medical services of competent practitioners. These nurses were American citizens, high school graduates, graduates of state accredited schools whose hospitals had at least 50 daily average patients, registered, and of good health and character.

Two important new methods were used to increase the nurse supply—the Vassar Training Camp for college graduates and the Army School of Nursing. The Army School, of which Annie W. Goodrich was the first Dean, had branches in several major hospitals and camps. By 1924, the Army School had served its purpose and closed. The Vassar Training Camp had provided for a centralized preparatory course in nursing. Most of the more than 400 college graduates who had received the 3 months initial preparation at the Camp transferred to cooperating nursing schools for a somewhat shortened and accelerated program.

The nursing problems characteristic of this war—tetanus, aerial warfare and respiratory diseases—were responsible for 82 per cent of the deaths. Gas warfare, parasites and typhus fever added to the nursing problems. Shrapnel injuries necessitated new and daring experiments in plastic surgery. The Dakin-Carrel method of combating wound infections was devised. All of these demanded nursing skill and flexibility.

The more recent activities of women in the 4 military Nurse Corps associated with the Armed Services in World War II, the Korean War, the war in Vietnam, and others are found in Chapter 11.

While war is the curse of mankind, it has, until recently, called forth the highest patriotic devotion of both men and women. War has stimulated improved care of the sick and better prepration of nurses. And women, especially nurses, have demonstrated that they have a unique and irreplaceable service to give their country in times of war.

SECULAR INFLUENCE

In the normal development of community life, health care responsibilities came to be assumed by secular as well as religious groups. As towns developed, people lived under new conditions, the monasteries were no longer the centers of all activities, and the cloistered orders were no longer able to meet the need. Also, excessive restrictions that had come to be put upon many of the religious orders made it necessary to develop more democratic and freer types of organization for providing nursing to the people living under these new conditions. Also, as individuals and groups move toward democratic practices, they strive toward goals that they believe can be achieved best through their own self-directed efforts. Such movements constitute the secular influence on nursing. However, secular orders interested in social welfare and nursing also had religious motives. Their differences were more related to the lack of monastic restrictions and religious vows, and the nature of the control or auspices of the order.

Today, educational influences and secularization in society, as well as a return to the early Christian ideals and practices, are having a real influence on religious orders. Nuns are moving out of their convents to take positions outside of their religious orders and to provide Christian services in the communities in which they reside.

Secular Orders

During the Middle Ages, when man was taking an increasingly wider view of his world, questions were raised as to the necessity of the strict monastic rules and the isolation of members from humanity at large. An adherent of this broader ideal of service was St. Francis of Assisi (1182-1226), one of the most lovable of all the "nursing saints." Some claim that he was more important because of what he *was* than because of what he *did*. He believed that there must be a way for men and women to participate in nursing and social welfare work and continue with their own occupations, family life and civic responsibilities. The great surge of young people wishing to join his First Order—the Franciscan Friars, and the Second Order—the Clarissas, or Poor Clares, headed by St. Clarissa, brought about the formation of the secular Franciscan Tertiaries or Third Order of St. Francis, which was under religious control but without vows or monastic restrictions. These members did many of the same things that you see Red Cross volunteers and Junior League members doing today. They helped to transport patients to the hospitals, provided material relief and assisted the nurses with the care of patients.

Fig. 1-10. Sister of Charity, Mlle. le Gras, and St. Vincent de Paul. (Poste Vaticane)

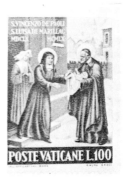

The best known of the Tertiaries was Elizabeth of Hungary, who built hospitals and gave care to patients in their homes and in her own palace. Beautiful legends have grown up around her beneficence and devoted care. She is an example of the interest shown in the care of the sick by royalty and the socially prominent throughout the centuries.

In the 17th century, Vincent de Paul of France (St. Vincent de Paul) was searching for new and better ways to care for the sick and the poor. Different experiments were tried, first that of enlisting the help of wealthy, prominent women to go as Dames of Charity into the Hotel Dieu and other hospitals to assist the nursing Sisters with their unbearable load. Interest waned, and husbands objected. Then they tried bringing young, strong country girls to Paris to work under the direction of the Dames. This also left much to be desired.

St. Vincent de Paul was most fortunate in securing the help of Mlle. le Gras (St. Louise de Marillac) with his ventures. Her travels and studies convinced both of them that carefully selected young women could succeed if they had common, systematic instruction and were housed together under supervision.

In addition to these early principles, Vincent taught moderation, encouraged the Daughters to substitute the patient's chamber of suffering for a nun's cell, and emphasized that this group, to fulfill its mission, must be secular—not cloistered. These Daughters must be able to go to the patient, wherever he was; they were to wear the everyday dress of the peasant woman with its gray-blue robe and great white coif; and they were to take the vows of poverty, chastity and obedience for only one year at a time. Mlle. le Gras became the first Daughter or Sister of Charity on March 25, 1634; and since then, on March 25, all Sisters renew their vows for another year if they so desire. These Sisters have rightfully been called the bridge between nursing as a religious vocation and as a secular occupation.

Secular Movements

Secular movements of the 19th and the 20th centuries in the USA and in other countries include the establishment of nurses' organizations, enactment of laws providing for registration or legal recognition of nurses and other legislation advantageous to nurses, promotion of economic security, and provision of channels whereby the nurses might speak for themselves through their official journals. These are discussed in later chapters. All of these secular movements have influenced the growth, the solidarity and the usefulness of nurses. Thus they have become able to conduct their own professional deliberations and to enact measures beneficial to themselves and the patients whom they serve.

EDUCATIONAL INFLUENCE

Learning through trial and error, through apprenticeship and through formal instruction has taken place in this order in many professions. Faint threads of a formal educational pattern in nursing had appeared by the Middle Ages.

Each young Augustinian novice was assigned to a Mother in Religion who taught her charge only what she herself knew. Sister Genevieve Boquet in the 17th century was brash enough to suggest that all novices should be taught alike. She was appointed Mistress of Novices, but this logical plan was hampered by resentment among the other Sisters.

Stronger threads of a common educational plan are evident in the Daughters of Charity of St. Vincent de Paul's 5-year curriculum, where regular classes and quiz sections were held. You will find quite prominent strands, similar to some of our present educational practices, already described in the section on the Kaiserswerth Deaconesses (p. 8). While the value of these early attempts at a teaching program is recognized, most historians date modern nursing education from 1860, the year when the Nightingale School, in London, England, opened. In this discussion, only the evolution of preservice programs will be sketched; postgraduate education will not be considered.

Nightingale Training School for Nurses

Concurrent with Miss Nightingale's efforts to aid the British soldiers was her other goal, the establishment of a new system of training for nurses. England's gift to her of £44,000 constituted her School's endowment. A residence was purchased, for without assurance of a carefully supervised home life no mid-Victorian Englishwoman of respectable family would have been permitted to leave her father's home. Since Mrs. Wardroper, the Matron of St. Thomas' Hospital, had developed better nursing care than existed in any other hospital in London, arrangements were made to use St. Thomas' and for Mrs. Wardroper to become the Matron of the School. The School opened on June 24, 1860, with 15 probationers.

Some of the points that would be examined by a modern accrediting group will be summarized. The Nightingale philosophy of nursing was that nursing was an art, the finest of the fine arts; that it demanded an organized, practical and scientific training; that a nurse could be as creative as an artist. Miss Nightingale believed that nursing was God's work and that it could be carried out as a secular vocation under secular auspices. As a result, the objectives of the School were to prepare "sick nurses" and "health nurses," and to send out those who were "trained to train" as matrons and sister tutors.

Students fell into 2 groups—the ordinary probationers and the educated probationers. The former had 1 year's training followed by 3 years of supervised practice at St. Thomas' in London and were paid a stipend. The educated probationers had 1 year's training and 2 years of supervised practice. This latter group was prepared to serve on the staff as teachers of probationers and also as matrons of hospitals or as superintendents of district nursing organizations. They paid fees for their training. The prime requisites for admission were maturity, culture and ability, and the number admitted was based on the clinical facilities available. Probationers were prepared for both hospital and home nursing.

Faculty were self-trained at first and were the best nurses available. Ward Sisters[7] were very important, since Miss Nightingale maintained that the one place to learn nursing was at the bedside. She urged the Ward Sisters to "learn the student" and to plan for her instruction. Without such instruction it was too easy for probationers to "potter and cobble out their year about the patient, and make not much progress in real nursing."[8] A Home Sister supervised the residence, the students' extracurricular activities and their study hours. The strict system of discipline was designed to protect the nurses as well as the patients. This discipline was an important factor in establishing respect and confidence in these new nurses. The matron had a high degree of power and was the ultimate authority. Yet Miss Nightingale urged that she be neither mistress nor servant but friend of every woman under her. Nurses and doctors who taught the probationers were paid from the Nightingale fund.

The formal curriculum was for the educated probationers only. It included 12 clock hours of anatomy and surgical nursing, 12 of physiology and medical nursing and 12 of chemistry, foods and sanitation. Limited to 36 hours, to be sure, yet the content was revolutionary—physical and biologic sciences, health sciences and nursing! In addition, talks on ethical and professional subjects were given. Miss Nightingale wrote an annual address to her nurses and gave it herself, when able. Clinical teaching was stressed with emphasis on what and how to think, what and how to observe. Lectures, quizzes, notes, case papers, library studies and diaries were all required of the probationers.

Miss Nightingale's principles of nursing education were 3: (1) the school

---

[7] The term "Sister" here refers to a nurse, not to a member of a religious order, although its usage derived from the Sisters of religious and secular orders.

[8] F. Nightingale. "Training of Nurses," in Richard Quain's *A Dictionary of Medicine,* New York. Appleton. 1895. p. 233.

should be associated with a medical school in a teaching hospital, (2) the Nurses' Home should be a place fit to form discipline and character and (3) the Matron must have final authority for the entire program, theoretical and practical instruction and experience, and living.

The School prospered and became the most influential force in nursing education in those times. Its graduates were sought for positions all over the world. Miss Nightingale gave consultation to her own graduates, and to doctors and nurses from many countries seeking to establish schools in the Nightingale pattern.

Early USA Schools

At the end of the Civil War, doctors were sure that there must be some better way of training nurses than they had seen. In 1869, the American Medical Association Committee on Training Nurses recommended that: (1) every large, well-organized hospital have a school, (2) county medical agencies establish district schools and (3) nurse societies similar to the American Medical Association be formed.[9] There is no evidence that the first 2 recommendations were ever followed in the pattern of nursing education in the USA.

During this same postwar period, powerful voluntary women's committees, which had been very active during the war, were seeking new projects. Fortunately, some of them turned their interest and energy toward reforming hospitals and starting training schools. Some were firm in their belief that while they expected that the presence of the school would improve patient care, the school did not exist primarily for this purpose but for the training of nurses. Others felt that schools should be established ". . . simply and solely because of the need of one of the great charity hospitals for better nursing."[10]

The New England Hospital for Women and Children Training School for Nurses (Boston) was established in 1872 and awarded the first American diploma in nursing to Linda Richards, a year later. However, it was not established on the Nightingale plan. Women doctors were in charge, and there was no Matron.

The authority given the Matron in the Nightingale schools was never accepted in the USA, and she was always subordinate to a hospital superintendent or some other individual or committee. Hence we speak of the modified Nightingale or the Bellevue system in the USA. The first school established on the modified Nightingale pattern was at Bellevue Hospital (New York) in 1873 and will be discussed as representative of these

[9] S. D. Gross. "Report of Committee on the Training of Nurses," *Transactions of the American Medical Association,* New Orleans (Philadelphia, Collins, Printer), 1869, pp. 161-174.
[10] L. Darche, "Proper Organization of Training Schools in America," in I. A. Hampton, *et al., Nursing of the Sick, 1893,* New York, McGraw-Hill, 1949, p. 94.

schools. An influential woman's committee, acting under the advice that Miss Nightingale gave to one of their strongest supporters — Dr. Gill Wylie — organized this school. They raised an endowment fund, secured clinical facilities at Bellevue, bought a residence and recruited a class of 26 from 73 applicants. Until almost the opening date, they had no Matron. At the very last moment a very able Anglican Sister (a British nurse who was visiting in the USA), Sister Helen, volunteered to help the school to get started. When it was decided that a uniform was needed, Sister Helen diplomatically sent the most beautiful and socially prominent student home to have her dressmaker design an attractive wash dress for her. Eagerly, her classmates asked to copy it, and the first uniform was adopted. Linda Richards, who had a genius for organization, became the first night superintendent and helped to develop policies and procedures fundamental to good nursing along Nightingale lines, in the principles of which she was a strong believer though not a graduate of a Nightingale school.

In 1872, there was only one school of nursing in the USA; in 1900, there were 400. As schools began to function, the outcomes previously recognized by the American Medical Association Committee became clearly evident: mortality rates in the hospitals were reduced, and costs of running the hospitals declined. With such desirable outcomes from the establishment of training schools, you cannot wonder that hospital administrators, after their first resistance and skepticism had passed, rapidly turned to this new method of saving lives and money. This saving of money immediately became, and continued to pose, the greatest threat to good nursing education.

At first, schools were run by Training School Committees, but the Committees' influence and high educational ideals decreased as hospital control increased. By the 20th century serious marks of deterioration were evident. The schools' educational function was submerged by the hospitals' manpower needs; essentials for teaching were not provided; students were denied the rights of students; their quality lessened; and the superintendent of nurses was in a state of constant conflict, torn between the needs of her students and the patients. The far-seeing M. Adelaide Nutting in 1908 made these educationally sound recommendations: (1) a preparatory course should be given outside the hospital in a central school, (2) clinical experience should be arranged by the central school, (3) the school should have a separate foundation, (4) students should pay tuition all the way and the school should be a part of a university scheme.[11]

How different the progress of nursing education would have been had these recommendations been followed in 1908 when they were proposed! The schools multiplied in good and in poor hospitals, in large general and in small specialized hospitals, until 2,155 existed in 1926. However, the figure in October, 1967, was 1,269. In 1926 there were 17,522 nursing

[11] M. A. Nutting, *A Sound Economic Basis for Schools of Nursing*, New York, Putnam, 1926, p. 38.

graduates while in 1967, despite the fact that there were fewer schools, there were 38,237 nursing graduates, an increase of more than 20,000![12, 13]

Evaluation of Nursing Education in the USA

The inadequate preparation of nurses in the USA, especially for community nursing, became very evident in the latter part of World War I. Friends and critics of nursing, nurses and doctors together began to investigate schools of nursing. Some highly significant reports of surveys made include: *Nursing and Nursing Education in the United States*, compiled by Josephine Goldmark in 1923 through the help of the Rockefeller Foundation; *Nurses, Patients and Pocketbooks*, in 1928; *Nursing Schools Today and Tomorrow*, in 1934, for the Committee on the Grading of Nursing Schools. Probably the most influential chapter in these surveys was Chapter 6 of the 1934 report, entitled, "The Essentials for a Basic Professional School," (published by the National League of Nursing Education). To us today its recommendations seem to be most limited. For instance, each school was to employ at least 1 full-time instructor, and a ratio of at least 1 staff nurse to 6 students was to be maintained. Even so, these recommendations were ahead of their times. For several reasons, schools were never graded.

Two surveys appeared after World War II. Esther Lucile Brown's *Nursing for the Future*, 1948, shook the whole structure of nursing education and hospital administration because she dared to suggest that, in the next half-century, professional nurses must be prepared in institutions of higher education. The American Nurses' Association's Goal Three, concerning the education basic to the professional practice of nursing, which was proposed in 1962, did the same thing but envisioned it within the next 20 to 30 years.

The other very significant survey, *Nursing Schools at the Mid-Century*, prepared for the National Committee for the Improvement of Nursing Services by Margaret West and Christy Hawkins, depicted in detail the very uneven progress made by the 1,193 state accredited schools of nursing in the USA. On a basis of 100 points, schools were rated on 6 criteria, such as curriculum and teaching staff. The highest fourth, Group I, scored between 96 and 60 per cent; the middle half, Group II, went as low as 40 per cent; the poorest 4th could score only 39 to 15 per cent on the criteria. The names of the schools in Groups I and II were published, providing the very first comprehensive classified list of schools (1950).

One of the most significant events affecting nursing education in recent years occurred when the ANA published its "Position Paper" on nursing education in 1965. The Association forthrightly asserted its position that: "Education for those who work in nursing should take place within the

[12] M. A. Burgess, *Nurses, Patients, and Pocketbooks*, New York, Committee on Grading of Nursing Schools, 1928, p. 35.
[13] M. B. Harty, "Trends in Nursing Education." *American Journal of Nursing*, **68**:767-772, Apr. 1968.

general system of education."[14] Despite the flurry of controversy which followed the publication of the position paper, there has been considerable movement toward the placing of nursing education in educational institutions. Since 1965, regional and state nursing groups have been engaged in interpreting the ANA position and in promoting the orderly transition of nursing education into institutions of higher education.[15] While it is too early to measure the full impact of the association's stand on the education of nurses at all levels of preparation, there is no question but that it has given the necessary impetus to accomplish the goal recommended by Esther Lucile Brown in 1948.

Accreditation

As the last section indicates, attempts in the USA to evaluate schools and differentiate the good from the poor had begun. Although the Association of Collegiate Schools of Nursing asserted that it was not an accrediting agency, the standards required for membership in this organization, formed in 1932, accomplished the same thing for educational programs in institutions of higher education. Membership was greatly coveted, and this small, influential group, now extinct, gave the impetus to many of the forward-moving practices in higher education nursing.

The former National League of Nursing Education started in 1939 to accredit schools of nursing that met their criteria, publishing its first list on June 1, 1941. For years the former National Organization for Public Health Nursing had approved public health nursing programs for graduate nurses. The Council on Nursing Edcuation of the Catholic Hospital Association of the USA and Canada had begun to accredit programs in 1938. The accrediting movement gained great momentum when the nursing organizations joined forces. The schools appearing on their approved lists, including those from the Catholic Association, constituted the initial 190 accredited schools of the newly formed National Nursing Accrediting Service in 1948. Thus, duplication of visits and multiplicity of standards were eliminated. Groups of visitors and Boards of Review competent to look at all aspects of the offerings of educational units in nursing were established. The major effect was directed toward school improvement; a secondary objective was the publication of a list of schools that had achieved high standards of educational practice.

At the time of the reorganization of the 5 national nursing organizations in 1952, accreditation of educational programs was allocated to the new National League for Nursing. Criteria were established for the various types of programs, and policies and procedures were formulated. These are

[14] American Nurses' Association, *Educational Preparation for Nurse Practitioners and Assistants to Nurses, A Position Paper*, New York, The Association, 1965, p. 5.

[15] L. E. Notter, and K. M. Smith, *Community Planning for Nursing Education. The Experiences of Two State Nurses' Associations in Planning for Nursing Education in Their Areas*, New York, American Nurses' Association, 1968.

under constant scrutiny, evaluation and revision and are designed to encourage experimentation in nursing education. Accredited schools are listed annually in the periodical, *Nursing Outlook*. As of January 1968, 770 of the 1,296 nursing education programs were accredited by NLN.[16]

Types of Schools

Over the years, the length of American educational programs in nursing changed, and new types developed. The early, 1-year diploma programs in hospital schools of nursing lengthened to 2 years, and on Isabel Hampton Robb's advice to 3 years. Students from these programs continued to provide a very substantial amount of service to the hospital. Attempts to improve these programs included affiliations, sciences taught at nearby institutions of higher education, improved faculty preparation, increased class instruction and decreased repetitive work on hospital wards. Some diploma schools were under the jurisdiction of universities. The University of Minnesota School of Nursing, opened in 1909, was the first. Today, in some hospital schools the students maintain themselves; consequently, their clinical experiences may be selected to meet course objectives rather than the hospitals' needs. Some are operating on an academic year pattern while others have shortened their programs to 2 rather than 3 years.

During the period of World War I, a few colleges and universities began programs leading to bachelor's degrees. The oldest program, which began as a 5-year curriculum and is still in existence, was the Cincinnati University School of Nursing, founded in 1916. Many types of patterns developed. Some nursing units were in medical schools, departments of education or hygiene, and some were autonomous. In some early programs the students completed a major in a subject other than nursing, such as psychology, botany, or physiology, and were given "blanket credit" for their nursing education. In other programs, nursing was called the major, but in many cases the degree students had their nursing classes and experiences with the diploma students.

The Yale School of Nursing offering a preservice program under the leadership of Annie W. Goodrich, the "dean of American Nursing," was endowed by the Rockefeller Foundation and required college graduation for admission. It opened in 1924 and forged new patterns in nursing education.

A tremendous evolution has taken place during the last half century in baccalaureate degree programs. Now, general education constitutes about half the degree requirements, nursing is an accepted major, the students are active participants in college life and maintain themselves as do other college students. Public health nursing is a component part of their education. The percentage of students in baccalaureate programs has gradually risen from 5 in 1947 to 25.8 in 1967. The importance placed on baccalaureate education by the Surgeon General's Report, *Toward Quality in Nursing*, 1963,

[16] See also the section on "Accreditation" in Chapter 21, "National League for Nursing."

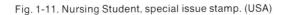
Fig. 1-11. Nursing Student, special issue stamp. (USA)

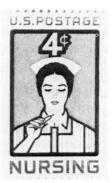

and by the ANA's 1965 position paper on nursing education assigns priority to these educational programs. They will prepare the broadly educated, highly competent nurses who can function as skilled practitioners, team leaders, public health nurses and, with experience, head nurses. From this group will come the graduate students who are preparing as clinical specialists and for teaching, supervision, administration, consultation and research.

The newest trend in nursing education is the development of programs in junior or community colleges with the goal of preparing the technical nurse. The programs, originated by Mildred Montag in 1952, go on the premise that competent nurses can be prepared in a shorter time by integrating many of the science and nursing courses, and by selecting clinical experience purely for its value in meeting course objectives. This trend places technical nursing education in the higher educational system and opens these courses to a segment of population that is wider in age range and marital status than do the typical diploma programs. It also seems to attract more men than do the other types of nursing programs.

Nursing education began with an apprenticeship type of training. The educational value decreased as the value of the learner to the hospital system became more and more evident. Finally, nursing education secured a place in the university and community college systems of the country. Nursing's place in the general educational institutions seems to be assured, and you can expect more nurses of the future to be prepared in junior and senior colleges along with other technical and professional workers in all fields.

COMMENTARY

Nursing has earned its present role in society through the hard work and vision of countless men and women working within organized nursing groups, the ANA and the NLN, as well as within civic and government groups or acting as individuals. This brief chapter brings you only a part of all of the influences which have affected the course of nursing. Religion, war,

self-determination and education were major influences in the past. However, they may seem to provide a limited frame of reference now if we
accept history as a dynamic expression of the time in which it occurs.
For example, while Christianity might have had considerable effect on our
system of nursing, the eastern cultures also had systems of patient care
which, though called medicine, were also often predominantly nursing in
nature. The Hebrew, Oriental and Indian cultures provided principles basic
to today's nursing care, for example, the work of Moses in developing laws
of sanitation. You might find it interesting to study the contribution of one
of these cultures to present day health care.

Indeed, nursing as the valuable institution it is today has been influenced,
and in turn has influenced, approaches to health care throughout history
and throughout the world. Presently it is an integral, interrelated part of
society and a vital force in all programs directed toward the care of the sick
and the disabled, the prevention of disease and the promotion of health.
Some of the present day influences on nursing include the rapid advance of
science and technology; the advent of space medicine; developments in
communications; advances in education; social progress, especially with
respect to the status of women throughout the world; and the emphasis
on assistance to developing countries and areas.

Tomorrow's nurses will need to be even more responsive to the health
care requirements of society, assisting in the determination, promotion and
attainment of those goals which modern science has made and will make
possible.

PROBLEMS

1. Summarize in a paper of about 1,000 words the contribution you feel
one person, selected from the following list, made to nursing. The paper
should include more than biographical material; it should be a report of
your interpretation of the difference that this person made in the development of nursing.

Nursing Education: Genevieve Bixler, Annie W. Goodrich, Nellie X.
Hawkenson, Elizabeth L. Kemble, R. Louise McManus, Florence Night-
ingale, M. Adelaide Nutting, Linda Richards, Isabel Hampton Robb,
Ruth Sleeper, Isabel M. Stewart and Margaret Tracey.

Red Cross Nursing: Clara Barton, Mary Beard, Jane Delano, Anne Magnussen and Clara D. Noyes.

Military Nursing and Federal Services: Edith Cavell, Dorothea Dix,
Annie W. Goodrich, Lucile Petry Leone, Pearl McIver and Julia Stimson,

Organization Work: Ella Best, Anna Fillmore, Janet M. Geister, Agnes
Gelinas, Adelaide A. Mayo, Blanche Pfefferkorn, Alma H. Scott and
Effie J. Taylor.

Public Health Nursing and Midwifery: Mary Breckenridge, Ruth Freeman, Mary Gardner, Annie W. Goodrich, Pearl McIver, Marion W. Sheahan and Lillian Wald.

Legislation: The Honorable Frances Payne Bolton, Elizabeth C. Burgess, Adda Eldridge and Lillian Wald.

Historian: Anne L. Austin, Lavinia Dock, Josephine Dolan, Virginia Dunbar, Sophia F. Palmer, Mary M. Roberts and Mabel K. Staupers.

Journalism: Sophia F. Palmer and Mary M. Roberts.

2. How have the following wars influenced health services and nursing: (a) World War II, (b) Korean War, (c) Vietnam War?

3. Compare earlier and modern practices in a selected field of nursing. What common strands do you find, and what marked differences in the 2 areas? (a) Curriculum of Kaiserswerth Deaconess Order vs. that of a modern diploma program. (b) Curriculum of the Nightingale School vs. that of a modern baccalaureate degree program. (c) Work of the Beguines vs. that of a modern public health nurse. (d) Work of the Augustinian Sisters vs. that of a modern hospital nurse. (e) Work and organization of the Knights of St. John of Jerusalem vs. that of the modern Army Nurse Corps. (f) Work of the Franciscan Tertiaries vs. that of the modern hospital volunteer. (g) Care of the insane in the 19th and the 20th centuries. (h) Military hospitals of the Civil War vs. a modern military hospital. (i) Midwifery of the Middle Ages vs. the Frontier Nursing Service. Prepare your material for oral class presentation.

4. Trace the major influences on graduate education for nursing in the USA beginning with the establishment of the nursing education program at Teachers College, Columbia University in 1899.

5. Trace the influence of the status of women generally on developments and progress in nursing.

SUGGESTED REFERENCES*

GENERAL

Atherton, W. H. *The Saintly Life of Jeanne Mance, First Lay Nurse in North America.* St. Louis, Catholic Hospital Association, 1945. Reprinted from *Hospital Progress,* June, July, and August, 1945, as Bulletin 282.

Austin, A. L. *History of Nursing Source Book,* New York, Putnam, 1957.

Bishop, W. J. "Florence Nightingale's Message for Today." *Nursing Outlook,* 8:246-249, May 1960.

Bullough, V. L. and Bullough, B. *The Emergence of Modern Nursing.* New York, Macmillan, 1969.

* Christy, T. E. "Portrait of a Leader: Lavinia Lloyd Dock." *Nursing Outlook,* 17:72-75, June 1969.

* _____. "Portrait of a Leader: Isabel Hampton Robb." *Nursing Outlook,* 17:26-29, Mar. 1969.

---

* In each chapter, all references used as citations are footnoted and are not included here. All starred references are recommended for additional reading.

* _____. "Portrait of a Leader: M. Adelaide Nutting." *Nursing Outlook,* **17**:20-24, Jan. 1969.

Disselhoff, D. "The Deaconesses of Kaiserswerth: A Hundred Years' Work." *International Nursing Review,* **9**:19-28, 1934.

Dock, L. L. *A History of Nursing,* vols. III and IV. New York, Putnam, 1912.

Dolan, J. A. *History of Nursing.* Philadelphia, Saunders, 1968.

Hampton, I. A., *et al. Nursing of the Sick, 1893.* New York, McGraw-Hill, 1949.

Kernodle, P. B. *The Red Cross Nurse in Action.* New York, Harper, 1949.

Nightingale, F. *Notes on Nursing.* New York, Appleton-Century, 1946. Facsimile of 1860 edition.

Norman, G. *Dorothea Lynde Dix.* New York, Putnam, 1959.

Roberts, M. M. *American Nursing.* New York, Macmillan, 1954.

* Stewart, I. M., and Austin, A. L. *A History of Nursing.* New York, Putnam, 1962.

Strachey, L. "Florence Nightingale" in *Eminent Victorians,* New York, Harcourt-Brace, 1918.

Wald, L. *The House on Henry Street.* New York, Holt, 1938.

* _____. *Windows on Henry Street.* New York, Little-Brown, 1934.

Woodham-Smith, C. *Florence Nightingale.* New York, McGraw-Hill, 1951.

* Woolsey, A. H. *A Century of Nursing.* New York, Putnam, 1950.

MILITARY

* Barber, H. J. "The Symbol of the Cross as Used in Nursing." *American Journal of Nursing,* **37**:788-792, July 1937.

Boardman, M. T. *Under the Red Cross Flag at Home and Abroad.* Philadelphia, Lippincott, 1915.

Cumming, K. *Kate: The Journal of a Confederate Nurse.* Edited by Richard Barksdale Harwell. Baton Rouge, Louisiana State University Press, 1959.

Dunant, H. *Un Souvenir de Solferino.* New York, Winston, 1911. Translated from the French by Mrs. David H. Wright.

Epler, P. H. *The Life of Clara Barton.* New York, Macmillan, 1927.

Greenbie, M. B. *Lincoln's Daughters of Mercy.* New York, Putnam, 1944.

Gumpert, M. *Dunant, The Story of the Red Cross.* New York, Oxford, 1938.

* Judson, H. *Edith Cavell.* New York, Macmillan, 1941.

Leech, M. *Reveille in Washington, 1860-1865.* New York, Harper, 1941, pp. 204-233.

Marshall, H. E. *Dorothea Dix: Forgotten Samaritan.* Chapel Hill, University of North Carolina Press, 1937.

Pember, P. Y. *A Southern Woman's Story.* Jackson, Tennessee, McGowat-Mercer, 1959.

* Roberts, M. M. *The Army Nurse Corps Yesterday and Today.* Washington, D.C., The United States Army Nurse Corps, 1957.

* Ross, I. *Angel of the Battlefield: The Life of Clara Barton.* New York, Harper, 1956.

EDUCATIONAL

* American Nurses' Association. *Educational Preparation for Nurse Practitioners and Assistants to Nurses: A Position Paper,* New York, The Association, 1965.

Bridgman, M. *Collegiate Education for Nursing.* New York, Russell Sage Foundation, 1953.

Brown, E. L. *Nursing for the Future.* New York, Russell Sage Foundation, 1948.

Columbia University. Teachers College. Division of Nursing Education. *Education for Nursing: Past, Present, and Future.* New York, National League for Nursing Exchange, 1959.

Committee on the Grading of Nursing Schools. *Nursing Schools Today and Tomorrow.* New York, The Committee, 1934.

* Goldmark, J. *Nursing and Nursing Education in the United States.* New York, Macmillan, 1923.

* Koch, H. B. *Militant Angel (Annie W. Goodrich).* New York, Macmillan, 1951.

* McKay, R. "A Comparative Approach to the Development of Nursing Education." *Nursing Science,* 2:125-137, April 1964.

Montag, M. L. *Community College Education for Nursing.* New York, McGraw-Hill, 1959.

National League for Nursing. *Three Score Years and Ten, 1893-1963.* New York, The League, 1963.

Richards, L. *Reminiscences of Linda Richards.* Boston, Whitcomb-Barrows, 1911.

Rogers, M. E. *Reville in Nursing.* Philadelphia, Davis, 1964.

_____. *Educational Revolution in Nursing.* New York, Macmillan, 1961.

* Russell, C. H. "Liberal Education and Nursing." *Nursing Research,* 7:116-126, Oct. 1958.

Seymer, L. R. "The Nightingale Training School: One Hundred Years Ago." *American Journal of Nursing,* 60:658-661, May 1960.

Spalding, E. K. "Trends and Problems in Advanced Nursing Education." *American Journal of Nursing,* 47:113-115, Feb. 1947.

* Stewart, I. M. *The Education of Nurses.* New York, Macmillan, 1943.

* U. S. Department of Health, Education, and Welfare. *Toward Quality in Nursing: Needs and Goals.* Report of the Surgeon General's Consultant Group on Nursing. Washington, D.C., Government Printing Office, 1963.

* West, M., and Hawkins, C. *Nursing Schools at the Mid-Century.* New York, National Committee for the Improvement of Nursing Services, 1950.

"What's Happening to Proposed Goal III?" *American Journal of Nursing,* 64:94-95, Mar. 1964.

CHAPTER

2

Professional Nursing in Its Present Social Setting

The most striking characteristic of our present society is change. The speed and the amount of this change affect all aspects of our lives—physical and emotional, social and economic. We seem to be in transition, moving from an abandoned past toward a future we are as yet unable to comprehend. The goals of our time are complex and technical. Nursing, along with other professional services to society, is not self-contained but modifies and is modified by its social setting. Many of the issues that confront nursing are only reflections of issues that face many other groups. For some of these issues to be resolved, first there must be changes in the structure and the functioning of our society. Similarly, many of the changes that seem to be unique to nursing have resulted, wholly or in part, from forces that have their origins outside of nursing and represent the ways in which nursing has adapted itself to the conditions created by these forces.

A major problem today is that of adaptation to the pace of change. It is important that you, as a future nurse, be aware of the influences that have helped to shape nursing as it now exists, and that you be alert to signs of impending shifts in the currents that may affect its future course. It is only through such awareness on the part of its members that nursing will be able to adapt itself to or even to change conditions in the manner that is best for the society which it serves.

SOME DISCERNIBLE TRENDS

It would, of course, be impossible within the scope of this book to delve into all of the forces that have made nursing what it is today and that have potentialities for influencing its future development. We shall mention a few here in the hope that you will be stimulated to search for others.

Consider, for example, the following sociological and economic facts and trends in the USA and their impact on nursing service and nursing education during the coming 5 to 10 years:

1. Increasing involvement of the Federal Government in health, education and welfare

2. The trend toward higher education for increasing numbers of the general population

3. A continuing rise in the standard of living while huge poverty areas also continue

4. The trend toward development of programs for removing or decreasing poverty

5. Experimentation with methods of distributing health care

6. Growth of prepaid health insurance by government and private agencies (Medicare and Medicaid, for example) as a way of meeting increasing health costs

7. The trend toward greater interest in solving the problems of aging

8. The emergence of black power and all of its implications

9. The growing demands of students in colleges and universities for greater participation in determining university policies, practices and programs

10. The movement toward elevation of civil disobedience to a civil virtue

11. The search for ways to create new jobs for the uneducated and the poor in lieu of expanding welfare programs

12. The international involvement of the USA, both in aid programs for developing countries and in wars

13. Effects on society resulting from the Korean and Vietnam wars

14. Effects of mass communications on our society, for example, the influence of newspapers and television on formulating and changing public opinion

15. Effects of studies on the use of tobacco and additive substances

16. The fantastic increase in the use of psychedelic and similar habit-forming drugs

17. Influence of such groups as the hippies and the yippies on family living and school life

18. The advent of regional planning for social, economic, educational and health endeavors

19. Shifts in the settings in which health care is given—the trend toward greater use of outpatient and extended care facilities

20. The increasing use of automation in hospitals and other health agencies

21. The expansion of knowledge about, and interest in, the behavioral sciences

22. The growing awareness of the importance of research and the development of research methods

23. Nuclear research and space explorations

Again, it would require a whole book to investigate the many repercussions that these trends have had and may have on nursing. The discussion here will be limited to a few of the effects on the role of nursing, the volume of nursing care, the organization of nursing services, the relationships between nursing and the other health professions and nursing education. All of these topics, of course, have a distinct bearing on the practice of nursing.

ROLE OF NURSING[1]

One of the chief characteristics of nursing today, and one which has created conflicts yet to be resolved, is the expanding and changing role of nursing in our society. Nursing is a major community health service, giving highly personal service in the care of individual patients. This role has been, and continues to be, greatly influenced by developments in modern science, technology and health legislation.

Some Conflicts About the Role of Nursing

Perhaps no health worker has been expected to assume so many and such diverse functions as has the nurse. While most nurses continue to work in hospitals, others can be found in many different settings — outpatient departments, extended care facilities, community health services, industry and schools, to mention some of the more traditional settings aside from hospitals. Today nurses can also be found working with regional medical programs, alcoholism and drug addiction programs, programs in poverty areas in this country and programs in the developing countries abroad. Nurses in these various settings may, in addition to having responsibility for their own practice, be carrying various amounts of supervisory, administrative, or teaching responsibility.

Nurses are also taking on a variety of new responsibilities in the hospital itself, in such situations as nursing in intensive care and coronary care units.

In viewing all of the varied responsibilities carried by nurses and the trend toward their assumption of additional functions, the complexity of the role of nursing can be seen. The question is frequently raised: What is

[1] The role of nursing is considered in a general way in this section. See Chapter 4, "Responsibility for Nursing Practice," for a more comprehensive discussion of the practice of nursing.

nursing? There would seem to be two main camps of thought about what the nursing role should be. The first group concentrates on the "nurturant" role of the nurse and believes nurses should confine their activities to this role.[2] The second group looks upon the nurse as the one best able to take over some of the physician's traditional functions in the hospital, in the patient's home and in the physician's office.[3]

It is perhaps inevitable that in a period of rapid and far reaching social and technological change there should be conflict about what the role of nursing in society should be. However, there can be no doubt that nursing will play an increasingly important role in the provision of health care. It remains in the hands of nurses themselves to evaluate the forces around them in order to plan the most effective nursing course and to attain the broad goal of improved health care in addition to the actual care of individual patients. According to Marian Sheahan:

Nurses, wherever they live and wherever they work, must understand the community aspects of the health care problem in its social, economic, and medical care aspects. The point of view of nurses as professionals and civic-minded citizens is important in community planning. Their views will be respected and sought to the extent the nurse is knowledgeable of the trends and of the interprofessional relationships involved in the complicated society in which we live.[4]

Growth of Modern Science and Technology

The second half of the 20th century is witnessing phenomenal advances in medical care as a result of the growth of modern science and technology in this country. The resulting changes in medicine and in the organization and administration of health services have and will continue to have a major effect on nursing.

At the same time that the teaching role of the nurse was recognized, there began to be a corresponding expansion of her independent functions. Today, the nurse is expected to determine the nursing needs of her patients, often referred to as "nursing diagnosis"; she is taking on increasing responsibilities from physicians; she performs more highly specialized tasks; she is more often expected to exercise independent judgment; and she is called on to use initiative in instituting emergency measures. In addition, the nurse continues to have an ever growing responsibility for the teaching and direction of a variety of auxiliary nursing personnel.

In recent years there has been increasing evidence of the influence of developments in modern science. The growth of research in nursing shows recognition of the need for scientific investigation to improve nursing

[2] V. Henderson, *The Nature of Nursing*, New York, Macmillan, 1966, and A. Baziak, "What Constitutes Clinical Practice?" *Nursing Forum*, 7:98-109, Winter 1968.

[3] J. P. Connelly, *et al.*, "The Physician and the Nurse—Their Interprofessional Work in Office and Hospital Ambulatory Settings," *New England Journal of Medicine*, 275:765-769, Oct 6, 1967.

[4] M. Sheahan, "Through Community Action: A Health Commission Reports," *American Journal of Nursing*, 66:1302, June 1966.

practice. The idea that nursing encompasses not only practice by the practitioner and teaching by the nurse educator, but also research by the nurse scientist, is slowly gaining ground.

Influence of Health Legislation

In 1965 some of the most significant health legislation of this century was passed—legislation which has deeply affected our system of health care in all of its aspects, including nursing. Two bills in particular are of great interest to nursing, *Public Law 89-97*, popularly known as Medicare, and *Public Law 89-239*, which established the regional medical programs.

The influence of Medicare on the character of health care services in terms of both quantity and quality was almost immediate and will continue. Of particular interest is the greatly expanded need for extended care facilities and home health agencies which meet the standards set for participation in the programs—facilities and agencies where nursing is of the utmost significance. The emphasis in these programs upon continuity of care has done more than all previous efforts of nurses to effect greater interrelation of nursing care between the hospital and the home care agency (see section on "Continuity of Care" later on in this chapter).

Nursing is also deeply involved in the institution of regional medical programs. Many nurses have served on advisory and planning committees for these programs, and have been employed on the staffs of specific regional projects. Educational programs for nurses in the care of heart, stroke and cancer patients have been initiated under these regional programs. It would be of interest to you to determine in what way nursing has participated in the regional medical programs in your state and the reciprocal influence of this program on nursing.

Concept of Health

We no longer think of health as merely the absence of disease. Instead, we regard it as a state of physical, mental, emotional and spiritual well-being in which the individual is able to function to the optimum extent of his potentialities. As a result of this broadened concept of health, rehabilitation and the promotion of health have become major objectives of health care, including nursing care. Emphasis on these goals has underlined the teaching role of nursing. To help a young mother to start her child toward healthy adulthood, or to assist a cardiac patient in understanding and accepting the need for limiting his activities, the nurse must be far more of a teacher than when she was concerned merely with ministrations directed toward making the patient comfortable and curing him of disease.

At the same time that teaching was being recognized as one of the most important dimensions of modern nursing, educational science was shedding new light on the nature of the teaching-learning process. Increasing emphasis was being placed on the fact that the learner must be an active participant in this process, not a passive receptacle for information.

This concept of teaching carries tremendous implications for nursing. Nursing care is conceived of not only as doing things *to* and *for* a patient but also as doing things *with* him; and of assisting him to learn to do as much *for himself* as possible, thus maintaining his independence. The idea of self-care as a part of rehabilitation and health maintenance is a recognized component of this concept. Such a concept obviously requires that the nurse and the patient have feelings of regard for and confidence in each other. Thus, the establishment of effective patient-nurse-physician relationships, in which the patient, the nurse, and the physician can come to agreement on the patient's health goals and cooperate in their achievement, is now recognized as one of the most important foundation stones of modern nursing practice.

VOLUME OF NURSING CARE AND GROWTH OF ORGANIZED SERVICES

Coincident with the expanding role of nursing, forces were at work which challenged and temporarily interfered with its fullest realization. Obviously, the pattern of nursing service most conducive to the establishment of close nurse-patient-physician relationships is that found in the private practice of nursing. In it, a nurse remains with the patient throughout the period when he requires nursing care, either in his own home or, as his companion and friend, in the strange world of the hospital. Since there is no intermediary nurse-employer between the nurse and the patient, and since they have a certain amount of freedom in selecting each other, a feeling of mutual trust and confidence tends to be fostered.

Private practice is no longer the dominant pattern of nursing service. One reason is that the patient can no longer bear the cost of private nursing care. Another reason is the mobility of our population. For people who move from one community to another, there is no "family doctor" and "family nurse" who, in former times, often knew their patients from birth and were intimately acquainted not only with their economic situations and medical histories but also with those of their sisters and their cousins and their aunts. Furthermore, nurses themselves found more economic security and opportunities for professional advancement in employment in organized services.

Increased Interest in Health

An even more important factor in the dwindling prevalence of private nursing practice was the explosion in the volume of demand for nursing services in hospitals and related health care facilities and agencies. With the rapid increase in the ratio of population to land, a man's talents and abilities became a most important, and in many instances, his only income-producing asset. Therefore, it behooved him to take the best possible care of himself. Others, too, recognized that they had a stake in his health for economic reasons, if for no other. His employers, realizing the relationship between his health and his efficiency as a worker, became convinced of the value of commercial and industrial health services. His fellow citizens recognized that it was to their interest that he remain or become a fully productive member of society, and they saw the advantages that would accrue from publicly supported health services of various kinds. At the same time, the increasing productivity of our economy made it possible for people, both individually and collectively, to purchase more health care than had previously been within their means. The growth of private health-care insurance and the introduction of Medicare and Medicaid which have acted to increase purchasing power by spreading the risk, also have served to increase the demand for service. With the desire for more health services burgeoning and the financial means for developing them at hand, their swift multiplication was inevitable.

New Patterns of Services

Obviously, a pattern of nursing service built on a one-to-one relationship between patient and nurse could not meet this multiplied demand for health care. There simply would not be enough nurses to go around. Under the circumstances, it was inevitable that the private practice of nursing would, to a large extent, be superseded by patterns of nursing service in which one nurse's services could be divided among several patients. In 1966, 65.3 per cent of all employed nurses worked in hospitals.

Other reasons undoubtedly exist for the growth of organized nursing services: the pleasure that many people experience from working in groups; the opportunities that group work gives an individual to rise to a leadership position; and the desire on the part of many people, including nurses, for the security afforded by a regular pay check, paid vacations and sick leaves and insurance and retirement benefits. However, these last-mentioned reasons seem to be less compelling to a profession with the social conscience of nursing and are probably secondary to the first one: recognition of the responsibility for distributing available nursing services according to the exigencies of each person rather than according to his ability to pay for them.

Despite the wider dispersion of nursing services that was achieved through this re-patterning, the demands for nursing care continued to outstrip the supply. Advances in the health sciences made nursing care by trained people essential for many patients who formerly would have been cared for by members of their families. Besides, the family reservoir of nursing care — the mothers and the sisters and the maiden aunts — had, in many instances, been drained off into offices and professional careers of their own. Also, the gap between "services demanded" and "services available" had been further widened by the shortening of the workweek for all workers, including nurses.

Increase in Number of Nurses

It soon became apparent that, to close the gap between services demanded and services available, all obtainable human resources must be utilized. As a result of several social trends, these resources were expanding. First, unmarried women joined the working population in large numbers. Later, it was not unusual for them to continue their careers after marriage and to resume them when their family responsibilities were lightened. The increase in the number of female workers was particularly significant to professions like nursing that have a special appeal for women. So, also, was the trend toward education for all according to their abilities. The expansion in the number of high school graduates swelled the reservoir of potential students of nursing, and larger and larger proportions of these graduates made plans for continuing their education. Efforts have been made to increase the percentage of these graduates who enter nursing and to direct these potential nursing students into programs for which they are best suited. Minority racial groups, hitherto denied many career and educational opportunities, were welcomed into many professions, including nursing. It might be noted that as a result of the wider educational opportunities becoming available to Negroes, the supply of candidates for nursing careers should continue to increase, though in 1966 to 1967 only 4 per cent of all of the girls graduating from high school were recruited into nursing programs. It would seem important at this time to intensify recruitment of racial minority groups and men into nursing.

In the past few years great emphasis has been placed upon helping the inactive nurse return to nursing. Special inducements include refresher courses, part-time work, provision of nursery school facilities, and the like. With funds from the U.S. Department of Labor and the Bureau of Health Manpower, Division of Nursing of the Public Health Service, the ANA in 1967 spearheaded a national refresher course project in which a number of the states participated.[5] In 1968, the Federal Government released $1 million in additional funds for the ongoing refresher programs.[6]

By capitalizing on these social trends, nursing was able to increase the number of employed registered nurses from slightly over 100,000 in 1920 to about 593,694 in 1966. It is interesting to note that 63.5 per cent of these employed nurses were married. Yet even this increase in personnel was insufficient for the mounting demands of our health-conscious population. It has been suggested that we will need 1 million nurses by 1975.[7] All of our best efforts will be required to increase our numbers to this amount. The

[5] "ANA Begins Promotional Campaign for National Refresher Course Project," *ANA in Action,* 1:4, Sept.-Oct. 1967.

[6] "$1 Million Released for Refresher Courses," (At Press Time) *American Journal of Nursing,* **68:**939, May 1968.

[7] U.S. Department of Health, Education, and Welfare. Public Health Service, *Nurse Training Act of 1964: Program Review Report,* Washington, D.C., Government Printing Office, 1967.

fact is that this is one of the most serious challenges nursing has to face in the next few years.

Auxiliary Nursing Personnel

Nurses are trying to meet this challenge. They take the stand that nursing is much broader than a profession; it is an occupation that embraces activities requiring less than professional knowledge and skill. Therefore, it can assimilate into its services people who are not registered nurses, thereby extending the human resources from which it draws its personnel.

This has been a very difficult step for so young a profession to take. It has not yet had time to define fully its unique professional functions, to clarify its relationships with the other health disciplines or to come to grips with many of its educational problems. To these unsolved problems it is now adding others: the differentiation of the tasks that could be performed by several types of workers, the training of these new workers, and the organization of nursing services in such a way that each worker can assume his appropriate responsibilities.

The preparation, organization and use of the auxiliary nursing groups have proven to be an enormous and sometimes impossible task. Yet, it is one of great significance. The solving of the problems and issues involved should have the highest priority for the nursing profession if nursing practice is to be improved. For example, adequate teaching and supervision of auxiliary personnel is a serious problem. The mounting pressure from society and government to plan for upward mobility among the various groups in nursing, including the auxiliary groups, is posing another serious problem and one most difficult to solve.

ORGANIZATION OF NURSING SERVICES

As has been pointed out, one of the fundamentals of modern nursing practice is the existence of a close relationship between the patient and his nurse. The shift in the settings in which health care is given, particularly affected by the growth of hospitals, ambulatory services, extended care facilities and home health agencies, has had a marked effect on the practice of nursing. As nursing became institutionalized, the patient has been confronted with a succession of strangers; similarly, the nurse has had to become acquainted with the nursing problems of many patients. One of the major problems of nursing has been, and continues to be, adjusting to its institutionalization in such a way that effective patient-nurse-physician relationships can be maintained. On the other hand, the employing health agencies have a tremendous responsibility to recruit competent nursing personnel, to organize nursing services in such a way as to provide adequate nursing service at all times, and to continuously improve that service through appropriate inservice education, on-the-job training, supervision, and the use of sound administrative policies and practices.

Continuity of Care

One approach to coordination of services has been to establish relationships between the different kinds of nursing services. The multiplicity of patient-nurse-physician relationships is partially caused by the variety of settings in which nursing services are offered. As an example, the nursing care of an industrial worker may begin in an occupational health service and be continued first in a hospital, then in a convalescent home, and finally with the care provided by a public health nursing agency in his own home. Nurses associated with 4 different agencies have been involved in his care. How can he be helped to feel less like a stranger with each new nurse whom he meets? And how can his care be made continuous so that there is no loss of gains in his progress toward rehabilitation or health?

One way, as you know, is for each nurse to learn about the patient's problems and needs from her predecessor. Then, when she first meets the patient, he is less of a stranger to her. Also, just as we become acquainted more quickly with people who have heard about us from our friends, the patient can accept the nurse more rapidly. Adequate referral systems between institutions and agencies that provide nursing care therefore can constitute an important means of furthering the quick establishment of relationships between nurses and patients. While referral systems have been advocated for a number of years as a means of providing for continuity of care, progress has been slow in their development. With the myriad of services patients are involved in from hospital, to extended care facility, to home care, and to ambulatory care, it is crucial that a plan be made for continuity of care. A large share of the responsibility for leadership in developing a system whereby continuity is assured belongs with nursing.

Staffing Patterns

The problem of staffing is not only one of securing interorganizational continuity of care. Within each agency, the patient must be helped to feel close enough to one nurse to be able to tell her about his problems and talk over his future course of action with her. While he may have nursing care from a number of different people, he should be able to identify one of them as "my nurse." While there are a few isolated instances where patients may be able to identify and relate to their own nurse, in most situations today no patient can be assured of this. This is a major and serious situation.

In the hospital, however, where nursing care is not by appointment, it is obviously impossible to assure each patient that one particular nurse will be available each time he needs attention. This is true in all types of nursing service, including home health agencies. Nursing personnel in hospital services have always been in short supply, and sometimes nursing activities have been organized so as to get the job done rather than to get it done well. When the practice of nursing was regarded as mainly consisting of the performance of technical procedures, it was not unusual to find an assembly-line division of labor with one nurse taking temperatures, another changing dressings, a third giving medications and so on. Under this system of "functional assignment," patients did not appear like people to some nurses but rather were recognized as "the leg in Ward 8" and "the heart in Ward 2." From the patient's point of view, these nurses seemed like machines. Since a leg can scarcely be expected to develop any feeling for a machine or vice versa, such arrangements were scarcely conducive to the establishment of anything like a nurse-patient relationship. On the other hand, under the "patient assignment" method, one nurse might have to give all the nursing care to so many patients that she scarcely had time to find out their names, much less to become acquainted with each one of them.

The advent of practical nurses and nursing aides as well as the use of many volunteer workers in hospital nursing services has relieved the personnel shortage considerably, but it has made the organizational problems more complex. Since these allied nursing personnel cannot perform all nursing activities, each worker cannot be given responsibility for the total care of a given number of patients. Nor, fortunately perhaps, is the functional-assignment method suitable. The giving of a bath or an enema to certain patients might appropriately be assigned to an aide or a practical nurse. However, this would not be safe in the case of other patients.

Therefore, hospital as well as other types of nursing services have been experimenting with different staffing patterns. The one that has received most attention thus far is the nursing-team method, in which a group of nursing workers of various categories, under the leadership of a professional nurse, is assigned responsibility for the total nursing care of a group of patients. The team leader is responsible for identifying the nursing problems of each patient; for determining, with the patient, the nursing objectives; for developing a program of individualized nursing care; and for assigning appropriate tasks to each of the other workers. She might be likened to the mother of a large family who has help from other people but does not relinquish the role and the full responsibility of motherhood. Similarly, the team leader works through others whenever possible, but when direct care of a professional nature is needed, she is able to "take over." In other words, she is still the patient's nurse and is recognized by him as such, even though she often calls upon others for help in providing him with all of the care that he needs.

It has not been determined whether the nursing-team plan is the best solution, one of many appropriate solutions, or no solution to the problem of organizing nursing services in such a way that patients may have modern nursing care. The evaluation of this method and experimentation with other methods are among the tasks that face you and others among the coming generation of nurses. Other ways of organizing nursing care that are in common use today are, of course, "intensive nursing care," "recovery room care" and "progressive patient care," with emphasis on "self care", the use of clinical nursing specialists and the use of unit managers. Chapter 4, "Responsibility for Nursing Practice," will go into these various methods of organizing care in greater detail.

RELATIONSHIP OF NURSING TO OTHER HEALTH DISCIPLINES

As a result of the tremendous advances in scientific knowledge and technology that have occurred during the past few decades, there has been a great trend toward specialization throughout our entire society. This trend has been particularly apparent in the health field, which has been affected so greatly by scientific developments. One of its results has been the creation of the *health team*. For example, no one person could be expected to be conversant with the intricacies of such fast-growing bodies of knowledge as pharmacology and nutrition, but by bringing together experts in these and other fields, the hospital can give the patient the advantage of their combined knowledge and skills.

The Nurse as Coordinator

The advent of so many specialists and specialized services in the hospital has created a new responsibility for nursing—that of coordinating all of the activities that involve contact with the patient. Although many other members of the health team work directly with the patient, they do so only at intervals. Since nursing is the only service that is continuously at the patient's side, those responsible for these other services must rely on the nurse to observe the patient in all situations and to report significant occurrences to appropriate personnel. For example, the physician and the nutritionist may prescribe and plan a dietary regimen, but it is the nurse who needs to see that the patient gets the right foods, who observes which foods the patient refuses to eat and who finds out the reasons for this rejection, determining whether the rejection and the reasons for it should be reported. Moreover, she is aware of the services that have been given to the patient by others and can raise questions when she has reason to believe that the objectives of these services contradict rather than complement each other.

Poor Utilization of Nursing Personnel

Unfortunately, the coordinating and collaborative functions of nurses have often been misinterpreted as assisting roles. This misunderstanding possibly had its origins in the days when the health team was limited to the nurse and the physician and sometimes the members of the patient's family. At that time the nurse was inclined to think of her responsibilities as embracing all of the tasks required to further the patient's health that were not done by the rest of this small team. She served in such roles as manager of the patient's environment, supervisor of his nutritional requirements, recreational therapist and social worker. Although these roles have since been taken over by specialized personnel, because of her understanding of them the nurse frequently has been expected to serve as a stand-in. At a time when there is a desperate need for personnel to fulfill important nursing responsibilities, nurses still serve as nighttime hospital administrators, junior physicians, assistant housekeepers, pharmacists' helpers and clerical workers. Thus, the nurse who has a unique contribution to make to the health care of patients and is therefore as much of a specialist as any other member of the health team is frequently treated like a Jack-of-all-trades. Efforts are underway to change this practice.

Nurses have made a start in solving this problem by clarifying the functions that are unique to nursing. Some hospitals, recognizing this, have begun to provide around-the-clock, 7-day-a-week services in areas other than nursing. However, until there is wider acceptance by all health personnel, including nurses themselves, that the nurse's first responsibility is to fill the role for which she alone is prepared, nursing will not be able to realize its maximum potential contribution to the care of patients.

NURSING EDUCATION

Trends in Education for Other Fields

It is interesting to note the evolutionary stages through which various kinds of professional and technical education have passed in this country. In some instances the first step has been apprenticeship training in which the student helped the lawyer or the physician or the master craftsman, as the case might be, with his work, meanwhile learning from him the knowledge he was able to impart. While this form of education had the advantages of a one-to-one student-teacher relationship, the educational resources from which the student could draw reposed largely with a single person. Another fairly early stage was the autonomous, single-purpose school — the normal school that prepared only teachers, the medical school that prepared only physicians, and so on. While such schools could offer the student instruction from a variety of experts in his chosen field, few of them could provide the wealth and the variety of resources in related fields that are found in an institution of higher education. Accordingly, as the importance of scientific and humanistic foundations for all fields of work became recognized, most of these separate schools moved into such educational institutions. By and large, the trend of professional and technical education in this country has been toward amalgamation with institutions of higher learning.

Trends in Nursing Education

Nursing education followed this trend to a certain point. It began as a learning-through-service experience; then schools of nursing were developed. However, these schools were not autonomous institutions but were departments of hospitals. Nor did the majority of them move into multi-purpose educational institutions. When the need for instruction in the sciences and the humanities became apparent, the hospital school either supplied such instruction itself or made arrangements with an institution of higher learning for affiliated courses. Generally speaking, however, the hospital school has not been able to provide the broad cultural and scientific climate of the university or to give its students the benefits that come from association with students in other fields.

Some of these hospital schools, particularly those in university hospitals, have been closed or the universities have taken over responsibility for the schools. Other colleges, including junior colleges, have established programs in nursing at various levels. An important issue for these schools is the selection and control of the clinical setting for their students. Graduate education for nurses is recognized as belonging within the orbit of the university. During the last decade particularly, the growth of nursing programs in educational institutions has far exceeded that of hospital schools of nursing, which have in fact declined somewhat during the past few years. In the main, however, the preparation of registered nurses has remained under the control of service institutions outside the current of general education.

An Unresolved Issue

Although the question of appropriate control for educational programs in nursing has been debated widely for many years, until recently the issue has been largely an academic one. It has become a very live one in the past few years. Up to this time it is doubtful whether institutions of higher learning have been in a position to absorb a student body of approximately 140,000 students or whether these institutions and students of nursing could have borne together the full costs of nursing education. Furthermore, nursing has not been able to supply an adequate number of teachers with the academic qualifications for appointment to faculties in institutions of higher education.

Whether, in the absence of these barriers, nursing education would have followed the trend of other professional and technical education is a matter of speculation. It might be noted that practical nursing education, which has been less affected by these problems, has largely developed under educational auspices, but it came into existence at a time when the responsibility for almost all education had been assumed by educational institutions.

In any event, there are certain indications that these barriers may be removed. The capacity of publicly supported institutions of higher learning, particularly community colleges, is expanding rapidly. State legislatures are providing scholarships for students in fields of social importance such as nursing. In other words, there appears to be a trend toward public provision for higher education to all who can profit from it. Furthermore, under the impetus of both foundation and government grants, the supply of academically qualified teaching personnel is increasing. The Federal Government itself, through *Public Law 88-581* (The Nurse Training Act of 1964), provides assistance with construction or rehabilitation of school facilities, school improvement grants and student loans.

The effect of present efforts of the national nursing organizations, as well as of outstanding nurse educators, is evidenced by the growth in number and quality of nursing education programs in colleges and universities. By the end of 1967 there were 221 baccalaureate degree programs and 281 programs in community or junior colleges, as compared to 167 and 28 in 1957.[8] It will be interesting to watch the effect of the efforts of the ANA to implement their stand on education – that all who work in nursing should be educated in institutions of learning within the general system of education. Their position further states that minimum education for professional nursing should be a baccalaureate degree in nursing, and for technical nursing an associate degree.[9]

While much progress has been made in the movement of nursing education into educational institutions, the issue of education for nursing remains a live one. There are many who do not agree with the ANA position on preparation for professional and technical nursing practice. The resolution of the issue will take time and thoughtful, responsible action.

As a result of a recommendation made by the Surgeon General's Consultant Group on Nursing, a National Commission for the Study of Nursing Education was established in 1967. Organized as an independent, autonomous commission by the ANA and the NLN, it will study the present system of nursing education in terms of the levels of skill and responsibilities needed by the nurse to give high quality nursing care. It is anticipated that the work of the commission will take about 3 years and that the findings will provide the information and recommendations needed for effective future planning.

It is suggested that you study the report when it becomes available in 1970, especially the implications for programs preparing professional and technical nurses. Meanwhile, you will be interested in reviewing current trends and forces affecting nursing and nursing education in your own state or region in the past 5 years. During this same time what activities have been carried out by your state nurses association and state league for nursing with regard to nursing education? To what extent should nursing students themselves be involved in planning the direction of their preparation for future practice?

YOUR RESPONSIBILITY

As you review these issues and trends that have been discussed in this chapter and as you see the advantages that they have brought to your profession, and the problems that they have created for it, you will realize

---

[8] M. B. Harty, "Trends in Nursing Education," *American Journal of Nursing,* **68**:767, Apr. 1968.

[9] American Nurses' Association, *Educational Preparation for Nurse Practitioners and Assistants to Nurses: A Position Paper,* New York, The Association, 1965.

your responsibility as a nurse to study and deal with current and future trends. Here are a few guidelines about how to meet this responsibility.

1. Be alert to trends that seem to be appearing over the horizon. For example, there is a significant increase in the number of patients who require nursing-home care and a recognition that nurses are responsible for establishing and promoting acceptable standards of nursing care in these institutions. There is also increasing awareness of the importance of ambulatory and home-care services in most communities today, particularly for those with long-term illness or disability. Moreover, opinion is growing, particularly in the mental-health field, that many patients who are now in a hospital could be rehabilitated better in other environments. Take note of such trends; then think about how they might affect nursing services and nursing education.

2. Recognize that an occurrence may affect nursing in several ways. At the same time that it solves a problem it may create another. For example, while the increasing health-consciousness of the American public is, of course, eminently desirable, it has brought many problems to nursing. Therefore, if there is a choice as to whether nursing should go along with a particular trend, weigh carefully the advantages and the disadvantages of doing so. In any event, choice or no choice, be prepared to capitalize on the favorable results of any shift that may occur; at the same time, plan ways of meeting the problems that it may bring.

3. Do not assume that you or anyone else can predict all the developments that will occur. Build up your inner strengths so that you will be able to accept and deal with the unforeseeable with courage and confidence. This is probably the biggest and most important task that faces you as a future nurse and as a member of society.

Because nursing is predominately a woman's profession, the status of nurses and nursing is closely related to the status of women generally. In 1963, the Commission on the Status of Women, appointed by President Kennedy, issued its important report, *American Women*.[10] (See Figure 2-1.)

According to Miss Esther Peterson, vice-chairman of the Commission, we must upgrade the working conditions of women. The concept that it is normal for women to have a "working life" is an accepted fact, and in 1963 the average age of women who were working was 41 years, a marked contrast to the average age of 26 in 1900.[11] The need for continuing education and for opportunities for higher education for women was emphasized. Nurses face many of the same problems as do other professional women.

A report on the status of women, as of April 1968, indicated little change from 1963, with 28.7 million women workers in the USA 16 years of age and over, and with a median age of 40 years. As a matter of fact, almost

[10] Commission on the Status of Women, *American Women*, Washington, D.C., Government Printing Office, 1963.
[11] G. Gerds, "The Status of Women Today and Its Effect on Nursing." *American Journal of Nursing*, **63**:70-73, Nov. 1963.

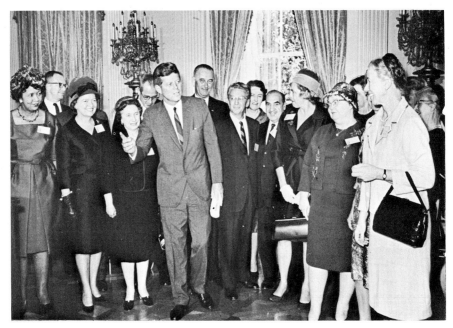

Fig. 2-1. President Kennedy holding the first copy of the report of his Commission on the Status of Women. Looking on (5th person to the President's left) is Mrs. Margaret Dolan, ANA President at that time (Picture by Harry Naltchayan, Staff Photographer, The *Washington Post*)

half of all women 18 to 64 years of age were working in 1968, with 3 out of 5 married and living with their husbands.[12]

PROBLEMS

1. Plan a symposium on "Current Social and Economic Problems of Society" which have a relationship to nursing. Include the following or similar topics: (a) Family Planning and the Nurse in Public Health; (b) The Role of the Nurse in Eliminating Housing Discrimination; (c) The Role of the Nurse in the Promotion of Anti-poverty Programs; (d) What the Nurse Should Know and Do to Combat Disease Caused by the Use of Tobacco; (e) The Responsibility of the Nurse in Dealing with Teenage Drug Users.

2. In spite of the number of commissions and committees on human rights there has been intensified violence and brutality. What role can nursing organizations take in mobilizing public opinion against such violence?

3. One of the most striking phenomena of the past several decades has

[12] U.S. Department of Labor, Wage and Labor Standards Administration, *Background Facts on Women Workers in the United States,* Washington, D.C., The Department, Sept. 1968, p. 1.

been the increased longevity of the population in the USA. In 1969 approximately 1 in 10 of the population were 65 and older. By 1975 it is estimated
that the increase will be 2 to 3 per cent greater. What effect does this have
on the ability of the aging person to meet his economic and health needs?

4. Learn the objectives and programs of national and community groups
which are concerned with: (a) problems of the aging, (b) human relations,
(c) civil rights, (d) civil disorders.

5. Of what significance is the passage of *Public Law 89-749*, The Comprehensive Health Planning Act, to the provision of patient care in this country?

6. What impact do the Medicare and Medicaid programs have upon the
nursing profession? the medical profession? the health services supplying
patient care?

7. Evaluate the values and roles of nursing in extended care facilities.

8. What effects have the Associate Degree programs in nursing had upon
nursing practice?

9. Review the 1963 Report of the Surgeon General's Consultant Group
on Nursing (Public Health Service), *Toward Quality in Nursing: Needs
and Goals*. List the steps taken by the nursing profession to carry out its
recommendations.

10. Discuss the 1965 position paper of the ANA on *Educational Preparation for Nurse Practitioners and Assistants to Nurses*.

11. Most health services used for beginning student field experience in
nursing by institutions of higher education are controlled by the service
institutions and agencies and not by the educational institution offering the
program. What impact does this have upon the student's ability to learn
effective nursing practice? What new fundamental pattern in nursing education could be developed that would use to the utmost the wealth of nursing
capabilities of student nurses in addition to the resources of the educational
institutions offering the program?

12. Many people are discussing "situation ethics." What does this mean?
How is this concept influencing 20th century morality? 20th century
nursing?

SUGGESTED REFERENCES*

POLITICAL, SOCIAL, AND EDUCATIONAL TRENDS

* American Federation of Labor and Congress of Industrial Organizations. *The
  AFL-CIO Platform Proposals to the Republican and Democratic National
  Conventions 1968*. Washington, D.C., the Federation and Congress, 1968.
* Commission on Human Rights Year. *To Deem Our Commitment, The President's
  Commission for the Observance of Human Rights Year 1968, Interim Report*.
  Washington, D.C., Government Printing Office, 1968.

---

* In each chapter all references used as citations are footnoted and are not included here.
All starred references are recommended for additional reading.

Drumheller, S. J. "The Schools Responsibility to Society and to the Individual." *Educational Horizons,* **46**:65-67, Winter 1967-1968.

* *Facts on File: A Weekly Digest of World Events: With a Cumulative Index, 1940-   .* New York, Persons Index—Facts on File, 1940-   .

* Herzog, E. *About the Poor: Some Facts and Some Fictions.* Washington, D.C., Government Printing Office, 1968.

Jencks, C., *et al.* "The War Between the Generations." *Teachers College Record,* **69**:1-21, Oct. 1967.

* The Kiplinger Washington Editors. *The Kiplinger Washington Letter.* (weekly) 1729 K. St., N.W., Washington, D.C., The Editors.

Marris, P. and Rein, M. *Dilemmas of Social Reform.* New York, Atherton, 1967.

* National Education Association of the United States. Department of Higher Education. *Current Issues in Higher Education.* Washington, D.C., The Association. Published annually.

* Paul, Pope. *Regulation of Birth:* trans. of *Humanae Vitae.* Washington, D.C., U.S. Catholic Conference, 1968.

Paul, Pope. *On the Development of Peoples. Populorum Progressio.* Boston, Daughters of St. Paul, 1967.

Political Handbook of the World, 1927-   . New York, Council on Foreign Relations, 1927-   .

* *Public Affairs Information Service Bulletin, 1915-   .* New York, Public Affairs Information Service, 1915-   .

* *Social Legislation Information Service: A Periodical.* Washington, D.C., Social Legislation Information Service, Inc.

U.S. Congress. *Congressional Record, 1873-   .* Washington, D.C., Government Printing Office, 1873-   .

————. *Official Congressional Directory, 1809-   .* Washington, D.C., Government Printing Office, 1809-   .

U.S. National Archives. *Federal Register, March 14, 1936-   .* Washington, D.C., Government Printing Office, 1936-   .

U.S. Office of Government Reports. *United States Government Manual, 1935-* Washington, D.C., Government Printing Office, 1935-   .

Yearbook of the United Nations, 1946-   . New York, United Nations, Department of Public Instruction, 1946-   .

See also, regularly 1 or 2 current periodicals on public affairs.

20TH CENTURY MORALITY

Barrett, D. *Values in America.* Notre Dame, Ind., University of Notre Dame, 1961.

* Cox, H., Ed. *The Situation Ethics Debate.* Philadelphia, Westminster, 1968.

Curran, C. *Absolutes in Moral Theology.* Washington, D.C., Corpus Instrumentorum, 1968.

Findlay, J. *Values and Interests: Study in the Value Theory and the Philosophy of Mind.* London, Macmillan, 1961.

* Fortas, A. *Concerning Dissent and Civil Disobedience. We Have an Alternative to Violence.* New York, New American Library, 1968.

* Hershey, N. "Questions of Life and Death." *American Journal of Nursing,* **68**:1910-1912, Sept. 1968.

"Papal Encyclical Gets Mixed R.N. Reaction." *American Journal of Nursing,* **68**:1835-1868, 1874, Sept. 1968.

* Raths, L. *Values and Teaching: Working with Values in the Classroom.* Columbus, Merrill, 1966.

* Rogers, E. S. "Public Health Asks of Sociology . . . Can the Health Sciences Resolve Society's Problems in the Absence of Human Values and Goals?" *Science,* **159**:506-508, Feb. 1968.

Shurtleff, R. F. *Academic Dishonesty: A Bibliography*. Boston, North Eastern University, 1966.
* *Storm Over Ethics: Collection of Essays*. Philadelphia, United Church Press, 1967.

FAMILY PLANNING

Arnold, E. "Individualizing Care in Family Planning." *Nursing Outlook*, **15**:26-27, Dec. 1967.
Martin, R. M. "Teaching Family Planning: A Survey." *Nursing Outlook*, **15**:32-35, Dec. 1967.
* Milton, I. C. "Contraceptive Practices: Past and Present." *Canadian Nurse*, **63**:29-31, Oct. 1967.
* Noonan, J. T. "Contraception: the Shaping of the Catholic Doctrine." *The Catholic Nurse*, **16**:15-27, 62-63, Dec. 1967.

STATUS OF WOMEN

* Commission on the Status of Women. *American Women*. Washington, D.C., Government Printing Office, 1963.
Lind, N. "Politics, a Developing Field for Women." *Tidsskrift for Sygeplejersken* (Denmark) **67**:346-347, Aug. 1967.
Scotford, H. "The Professional Woman." *Australian Nurses Journal*, **65**:245-248, Dec. 1967.
Stahl, V. "Studies on Various Aspects of Women's Work." *Munca Sanitaria* (Rumania), **15**:729-732, 1967.
* U.S. Department of Labor. Women's Bureau. *Continuing Education Programs and Services for Women*. Washington, D.C., Government Printing Office, 1968.
* _____. *Trends in Educational Attainment of Women*. Washington, D.C., Government Printing Office, 1967.
* U.S. Interdepartmental Committee on the Status of Women. *American Women 1963-1968*. Washington, D.C., Government Printing Office, 1968.

HEALTH, MEDICAL AND HOSPITAL TRENDS

American Hospital Association. *Mental Health Facilities*. Chicago, The Association, 1968.
_____. *Hospitals as Educational Institutions*. Chicago, The Association, 1966.
* Bugbee, G. "Appraising of the New Forces in Health Care Planning and Delivery." *Hospitals*, **12**:71-74, Feb. 1968.
Caswell, J. E. "A Brief History of Coronary Care Units." *Public Health Reports*, **82**:1105-1107, Dec. 1967.
"Comprehensive Planning of Health Facilities and Services." *Journal of the American Medical Association*, **204**:808-810, May 1968.
Conley, V. L. and Olson, S. W. "Regional Medical Programs." *American Journal of Nursing*, **68**:1916-1926, Sept. 1968.
Cornely, P. B. "The Health Status of the Negro Today and in the Future." *American Journal of Public Health*, **58**:647-654, Apr. 1968.
Esty, G. W. "The Psychoeconomics of Family Mental Health and Living Space." *Journal of School Health*, **38**:9-15, Jan. 1968.
Facts About the Hill-Burton Program July 1, 1947-June 30, 1968. Silver Springs, Md., U.S. Public Health Service, 1968.
* Fenninger, L. D. "Education in the Health Professions." *Nursing Outlook*, **16**:30-33, Apr. 1968.
Goeppinger, J. "Why a Home Health Aide." *American Journal of Nursing*, **68**:1513-1516, July 1968.

* Goerke, L. S. "Changes in Preventive Medicine." *Journal of School Health,* **38**:1-8, Jan. 1968.
* Gregg, M. B. "Communicable Disease Trends in the United States" *American Journal of Nursing,* **68**:88-93, Jan. 1968.
Harvey, J. D. "This I Believe About the Health Crisis." *Nursing Outlook,* **16**:53-56, Jan. 1968.
Hornstra, R. K. "Elements of Comprehensive Mental Health Care." *Hospitals,* **42**:42-46, Feb. 1968.
Hudson, C. L. "The Changing Medical Climate of America." *Missouri Medicine,* **64**:965-969, Dec. 1967.
Ingles, T. "A New Health Worker." *American Journal of Nursing,* **68**:1059-1061, May 1968.
Jarvis, M. A. "Health Larnin in Appalachia." *American Journal of Nursing,* **67**:2345-2347, Nov. 1967.
* Lambertsen, E. C. "The Emerging Health Occupations." *Nursing Forum,* **7**:87-97, Winter 1968.
Lifson, S. S. "Our Changing Society—the Years Ahead: the Outlook for Health Education Practice." *American Journal of Public Health,* **58**:678-683, Apr. 1968.
"The Meaning of Community Medicine." *New England Journal of Medicine,* **278**:44-45, Jan. 1968.
Mendelsohn, R. S. "Comprehensive Care for the Hard to Reach Family." *Journal of the American Medical Association,* **203**:304-322, Jan. 1968.
Milio, N. "Making Health Care Relevant to Life in a Low Income Neighborhood." In *ANA Regional Clinical Conference,* New York, The Association, 1967, pp. 86-94.
Moxley, J. H. "The Predicament in Health Manpower." *American Journal of Nursing,* **68**:1486-1490, July 1968.
Mylinger, R. E. *Innovation in Local Health Services.* Washington, D.C., Government Printing Office, 1968.
Olson, E. V. "Health Manpower Needed: a Shake Up in the Status Quo." *American Journal of Nursing,* **68**:1491-1495, July 1968.
Phaneuf, M. C. and Lowinger, P. "Healers in a Sick Society." *American Journal of Nursing,* **68**:1283-1284, June 1968.
Sanders, A. A. "The Church and the Care of the Sick." *Hospital Progress,* **48**:34-37, Dec. 1967.
Secretary's Advisory Committee on Hospital Effectiveness. Washington, D.C., U.S. Department of Health, Education, and Welfare, 1968.
Stewart, W. H. "New Dimensions of Health Planning." *Hospital Topics,* **45**:27-28, Sept. 1967.
* Wensley, E. E. *Nursing Service Without Walls.* New York, National League for Nursing, 1963.
Yerby, A. S. "Improving Care for the Disadvantaged." *American Journal of Nursing,* **68**:1043-1047, May 1968.
See also annual reports of the World Health Organization and the World Federation of Mental Health.

TRENDS IN EXTENDED CARE FACILITIES

* American Hospital Association. *Developing Policies and Procedures for Long-Term Care Institutions.* Chicago, The Association, 1968.
* American Nurses' Association. *Standards for Organized Nursing Services in Hospitals, Public Health Agencies, Nursing Homes, Industries, and Clinics.* New York, The Association, 1965.
* Baltz, F. L., *et al.* "Nursing Homes—a Review." *Nursing Outlook,* **16**:46-47, Jan. 1968.

Becker, C. A. "What the Extended Care Facility Expects from the Physician and the Nurse." *Wisconsin Medical Journal*, **67:**136-138, Feb. 1968.

Bernstein, R. "Patients' Families and Nursing Homes." *Professional Nursing Home*, **10:**37-39, Feb. 1968.

* Boone, B. "The Role of the Extended Care Facility in Providing Health Care." *Hospital Management*, **104:**52-53, Aug. 1967.

Cantland, L. "The Home Care Administrator." *Nursing Outlook*, **16:**30-33, Jan. 1968.

* Dornblaser, B. M. "Hospital-Based Extended Care: a Social Model of Extended Care." *Hospitals*, **42:**103-110, June 1968.

* Karen, Sister. "Reorganizing for Extended Care." *Hospital Progress*, **49:**56-70, May 1968.

* National League for Nursing. *Guide for Assessing Nursing Services in Long-Term Care Facilities*. New York, The League, 1968.

* Nelson, G. W. "The Church Home for the Aged: Where is It Headed?" *Professional Nursing Home*, **9:**13-16, Oct. 1967.

* Rourke, A. J. "Hospital Should Offer Extended Care Service." *Modern Hospital*, **109:**130, Aug. 1967.

Sherman, J. B. "Categories of Nursing Care." *Nursing Homes*, **16:**22-24, Dec. 1967.

NURSING TRENDS

* American Nurses' Association. *Facts About Nursing: A Statistical Summary*. New York, The Association, Current Edition.

* _____. Committee on Education. "American Nurses' Association First Position on Education for Nursing." *American Journal of Nursing*, **65:**106-111, Dec. 1965.

Cohen, H. "Accreditation of Community Nursing Services." *American Journal of Public Health*, **57:**2138-2142, Dec. 1967.

* Commission to Study Nursing Education." *American Journal of Nursing*, **67:**1181-1182, June 1967.

Deakin, B. M. "Nursing Education in Relation to Current Social Problems." *International Nursing Review*, **14:**53-64, Aug. 1967.

Dickey, F. G. "Looking at Accrediting in the Future." In *National League for Nursing Conference Papers*. New York, The League, 1969, pp. 58-62.

Dustin, L. C. "Education for Nursing: Apprenticeship or Academic." *Nursing Outlook*, **15:**26,28,30, Sept. 1967.

* Education Study Commission Announces Members and Staff." *American Journal of Nursing*, **67:**2011-2012, Oct. 1967.

Elliott, J. E., *et al*. "A Conversation on: Nursing Services, Nursing Education and Economic and General Welfare." *American Journal of Nursing*, **68:**792-799, Apr. 1968.

* "Epilogue to '68 – Prologue to '69." *American Journal of Nursing*, **69:**81-88, Jan. 1969.

"Federal Funds for Nursing Education." *American Journal of Nursing*, **68:**312-315, Feb. 1968.

Johnson, D. E. "Competence in Practice: Technical and Professional." *Nursing Outlook*, **14:**30-33, Oct. 1966.

Kelly, C. "Health Care in the Mississippi Delta." *American Journal of Nursing*, **69:**759-763, Apr. 1969.

Kelly, C. W. *Dimensions of Professional Nursing*. New York, Macmillan, 1968, pp. 479-477.

Lambertson, E. C. "The Nature and Objectives of Intensive Care Nursing." *Nursing Clinics of North America*, **3:**3-6, Mar. 1968.

Larson, C. B., *et al.* "Dialogue on Nursing Schools." *New England Journal of Medicine,* **278:**1293-1295, June 6, 1968.
* Levine, E. "Nurse Manpower; Yesterday, Today, and Tomorrow." *American Journal of Nursing,* **69:**290-296, Feb. 1969.
Lewis, E. P. "USA: Nursing Education in Ferment, Part I." *International Nursing Review,* 15:50-58, No. 1; "Part II." **15:**121-132, Apr. 1968.
Lewis, E. R. "Role of the State Nurses' Association in Effecting Change in Nursing Education." *Tar Heel Nurse,* **30:**38-46, 87, June 1968.
* *Medical and Nursing Practice in a Changing World: Proceedings of First National Conference for Professional Nurses and Physicians Sponsored by the American Nurses' Association and the American Medical Association, Feb. 13-15, 1964, Williamsburg, Va.* New York, The American Nurses' Association, 1964.
Pellegrino, Edmund D. "Rationale for Nursing Education in the University." *American Journal of Nursing,* **68:**1006-1009, May 1968.
Ramphal, M. "Needed: A Career Ladder in Nursing." *American Journal of Nursing,* **68:**1234-1237, June 1968.
Reinkemeyer, Sister Agnes M. "It Won't Be Hospital Nursing." *American Journal of Nursing,* **68:**1936-1940, Sept. 1968.
Reinkemeyer, Sister Mary Hubert. "A Nursing Paradox." *Nursing Research,* **17:**4-9, Jan./Feb. 1968.
"RN Survey: The Nurse Today." *RN,* **31:**31-46, July 1968.
Schmitt, M. H. "Role Conflict in Nursing: Is It Based On a' Dubious Dichotomy?" *American Journal of Nursing,* **68:**2348-2350, Nov. 1968.
Schulman, D. P., *et al.* "The Nurse as a Catalyst." *American Journal of Nursing,* **68:**1890-1894, Sept. 1968.
Scott, J. M. "Three Years with the Nurse Training Act." *American Journal of Nursing,* **67:**2107-2109, Oct. 1967.
Sheldon, A., *et al.* "The Developing Role of the Nurse in a Community Mental Health Program." *Perspectives in Psychiatric Care,* **5:**272-279, Nov./Dec. 1967.
The Sick Person Needs....: Report of the Third National Conference for Professional Nurses and Physicians, Coronado, Calif., Feb. 23-25, 1967. Sponsored by the American Medical Association and the American Nurses' Association. New York, American Nurses' Association, 1967.
Towner, A. M. "No More Supervisors." *Nursing Outlook,* **16:**56-58, Feb. 1968.
"Transition in Nursing Education." *American Journal of Nursing,* **67:**1211-1223, June 1967.
U.S. Department of Health, Education, and Welfare. Surgeon General's Consultant Group on Nursing. *Toward Quality in Nursing: Needs and Goals.* Washington, D.C., Government Printing Office, 1963.
Waters, V. H. "Distinctions are Necessary." *American Journal of Nursing,* **65:** 101-102, Feb. 1965.
Wilansky, E. "Nursing Vista." *American Journal of Nursing,* **69:**991-993, May 1969.
See also, Annual Reports on Admissions, Enrollments and Graduations in Practical, Associate Degree, Diploma, Baccalaureate Degree and Graduate Programs in Nursing which appear annually in one of the Fall issues of *Nursing Outlook.*

AGING

Bucke, M. "The Contribution of Voluntary Bodies to the Welfare of the Aged." *Gerontologia Clinica* (Basel), **9:**217-229, 1967.
Cohen, I. J. "Practical Methods for Meeting the Social Needs of the Elderly." *Hospitals,* **41:**90-92, Dec. 1967.

Council of Churches in Oakland, California. *What Churches Can Do: Designs for Action for Older Americans*. Washington, D.C., Government Printing Office, 1968.

Dominick, J. R., *et al*. "The Adjustment of Aged Persons in Nursing Homes." *Journal of the American Geriatric Society*, **16**:63-77, Jan. 1968.

* Koller, M. R. *Social Gerontology*. New York, Random House, 1968.

* Meeting the Needs of the Aging." *American Journal of Nursing*, **68**:49, Sept. 1968.

Moon, D. A. "Boarding Out Elderly People." *District Nursing*, **10**:230-232, Jan. 1968.

* President's Council on the Aging. *A Time of Progress for Older Americans*. Washington, D.C., Government Printing Office, 1968.

Suggested Periodicals on Aging:

Aging. Washington, D.C., Government Printing Office.

Current Literature on Aging. Quarterly. 315 Park Avenue, South, New York, Council on Aging.

Geriatric Focus. Semi-monthly. 2501 Mayzata Blvd., Minneapolis, Miller Publishing Co.

Geriatric Times. Monthly. 342 Madison Ave., New York, Edwill Publications.

Journal of the American Geriatric Society. Monthly. 10 Columbus Circle, New York, American Geriatric Society.

Journal of Gerontology. Quarterly. 660 S. Euclid St., St. Louis, Gerontological Society.

Senior Citizens News. Monthly. 1726 K. St., N.W., Washington, D.C., National Council of Senior Citizens.

MEDICARE AND MEDICAID

Fonseca, J. D. "The Effect of Medicare on 200 Agencies." *Nursing Outlook*, **16**:42-45, Jan. 1968.

Lipscomb, W. R. "The Impact of Medicare on Psychiatry." *American Journal of Psychiatry*, **124**:910-916, Jan. 1968.

Pope, I. "Medicare: Impetus for Change." *Nursing Outlook*, **16**:34-35, Jan. 1968.

* U.S. Department of Health, Education, and Welfare. Social and Rehabilitation Service. Medical Services Administration. *Questions and Answers: Medical Assistance — Medicaid*. Washington, D.C., Government Printing Office, June 1968. Revised when changes are made in legislation.

* U.S. Department of Health, Education, and Welfare. Social Security Administration. *Your Medicare Handbook*. Washington, D.C., Government Printing Office, May 1968. Revised when changes occur in the medicare legislation.

* _____. *A Brief Explanation of Medicare: Health Insurance for People 65 or Older*. Washington, D.C., Government Printing Office, Feb. 1968. Revised when changes are made in legislation.

DRUGS, TOBACCO, AND ALCOHOL

Bowers, M. "Student Psychedelic Drug Use — An Evaluation by Student Drug Users." *International Journal of the Addictions*, **4**:89-99, Mar. 1969.

Byrne, M. "Resocialization of the Chronic Alcoholic." *American Journal of Nursing*, **68**:99-100, Jan. 1968.

Dana, A. H. "Participation as a Vital Fact in Adoption of Company Alcoholism Program." *American Association of Industrial Nurses Journal*, **16**:13-18, Feb. 1968.

Debold, R. C., *et al. LSD, Man and Society*. Middletown, Conn., Wesleyan University Press, 1967.

* A Digest of the Federal Trade Commission Cigarette Report to Congress." *Journal of School Health*, **38**:27-32, Jan. 1968.

"Drug Problems in the Haight-Asbury." *American Journal of Nursing*, **68**:1686-1689, Aug. 1968.

Einstein, S. "The Addiction Dilemma: Gaps in Knowledge, Information-Dissemination, Service and Training." *International Journal of the Addictions*, **4**:25-44, Mar. 1969.

Fodor, J. R., *et al.* "Smoking Behavior, Cognitive Skills and Educational Implications." *Journal of School Health*, **38**:94-98, Feb. 1968.

Lemin, B. "Smoking in 14-Year Old School Children." *International Journal of Nursing Studies*, **4**:301-309, Dec. 1967.

* Moredock, G. E., Jr. "Alcohol Usage and Drinking Patterns in Our Society." *American Association of Industrial Nurses Journal*, **16**:7-12, Feb. 1968.

* Nowlis, H. H. "Why Students Use Drugs." *American Journal of Nursing*, **68**:1680-1685, Aug. 1968.

Pienar, A. J. "Alcoholics Can Recover." *South African Nursing Journal*, **34**:10-11, Sept. 1967.

Shachter, B. "Psychedelic Drug Use by Adolescents." *Journal of the National Association of Social Workers*, **13**:33-39, July 1968.

* U.S. Children's Bureau and the National Institute of Mental Health. *Thinking About Drinking*. Washington, D.C., Government Printing Office, 1968.

* U.S. Department of Health, Education, and Welfare. Public Health Service. *The Health Consequences of Smoking*. Washington, D.C., Government Printing Office, 1968.

RACE RELATIONS

* Marx, G. T. "Document With a Difference." *Trans-Action*, **5**:56-58, Sept. 1968.

"Negroes in the New World: Anthropologists Look at Afro-Americans." *Trans-Action*, **5**:49-75, July/Aug. 1968.

* Phaneuf, M. C., *et al.* "Healers in a Sick Society." *American Journal of Nursing*. **68**:1283-1284, June 1968.

Schutt, B. G. "Confrontation." (editorial) *American Journal of Nursing*, **68**:97, May 1968.

* Staupers, M. K. *No Time for Prejudice*. New York, Macmillan, 1963.

"Untouched in the Holocaust." *American Journal of Nursing*, **68**:508-509, Mar. 1968.

* U.S. National Advisory Commission on Civil Disorders. *Report of the National Advisory Commission on Civil Disorders*. Washington, D.C. Government Printing Office, 1968.

CHAPTER

3

Nursing
as a
Profession

Before you really can be a good professional worker, you need to know what total nursing is and what it should achieve for the good of society. You need to be much like an artist: have a general idea of what you expect to accomplish, then start putting the idea into effect, standing off occasionally to look over your work to see where you can improve it, perhaps to erase some blemishes or add some other strokes of beauty. In other words, once knowing what you wish to do, occasionally you must recollect, contemplate and evaluate.

All that you do needs to be weighed in the light of standards of good nursing and ultimately of the standards of good living. We should take time out once in a while to think about what we believe nursing is and ought to be. You might ask yourself these questions: Do I overvalue some things, undervalue others and completely overlook still others? What should I, as a good nurse, citizen and person, know, do and be?

CRITERIA OF A PROFESSION

It is generally accepted that the professions serve society and not the ends of any particular interest group. The aims of a profession are therefore altruistic rather than materialistic.

It would be less than candid to say that all nurses who are called professional today are really professional. As used throughout this chapter "professional" refers to the nurse who has acquired the art and skill of nursing and who interprets her role in nursing in terms of the social ends for which it exists—the health and welfare of society.

Many writers have listed criteria of professionalization. It is generally agreed that to be a professional person you must: (1) have a grasp of fundamental truth—a kind of truth that will make you free to think and act, (2) have the ability to apply truth in dealing with new problems for which there is no precise answer at the moment and (3) be able to meet the perplexities of changing basic knowledge, demands, social conditions or personal upsets courageously and wisely.

The criteria of a profession as listed by William Shephard are:

1. A profession must satisfy an indispensable social need and be based upon well established and socially accepted scientific principle.

2. It must demand adequate pre-professional and cultural training.

3. It must demand the possession of a body of specialized and systematized knowledge.

4. It must give evidence of needed skills which the public does not possess; that is, skills which are partly native and partly acquired.

5. It must have developed a scientific technique which is the result of tested experience.

6. It must require the exercise of discretion and judgment as to time and manner of the performance of duty. This is in contrast to the kind of work which is subject to immediate direction and supervision.

7. It must be a type of beneficial work, the result of which is not subject to standardization in terms of unit performance or time element.

8. It must have a group consciousness designed to extend scientific knowledge in technical language.

9. It must have sufficient self-impelling power to retain its members throughout life. It must not be used as a mere steppingstone to other occupations.

10. It must recognize its obligations to society by insisting that its members live up to an established code of ethics.[1]

Additional criteria, as a basis for determining professional activities in nursing, are:

1. A profession has the responsibility for determining its own goals and responsibility for meeting society's needs for its services. In deciding its own goal, consideration must be given to its role and function in relation to the other health professions.

2. It needs to decide its own specific functions and responsibilities as a unique profession and as a member of the interdisciplinary group composed of the allied health professions.

3. It needs to include in its code of ethics what the particular pro-

[1] W. Shephard, "The Professionalization of Public Health," *The American Journal of Public Health and The Nation's Health,* **38:**146, Jan. 1948.

fessional group ought to know in order to have an understanding of the ethical principles which govern professional practice. Another important point to stress is the ethical obligation of the professional person to give service to the public above all – above personal considerations such as remuneration, although, of course, "the laborer is worthy of his hire."

In an article discussing the professional status of nursing, Genevieve K., and Roy W. Bixler have said that a profession:

1. Utilizes in its practice a well-defined and well-organized body of specialized knowledge which is on the intellectual level of the higher learning.

2. Constantly enlarges the body of knowledge it uses and improves its techniques of education and service by the use of the scientific method.

3. Entrusts the education of its practitioners to institutions of higher education.

4. Applies its body of knowledge in practical services which are vital to human and social welfare.

5. Functions autonomously in the formulation of professional policy and in the control of professional activity thereby.

6. Attracts individuals of intellectual and personal qualities who exalt service above personal gain and who recognize their chosen occupation as a life work.

7. Strives to compensate its practitioners by providing freedom of action, opportunity for continuous professional growth, and economic security.[2]

How well does nursing measure up to these various criteria? Nursing has been moving over the years toward greater professionalization. In the last decade or so, activities in research toward the identification and elaboration of scientific knowledge in nursing; the development of programs for the preparation of nurse scientists; the general acceptance by the profession of the long-term goals to stimulate research and experimentation by nurses and other specialists in order to enlarge the scientific principles on which nursing rests and to encourage the application of these findings to nursing practice; as well as the position taken by the ANA on preparation for the practice of professional nursing[3], all point to a growing professionalization.

However, the growth toward professional status has been uneven. Despite the ANA position paper, one of the most troublesome spots has been in education. The great majority of nurses continue to graduate from programs in hospital schools of nursing.

Nurses throughout the years have been strongly conscious of their ethical responsibilities. To this end, they have developed a code of ethics and in recent years groups within the professional association have been focusing on the development of professional standards of practice.

[2] G. K. Bixler and R. W. Bixler, "The Professional Status of Nursing," *American Journal of Nursing*, **59**:1142-1146, Aug. 1959.

[3] American Nurses' Association, *Educational Preparation for Nurse Practitioners and Assistants to Nurses: A Position Paper*, New York, The Association, 1965.

CODES OF ETHICS OF THE NURSING PROFESSION

Codes of ethics serve a variety of purposes. They serve as one basis for developing preservice curricula for the particular professional group. They help to orient the new practitioner to his professional responsibilities, rights and privileges. They furnish the basis for distinguishing scrupulous and unscrupulous conduct. They serve as a basis for regulating the relationship of the practitioner to consumers of the professional service, to the profession itself, to society and to co-workers within and outside the profession. They provide the profession with a basis for excluding the unscrupulous or the incompetent practitioner and for defending the practitioner who is unjustly accused of wrong-doing. They serve as a guide to the public for understanding the characteristics of professional conduct.

The Code of the ANA, adopted in 1950 and revised in 1960 and 1968, is one of the most important statements of the ANA. It serves all nurses as a guide to standards of conduct, relationships, and practice. The following is the Code as revised in 1968:

1. The nurse provides services with respect for the dignity of man, unrestricted by considerations of nationality, race, creed, color, or status.

2. The nurse safeguards the individual's right to privacy by judiciously protecting information of a confidential nature, sharing only that information relevant to his care.

3. The nurse maintains individual competence in nursing practice, recognizing and accepting responsibility for individual actions and judgments.

4. The nurse acts to safeguard the patient when his care and safety are affected by incompetent, unethical, or illegal conduct of any person.

5. The nurse uses individual competence as a criterion in accepting delegated responsibilities and assigning nursing activities to others.

6. The nurse participates in research activities when assured that the rights of individual subjects are protected.

7. The nurse participates in the efforts of the profession to define and upgrade standards of nursing practice and education.

8. The nurse, acting through the professional organization, participates in establishing and maintaining conditions of employment conducive to high-quality nursing care.

9. The nurse works with members of health professions and other citizens in promoting efforts to meet health needs of the public.

10. The nurse refuses to give or imply endorsement to advertising, promotion, or sales for commercial products, services, or enterprises.[4]

It is suggested that you read and discuss the official interpretation of the Code and its implications for nursing practice. Also consider whether the

[4] American Nurses' Association, *Code For Nurses with Interpretative Statements,* New York, The Association, 1968.

ANA Code should place emphasis on the responsibility of the nurse as a teacher. What additional points, if any, would you include in the Code? To help you understand the ethics of the nursing profession, it is urged that you relate your study of the Code to the evaluation of the history of nursing. It is also suggested that you read the International Council of Nurses Code of Ethics as adopted in 1965 and reported in Chapter 25.

MAINTAINING PROFESSIONAL STANDARDS

According to Robert K. Merton, "The foremost obligation of the [professional] association is to set rigorous standards for the profession and to help enforce them. . . ."[5] He goes on to say that "The association must be in the vanguard. The standards it sets must be more exacting than those with which the lay public might be content."[6]

The establishment of standards of professional practice and conduct is, however, but one aspect of the profession's concern. The professional association is also concerned with the enforcement of the code and the maintenance of the standards of practice set. Each nurse carries individual responsibility for her own conduct and practice. However, as in any profession, there are in nursing, too, individuals who are not committed to the ideals of the profession. The activities of the ANA Divisions of Practice are directed toward the goal of improvement of nursing practice.

We suggest that you read Margaret Lindsey's article, "Professional Standards—Whose Responsibility?" in the November 1962 issue of the *American Journal of Nursing*.

MEANING OF PROFESSIONAL NURSING

What Is Professional Nursing?

Professional nursing is an art and a science dominated by an ideal of service in which certain principles are applied in the skillful care of the sick in appropriate relationship with the patient and the physician and with others who have related responsibilities. It is concerned equally with the prevention of disease and the conservation of health. Skillful care embraces the whole person—body, mind and soul—his physical, mental and spiritual well-being. Nursing encompasses:

1. Caring for the sick and injured, bringing to bear the resources of the patient, his family and environment and the services of available cooperating personnel to facilitate his recovery and rehabilitation in

[5] R. K. Merton, "Functions of the Professional Association," *American Journal of Nursing*, **58**:52, Jan. 1958.
[6] *Ibid.*

accordance to the diagnosis made and treatment prescribed by a licensed physician.

2. Helping an individual and his family to take positive action in relief of illness and improvement of his individual, family and community health needs.

3. Training students and auxiliary personnel to function as members of the nursing team.

4. Adapting nursing service to cooperate with responsible planning authorities in emergencies due to disaster caused by disease and natural causes or war.

5. Evaluating and conducting research to continually improve methods whereby nursing in particular and health medical care adequately meet society's needs.

6. Sharing with others in the dissemination of general health information to individuals and community groups to further the cultivation of health.[7]

What you call nursing is much less important than what you make it. How well you serve society as a citizen and how well you live as a human being are not determined solely by your avocations and your use of leisure but largely by that part of your life to which you devote your major time, energies and interests – your life's work.

Every nurse has the opportunity to be a professional person regardless of the assigned status of nursing as a profession today. Harking back to the criteria of a profession as described in an earlier section of this chapter, how shall we describe the truly professional nurse? The following check list is a modification of one suggested by Erline Perkins:

1. Do the nurse's actions involve intellectual operations or are they purely mechanical? What is the quality of her judgments? Does she depend on routines?

2. Does the nurse make practical application of what she has learned? What is the quality of decisions regarding these applications? How broad are the applications made? Do they include concern for society?

3. Does the nurse keep up with trends in nursing and health care, generally?

4. Does she share this knowledge and information with others in her own and related fields?

5. Does she show concern for the human element in nursing?

6. Does she belong to and participate in her professional organization?

7. Does she interpret the nursing profession to the public?

8. Is she committed to nursing as a life profession (even though she may not be always actively practicing nursing), or does she see it only

---

[7] R. L. McManus, "Society's Demands of Nurses That Influence Nursing Education," *Problems of Graduate Nurse Education: Report of Work Conference,* New York, Bureau of Publications, Teachers College, Columbia University, 1952, pp. 12-13.

as something to work at? Does she feel responsible for keeping the ideals of nursing ahead of financial returns, while at the same time promoting the goal of adequate remuneration for the services of nurses?

9. Does she, through observation, questioning, study, or research, add to the knowledge basic to the profession?[8]

Scope of Functions of Professional Nursing

According to Tead and Metcalf, "a function is a nucleus of activities, responsibilities, or duties so homogeneous in character as to fall logically into a unit for purposes of execution."[9]

Professional groups have distinctive functions to perform. It has not been easy to identify functions for the nursing profession. However, Lesnik and Anderson have identified and listed 7 areas of functions in professional nursing, based on legislative and judicial decisions. Six of these are classified as independent areas and one as a dependent area. The 6 independent areas of functions are:

1. The supervision of a patient involving the whole management of care, requiring the application of principles based upon the biologic, the physical and social sciences.

2. The observation of symptoms and reactions, including symptomatology of physical and mental conditions and needs, requiring evaluation or application of principles based upon the biologic, the physical and the social sciences.

3. The accurate recording and reporting of facts, including evaluation of the whole care of the patient.

4. The supervision of others, except physicians, contributing to the care of the patient.

5. The application and the execution of nursing procedures and technics.

6. The direction and the education to secure physical and mental care.

The dependent function is:

7. The application and the execution of legal orders of physicians concerning treatments and medications, with an understanding of cause and effect thereof.[10]

Some authorities in nursing are now suggesting that all of the nurse's functions are independent. How would you defend this position?

[8] E. W. Perkins, "The Registered Nurse—A Professional Person?" *American Journal of Nursing,* **63**:92, Feb. 1963.

[9] O. Tead and H. C. Metcalf, *Personnel Administration,* New York, McGraw-Hill, 1933, p. 350.

[10] M. J. Lesnik and B. E. Anderson, *Nursing Practice and the Law,* Philadelphia, Lippincott, 1962, pp. 259-260.

Studies of Functions of Nursing

The former occupational sections of the ANA developed statements of functions for the various types of positions in which nurses are employed. Studies of functions of nursing have and are being made by other groups, nursing service and nursing education. Sociologists have assisted with some of these studies. You will wish to keep up to date with these studies by reading about them in current nursing and related periodicals and by reviewing the reports of such studies. But, more important, why could you not do some studies of your own on the functions and the activities of nurses?

QUALIFICATIONS AND ABILITIES OF A PROFESSIONAL NURSE

What should you, as a good nurse, be? Know? Be able to do? As a good nurse you should:[11]

Have faith in the fundamental values that underlie the democratic way of life; for example: you should have respect for the individual dignity of every human being, practicing self-sacrifice for the common good, participating and allowing participation of others in matters affecting both the individual and the group and having a strong sense of responsibility for bearing full share in solving the problems of society. As Arthur Corey has so ably stated: "No group of specialized workers can dare to dream of making its calling pre-eminent unless the significance of its social contribution is so compelling that pre-eminence is imperative."[12]

Have a sense of responsibility for understanding those with whom you work or associate through use of the following skills: (1) skill in utilizing pertinent basic concepts of psychology and (2) skill in handling yourself so that you and others may work effectively together.

Have faith in the reality of spiritual and aesthetic values and awareness of the value and the pleasure of self-development through the pursuit of some aesthetic interest.

Have the basic skill and knowledge necessary to apply to present-day social problems realistic, incisive and well-ordered thought through use of the following skills: (1) skill in securing, appraising, and organizing evidence; (2) skill in inductive analysis of social problems in terms of their origins; and (3) skill in using basic concepts and generalizations for deductive analysis.

---

[11] The following has been modified from these references: E. D. Smith, *Materials on General Education, Professional Education and Teaching,* New York, Bureau of Publications, Teachers College, Columbia University, n.d., pp. 2-3. Mimeographed. E. Johns and B. Pfefferkorn, *An Activity Analysis of Nursing,* New York, National League of Nursing Education, 1934, pp. 40-41.

[12] A. Corey, "The Professional Standards Movement in Education," *The Journal of Teacher Education,* 6:224, Sept. 1955.

Have skill in using written and spoken language, both to develop your own thoughts and to communicate them to others.

Understand and appreciate the importance of good health.

Have emotional balance.

Like hard work and possess a capacity for it.

Appreciate high standards of workmanship.

Accept and try to understand people of all sorts, regardless of race, religion or color.

Know nursing so thoroughly that every person you nurse will receive excellent care.

PROFESSIONAL EDUCATION

As has been indicated earlier in this chapter, one of the earmarks of a profession is that preparation for it involves an extended period of specialized study, ordinarily in an institution of higher education. However, the history of professional education shows that for any given profession the educational program may evolve through several stages: (1) the apprentice stage, (2) the proprietary school stage, (3) the university school stage, (4) the pre-professional stage and (5) the general education stage. Some professions, for example medicine and dentistry, have passed through all of these stages. Others may not find this necessary. In any single profession one may often find several stages existing at the same time.[13] This is true of the nursing profession today. Can you identify the various stages in nursing education?

There are 3 general types of professional nursing education: undergraduate education for preservice students, generalized education for the graduate nurse leading to a baccalaureate degree (this is also undergraduate and is being discontinued rapidly in favor of one preservice program) and graduate education for nurses. Only these 3 types of education for nursing are described in this chapter. Other current types are described in Chapter 10.[14]

Undergraduate Education in Nursing

There are common considerations in the development of any undergraduate professional curriculum. McGlothlin has said that professional education must help the student to achieve 5 sets of attributes:

1. Competence to practice his profession, with sufficient knowledge and skill to satisfy its requirements

[13] E. J. McGrath, *Liberal Education in the Professions,* New York, Teachers College Columbia University, 1957, pp. 28-34.

[14] Plans have been made for a comprehensive study of nursing education by the profession. Following the report of the Surgeon General's Consultant Group on Nursing, the boards of directors of the ANA and the NLN planned jointly in the establishment of a commission, an autonomous body, to study the present system of nursing education. The commission, under the presidency of W. Allan Wallis, president of the University of Rochester, and the direction of Dr. Jerome P. Lysaught, began work in 1967. See "Commission to Study Nursing Education," (News) *American Journal of Nursing,* **67:**1181-1182, June 1967.

2. Social understanding, with sufficient breadth to place his practice in the context of the society which supports it, and to develop capacity for leadership in public affairs

3. Personality characteristics which make possible effective practice

4. Zest for continued study which will steadily increase knowledge and skill needed by practice

5. Competence in conducting or interpreting research so that he can add to human knowledge either through discovery or application of new facts[15]

There should be a sound combination of general liberal education and occupational preparation which aims at laying a foundation for practice, for growth and for future graduate education. Nursing education is the process that transforms an individual from a high school graduate to nursing student to competent practitioner. During this time the student must learn the necessary skills, proper at all times, and the values and expectations of the professional role.

In addition to the specific technical or professional preparation for practice, the student of nursing needs a good understanding of man, of her own motivations, of society, of human needs and their spiritual and social expression, and with skill in interpersonal relations. Needed also is training in the intellectual skills of analysis and interpretation and in the ability to use the written and spoken language effectively as a method of communication. Education that includes the liberal arts is offered not just to enrich the professional program but to produce a more broadly educated woman or man.

The major areas of learning experience in nursing are derived from: (1) the major health problems of society—local, national and international; (2) health problems of all age groups; (3) all phases of health work—promotion, maintenance, detection and cure of illness and rehabilitation; and (4) consideration of normal health conditions and deviations from these. Learning experiences include practicing in nursing situations where health problems are dealt with—in homes, industries, hospitals, nursing homes, and community health agencies, both rural and urban.

To acquire the skills necessary for serving society involves learning and using the fundamental concepts of history, biologic and physical sciences, political science, government and economics, psychology, social psychology, sociology and statistics. Some educators have suggested that half of the curriculum should be devoted to liberal education subjects. Mildred Newton in an address to a group of nursing students indicated the following 6 outcomes of the preservice baccalaureate program as important:

1. Changed behavior—changes in ability, goals, philosophy and personality—and ability to change as nursing changes

2. Ability to see an increasing number of alternatives in approaching the solving of problems

---

[15] W. J. McGlothlin, *Patterns of Professional Education*, New York, Putnam, 1960, p. 7.

3. Ability to think effectively
4. Ability to communicate effectively
5. Ability to make relevant judgments
6. Ability to discriminate among values[16]

Since nursing is accomplished by one human being dealing with another human being or group of human beings, the nurse should understand the complex of relationships of nurses to patients, nurses to physicians and all others in the various settings where nursing care is given. Complete patient services can be given only if relationships are understood. This calls for the understanding needed and essential skills in working with people of different cultural, religious, social and economic backgrounds and the understanding of the effects of family relationships in patient care. To acquire foundational experience so as to be helped in self-direction to the end that the nurse and others may work effectively together, the following areas are important to stress: cultural and social anthropology, general sociology, social psychology, the community and contemporary society, the framework of health services, interpersonal and interprofessional relations, mental health, psychiatric principles and professional ethics.

The nurse needs to be able to recognize that patients' needs are complicated and that at various times different needs are evident—sometimes physical, sometimes emotional, sometimes spiritual—or there may be a whole combination of needs evident at one time. Therefore, ample opportunity should be provided for the student of nursing to be responsible for the comprehensive care of patients while learning nursing so as to learn how to apply sound principles of nursing practice along with sociologic, public health and other important principles to promote recovery, rehabilitation and continued health.

Programs participated in by all health workers and incorporating basic elements of plans of patient care with nursing care as an integral part are a universal basic need. Nurses must understand patient care in its broadest terms and know the relationship of nursing to the total patient-care plan.

The nurse needs to understand the physical and emotional development of people at different stages in life—infancy, childhood, adolescence, adulthood, old age—in relation to environment. Therefore, the nurse should be helped to understand a patient as a human being in all phases of growth and development, including characteristics of various stages of life, emotional problems, minor deviations and serious maladjustments.

Emphasis needs to be placed on fundamental understanding in the areas of anatomy and physiology, microbiology, chemistry and physics as a basis for learning the scientific principles underlying nursing.

The student in preparing to live her life well should be helped to understand spiritual values, to pursue some aesthetic interest and to gain skill in

[16] M. Newton, "The Nurse in the University Community," *First Annual Viana McCown Lectureship in Nursing, April 17, 1964,* Columbia, South Carolina, The University of South Carolina School of Nursing, pp. 3-7.

the appreciation of some field of beauty so that after graduation she will continue to turn to it for relaxation and for the enrichment of life. Toward this end, philosophy, religion, literature, art and music are important. Consideration of relevant social, economic, historical and ethical questions provide opportunity for the student to consider herself and her goals with a broader perspective.

Instructional methods that will assist students in their integration of all learning experiences are essential. It is of more value for the student of nursing to care for a certain number of patients throughout the entire cycle of illness than to have a large variety of isolated experiences. In general, learning should be by wholes. Students should be introduced to total nursing situations. The learning may take place through a variety of methods — reading, demonstration, conference, observation, interview, lecture, case discussions and others. Learning really takes place through the actual care of patients and families. The student needs to be a participant in her own education, and learning should be a cooperative enterprise of patient, teacher and student. It is important for a student as far as possible to gain generalized concepts through her own deductions from clearly understood instances and to strengthen her understanding of these concepts by putting them to use in solving concrete problems.

Program for Nurses Leading to a Baccalaureate Degree

It is now general practice for the graduate of hospital schools of nursing, or of the 2-year associate degree programs, to enter undergraduate baccalaureate degree programs for preservice students in nursing. In some instances these nurses can obtain advanced standing by taking subject examinations in the liberal arts and, in a few instances, proficiency examinations in the nursing subjects.

A few universities continue to offer the generalized program for nurses leading to a baccalaureate degree. This program aims to round out the preparation of the graduate from a hospital school of nursing or from an associate degree program in nursing. This program is sometimes called a supplementary or continuation program in nursing. The general goals of this program are: (1) to broaden the understanding of the nurse about the scope and the role of nursing in a dynamic society, (2) to broaden her knowledge of professional practice and to increase her ability to function as a professional nurse and (3) to provide her with a foundation for graduate study.

The generalized program is undergraduate education that includes essential liberal education and special education in nursing. It provides the broad understandings of human communications, social developments, scientific method and essentials of nursing practice as a basis for helping the nurse to perform as a professional worker.

There is a growing trend for universities to admit nurses directly into undergraduate programs for preservice students in nursing rather than into special generalized programs for graduate nurses. What is your idea about this?

Graduate Education for Nurses

Graduate education for nurses leads to such higher degrees as master's and doctor's. It begins where undergraduate education in nursing ends. It is assumed that graduate education builds on the baccalaureate program in nursing, which prepares for professional nursing practice. A graduate program prepares the nurse for a specialized professional role — expert clinician, teacher, supervisor, administrator, consultant, or research worker. Each program provides for the development of understanding of the theory in the specialized role or roles, and for competence in practice.

The curriculum design and content for graduate programs for nurses vary somewhat in accord with the philosophy and the purposes of the different educational institutions offering these programs. In general, the curriculum pattern for preparation for positions in either nursing education or nursing service falls into similar areas: (1) foundation courses for all students as specified by the faculty of the specific educational institution; (2) trends and relationships in nursing; (3) research (study-making and research interpretation); (4) content related to the function or functions of expert clinical practice, teaching, curriculum development and improvement, supervision, administration, research, or various combinations of these; and (5) special interests.

The extent and the kind of research education to be required for all nurses in graduate education constitute a moot question. Many nurse educators concede that the research courses in all graduate programs for nurses on the level of the master's degree should give the student an opportunity to investigate and use research findings in the solution of complex nursing problems in the specialized area for which she is preparing. The doctoral student is expected to carry out an independent, scholarly study. Many nurses continue to obtain their doctoral degree in fields other than nursing, such as education, sociology, psychology, and so forth. Nurse-scientist programs provide for both nursing and another field such as sociology, anthropology, physiology, and so forth. Today, an increasing number of programs provide a doctoral program in nursing.

Functions, qualifications and preparation of graduate nurses for work in special fields are discussed in some detail in Chapters 9 and 10. The overall current system of education for nursing is discussed in Chapter 16.

IMPORTANCE OF A PERSONAL PHILOSOPHY

Why should you have a definite working philosophy? To answer this question adequately it would be necessary to discuss the meaning and the function of philosophy, a lengthy task. However, a few brief comments may serve to reintroduce you to this important and challenging subject.

Philosophy is the study of reality through ultimate causes by the light of human reason. It explains the origin, the nature and the destiny of man and the purpose of life. It helps to direct activities, weigh values and make sound decisions; it also helps to detect order that already exists, as well as to create order where it should, but does not, exist. Such being the case, nurses need a philosophy of nursing; they need to formulate the reason for nursing, the nature of nursing and the end to be achieved by it.

You might ask yourself these questions to help you formulate a philosophy of nursing: How do I define nursing in terms of responsibilities and scope? What do I believe are major concepts basic to good nursing care? Who should nurse? Should there be a splitting of nursing functions among various types of workers? If so, on what basis? Where should nursing take place? How does work setting influence the nature of nursing services and nursing practice? What do I consider to be my relation with my colleagues, with allied nursing personnel and with other workers in the health field? How do I expect society to benefit by my nursing? What kind of person, worker and citizen should I be in order to fit into the system of nursing service described in my answers to these questions?

You cannot solve problems successfully until you first have defined your philosophy of life in general. The answer to every nursing question is influenced by your philosophy of nursing. It influences not only the selection of what you will do, how you will do it, when you will do it and what sources you will use to help you make decisions, but it is also the essence of your whole plan of nursing.

Whether we realize it or not, we all have some sort of philosophy of life, of nursing and of education. It is highly important that our philosophy be sound and that we be actively and consistently aware of it as a directing force – in other words, that we express it vividly and attempt to live it always.

PROBLEMS

1. There are different meanings given to the word "profession" by various occupational groups and in different countries of the world. Try to locate as many of these definitions as you can.

2. Examine the issues discussed, for the last 5 years, in the *International Nursing Review* and the USA nursing periodicals and locate articles on the "professional status of nursing." Review these articles and use as a basis for discussion with a group of your classmates.

3. It is suggested that you analyze the current edition of the ANA Code of Ethics for Nurses. (a) What additional planks, if any, would you include in this "Code"? (b) Compare the "ANA Code" with that of the ICN.

4. How can a registered nurse who has not graduated from a professional school obtain full professional status?

5. State, in writing, your philosophy of life. As you grow in your thinking, bring it up to date.

6. (a) What kinds of simple, practical questions about professional values

can you ask yourself when you are graduated, in order to evaluate yourself and your work? (b) Could you begin to apply these criteria now?

SUGGESTED REFERENCES*

PROFESSIONAL EDUCATION

Allyn, N. C. "College Credit by Examination." *Nursing Outlook,* **17:**44-46, Apr. 1969.

Arnold, M. F. "Our Changing World: Comments on Philosophy and Concepts of Public Health Education in Medical Care." *American Journal of Public Health,* **58:**238-245, Feb. 1968.

Aydelotte, M. K. "Issues of Professional Nursing; the Need for Clinical Excellence." *Nursing Forum,* **7:**72-86, Winter 1968.

Campbell, J. *Master's Education in Nursing.* New York, National League for Nursing, 1964.

"Characteristics of Baccalaureate and Graduate Education in Nursing." *Nursing Outlook,* **16:**36-37, July 1968.

* Dudas, S. "The RN in the Baccalaureate Program." *Nursing Outlook,* **16:**51-53, July 1968.

"Let's Examine – Science and Nursing Knowledge of Graduate Students." *Nursing Outlook,* **15:**53, Dec. 1967.

Millard, R. Jr. "Liberal and Professional Nursing Education." *Nursing Outlook,* **16:**22-25, July 1968.

* Mussalem, H. K. "The Changing Role of the Nurse." *American Journal of Nursing,* **69:**514-517, Mar. 1969.

* National League for Nursing. Department of Baccalaureate and Higher Degree Programs. *College Education: Key to Professional Careers in Nursing.* New York, The League, 1968.

* _____. *Characteristics of Graduate Education in Nursing.* New York, The League, 1968.

Pitel, M. "Current Trends in Nursing Education with Implications for Nursing Service." *Kansas Nurse,* **44:**2-4, Feb. 1969.

* Reiter, F. "Preparation For Professional Nursing Practice." *Johns Hopkins Alumnae Magazine* (Nursing), **66:**49-50, Sept. 1967.

Shryock, R. H. "Nursing Emerges as a Profession: The American Experience." *Clio Medica,* **3:**131-147, 1968.

Teachers College, Columbia University. Division of Nursing Education. *Problems of Graduate Nurse Education: Report of Work Conference:* New York, Bureau of Publications, Teachers College, Columbia University, 1952, pp. 8-21.

PROFESSIONALISM

* Anderson, B. E. "Accepting Responsibility for Achieving Professional Status." *Bulletin Tennessee Nurses Association,* **31:**10-18, Summer 1967.

Arnold, M. "Professionalism and Changing Concepts of Administration." *Journal of Nursing Education,* **7:**5-10, Jan. 1968.

Babich, K. S. "Perception of Professionalism: Equality." *Nursing Forum,* **7(1):** 14-20, 1968.

---

* In each chapter all citations are footnoted and are not included here. All starred references are recommended for additional reading.

Brown, E. L. *Nursing for the Future*. New York, Russell Sage Foundation, 1948, pp. 73-75, 138-173.

Clark, A. R. "Candidly Speaking on Nursing and Professionalism." *Nursing Forum*, 7:10-13, Winter 1968.

"Code for Nurses." *American Journal of Nursing*, **68**:2581-2585, Dec. 1968.

Davis, F., Ed. *The Nursing Profession: Five Sociological Essays*. New York, Wiley, 1966.

Dock, L. L., *et al*. *A Short History of Nursing from the Earliest Times to the Present Day*. New York, Putnam, 1938, pp. 353-379.

Ferguson, C. M. "Professions, Professionals and Motivation." *Journal of the American Dietetic Association*, 53:197-201, Sept. 1968.

Hall, R. N. "Professionalization and Bureaucratization." *American Sociological Review*, **33**:99-104, Feb. 1968.

Lindsey, M. "Professional Standards: Whose Responsibility?" *Mississippi RN* **30**:21-25, July 1968.

Marston, J. "Hallmarks of a Profession." *Public Relations Journal*, **24**:8-10, July 1968.

Mayes, N., *et al*. "Commitment to Nursing: How is It Achieved?" *Nursing Outlook*, **16**:29-31, July 1968.

* "The Nurse in Research: ANA Guidelines on Ethical Values." *American Journal of Nursing*, **68**:1504-1507, July 1968.

* Pellegrino, E. D. "Ethical Implications in Changing Practice." *American Journal of Nursing*, **64**:110-112, Sept. 1964.

Scotford, H. "The Professional Woman." *Australian Nurses Journal*, **65**:245-248, Dec. 1967.

"Sociologist Describes Nursing as a Reluctant Profession." *Hospital Topics*, **46**:23, Apr. 1968.

Ten Brink, C. L. "The Process of Socialization into a New Role: the Professional Nurse." *Nursing Forum*, 7:146-160, 1968.

Walsh, J. L., *et al*. "Professionalism and the Poor Structural Effects and Profes sional Behavior." *Journal of Health Social Behavior*, **9**:16-28, Mar. 1968.

"Who's Professional?" (editorial) *Delaware Medical Journal*, **40**:260-261, Aug. 1968.

See also, references on "What's in Our Code" in the *American Journal of Nursing*, 1952 through 1963.

CHAPTER

4

Responsibility for Nursing Practice

Responsibility for nursing practice and its improvement is a major concern of many persons within both the nursing profession and other professional and lay groups. This concern has been increasingly voiced in professional and popular literature; even newspapers occasionally carry editorials and feature stories on this significant topic.

Although nurses have direct responsibility for nursing practice, people in other professions, institutions and agencies, as well as society as a whole, share responsibility for providing and maintaining the system of health services through which nursing care is provided. For example, the educational system for nursing is concerned with the preparation of nurse manpower; the employing institutions or agencies are responsible for utilizing personnel to best advantage; other health professions, along with nursing, help to develop new health programs; and society helps to determine policy and payment.

DEFINITION OF RESPONSIBILITY

Responsibility rests upon the particular set of standards and values held by the individual or group involved. True responsibility lies within the individual and includes both commitment to fulfill one's trust and accountability for one's actions. It does not mean being compelled to do a job solely by rules and regulations. Instead, true responsibility is dependent upon knowledge, discretion, judgment and ability to make decisions about one's work. Furthermore, a truly responsible person works for her own self-improvement as well as for the development of sound methods that work in whatever situation she finds herself. Her commitment is to achieve excellence.

It may not always be easy to decide one's responsibility or, once having made the decision, to carry it out. Take this instance for example. In a particular hospital it was standard to administer intermittant positive breathing treatments 4 times a day. The physician in charge of making rounds found that the assigned nurse had instituted the treatment only once. When queried by the physician the nurse said: "With only one nurse on duty he is lucky to get it once a day." This example reflects one response toward responsibility in the face of difficulties—lowering standards and lack of commitment to the trust inherent in the nurse's responsibility to the patient. This negative example is given only because one so often hears complaints of shortages of nursing personnel with resulting inability to provide adequate care. Admittedly, it is easier to assume professional responsibility for good care when situations are ideal. However, since one seldom finds ideal situations in real life, one must be able to carry out one's professional responsibility in numerous less-than-ideal situations.

How would you cope with patient care in the face of too few nursing personnel? Is it possible that the nurse in this situation might have planned patient care on her unit so that essential care was guaranteed? To plan well, the nurse must know certain facts and make evaluations about the essential needs of each patient and the components of good care. She must have the ability to assess the relative importance of care needed and to determine priorities. In addition, maintaining a belief in oneself and in the importance of one's work will prevent the job from becoming routine or merely a case of "getting the work done."

SOME CONCEPTS OF NURSING PRACTICE

The word "nurse" denotes a person who performs or practices nursing, that is, gives nursing care. Most people, including the public, nurses themselves, and other health professionals would agree with this concept. However, when one goes a bit deeper and asks what nursing practice actually is, much less agreement is found. As students of nursing you may already have noted differences in what is expected from a nurse by patients and their families, by nurses in practice, by your teachers, and by other health professionals, such as physicians and dentists.

In order to become a responsible practitioner, each nurse must be crystal-clear about what nursing practice means to her. Without such understanding she will be unable to perform effectively, or to interpret her practice adequately to others.

What is your definition of nursing? You might, for example, consider some of the following questions in class discussion: To what extent is nursing the actual giving of physical care and treatment to patients and to what extent is it the supervision and guidance of auxiliary personnel in providing this care? Some nurses define nursing as care, cure and coordination. How do you react to this? What about the concepts of prevention of disease and the promotion of health as aspects of nursing care? Nursing practice can be defined in relation to the care of individual patients. How do you define practice as it encompasses community health? Nursing has been called both an art and a science. Do you believe it is both an art and a science? If so what are its characteristics as an art? As a science? One's concept of nursing needs to be reexamined periodically in light of new knowledge and changes in the nursing profession, in the health field and in society.

While it may be rather difficult today to find a definition of nursing practice acceptable to everyone, attempts have been and are being made to do this. One definition is the legal one that is used to describe nursing in nurse practice acts. Another definition is that developed by the nursing profession itself. Still other definitions of nursing are based upon personal philosophies of nursing care.

Legal Definition

In the various states there are nurse practice acts which define the conditions under which nurses may practice their profession. These acts have been established by law to protect the public against unauthorized nursing practices. Therefore, they contain definitions of nursing practice. Chapter 6 discusses the legal definition of nursing in some detail.

The Profession's Definition

In a position paper on nursing education, the ANA defined 2 types of nursing practice: professional and technical. These definitions are related to the educational preparation of the nurse. Baccalaureate education is proposed as the minimum preparation for professional nursing practice, whose components are listed in the paper as care, cure and coordination. The central idea of baccalaureate education is to provide a student with the knowledge needed for making sound judgments about patient care, both for herself and for those auxiliary nursing personnel for whom she has teaching and supervisory responsibility. Technical nursing practice, on the other hand, is defined as purely the performance of nursing measures and medically delegated procedures. According to the ANA paper, preparation for this latter type of practice should be obtained in associate degree programs.[1]

[1] American Nurses' Association, *Educational Preparation for Nurse Practitioners and Assistants to Nurses: A Position Paper,* New York, The Association, 1965, pp. 5-9.

Definition Related to Personal Philosophy

In attempting to describe what nursing practice is, much attention has been given to a determination of the unique aspects of this practice. The ANA definitions of professional and technical nursing practice are one such attempt. Some nurses are deeply concerned about the need to examine clinical nursing practice, with emphasis on the nurturant role. Some emphasize the expanding role (generally meaning the assumption of functions formerly belonging to physicians) of nurses. Others believe there needs to be emphasis on the role of the nurse in encouraging self-help by the patient in accordance with his abilities and capacities.

A noted nurse educator describes her own personal concept of the essential function of the nurse in any setting as follows:

The unique function of the nurse is to assist the individual, sick or well, in the performance of those activities contributing to health or its recovery (or to peaceful death) that he would perform unaided if he had the necessary strength, will or knowledge. And to do this in such a way as to help him gain independence as rapidly as possible. This aspect of her work, this part of her function, she initiates and controls; of this she is master. In addition she helps the patient carry out the therapeutic plan as initiated by the physician.[2]

Another nurse educator, working independently of Henderson, has proposed the following concept of nursing:

Nursing is assistance to persons in particular life situations in the achievement of health results or in a more effective way of living through continuing daily self-care based upon scientifically derived knowledge of health and disease and known effective self care practices, into which is incorporated the medical orders of the person's physician. The adult person assisted is in whole or in part unable to act for himself without assistance because of his health state, or health needs. The child who requires nursing is unable to provide himself care because he is a child and his parents or guardians are not able to care for him effectively because of his health state or needs.[3]

Whenever there are discussions of non-nursing activities, there is probably little or no disagreement about what nursing practice is *not*. There is general agreement that nurses in hospitals or clinics should not be performing housekeeping, dietary, pharmaceutical, or even business office activities. For far too long nursing personnel, because they are present around-the-clock, have assumed responsibility for many such functions, taking valuable nursing time away from patient care. These functions should be the responsibility of the various departments within the institution created for these services. You may, however, find yourself in situations where failure of a department to assume its rightful responsibility hampers your nursing care. In such instances, you will need to seek help through administrative channels, such as your supervisor or a nursing care committee, in order to affect change. This process will take time and often diplomacy and tact as well.

---

[2] V. Henderson, "The Nature of Nursing," *American Journal of Nursing*, **64**:63, Aug. 1964.
[3] D. E. Orem, *Foundations of Nursing and Its Practice*, New York, McGraw-Hill, (Manuscript in process of publication), p. II, 17.

In some situations, especially in small hospitals, there may really be no department to take over some of these non-nursing functions; compromises to protect the care of the patients may have to be made temporarily.

It is argued by some that the nurse should be relieved of certain management functions at the division or ward level. Unit managers have been employed effectively in some hospitals.[4]

There are areas of nursing practice that overlap with the practice of the physician. Called "gray areas of practice" by some, these activities, such as closed chest cardiac massage, are of concern to both physicians and nurses. Some nurses and doctors believe it is logical for nurses to assume increasing responsibility for certain acts which formerly were the exclusive function of doctors. Nurses in intensive care units, including coronary care units, are fulfilling some of these functions daily, for example, identifying the need for and carrying out life-saving procedures for coronary care patients. Other expansions of the nurse's role, such as "pediatric-nurse-practitioner" in pediatric clinics or her counterpart in geriatric clinics, where realignment of the functions performed by physicians and nurses is being tried out, are the subject of much debate.[5,6]

Encouraged by the ANA, various state nurses associations are collaborating with state medical and hospital associations and state associations of hospital pharmacists to determine the functions of nurses, doctors and pharmacists in the "gray" areas. As a result of these joint efforts, statements have been adopted concerning such procedures as closed chest cardiac resuscitation, administration of investigational drugs, and the care of patients with cardiovascular disease in coronary care or intensive care units. In addition, various institutions, hospitals and health agencies are establishing advisory committees of physicians, nurses and administrators whose functions are to review developments and changes in medical and nursing practice and to develop written policies outlining the responsibilities of physicians and nurses in the performance of certain procedures.

An interesting development in recent years has been the nurse-clinician or clinical nurse-specialist role. Frances Reiter, a leading proponent of nurse-clinicians, states that she believes personal care of patients is the heart of nursing practice. Her idea is that clinical competence has 3 dimensions: range of function, depth of understanding, and breadth of services. Range of function refers to care, cure and counseling. Nurses prepared as clinicians not only would know how to practice nursing in a special field but would have a broad preparation in the sciences involving the specialty area. Such a practitioner would be able to assess a patient's need for nursing care and plan a therapeutic regime for him. Miss Reiter's definition of

[4] See W. M. Brooks, "A Pattern for Unit Management," *Hospital Progress*, **48**:124-128, May 1967, and L. T. Mercadante, "The Functions and Benefits of the Unit Manager," *Hospital Progress*, **47**:114-117, Jan. 1966.

[5] H. K. Silver, *et al.,* "The Pediatric Nurse-Practitioner Program," *Journal of the American Medical Association,* **204**:298-302, Apr. 22, 1968.

[6] C. E. Lewis and B. A. Resnik, "Nurse Clinic and Progressive Ambulatory Patient Care," *New England Journal of Medicine,* **277**:1236-1241, Dec. 7, 1967.

breadth of service includes coordination, continuity and collaboration; this is, coordination of the various services directly related to the patient's welfare, provision for continuity of care and collaboration with the physician responsible for the patient. The nurse-clinician is, in fact, seen as a master practitioner bringing to the patient the very finest personal and professional nursing service.[7]

The number of nurse-clinicians employed in hospitals, particularly in large medical centers, and in public health agencies has grown appreciably. Generally speaking, in hospitals and agencies where clinical specialists are working, you will find that staff nurses tend to have more autonomy in planning for, and carrying out their nursing care responsibilities. A clinical specialist usually has her own case load of patients, but also observes other patients on the unit and acts in a consultative capacity to the rest of the nursing staff with regard to clinical nursing problems. In some situations there no longer are head nurses; an administrative nursing supervisor or assistant director in nursing service is responsible for overall administration, and a unit manager or unit coordinator handles the managerial functions of the unit, such as ordering supplies, running messenger services and so forth.

At this point, we should reemphasize that our concept of nursing is *not* confined only to nursing carried out within hospitals. Modern nursing also embraces concern for patients in ambulatory services, nursing homes and other extended care facilities and all types of community health agencies. The walls of the hospital are coming down, and the importance of continuity of care as a responsibility of nurses in institutions, clinics and homes is becoming increasingly clear. As you noted in Chapter 2, social forces, legislation and changes in technology and science have greatly influenced the scope of nursing practice.

A statement on concepts of nursing practice made by the editor of the *American Journal of Nursing* would seem to be most appropriate to consider here:

How can anyone distinguish in a few understandable words the activities of a group as vast as nursing, serving so many different kinds of patients in such diverse ways: nurturing children and parents in neighborhood health centers, helping the alienated search for identity in group psychotherapy, detecting and converting arrhythmias in sophisticated cardiac units, patiently training the mentally retarded, manning trauma units, rekindling the sense of safety in the elderly, bolstering the trust of the preoperative, and many more.[8]

You may well ask at this point: By what standards do I consider the various concepts of nursing practice? How do I arrive at my own concept? There is perhaps no easy answer, but as a result of your clinical experiences as a student and your readings and observations, you will draw certain

    [7] F. Reiter, "The Nurse-Clinician," *American Journal of Nursing,* **66**:274-280, Feb. 1966.
    [8] B. G. Schutt, "The Promise in Practice," (editorial), *American Journal of Nursing,* **67**:2515, Dec. 1967.

conclusions that will help you to develop your concept. Then, too, one of the goals of class discussions will be to develop and refine this concept. As a class you might discuss how, as a graduate nurse, you might handle problems you may encounter in the real-life situation of the hospital or other health agency in the community. We have implied that one of your functions as a graduate nurse may be that of an agent of change. While this chapter cannot go into the processes involved in affecting change, this is another area for consideration in your class sessions.

In addition to acquiring a clear concept of nursing practice, developing responsibility also is dependent upon an understanding of the characteristics of this practice. The next unit deals with some of these characteristics.

SOME CHARACTERISTICS OF NURSING PRACTICE

Patient-, Family- and Community-Centered Practice

What are the important characteristics of nursing practice? Perhaps any attempt to develop a list would be inadequate. However, at the top of any list would be the focus on the patient, family, or community needing nursing service – in other words, the individualization of nursing care. For the patient and his family this involves the goal of meeting physical, psychological, emotional, social and spiritual needs regardless of age, stage of illness, or the environment where the care is given.

One possible result of changes in society and in health care today is increasing depersonalization. Technological advances creating more opportunities to mechanize activities in our society tend to promote this depersonalization unless steps are taken to prevent it. In the hospital, it is easy to see this trend in the type of equipment now in use in intensive care and coronary units, the so-called "heart machines, lung machines, kidney machines and the like." Even though the depersonalizing effect of organizing nursing services around institutional rather than patient care needs may be, perhaps, less obvious to the casual observer, such a method of organization can have exactly the same effect as machines are having. Because it is new to hospitals, the effect of using data processing equipment in planning and giving patient care is not yet known, but the use of this tool could well add to the problem of depersonalization if great care is not given to prevent such a reaction.

In years gone by, it was relatively simple to individualize care. Today, a nurse will find it necessary to develop a plan whereby she determines the needs of each patient or family and the methods she will employ to help the patient or family meet these needs from the available resources. When you are working on a busy unit you may sometimes feel that you do not have time for talking with and listening to patients in order to learn their needs or you may begrudge the time it takes to develop a nursing care plan. But cutting corners in this area will lead to ineffective nursing care and only add to, rather than help solve, your problems. Genuine interest, as expressed in your conversation with patients and in careful listening, is essential for sound planning for and with patients and their families.

The Importance of Observation in Nursing

The quality of nursing practice is related in no small part to the nurse's assessment of the needs of her patients. This assessment, or "diagnosis" as it is sometimes termed, is in turn related to a nurse's ability to observe accurately. Observational skill is a primary factor in obtaining the data needed for a comprehensive medical and nursing evaluation or diagnosis. It not only involves the ability to *see* the patient's symptoms and reactions to medical and nursing care, but also the ability to *hear* him, thereby helping him share his feelings and problems.

How do you go about making accurate observations? One method has already been mentioned in the previous section: talking with and listening to patients. It is suggested that you read Dumas, Orem, Orlando, and Wiedenbach who discuss how you might go about improving your ability to determine patients' needs through these means.[9]

Visual observations of the patient, the actual family situation and the community environment are also important. Perhaps one way to sharpen your ability is to check your observations against those of someone else to see how much agreement there is between you.

Among other methods available for improving observational skills is taking a nursing history. Nurses at the University of Florida devised a method of this kind "to systematically, concisely, and economically collect information relevant to nursing practice from patients and families." Dorothy Smith, in reporting on nursing histories, goes on to say that it is a "tool for thinking clinically" and that "it may provide a basis for badly needed clinical nursing research."[10] Nurses collect data about patients on specially prepared forms, asking specific questions and noting nonverbal as well as verbal responses.

Recording—An Aid to Diagnosis and Care

Of equal importance to nursing practice is the systematic and accurate recording of nurses' observations of patients and of nursing care given. A good history has little value if it is not recorded properly. Good recording provides data for diagnostic and nursing evaluation as well as for clinical research. The use of data processing methods to record nurses' notes is just

[9] See R. Dumas, *et al.*, "Validating a Theory of Nursing Practice," *American Journal of Nursing,* **63**:52-55, Aug. 1963; D. E. Orem, *Foundations of Nursing and Its Practice,* New York, McGraw-Hill, when published; J. I. Orlando, *The Dynamic Nurse-Patient Relationship, Functions, Process and Principles,* New York, G. P. Putnams Sons, 1961; and E. Wiedenbach, *Clinical Nursing. A Helping Art,* New York, Springer, 1964.

[10] D. Smith, "Nursing Care—Quality and Quantity," *Mississippi RN,* **30**:18, Apr. 1968.

around the corner. The rise of this new technology will require a nurse to focus much more sharply upon her observational and recording skills.

In some diseases certain physical phenomena dictate medical and nursing procedures. Therefore, recordings must relate to these symptoms or they have little value. How often have you seen on changing shift summaries a note only that the patient has had a good or a bad night or that his condition is critical, poor, satisfactory, or good? This tells nothing about vital signs, intake or output, nausea, I.V. flow, or other items of significance. The physician needs records that will help him in diagnosis and medical treatment. The nurse coming on to care for the patient needs records that will help her to know whether certain procedures should be stopped or continued or whether different nursing measures should be instituted.

Nurses' notes are important not only for developing an initial nursing diagnosis and nursing care plan, but also for continuing the plan of care. These notes are equally necessary in evaluating care and in determining future nursing goals. Last but not least, nurses' notes are of vital importance to the attending physician for evaluation of the patient's condition and as one basis for diagnosis and therapy.

To serve these purposes, a record should include an objective picture of nursing needs, of measures instituted to meet these needs, including teaching or guidance given, of responses to the nursing care measures and of plans for future care. Skill in recording requires practice. Evaluate your own nursing notes in terms of what they do and do not include about what you know or have observed about a patient, as well as what facts you require but have not yet obtained through observation. Then rewrite the notes in an effort to present a clearer picture.

Communications and Relationships in Nursing Practice

The ability to communicate is essential in nursing practice. There is little that the nurse does which does not involve communicating with: (1) the patient and his family, (2) the various members of the nursing team, (3) nursing and other administrative personnel, (4) physicians, (5) other personnel in the situation and (6) the general public or consumers of nursing. Unfortunately, the evidence too frequently points to the lack of communication between the nurse and these various groups.[11]

Good communication is characterized by the ability to express oneself well, to listen with empathy toward others and to maintain good interpersonal and interprofessional relationships. How do you develop these qualities? One objective of your educational program has been to help you develop the ability to express yourself well both orally and in writing. One of your own goals should be to continue to focus on improving these skills through practice and perhaps through further education after graduation.

[11] R. S. Duff and A. B. Hollingshead, *Sickness and Society,* New York, Harper and Row, 1968, pp. 217-247.

"Empathy" is a quality based upon the ability to "feel with others." You will need to assess how much you can put yourself in the place of another. Respect for the dignity and rights of all persons is a basic ingredient of this characteristic. In order to develop empathy for your patients and families, it will be necessary for you to examine your own feelings about them and then to make a serious attempt to understand them.

Good interpersonal relationships between nurse and patient often require that the nurse take the initiative in establishing the relationship. Many, if not most, patients are desperately in need of understanding, kindness, and empathy from the nurse. Time and again, it has been pointed out that no amount of skill in carrying out procedures is enough when there is lack of warmth, respect, and understanding on the nurse's part. This is not to say that technical skill is not important; it simply is not sufficient if the patient requires attention to more than his physical needs.

Time spent talking with a patient, listening to him, making an assessment of his needs, and checking on this assessment will pay enormous dividends in improved care for the patient and in satisfaction for the nurse. She can then identify with the patient and truly individualize his care. For example, you answer a patient's call bell and he tells you he has a headache. You think first of all about the patient's diagnosis and his physician's orders. The patient has had gastric surgery and has an order for medication for pain. You observe his worried expression and pause to straighten his pillow, helping him adjust to a better position. As you do this, you might ask him if everything else is all right. If he senses your interest, he may then tell you his worries about his family and his own future. He is a traveling salesman and his chief concern may be about the way he is going to be able to manage his diet. Just listening to him and, when he has told you what he is worried about, answering his questions and reassuring him by telling him that he will be receiving guidance on this may be better nursing care than quick acceptance and treatment of such a symptom as a headache. The essence of professional nursing practice lies in this kind of assumption of individual responsibility for your patient.[12]

Good interpersonal relationships with co-workers — other nurses, licensed practical nurses, and nurses' aides — are based upon respect for and understanding of the contributions of each one. In other words, in order to build sound relationships you need to learn about the functions and responsibilities of these other nursing personnel, have a genuine respect for them as human beings, and have a sincere willingness to work with them. Showing courtesy and friendliness will also help you to promote good relationships.

Although effective nursing requires communication and cooperation with many people, it demands special attention to communication and cooperation with the physician. Some nurses and nursing students seem to be afraid of physicians, especially in hospitals. Is this due perhaps to a lack of understanding of how to discuss patients' problems and concerns with the physi-

[12] See references listed in footnote number 9.

cian? Or does the nurse's work load and other administrative policies and conditions prevent her from spending sufficient time with physicians in order to establish good relationships? In some hospitals it is a rare occurrence for a nurse to accompany a physician on his visits to patients. Recently, a head nurse asked a number of nurses this question: "With how many physicians have you established a good and helpful relationship?" Very few of them could say that they had established such relationships.

Because of the technological and scientific advances in health care, nurses in the future will be carrying much greater independent responsibility for patient care. For example, when one contemplates the responsibility of nurses in extended care facilities and in neighborhood or so-called storefront family clinics, it becomes increasingly clear that nurses must develop collaborative roles with physicians.

Establishing good working relationships with physicians may be a bit more difficult for a young graduate. The ability to do this will not be learned overnight. However, again, the basis is mutual respect and understanding. Equally important is self-respect and a belief in the value of the contribution which nurses have to make to the care of patients and families. If you have this much to start with you will be able to build upon it as an experienced nurse. The process of developing and maintaining relationships is never finished; it is something we continue to work at all of our lives. To maintain good relationships requires that we evaluate and learn from our successes and failures and then try again.

Despite the problems involved because physicians and nurses are extremely busy people, there is evidence that both physicians and nurses value collaboration and are studying ways in which this can be better achieved. One physician has suggested the following ways for promoting interprofessional cooperation: (1) patient care committees in hospitals, related institutions, and agencies; (2) appointment of liason doctors and nurses whose function is to create and open channels of communication; (3) institutional and service-oriented interprofessional conferences at local, state and national levels; and (4) interdigitation of medical and nursing education in medical centers.[13]

Clinical Competence

In our discussion of some of the characteristics of nursing practice, we have highlighted the importance of individualized care, of accurate observation and recording, of skill in communicating and of the development of good interpersonal and interprofessional relationships. We have pointed out the growing importance of the nurse's collaborative role vis-a-vis the physician. We have not dealt with skill in clinical practice, but it goes without saying that this is a major characteristic of nursing practice.

[13] E. D. Pellegrino, "What's Wrong With the Nurse-Physician Relationship in Today's Hospitals," *Hospitals*, **40**:70, 77-79, Dec. 1966.

A principal objective of your educational program has been the development of the knowledge and skill you will need to practice nursing. You have been acquiring the basic scientific principles and the broad general background upon which you will draw in your practice as a graduate nurse. This practice will include manual skills but, as stated before, these are not enough without the other characteristics we have discussed.

Furthermore, we would be less than truthful if we said that you will be a finished product when you complete your education program. You are ready to *begin* the practice of nursing. It will be up to you to further develop your knowledge and skill. Many of you will possibly go on to graduate education in your effort to increase your clinical competence.

Such interest in improving clinical competence and, in turn, patient care will also lead you into the realm of research in nursing. As a professional practitioner you have a responsibility to be familiar with and make use of the findings of research. You will be constantly looking for new and better ways of practicing. You may even be called upon to assist in nursing research. A few of you will eventually become the nursing researchers of the future.

The Importance of Social Amenities

One final word might be said before leaving the subject of characteristics of nursing practice. One of the ingredients of nursing practice which patients often comment upon is whether or not the nurse was pleasant, kind and interested. Esther Lucile Brown calls these the amenities of nursing.[14] Much of the happiness and contentedness of a patient will depend upon whether he receives prompt, pleasant attention. Pleasantness and genuine interest on the nurse's part in all of her relationships may serve to set the stage for understanding and for the kind of interpersonal relationships essential to good practice.

TEAM NURSING

Perhaps one of the most important influences in recent years on the delivery of nursing services has been the introduction of team nursing. The idea, initiated some 15 to 20 years ago, was conceived as a method of improving patient care by coordinating and improving the services of the various persons providing nursing care, that is, the registered nurse, the licensed practical nurse and the nurse's aide. Begun as a means of distributing nursing service to hospital patients, it is now utilized in a number of extended care facilities and public health agencies as well.

The core of team nursing lies in its major characteristics: (1) the leader-

---

[14] E. L. Brown, "As I See Nursing: Its Present and Its Future," *New Jersey Nurse*, **23**:3-12, Dec. 1967.

ship of a well-qualified professional nurse, (2) a written nursing care plan, (3) planned assignments for each member of the team and (4) the nursing team conference. The value of the method lies in its team approach — sharing observations of patients' needs and pooling knowledge and skills in providing for those needs. While the patient has not generally been considered a member of the team, there is growing belief that he should assume a more active role on the health team — that his ideas, opinions and cooperation should be actively sought both by the total health care team and by the nursing team in making decisions about his care. Understanding and working with both the patient's and the physician's goals enhances patient care.

It must also be remembered that the nursing team, just as other forms of organized care, can result in use primarily benefiting nursing personnel and giving little thought to the patient or his family. To be truly successful in improving patient care, the team must keep their focus on the needs of the patient or his family rather than on factors important only to the nurses or to the running of the unit or agency. Considering the patient as the primary team member places him where he rightly belongs, at the center of the team's activities. As a nurse you may have an opportunity to serve as a staff member and later as a leader of a nursing team. Your concept of the team's function will be crucial to its success in providing quality patient care, whether in a hospital or in a public health nursing agency.

PREPARATION FOR NURSING PRACTICE

The major purpose of nursing education is preparation for nursing practice. As we have indicated before, upon graduation you are ready to begin nursing practice but you are not a finished product. When you begin to work as a graduate nurse, you have a right to expect an orientation to the policies and practices of the institution or agency which employs you. Today, many institutions and agencies provide for the orientation of all new nursing employees. In addition, they provide for continuing inservice education of all nursing personnel, including general staff nurses, licensed practical nurses and nurse's aides, as well as for nurses in various administrative categories. While your preservice education prepares you for beginning practice, you will still be greatly lacking in experience when you graduate. As a newly graduated nurse you will require intensive supervised experience before taking on major responsibilities as a staff nurse or team leader. You should not be expected to manage a team or administer a busy unit right away. It would perhaps be prudent for you to look for experience as a general staff nurse for the first 5 or 6 months before serving as a team leader or head nurse. The experience gained will serve you well later on.

As a registered nurse you will eventually be responsible for assisting in the orientation and inservice education of auxiliary nursing personnel, or even for helping with their on-the-job training. You will also be responsible for planning and supervising their work. It will be important for you to remember that they should not be expected to perform activities for which they are not adequately prepared through training and supervised practice. As with your own services, the law defines the practice of the licensed practical nurse and this definition guides the assignment of their functions. As with registered nurses and physicians, there is some overlap between the functions of registered nurses and those of licensed practical nurses. You should become familiar with the limits of accepted practice for the licensed practical nurse in the state where you work. Active participation in your state and local nurses' association is one way of keeping informed about changes in areas of practice of both the registered nurse and the licensed practical nurse, as well as of the acceptable functions of nurses' aides.

When work pressures are great, you may be tempted to permit auxiliary personnel to perform functions that are not within the legal bounds of their practice. However, you do this at great risk to the patient, to the auxiliary personnel and to yourself. There is a trend toward forming nursing practice committees in hospitals and community health agencies whose responsibility is to study and determine the limits of practice of their various groups of nursing personnel. In institutions with such committees you would discuss problems of changing functions in these committees. In places without such committees, you could be instrumental in instituting them.

RESPONSIBILITY OF CONCERNED GROUPS FOR NURSING PRACTICE

Responsibility of the Employing Institution or Agency

The institution or agency created to offer patient care has the responsibility to provide or aid in providing an environmental situation that will assist a patient to meet appropriate health goals. How nursing service is delivered depends on the philosophy of the particular health service within which the nursing is provided. Hospital administrators, for example, say to the public: "Our patients are provided with nursing care along with other required services." The patient's hospital charges include those for nursing care. Therefore, hospitals have an obligation to provide competent nurses and to have policies that promote good nursing practice. The professional nurses in the institution must be permitted by the administrator to set the standards for nursing practice and its improvement. As a new graduate you will probably not be expected to carry major responsibility for setting these standards. However, as you grow in ability and in responsibility you may serve on agency or hospital committees, or on state and national association committees establishing standards of practice.

The health service institution or agency should have the same type of standards of employment for nurses that are in effect for such other professional health workers as physicians, social workers and dietitians. Nursing personnel should be employed on the basis of job descriptions tailored to fit the specific nursing position. In exploring potential positions, you might ask yourself whether or not you wish to work in a place where all types of nursing positions have the same job descriptions.

Some of the major problems in hospital nursing today stem from unprepared personnel. No health service institution or agency should operate on the premise that, unable to employ competent nurses, they will employ almost anybody, teach them a few procedures and then place them in a nursing situation with little or no on-the-spot training and supervision. All too frequently one finds, not the professional nurse, but the licensed practical nurse and the aide as the ones who are closest to the patient in the hospital. This situation needs immediate correction if appropriate nursing practice is to be delivered to patients. If the institution or agency employs different kinds of nursing personnel, assignments should be commensurate with each one's preparation and experience.

Assignment of nursing personnel — one important responsibility of a hospital — is related to the institution's philosophy of care. A patient requires care from the time of admission to the time of discharge and he should be provided with this care by appropriate nursing personnel. Some hospitals have a practice which places emphasis on what is called "patient-assignment equity." This means that every member of the nursing staff is responsible for exactly the same number of patients, regardless of the various factors involved. Also, in some hospitals members of the nursing staff may be constantly assigned to different patients. Neither of these practices leads to individualized patient care. As a new staff nurse you may not be able to do much about these practices. However, should you be in a position of more authority you may be able to exert influence to change the situation. Many agencies and institutions today base the kind and amount of nursing personnel staffing on the specific nursing needs of patients in the unit. Some institutions are experimenting with the use of data processing methods to determine staffing needs.

Responsibility of Society to Nursing

Society, in general, has accepted the responsibility to help those who cannot help themselves because of their state of health. More advanced communities realize that the health of all people depends upon the health of each individual in the community and that no society can afford to fail in promoting and maintaining the health of its citizens. Nor can a community neglect to provide for the ill, the infirm and the aged. In many communities, people recognize that nursing is an important and much needed health service. All citizens, along with nurses, have the obligation to find appropriate answers to such questions as: "What quality and quantity of nursing is available to a community? What are the costs involved in providing nursing in a community? What does a person have to pay [for] nursing? How can nursing be secured? ... How can [the] community fulfill its needs for nurses?"[15] Some state nurses' associations are promoting the development of citizens' groups whose purpose is to determine local needs and ways to help meet them. As individual citizens, all nurses have a responsibility to interpret nursing and the need for nursing services for interested civic and social groups within their communities.

Citizens also share in determining the estimated number and kind of nurses needed during the promotion or approval of the development of new health services, such as hospitals and clinics or the introduction of new ways of financing health care, such as Medicare. Nurses, as citizens with special know-how, must be also active here and assist in the deliberations and decisions affecting health care. In this instance, the welfare of the community should be the focus of their activities, not just the special interests of nurses.

Other ways in which a community can share responsibility in providing adequate nursing are: (1) promoting nursing as a desirable career and (2) protecting its citizens from incompetent and unqualified nurses by passing strong nursing practice acts and approving educationally sound programs for the preparation of all types of nursing personnel. When a community is assured that the nursing profession wishes to serve the public rather than its own private interests, the community will be more likely to promote and engage in activities which will provide quality nursing.

Responsibility of the Patient for His Nursing Care

As mentioned elsewhere, the patient should be made a member of the health and nursing care teams for the purpose of participating in his own care. Orem describes the patient's role in his care as: (1) receiving and accepting needed care; (2) giving self-care, whenever possible; (3) seeking and receiving advice; (4) seeking direction and receiving supervision; (5) receiving physical and psychological support; (6) securing information, receiving and utilizing resources; (7) using the physical and social resources within an environment and becoming a contributor to the promotion of growth and developmental factors in an environment; and (8) learning motivation to acquire self-care skills, to place realistic values on self-care and to overcome temporary and long-term personal and environmental obstacles to self-care.[16] In addition, the patient or his family also pays for his care, either directly or indirectly.

The patient and his family also have a responsibility to become familiar with the available kinds of nursing service, public and private, if appropriate choices are to be made. A patient may have to decide whether to use the nursing service provided by a hospital or extended care facility, whether to employ a nurse, nurses, or auxiliary worker in the home, or whether to use

---

[15] D. E. Orem, *Foundations of Nursing and Its Practice*, New York, McGraw-Hill, (Manuscript in process of publication, p. II, 3).

[16] Modified from D. E. Orem, *Ibid.*, pp. 15-16.

the services of a public health agency. Nurses and physicians are frequently sources of information about the available care that the patient or family requires. Most frequently it is the nurse who serves to insure continuity of nursing care from hospital to home through appropriate referrals for nursing care.

Nurses and doctors are also often asked for information about health-care insurance. Much of this information may be obtained from insurance brokers, but nurses, particularly those in community agencies, are increasingly called upon to help individuals understand the benefits of insurance, especially Medicare and supplementary health insurance. If a person is unable to pay for such insurance, information will be needed about nursing services available through welfare and similar agencies.

Responsibility of the Nursing Profession

The ANA has a responsibility to foster high standards for nursing practice and to promote the education and welfare of nurses so that all people have good nursing care. The ANA, through its 5 divisions on practice, is currently developing standards for practice in several clinical areas of nursing—community health, geriatric, maternal and child health, medical surgical, psychiatric and mental health nursing.[17] You will want to become familiar with these standards and make sure that your own practice measures up to or exceeds them. It may be that in some instances you will want to suggest revisions.

For a more complete description of the responsibility of the nursing profession for the maintenance of effective nursing practice and its improvement, review the chapters in "Part Four: Organizations and Related Activities," especially the chapters on the ANA, the NLN and the ANF.

YOUR RESPONSIBILITY FOR NURSING PRACTICE

Many of your nursing practice responsibilities have been referred to throughout this chapter. In this section we will summarize and comment on some of your major responsibilities.

It is common practice for some nurses to be concerned primarily with carrying out the physician's orders, and carrying out these prescribed measures is a major responsibility. However, nursing practice involves more than this. There are specific nursing measures that can be planned with the patient or family as a continuous process. Judgments about nursing measures need to be based upon a knowledge of standards of practice, taking into consideration the needs of the patient or family within the particular physical and social environment. Without such a plan of care there can be

---

[17] "Establishing Standards for Nursing Practice," *American Journal of Nursing,* **69:**1458-1463, July 1969.

no effective nursing. The nursing student and the nurse practitioner need to learn early to identify the patient's or family's needs and requirements and to set priorities within the nursing plan.

The effective nurse is always looking for ways to promote learning for the patient. For example, the nurse who is giving a bath, rubbing a patient's back, or with him at meal time is providing an opportunity for him to ask questions which he might not think of at other times. A nurse, by explaining how and why she performs a nursing measure that the patient will have to perform later for himself, may be able to stimulate his interest so that he observes, listens, and asks pertinent questions. Under certain conditions, group teaching may stimulate some patients to become more effective in their self-care as a result of group motivation and the universal need for social approval.

It is up to nurses, particularly professionally educated nurses, to bring about the changes that will permit them to provide competent nursing care to patients. In any nursing service situation this requires an understanding of human limitations in nursing practice, in teaching, supervisory and administrative procedures and in the formal organization structure. An appreciation of the importance of setting priorities and of developing a plan for nursing care also leads to greater competence.

When you graduate and become a nurse, you will be assuming responsibility not only for your own practice but eventually for the supervision and coordination of the services of others on the nursing care team. You will also have a role on the total health team which includes members of the various health professions. You will be called upon to interpret your role to each of the other team members as well as to the patient and the general public. Probably your greatest individual responsibility will be to develop a philosophy of nursing that embodies respect for the rights of others and that values the maintenance of excellence in practice as a goal to be constantly sought. The quality of nursing care in the future depends heavily on your philosophy of nursing, on the breadth of your concept of nursing care and, finally, on your acceptance of responsibility for the quality of patient care.

PROBLEMS

1. Read *The Nature of Nursing* (1966 edition) by Virginia Henderson. Give your reasons for agreeing or disagreeing with her concept of nursing practice.

2. Review the concepts of nursing and supporting propositions of Florence Nightingale, Isabel A. Hampton, *et al.*, Virginia Henderson and Dorothea Orem (these books are listed at the end of this chapter or in footnotes). Some of these concepts have emerged over a span of 75 years. Decide in what way the concepts are alike and in what ways they differ.

3. Describe your concept of nursing as an assisting art that helps the individual patient (adult or child) to maintain health and to prevent or cure disease. In connection with this assignment read *Foundations of Nursing and Its Practice* by Dorothea Orem, Chapters I and II (when published), or *Clinical Nursing. A Helping Art* by Ernestine Wiedenbach.

4. As a class project each student asks 5 hospital patients to list the incidents involving nursing practice that gave them aid or satisfaction and those that displeased them or made them unhappy. Study these incidents and identify the standards of nursing practice that were observed and those that were violated. Make recommendations for improvement of nursing practice in the situations reported.

5. Discuss the ethics of assigning a nurse or an auxiliary worker to care for a patient regardless of the patient's nursing requirements or the ability of the particular nurse or auxiliary worker to provide the care required.

6. Engage in a discussion of the demands on and the functions of the nurse in various areas of nursing practice, such as the care of: (a) the newborn, (b) the premature infant, (c) children with deformities, (d) the mentally ill, (f) the chronically ill, (g) the aging, (h) the confused patient and (e) the dying. You could add areas to this list.

7. Plan a symposium on "Nursing Team Leadership" using the following or similar topics: Meaning of Leadership; Attributes and Demands of Good Nursing; The Basic Needs of Team Members; The Limits of Supervisory Responsibility; Planning of Nursing Care; Communication Essentials as a Prime Factor; Legal Responsibilities of the Team Leader.

SUGGESTED REFERENCES*

NURSING PRACTICE: GENERAL AND SPECIAL

Anderson, B. E. "Accepting Responsibility for Achieving Professional Status." *Bulletin Tennessee Nurses' Association,* **31:**10-18, Summer 1967.

Asplund, B. "The Nurse's Role Tomorrow." *International Nursing Review,* **13:** 25-33, Nov.-Dec. 1966.

* Aydelotte, M. K. "Issues of Professional Nursing: The Need for Clinical Excellence." *Nursing Forum,* **7:**72-86, Winter 1968.

Baziak, A. T. "What Constitutes Clinical Practice?" *Nursing Forum,* **7:**98-109, Winter 1968.

Bird, H. C. "Nursing Services in General Practice." *British Medical Journal,* **1:**378-379, Feb. 10, 1968.

Brodie, D. C. "Trends in Pharmaceutical Education." *American Journal of Nursing,* **68:**1948-1951, Sept. 1968.

Brown, E. L. "Nursing and Patient Care." In *The Nursing Profession: Five Sociological Essays.* Edited by F. Davis. New York, John Wiley, 1966, pp. 176-203.

---

* In each chapter all citations are footnoted and are not included here. All starred references are recommended for additional reading.

* Burnside, I. M. "The Patient I Didn't Want." *American Journal of Nursing,* **68:**1666-1669, Aug. 1968.

Byers, V. B. *Nursing Observation.* Dubuque, Wm. G. Brown, 1968.

Cambell, E. B. "Not Education, Not Service, but Nursing. The Process of Change." *American Journal of Nursing,* **67:**990-994, May 1967.

Campana, L. M. "R.N.—Patient Describes Neglect on Ward." *American Journal of Nursing,* **68:**1654-1657, Aug. 1968.

* Carl, M. K. "Decision Making: An Essential Process in Nursing Care." *Maryland Nursing News,* **36:**21-23, Spring 1968.

Carn, I. "The Nursing Audit as a Learning Tool for Undergraduates." *Nursing Clinics of North America,* **4:**351-358, June 1969.

Conant, L. H. "Closing the Practice-Theory Gap." *Nursing Outlook,* **15:**37-39, Nov. 1967.

Dyer, E. "Factors Affecting Nursing Performance." *Utah Nurse,* **18:**17-18, Autumn 1967.

Edelstein, R. P. "Automation: Its Effect on the Nurse." *American Journal of Nursing,* **66:**2194-2198, Oct. 1966.

Ewell, C. M. "What Patients Really Think About Their Nursing Care." *Modern Hospital,* **109:**106-108, Dec. 1967.

Farrisey, R. M. "Clinical Nursing in Transition." *American Journal of Nursing,* **67:**305-309, Feb. 1967.

Greenough, K. "Determining Standards for Nursing Care." *American Journal of Nursing,* **68:**2153-3157, Oct. 1968.

Hagerman, Z. J. "Teaching Beginners to Cope With Extreme Behavior." *American Journal of Nursing,* **68:**1927-1929, Sept. 1968.

* Hall, L. E. "Another View of Nursing Care and Quality." *Maryland Nursing News,* **36:**2-12, Spring 1968.

* Hampton, I. A., *et al. Nursing of the Sick, 1893.* New York, McGraw-Hill, 1945.

Henderson, C. "Can Nursing Care Hasten Recovery?" *American Journal of Nursing,* **64:**80-83, June 1964.

* Henderson, V. *Basic Principles of Nursing Care.* London, International Council of Nurses, 1960.

Hershey, N. "Scope of Nursing Practice." *American Journal of Nursing,* **66:**117-120, Jan. 1966.

Hilliard, M. E. "A Viewpoint on the Primary Focus of Nursing." *National League for Nursing Papers,* **23:**5-8, 1967.

Holdsworth, V. E. *Fundamentals of Bedside Nursing.* New York, Macmillan, 1968.

Huizenga, L. "Responsibility for Improving Nursing Practice." *Michigan Nurse,* **40:**5-8, Dec. 1967.

* Jacox, A. K. "Who Defines and Controls Nursing Practice." *American Journal of Nursing,* **69:**977-982, May 1969.

Johnson, B. S. and Campbell, E. B. "Its Time to be Realistic About the Work Load." *American Journal of Nursing,* **66:**1282-1284, June 1966.

* Johnson, D. E. "Competence in Practice: Technical and Professional." *Nursing Outlook,* **16:**30-33, Oct. 1966.

Kalkman, M. E. "Recognizing Emotional Problems." *American Journal of Nursing,* **68:**536-537, Mar. 1968.

* Keller, N. S. "Care Without Coordination: A True Story." *Nursing Forum,* **6:**280-323, Summer 1967.

Kennedy, E. "Bedside Nursing from the Viewpoint of the Private Duty Nurse." *American Journal of Nursing,* **30:**285-289, Mar. 1930.

* Kramer, M. "Collegiate Graduate Nurses in Medical Center Hospitals: Mutual Challenge or Duel." *Nursing Research,* **18:**196-210, May-June 1969.

Larson, K. H., *et al. Direct Care Nursing.* New York, Macmillan, 1968.

Lees, W., *et al.* "Progressive Patient Care." *Nursing Times,* **64:**Suppl:13-16, Jan. 26, 1968.

Leminen, A. "The Theory of Nursing." *International Nursing Review,* **14:**63-69, Dec. 1967.

* Lewis, E. P. "Four Nurses Who Wanted to Make a Difference." *American Journal of Nursing,* **69:**777-782, Apr. 1969.

Little, D. and Carnevali, D. L. *Nursing Care Planning.* Philadelphia, Lippincott, 1969.

MacGregor, F. C. Nursing in Transition: Challenge for the Future." *Journal of the American Medical Association,* **198:**174-175, Dec. 12, 1966.

Martucci, M. E. "Individual Counseling Conference as a Means of Dissolving Stressful Situations." *Journal of Psychiatric Nursing,* **6:**27-34, Feb. 1968.

McPhetridge, L. M. "Nursing History: One Means to Personalize Care." *American Journal of Nursing,* **68:**68-75, Jan. 1968.

Minkley, B. B. "The Multiphasic Human to Human Monitor (ICU Model). Nursing Observation in the Intensive Care Unit." *Nursing Clinics of North America,* **3:**29-39, Mar. 1968.

Moss, F. T. and Meyer, B. "The Effects of Nursing Interaction Upon Pain Relief in Patients." *Nursing Research,* **15:**303-306, Fall 1966.

Myers, E. and Pott, E. "An Internship for New Graduates." *American Journal of Nursing,* **68:**96-100, Jan. 1968.

* Nightingale, F. *Notes on Nursing: What it is and What it is not.* Facsimile of 1859 ed. Philadelphia, Lippincott, 1946.

* O'Connor, D. and Hagan, F. "Liaison Nurse." *American Journal of Nursing,* **64:**101-103, June 1964.

O'Koren, M. L. "Caring – The Basis of Responsibility." *Alabama Nurse,* **21:**8-12, Dec. 1967.

* Phaneuf, M. C. "Analysis of a Nursing Audit." *Nursing Outlook,* **16:**57-60, Jan. 1968.

Piepgras, R. "The Other Dimension: Spiritual Health." *American Journal of Nursing,* **68:**2610-2613, Dec. 1968.

Powers, M. E. and Storlie, F. "The Apprehensive Patient." *American Journal of Nursing,* **67:**58-63, Jan. 1967.

Ramphal, M. M. "The Patient is the Center of Nursing." *Maryland Nursing News,* **36:**13-20, Spring 1968.

* Reader, G. G. and Schwartz, D. R. "Joint Planning for Patient Care." *Journal of the American Medical Association,* **201:**364-367, Aug. 7, 1967.

Reeder, M. K. "Nursing Practice: A Student's Perspective." *Nursing Clinics of North America,* **3:**135-142, Mar. 1968.

* Resnick, B. A. "The Nursing Clinic: An Experiment in Ambulatory Patient Care." In *ANA Regional Clinical Conferences, 1967.* New York, Appleton-Century-Crofts, 1968, pp. 95-100.

Rothberg, J. S. "Why Nursing Diagnosis." *American Journal of Nursing,* **67:**1040-1042, May 1967.

Schulman, D. and Schulman, S. "The Coordinating Role of the Nurse is Well Known; Less Well Known is Her Important Role as a Catalyst." *American Journal of Nursing,* **68:**1890-1894, Sept. 1968.

* Schutt, B. (editorial) "Indictment: How Shall We Plead? *American Journal of Nursing,* **68:**1665, Aug. 1968.

* Smith, D. M. "A Clinical Nursing Tool." *American Journal of Nursing,* **68:**2384-2388, Nov. 1968.

* Smith, D. W. "Patienthood and Its Threat to Privacy." *American Journal of Nursing,* **69:**509-513, Mar. 1969.

Stringer, L. "Self-evaluation of Clinical Performance." *Nursing Outlook,* **15:**63-65, Nov. 1967.

Theis, C. and Harrington, H. "Three Factors That Affect Practice: Communications, Assignments, Attitudes." *American Journal of Nursing,* **68:**1478-1482, July 1968.

Ujhely, G. B. "What Is Realistic Emotional Support." *American Journal of Nursing,* **68:**758-762, Apr. 1968.

Verhonick, P. J. "The Nurse's Response to Human Suffering Today." *Bulletin Infirmieres Catoliques de Canada,* **34:**217-224, June 1967.

* Wagner, B. M. "Care Plans: Right, Reasonable, and Reachable." *American Journal of Nursing,* **69:**986-990, May 1969.

"What RN's Can Learn From Student Nurses." *RN,* **30:**37-42, Nov. 1967.

* Wooldridge, P. J., *et al. Behavioral Science, Social Practice, and the Nursing Profession.* Cleveland, Press of Case Western Reserve University, 1968.

RELATIONSHIPS

Bates, B. and Kern, M. S. "Doctor-Nurse Teamwork: What Helps? What Hinders?" *American Journal of Nursing,* **67:**2066-2071, Oct. 1967.

Berkowitz, N. H. and Malone, M. F. "Intra-Professional Conflict." *Nursing Forum,* **7:**50-71, Winter 1968.

* Brunclik, H., Thurston, J. R. and Feldhusen, J. "The Empathy Inventory." *Nursing Outlook,* **15:**42-45, June 1967.

Dake, M. A. "What's Wrong With the Nurse-Physician Relationship in Today's Hospitals. A Nurse's View." *Hospitals,* **40:**70-74, 122, Dec. 16, 1966.

* Hall, B. L. "Human Relations in the Hospital Setting." *Nursing Outlook,* **16:**43-45, Mar. 1968.

* Johnson, J. E. "Interpersonal Relations: The Essence of Nursing Care. *Nursing Forum,* **6:**324-334, Summer 1967.

Lyons, M. L. "The Creative Use of Self in Human Relations." *AORN Journal,* **5:**47-56, Feb. 1967.

Skipper, J. K. Jr., *et al.* "Some Barriers to Communication Between Patients and Hospital Functionaries." *Nursing Forum,* **2(1):**17,19, 1963.

Stein, L. I. "The Doctor-Nurse Game." *American Journal of Nursing,* **68:**101-105, Jan. 1968.

* Verwoerdt, A. and Wilson, R. "Communication with Fatally Ill Patients." *American Journal of Nursing,* **67:**2307-2309, Nov. 1967.

CLINICAL NURSE SPECIALIST

Anderson, L. C. "Clinical Nursing Expert." *Nursing Outlook,* **14:**62-64, July 1966.

Ayers, R., *et al.* "An Experiment in Nursing Service Reorganization." *American Journal of Nursing,* **69:**783-786, Apr. 1969.

Erickson, F. "Nurse Specialist for Children." *Nursing Outlook,* **16:**34-36, Nov. 1968.

* Fagan, C. M. "Clinical Specialist as a Supervisor." *Nursing Outlook,* **15:**34-36, Jan. 1967.

Gordon, M. "The Clinical Specialist as a Change Agent." *Nursing Outlook,* **17:**37-39, Mar. 1969.

* Johnson, D., *et al.* "The Clinical Specialist as a Practitioner." *American Journal of Nursing,* **67:**2298-2303, Nov. 1967.

Little, D. "The Nurse Specialist." *American Journal of Nursing,* **67:**552-556, Mar. 1967.

Peterson, S. "The Psychiatric Nurse Specialist in a General Hospital." *Nursing Outlook,* **17:**56-58, Feb. 1969.

Pitel, M. "Current Trends in Nursing Education with Implications for Nursing Service." *Minnesota Nursing Accent,* **40:**189-192, Dec. 1968.

Plaisted, L. M. "The Clinical Specialist in Rehabilitation Nursing." *American Journal of Nursing,* **69:**562-564, Mar. 1969.

Richards, J. F. "Integrating a Clinical Specialist into a Hospital Nursing Service." *Nursing Outlook,* **17:**23-25, Mar. 1969.

* Simms, L. L. "The Clinical Nursing Specialist." *Journal of the American Medical Association,* **198:**675-678, Nov. 7, 1966.

THE NURSING TEAM

Alman, B. "Patients Participate in Nursing Care Conferences." *American Journal of Nursing,* **67:**2331-2334, Nov. 1967.

Fielding, V. V. "New Team Plan Frees Nurses to Nurse." *Modern Hospital,* **108:**122-124, May 1967.

Frederick, M. "Team Nursing: A Great Potential." *Chart,* **64:**320-322, Dec. 1967.

* Heskett, L. "Team Leadership for Nurses' Aides." *Nursing Homes,* **17:**18-20, Feb. 1968.

Jimm, L. R., *et al.* "A Shared Experience in Leadership." *Nursing Outlook,* **15:**36-39, Oct. 1967.

Keys, M. L. "Our Team Includes the Private Nurse Practitioner." *Nursing Outlook,* **15:**32-33, Jan. 1967.

Kramer, M. "Team Teaching is More Than Team Planning." *Nursing Outlook,* **16:**47-50, July 1968.

Kron, Thora. *Nursing Team Leadership.* Philadelphia, Saunders, 1966.

* Lambertsen, E. C. "Defining the Right Roles Helps Assure the Right Team." *Modern Hospital,* **109:**128, Dec. 1967.

Little, D. and Carnevali, D. "Nursing Care Plans: Let's be Practical About Them." *Nursing Forum,* **6(1):**61-76, 1967.

Manthey, M. E. "A Guide for Interviewing." *American Journal of Nursing,* **67:** 2088-2090, Oct. 1967.

Martin, S. "Team Approach in Public Health." In *The Challenge of Changing Patterns.* Report of the First Conference of the NLN Western Region Committee on Community Nursing. New York, The League, 1968, pp. 12-14.

Parramore, B. and Yeager, W. "Team Nursing In Public Health." *Nursing Outlook,* **16:**54-56, June 1968.

* Peeples, E. H. and Francis, G. M. "Social-Psychological Obstacles to Effective Health Team Practice." *Nursing Forum,* **7:**28-37, Winter 1968.

Schwartz, D. "Some Thoughts on Quality in Nursing Service." *International Nursing Review,* **14:**29-34, Apr. 1967.

Swansburg, R. C. "An Experiment in Team Nursing." *Nursing Outlook,* Part I, **16:**45-47, Aug. 1968; Part II, **16:**42-43, Sept. 1968.

Tryon, P. A. "The Effect of Patient Participation in Decision Making on the Outcome of a Nursing Procedure." In *Nursing and the Patient's Motivations.* New York, The American Nurses' Association, 1962, pp. 14-18.

Westbury, S. A., Jr., *et al.* "Three Step Program Lets Night Nurses Get Back to Nursing." *Modern Hospital,* **110:**85-87, Jan. 1968.

UNIT MANAGEMENT

Blickensderfer, B. "Unit Manager Can Help in the O.R., Too." *Modern Hospital,* **108:**97-98, Jan. 1967.

Brady, N. A., *et al.* "The Unit Manager." *Hospital Management,* **101:**30-36, June 1966.

Corrigan, S. M., *et al.* "Head Nurse, Maternal or Executive?" *Nursing Research,* **15:**214-217, Summer 1966.

* Hourz, D. T. "The Unit Manager in the Hospital Organization." *Hospital Progress,* **47:**73-78, Feb. 1966.

Mauksch, H. O. "The Organizational Context of Nursing Practice." In Davis, F., ed. *The Nursing Profession: Five Sociological Essays.* New York, Wiley, 1966, pp. 133-135.

* Nellis, W. L. "Unit Managers Cut Patients' Complaints 50 Per cent." *Hospital Topics,* **46:**42-45, June 1968.

Reed, D. A. "Relieving the Nursing Shortage . . . What Administration Can Do." *Hospital Progress,* **47:**96-100, Apr. 1966.

Taylor, C. "How the Unit Manager System Works for Us." *Modern Hospital,* **99:**69-72, Aug. 1962.

Ware, A. V. "What is a Unit Manager?" *AORN Journal,* **4:**89-92, May/June 1966.

AUXILIARY NURSING

American Hospital Association. *Training the Nursing Aid: The Student Manual; The Instructor's Guide.* Chicago, The Association, 1965.

* "Code of Ethics for Licensed Practical Nurses: Adopted by the National Federation of Licensed Practical Nurses." *Bedside Nurse,* **1:**6, Mar./Apr. 1968.

Donovan, J. E., *et al. The Nurse Aide.* New York, McGraw-Hill, 1968.

Ginsberg, F. "The Problem of People: O R Aide and R.N." *Modern Hospital,* **108:**140, Mar. 1967.

Grant, M. "Health Aides Add New Dimension to Home Care Program." *Hospitals,* **40:**63-67, Dec. 1966.

* Hall, M. N. "The Indispensable Home Health Aide." *Nursing Outlook,* **16:**38-41, Jan. 1968.

* Hamil, E. M. "Effective Use of the LVN's Many Talents." *Bedside Nurse,* **2:**17-19, Jan./Feb. 1969.

Heath, A. M. "Health Aides in Health Departments." *Public Health Reports,* **82:**608-614, July 1967.

Johnson, U. R. "Practical Nursing — A Part of MDTA." *Nursing Outlook,* **15:**55-57, Nov. 1967.

* "The LPN's — Who They are, Where They Work, What They Do." *Bedside Nurse.* **2:**29-31, Jan./Feb. 1969.

* National League for Nursing. *Statements on Practical Nursing and Practical Nurse Education.* New York, The League, 1968.

* O'Brien, M. "The Ideal Practical Nurse." *Journal of Practical Nursing,* **17:**31, 34, Dec. 1967.

Ross, C. F. *Personal and Vocational Relationships in Practical Nursing.* Philadelphia, Lippincott, 1965.

PART 2

Legal, Professional
and Personal Problems
and Relationships

PREVIEW

Life has some of the characteristics of the drama. It has a beginning, rising action, climax and, finally, the ending. To act in such a way as to reach the final goal with true success, it is essential to have a long-view plan for life that includes both immediate and remote objectives, some notion of ways and means to achieve them, and some idea of expected accomplishments.

The aim of this entire book is to present some of the important considerations to help you reach personal and professional goals, but there has been no attempt to formulate individual plans for you. This task is yours.

Part Two, consisting of 3 chapters, is designed to help you to understand how to approach and solve the problems and situations that will confront you in nursing, in your search for security and in your striving for sound legal, personal and professional relationships. This part does not, by any means, include all the problems that you may encounter in your personal or professional life. Its message can be expanded considerably, depending on the additional problems and background of knowledge and experience you bring to the class group.

CHAPTER

5

Problem Solving: A Major Activity of the Professional Nurse

All of us seem to be beset every day by problems which must be considered and solved. Our problems cover a wide range in our daily lives. It is only by the satisfactory exploration of these daily problems that growth results and peace of mind is maintained.

It might be that in relation to your future you may have to make decisions concerning your personal as well as your professional objectives. There may be a conflict between these objectives. You may be concerned with how to get funds to continue your studies. You may be troubled about the progress you are making. You may be dissatisfied with certain practices in nursing. Many of these problems may stem from a lack of information and ability to use the problem-solving technique.

Many individuals could have saved themselves much difficulty had they tried to solve each problem systematically as it arose instead of waiting to do something about it until after they were in really serious trouble. Emotional aspects often are inherent in striving to achieve an objective. Problem solving as an objective approach can help to offset these and promote more effective approaches. Each person would be wise to give prompt attention to the solution of his problems and to recognize the fact that some problems which must be faced cannot always be solved immediately or even satisfactorily.

When we speak of problem solving in nursing we are defining problems as situations which the nurse faces and about which she must do something. In a sense, every patient poses such a situation or problem, and the solving of the problem leads to the provision of an individualized plan of care. Understanding the total situation is essential to its effective control. Seldom can a solution be reached until the problem has been defined in terms of specific subproblems or questions.

In all phases of life—personal, social, vocational, political, economic, educational, and religious—there is an increasing interest in the utilization of the problem-solving approach as a way of helping all of us to gain insight about and ability to solve our problems. Effective problem solving requires a sound philosophy of life, an acquaintance with helpful sources, a working knowledge of the steps and methods of problem solving, the accurate assessment of what the problem is, and whether the situation faced is a personal one or one regarding patient care.

USUAL STEPS IN PROBLEM SOLVING

The proper organization of ideas is important in problem solving. It involves reasoning or, as one authority put it, "the process of mental exploration undertaken in order to find or infer significant and practically useful relations between things already known and some new fact or experience whose existence or use constitutes a problem."[1] A good reasoner is such partly because of innate intelligence and partly because he has learned the skill of sound reasoning.

In addition to reasoning, imagination and judgment are essential for problem solving. Imagination may be brought to the aid of the reasoning process and used where there is need for creative work. Judgment tells when and how to act; good judgment usually comes from experience.

The study of problems differs in many respects depending on the types of problems to be investigated. Regardless of the type of problem, the problem solver follows somewhat the same procedure. There are 6 steps which usually can be followed in trying to solve any problem or to answer any question.

The 1st step is to be aware of and be concerned about the particular problem.

The 2nd step is to define the problem and identify the issues and the different aspects or questions involved in the problem. It is generally recognized that a problem well defined is half solved. Also involved here is the determination of what creates a problem: Why is it a problem? Who is affected by it? Why is there a need to do something about it? Why am I motivated to do something about it? Am I the one to attempt to solve it?

The 3rd step is to accumulate all the data that can throw light on the solution of the problem. You can utilize many or few sources for securing data, depending on the nature of the problem. In this 3rd step,

[1] O. Tead, *Human Nature and Management,* New York, McGraw-Hill, 1933, p. 83.

the problem solver also is concerned with deciding on appropriate methods for collecting the data.

The 4th step is to classify, analyze and interpret the data (all of the various kinds of information you can obtain), so as to formulate a tentative solution to the problem. There may be more than one possible solution, in which case select the one you find best.

The 5th step is to test and retest the tentative solution to see whether it works. Or, if it does not work and you have alternate possibilities, you will try these. In the end you may find that you will have to start all over in trying to solve the problem.

The 6th step in more formal problem solving is to prepare a report, so that others may use the conclusions or results of the investigation.

Sources of Data

Nursing-care problems may range from the very complex to the very simple. For example, a simple problem might be the provision of fluids for a normal postpartum patient. The provision of oxygen to a patient with a tracheostomy, however, may be very complex and require the use of special knowledge and skill. The solution of a nursing care problem may involve any or all of the following: (1) knowledge of the patient's diagnosis and his understanding of it; (2) an understanding of the patient's and his family's reactions, questions, and fears; (3) knowledge of the physician's orders and the reasons for these; (4) your own observations of the patient and of his family or friends; (5) appropriate use of the reports of tests or treatments the patient has had; (6) knowledge of the drugs the patient is receiving; (7) use of your own previous training and experience; and (8) use of reference materials. This is only a suggested list of the sources of your data, and is certainly not exhaustive. You may think of other sources.

In most problem solving, the intelligent use of the library to locate pertinent data related to the area under study will go far in leading you to the solutions you are seeking. The library search that you make should be sufficiently thorough to make sure that you have covered the field adequately. Scientific research calls for the most meticulous and exhaustive search of the literature. Other less involved problem solving may call for less exhaustive library search. However, knowing your way around in the library will make the job of finding the data you need easier.

Learning to use the library intelligently is one of the most important steps that you can take and one you should take early in your student career. Skill in the use of the library will bring to your fingertips the vast store of knowledge waiting there for you when you need it. You are no doubt familiar with some of the bibliographic tools available to you in locating materials. A number of the common reference books, including directories, indexes, encyclopedias, dictionaries, and other general references and guides are listed in Part One of the Appendix to this book. Your librarian can give you additional help in your search. She has been especially trained in the art of assisting persons in their way around the world of books and periodicals and is a good person to turn to when you are starting on your investigation.

A number of references on libraries are cited at the end of this chapter. Read those that are starred and as many others as you can — for better understanding of the library as a basic tool in problem solving.

EVERYDAY USE OF PROBLEM-SOLVING METHODS

Solving Personal Problems

Solving a personal problem is not unlike solving any other problem. The same problem-solving methods and steps can be used.

In solving a personal problem, sometimes you can get help by reading about persons who have had a similar experience and thereby get the viewpoints of others and acquire new insights. At other times, it may be desirable to take the problem to a trusted friend who is willing to listen and assist in guiding you, through the use of the problem-solving methods, to a satisfactory solution. Your priest or minister may be able to help. Professional counselors, if well selected, can be helpful. Sometimes people may be facing such vexing problems that the professional services of a clinical psychologist or a psychiatrist may be indicated. Merely thinking out loud before someone else may be all that is needed to clarify confused thoughts and ideas. However, it is wise to remember that sometimes a solution is not reached because the right question is not asked — in other words, be careful to define the problem, first.

The following story is told of a young man who once approached Benjamin Franklin and asked this question: "Dr. Franklin, how do you always manage to make such sound decisions?" Franklin replied that he did not make decisions at all; that he simply let facts decide for him.

When confronted with two courses of action, I jot down on a piece of paper all of the arguments in favor of each one; then, on the opposite side I write the arguments against each one. Then, by weighing the arguments pro and con and canceling them out one against the other, I take the course indicated by what remains.

Sufficient time in thinking about the problem is of such importance that it cannot be overemphasized. Give yourself plenty of time to tussle and come to grips with any problem, because good ideas do not often develop quickly. They are the products of effective and reflective thinking. Patience with the problem-solving process, persistence in thinking, tolerance with the results obtained and, sometimes, courage in the application of the solution reached are all important. It is advisable to think a while about a problem in all of its aspects, then forget about it and return to it later, probably from another point of view. Repeating this procedure sometimes lets the subconscious mind solve the problem, and you will find yourself following a definite path of action without realizing that a decision has been made.

Problems in Care of Individual Patients

In the care of individual patients, nurses need to solve nursing problems. This involves helping patients to solve their health problems. A nursing problem is defined as "a condition [or situation] faced by the patient or his family, which the nurse can assist him to meet through the performance of her professional functions."[2]

A patient's problem grows out of health needs centered around prevention, early detection, restoration or rehabilitation.

Some examples of nursing objectives, as you know, are: (1) to facilitate the maintenance of oxygen and nutrition in all body cells; (2) to maintain good body mechanics and prevent and correct deformities; (3) to maintain good hygiene and physical comfort; (4) to identify and accept the interrelatedness of emotions and organic illness; (5) to establish and maintain communications, especially with patients of different social or cultural background; and (6) to use community resources as an aid in resolving problems arising from illness.

Let us take one of these nursing objectives as an example of how the steps in problem solving can be used in determining how to meet the objective for a particular patient. For this illustration the authors have selected the use of community resources as an aid in resolving problems arising from illness. The suggested steps follow:

STEP 1. Be aware that the particular condition of the patient calls for some use of the resources of another or several community agencies, as for example, the patient with a speech condition, or one with postpartum psychosis, or a retarded child.

STEP 2. Break down the problem into its different aspects in terms of: (a) learning which community resources are available for helping in the specific situation, (b) planning with and preparing the patient and his family to accept the aid of the community resources and (c) learning how to reach the community agencies and to make appropriate referrals.

STEP 3. Accumulate information about the patient and his problem through the use of appropriate tools, such as review of records, observation, interviews and pertinent literature.

STEP 4. Analyze and classify this information for use in discussing the patient's problem with representatives of the community agency or agencies and in guiding the patient toward the solution of the problem. Involve the patient and family in the solution of the problem.

STEP 5. After the appropriate referrals about the patient have been made, check and recheck on the benefit or the lack of benefit being derived by the patient. If the plan that has been made for the patient as the result of the referrals does not work out, a new approach for solving the problem may have to be taken.

[2] F. G. Abdellah and E. Levine, *Appraising the Clinical Resources in Small Hospitals*, Washington, D.C., Government Printing Office, 1954, p. 3.

STEP 6. The 6th step, which involves the writing of a report, may not be essential in this instance. However, keeping an appropriate agency record would be important.

PROBLEM SOLVING IN BROAD STUDIES AND RESEARCH IN THE PROFESSION

Meaning of Research

Scientific research is the systematic study of a problem or a systematic attempt to answer a persistent question. It is an endeavor to discover, develop and verify knowledge or to add to the body of knowledge in a particular area through systematic investigation. Doing research involves clear organization of ideas and straight thinking. Research involves an intellectual process that has developed over the years, sometimes changing in form but always having the same over-all purpose — searching for the truth. According to one writer, it involves intellectual curiosity, the ability to question the obvious, nonconformity, independence of thought and judgment, persistence and a passionate need to solve a problem — to name a few of its characteristics.[3] Scholarly problem solving is a precursor to research.

Need for Research in Nursing

Systematic research is required to solve many of our professional problems and to build a scientific body of knowledge in nursing, a primary need of the profession today. According to the report of the Surgeon General's Consultant Group on Nursing, rapid changes in the biologic and social sciences and in patterns of medical care have increased greatly the need for nursing research and for nurse scientists to do the needed research. The report also pointed to the trend toward greater emphasis on patient-care research.

Some aspects of research for consideration of the professional nurse are discussed in the remaining part of this chapter. The discussion is very brief and in no way attempts to cover the topic of research in nursing. However, several excellent sources are cited at the end of the chapter to which you can and would need to refer for more intensive study.

In the acquisition of knowledge, nurses have sometimes used various sources of evidence, often without questioning how the knowledge came into existence or whether or not it has been verified. Certain types of knowledge have been accepted as valid because of custom, tradition, the dictates of various authorities or very limited experience. For example, the method in many nursing procedures has passed from one nurse to another, from

---

[3] F. C. Macgregor, "Research Potential in Collegiate Nursing Students," *Nursing Research,* **13**:260, Summer 1964.

generation to generation, without being questioned, even though these procedures have sometimes become outdated.

Today, however, with the idea of scientific research as a way of thinking, as Helen Bunge points out:

Nursing, as an increasingly independent occupation, is expected to find wise answers to its problems – to know what professional nursing is, and what scientific principles form the background of its practice. Professional nurses are being expected to assist and often take the leadership in the planning of patient care in hospitals and in communities. Because of these additional professional responsibilities more nurses must ask "why," if they are to make sound judgments on the direction in which nursing should move in the future.[4]

Some Historical Aspects of Research in Nursing

Nurses, like members of other professions, have engaged in research over a long period of time. There is evidence that the nursing profession has been interested in research ever since the time that Florence Nightingale lived. Her biographers, as well as her contemporaries, considered her an outstanding researcher and statistician.

Lavinia Dock, M. Adelaide Nutting and Isabel M. Stewart, leaders in the modern nursing education movement in the USA, have shown great interest in nursing research, particularly in the area of historical research.

Many major descriptive studies have been made in this country, and some have been made in other countries. These investigations have been carried on in national nursing and allied organizations, universities, educational foundations, government organizations and nursing service agencies, by graduate students of nursing, graduate students other than nurses, faculty members in nursing education programs and others. Psychologists and sociologists have been very active researchers in nursing in recent years.

If you wish to read about the development of nursing research, you will find the following references interesting and instructive:

Abdellah, F. and Levine, E. *Better Patient Care Through Nursing Research.* New York, Macmillan, 1965, pp. 3-29.

Bunge, H. "Research Is Every Professional Nurse's Business." *American Journal of Nursing,* **58:**816-819, June 1958.

McManus, R. L. "Today and Tomorrow in Nursing Research." *American Journal of Nursing,* **61:**68-71, May 1961.

———. "Nursing Research – Its Evolution." *American Journal of Nursing,* **61:** 76-79, Apr. 1961.

Meyer, B. and Heidgerken, L. E. *Introduction to Research in Nursing.* Philadelphia, Lippincott, 1962.

Newton, M. "As Nursing Research Comes of Age." *American Journal of Nursing,* **62:**46-50, Aug. 1962.

Simmons, I. W. and Henderson, V. *Nursing Research: A Survey and Assessment.* New York, Appleton, 1964, pp. 7-70.

As a result of the growing recognition of the need for research in nursing,

---

[4] H. L. Bunge, "Research Is Every Professional Nurse's Business," *American Journal of Nursing,* **58:**817, June 1958.

the ANA began a 5-year study of nursing functions in 1950. In 1955, it established the American Nurses' Foundation, the work of which is described in Chapter 23. In 1968, the ANA developed its statement on ethical values in research entitled. "The Nurse in Research: ANA Guidelines on Ethical Values."[5]

The Public Health Service of the U. S. Department of Health, Education, and Welfare has contributed greatly to research in nursing through its grants-in-aid to institutions and individuals for research projects, and through the studies conducted by its own personnel. The Division of Nursing has had a leadership role in research in nursing since its origin in 1949. It is suggested you read Ellwynne Vreeland's article "Nursing Research Programs of the Public Health Service" in *Nursing Research* (13:148-158, Spring 1964), for a description of this leadership.

In 1957, the army established a Department of Nursing at the Walter Reed Army Institute of Research in Washington, D.C., to conduct studies in all fields of nursing practice. This governmental agency has added to the body of knowledge in nursing through its investigations. Other nursing services of the Federal Government also have research programs. Early in 1963, the Veterans Administration began developing a program of studies and research in nursing. Nurses in VA hospitals are now doing research in clinical nursing as well as studying nursing service administrative patterns. In 1966, the Naval Medical Research Institute announced its newly established Nursing Research Division, charged with conducting investigations in nursing for the improvement of education and practice.

In addition to the research efforts of nurses in Federal services, a number of voluntary hospitals, particularly large medical centers, have developed programs of nursing research. A recent example is the establishment in 1968 of the Center for Experimentation and Development in Nursing within the Johns Hopkins Hospital in Baltimore. Its projects focus upon developing new concepts and roles for nurses and upon theoretical studies in nursing practice.

As research in nursing gained in momentum, nursing leaders became aware of a need to disseminate research findings more extensively. To this end, the launching of *Nursing Research,* in 1952, published and supported by the AJN Co., was the culmination of action initiated by the Association of Collegiate Schools of Nursing. The purposes of this magazine are fully discussed in Chapter 24.

The first unit for the conduct of research in nursing in an institution of higher learning is the Institute of Research and Service in Nursing Education of Teachers College, Columbia University, established in 1953. The institute carries on studies in nursing and also provides a learning situation for the preparation of research workers. Other centers of research have since been developed.

Most of the research that has been done in nursing, to date, has been

[5] "The Nurse in Research: ANA Guidelines on Ethical Values," *American Journal of Nursing,* **68:**1504-1507, July 1968.

descriptive in character. This trend is changing and today more experiments related to patient care are reported. There appears to be an urgent need for clinical, historical, philosophical and other types of research that will help us to clarify whence we have come in nursing and give us an indication of where we ought to go in the future.

RESPONSIBILITY OF THE PROFESSIONAL NURSE IN STUDIES AND RESEARCH

Every professional nurse has some responsibility for doing studies in nursing. The extent of this responsibility depends on a variety of factors. Some nurses prepare themselves as research workers. Many nurses will confine their efforts to carrying out simple studies in relation to their own work or to pointing out nursing problems that need to be solved. Mildred Newton has defined the roles that the professional nurse may assume in research as: data collector, student of research, teacher of research, researcher or project director, research expediter.[6] All professional nurses, wherever they may be employed, have the obligation to use the results of nursing research in improving their practices.

You will need to listen, read, discuss and think critically to get the research attitude and way of thinking and to gain new ideas.

In reading, at lectures, in discussing and in informal conversation, acquire the attitude of first asking "why" about every concept and procedure relative to nursing or nursing education and of then seeking supporting evidence. Follow clues and suggestions and ideas obtained in this way. You might develop the habit of carrying a pad of 3 by 5 inch slips or a notebook in which to jot down ideas as these are suggested to you. Evaluate, criticize and challenge what you read in books, in nursing and other professional periodicals and in reports of research studies. As a graduate nurse you will need to keep up-to-date regarding the reports of the best studies in your particular field. Follow up ideas that stem from completed research studies. Frequently, reports of studies indicate further research work that needs to be done.

Discuss problems with those who differ with your point of view. They may be right or they may be wrong, but they will stimulate you to think. Associate with the person who is research-minded and the intellectual person who likes to debate questions and to discuss research reports.

Explore areas of dissatisfaction in nursing. Listen to what others say they dislike about it. Find out why they are dissatisfied. Consider whether you are unhappy about conditions or practices in nursing. If so, could you investigate the problems suggested by your dissatisfaction?

If a professional or social issue is to be solved, you may wish to gather a group of interested persons to discuss it. Group discussion not only pro-

[6] M. Newton, "As Nursing Research Comes of Age." *American Journal of Nursing,* **62:** 46-50, Aug. 1962.

vides an opportunity to get the viewpoint of others, but it also brings forth a variety of ideas that usually result in increased knowledge and better insight for all.[7]

Every professional nurse needs to develop skill in evaluating the results of research if she is to use research findings for the improvement of patient care. Questions such as the following may serve as guidelines in the evaluation of a piece of research:

1. What problem was studied? Was it clearly stated? If the problem studied is not clear, then it will be difficult to relate the findings to it—a necessary step in evaluation.

2. What were the qualifications of the researcher? Did he, or she, appear to have the background to do research of the type undertaken?

3. Was the research methodology used. appropriate? For example, a study of attitudes of mothers toward their premature infants probably would not be made by means of a retrospective review of available hospital records. Attitude studies usually require a more direct study of the individual involved—for example, through such methods as interviewing, special questionnaires and projective tests.

4. What data were collected? Was the sample large enough? If comparisons were made between groups, were the groups really comparable? Were the data free of bias? Was the sample representative of the population studied?

5. Were the conclusions made in line with the findings? Were the conclusions presented cautiously, or were sweeping generalizations made? Much research is not based on sufficiently large samples to allow generalizations, but does permit suggestion of the direction toward which the findings point.

Once you have read a research report thoughtfully and have evaluated it, the next step is to consider its implications for nursing practice. Improvement of patient care is a major goal of nursing research.[8]

Ideas come from reasoning, reference sources, and association with people, places and things. A dearth of ideas may evolve from a dearth of experience. So it is wise to seek the widest possible range of desirable contacts and experiences. Organize your professional life on as broad a scale as possible. A knowledge that is comprehensive enough to cover the field of your endeavor is important in solving professional problems. Equally important is the will to learn and to advance. Experience, as well as hard, consistent work and critical thinking, is a factor in learning how to solve problems and to succeed in making a good professional adjustment as well as a good adjustment to life itself.

There is frequently an element in problem solving supplied by your own character which no amount of technical training can give you because it springs from deep sincerity, great charity, an unselfish viewpoint, high ideals,

[7] See Chapter 29, "Skills and Practices Which Aid in Professional Activities."

[8] For a more detailed discussion of evaluation of research see, "Nursing Research Is Every Nurse's Business," by L. Notter, *Nursing Outlook,* **11**:49-51, Jan. 1963.

an earnest and prayerful search for truth and a willingness to face truth no matter how unwelcome it may be. The wisest and most far-sighted persons possess these qualities. That is why their decisions are superior to those of persons who do not possess such qualities.

PROBLEMS

1. It is suggested that you try consciously to solve a simple problem by following the problem-solving steps. Select a professional problem which has confronted you during the last 6 months and seek a solution to it in the following manner: (a) state the problem, (b) list the sources used in solving it, (c) describe the procedure followed in solving it, (d) state the solution, (e) tell how you tested the solution, (f) list the bibliography.

2. Talk with your classmates and instructors to see what studies in nursing they think are needed. Add your suggestions and make a list of these studies for consideration of their significance by other members of your class.

3. Make a list of reports of studies in one of the following areas and report these in class: (a) nursing practice; (b) nursing education; (c) patterns of nursing service.

4. Select 1 report from the list you made of nursing studies and report on it to the class using the following outline; (a) statement of the problem; (b) significance of the problem; (c) sources and methodology used; (c) conclusions reached; and (e) the meaning of the study to you and how you would use the findings.

5. (a) Have a discussion with your classmates on the place and value of the National Library of Medicine to nursing; (b) What is MEDLARS? (c) Of what use is this tool to you?

6. Of what value are the Abstracts of Studies in Nursing? (See the "Abstracts" section in the current issue of *Nursing Research.)*

7. Identify the following persons by indicating their contribution to research in nursing: Faye Abdellah; Jeanne S. Berthold; Esther Lucile Brown; Helen Bunge; May Ayres Burgess; Ava Dilworth; David Fox; Josephine Goldmark; Elizabeth Hagen; Loretta E. Heidgerken; Virginia Henderson; Eleanor C. Lambertsen; Eugene Levine; Wanda McDowell; R. Louise McManus; Helen K. Mussalem; Lucille Notter; Doris Schwartz; Leo W. Simmons; Ouida Upchurch; Phyllis Verhonick; Ellwynne Vreeland.

SUGGESTED REFERENCES*

GENERAL

Abdellah, F. G. "Approaches to Protecting the Rights of Human Subjects." *Nursing Research,* **16:**316-320, Fall 1967.

* In each chapter all citations are footnoted and are not included here. All starred references are recommended for additional reading.

Abraham, G. E. "Promoting Nursing Research in an Organized Nursing Service." *American Journal of Nursing,* **68:**818-821, Apr. 1968.

Bunge, Helen. "The First Decade of *Nursing Research.*" *Nursing Research,* **11:** 132-137, Summer 1962.

Collins, R. D. "Problem Solving: A Tool for Patients, Too." *American Journal of Nursing,* **68:**1483-1485, July 1968.

Collins, V. "Implementation of Nursing Research." *Utah Nurse,* **19:**13-15, Fall 1968.

Davis, M. Z. "Some Problems in Identity in Becoming a Nurse Researcher." *Nursing Research,* **17:**166-168, Mar./Apr. 1968.

"Developmental Grants for Nursing Research. (editorial) *Nursing Research,* **17:**387, Sept./Oct. 1968.

Hawley, J. "Reconciling Nursing with Research." *Nursing Outlook,* **16:**34-35, June 1968.

Henderson, V. "An Overview of Nursing Research." *Nursing Research,* **6:**61-71, Oct. 1957.

Hochbaum, G. D. "The Nurse in Research." *Nursing Outlook,* **8:**192-195, Apr. 1960.

Kee, J. L. "Nursing in a Clinical Research Center." *American Journal of Nursing,* **67:**2110-2113, Oct. 1967.

Leone, L. P. *Workshop on the Improvement of Nursing Through Research, Catholic University of America, June 14, 1958.* Ed. by L. E. Heidgerken. Washington, D.C., The Catholic University of America Press, 1958, pp. 17-18.

Marvin, M. M. "Research in Nursing." *American Journal of Nursing,* **27:**331-335, May 1927.

McManus, R. L. "Today and Tomorrow in Nursing Research." *American Journal of Nursing,* **61:**68-71, May 1961.

_____. "Nursing Research—Its Evolution." *American Journal of Nursing,* **61:**76-79, Apr. 1961.

Nishio, K. "Creative Problem Solving." *Nursing Forum,* **6(4):**432-441, 1967.

Oram, P. G. and Routhier, W. R. "Research as Inservice Education." *Nursing Outlook,* **16:**20-22, Sept. 1968.

Roberts, I. "The Dissemination and Use of Research Reports." *International Nursing Review,* **14:**43-48, Oct. 1967.

Rogers, M. E. "Nursing Science: Research and Researchers." *Teachers College Record,* **69:**469-476, Feb. 1968.

Sanford, N. "Students and Studies." *American Journal of Nursing,* **68:**805-806, Apr. 1968.

Schwartz, D. R. "The Value of Small Local Nursing Studies." *American Journal of Nursing,* **66:**1327-1329, June 1966.

Verhonick, P. J. "Research in Nursing Practice." *Quarterly Review* (District of Columbia Nurses' Association), **34:**14-16, 21-22, Dec. 1966.

Verhonick, P. J. and Rowland, M. A. "Problem-Solving Approach to a Nursing Situation." *Military Medicine,* **125:**685-688, Oct. 1960.

Whaley, P. J. "Nursing Research: Limbo or Liberty." *American Journal of Nursing,* **67:**1675-1677, Aug. 1967.

RESEARCH METHODS

* Fox, D. J. *Fundamentals of Research in Nursing.* New York, Appleton-Century-Crofts, 1966.

* Fox, D. J. and Kelly, R. L. *The Research Process in Nursing.* New York, Appleton-Century-Crofts, 1967.

Johnson, J. E., *et al.* "Research Projects for Teaching Methodology." *Nursing Outlook,* **16:**27-29, Nov. 1968.

Levine, E. "Statistics: A Tool for Nurses." *International Nursing Review,* **15**:224-235, July 1968.

————. "Interpreting Statistical Data." *American Journal of Nursing,* **59**:230-233, Feb. 1959.

————. "The ABC's of Statistics." *American Journal of Nursing,* **59**:71-75, Jan. 1959.

See also current issues of *Nursing Research Report,* the bulletin of the ANF, published quarterly.

STYLE MANUALS

* Campbell, W. G. *Form and Style in Thesis Writing.* New York, Houghton-Mifflin, 1954.
* Hook, L. and Gaver, M. V. *The Research Paper: Gathering Library Material; Organizing and Preparing the Manuscript.* New York, Prentice-Hall, 1962.
* *A Manual of Style.* Chicago, University of Chicago Press, 1969.
* Turabian, K. L. *A Manual for Writers of Term Papers, Theses, and Dissertations.* Chicago, University of Chicago Press, 1967.

LIBRARY USAGE, ABSTRACTING, INDEXING AND PROOFREADING

Brandon, A. "Regional Libraries and Their Implications for Nursing." *League Exchange,* **83**:17-19, 1967.

Campbell, J. "Library Service in the Health Sciences." *League Exchange,* **83**:1-2, 1967.

* Cunningham, E. V. "A Critique of Two Indexes to Nursing Literature." *Nursing Forum,* **6**:352-362, Fall 1967.
* Doris, L. and Miller, B. M. *Complete Secretary's Handbook.* Englewood Cliffs, New Jersey, Prentice-Hall, 1960.
* Karel, L. "Nursing and the National Library of Medicine." *League Exchange,* **83**:3-5, 1967.

"MEDLARS: A New Bibliographic System for the Medical Literature with Implications for Nursing." *Nursing Research,* **12**:251-243, Fall 1963.

* Munson, A. H. "Make Friends With Your Library." *Nursing Outlook,* **11**:261-262, Apr. 1963.
* Munson, H. W. "Thanks, I Can Find It Myself." *Imprint,* **16**:10-13, Jan. 1969.

Parkin, M. L. "Library Services for Nurses: Current Trends." *Canadian Nurse,* **64**:49-50, Mar. 1968.

Pings, V. M. "Library Service in the Health Sciences." *League Exchange,* **83**:6-11, 1967.

————. *A Plan for Indexing the Periodical Literature In Nursing.* New York, American Nurses' Foundation, 1966.

Raybould, E. "Forming a School of Nursing Library." *International Nursing Review,* **14**:31-35, Aug. 1967.

* Taylor, S. D. "How to Prepare an Abstract." *Nursing Outlook,* **15**:61-63, Sept. 1967.

Warren, L. H. "Practical Suggestions for Reducing the Labor of Indexing a Text-Book." *Science,* **92**:217-218, Sept. 6, 1940.

Words into Type: A Guide in the Preparation of Manuscripts: for Writers, Editors, Proofreaders and Printers. New York, Appleton-Century-Crofts, 1964. Based on Studies by M. E. Skillin, R. M. Gay and Others.

See also "Sources: Reference Tools for Nurses" in the Appendix, and the references on "Writing" at the end of Chapter 29.

Definition of Professional Nursing by Legislation, Administrative Material and Case Law
Principles of Liability Related to Professional Performance
Additional Matters
Conclusion

CHAPTER

6

Legal Issues
in
Nursing Practice[1]

The purpose of this chapter is to describe the legal rules and doctrines that provide standards for the practice of professional nursing, and the principles applied in determining when liability may be imposed upon a nurse because of her performance of professional responsibilities. The focus is upon the legal issues related to the practice of individual professional nursing. Excluded from the scope of this chapter are legal matters of general applicability that pertain to nurses as members of the community, as well as those legal matters that, while they may have specific applicability to, or impact upon, the performance of professional nursing, do not directly apply to the practice of the individual professional nurse. Thus, although of interest to nurses, subjects such as Workmen's Compensation and basic principles of contract law, which fall within the first described exclusion, and the content of national health legislation, such as the laws establishing the Regional Medical Programs, Comprehensive Health Planning, Medicare and Medicaid, which fall within the second excluded area, are beyond the purview of this chapter. (For a discussion of these, see Chapter 27, "Legislation Affecting Nursing.")

[1] This chapter was prepared by Nathan Hershey, Esq., Research Professor of Health Law, Department of Public Health Practice, Graduate School of Public Health, University of Pittsburgh, Pittsburgh, Pennsylvania.

DEFINITION OF PROFESSIONAL NURSING BY LEGISLATION, ADMINISTRATIVE MATERIAL AND CASE LAW

Under the prevailing pattern of licensing in the USA, each state licenses a number of professions and occupations that it deems require such regulation. Some of the professions and occupations usually licensed are within the health care area and some are not. The avowed purpose of such licensing is the protection of the public from unqualified practitioners. Licensing legislation, in providing such protection, is an exercise of the state's police power.

There are 2 basic kinds of licensing laws for individuals, mandatory laws and permissive laws. *Mandatory laws* forbid any person from performing the activities and assuming the responsibilities of a particular licensed profession or occupation, unless he is legally licensed or is functioning within the proper scope of another licensed profession or occupation for which he has been granted a license. *Permissive laws* do not forbid unlicensed persons from engaging in the activities and assuming the responsibilities of the particular licensed profession or occupation, but they do forbid unlicensed persons from using the designation authorized by law for licensed individuals, such as "R.N." in the case of professional nurses, or from indicating to the public that they have been awarded licenses.

There are economic implications that can be derived from mandatory licensing. Under a mandatory law the state, in effect, grants a monopoly to those individuals who have been properly licensed to provide the kinds of services and engage in the activities that fall within the definition of the particular profession or occupation. This concept of the state permitting, if not assisting in, the establishment of a restriction on free-and-open competition seems contrary to one of our most cherished ideals. However, the justification for mandatory licensing legislation is that there is greater benefit to the public from preventing unqualified people from practicing or engaging in skilled activities, than there is harm to the public from the restrictive aspects of the situation that results.

At present, all but a few states have mandatory licensing legislation for professional nurses. A licensing law for professional nurses, usually called a *nursing practice act,* has 4 basic elements:

1. A definition of nursing practice or professional nursing
2. A provision establishing a board, sometimes, but not always, consisting of professional nurses exclusively, to implement and administer the law
3. An enumeration of criteria and qualifications for licensure, and procedures to be followed in granting licenses to qualified applicants and in renewing them
4. A description of conduct in violation of the law and of conduct that establishes a basis for suspension or revocation of a nurse's license

The 4 elements described above can be found in all licensing legislation for professional nursing. However, the state laws governing professional nursing are not identical; they vary somewhat from state to state. This variation is a direct result of our Federal system. Each state is free to decide which professions and occupations to license and whether a particular licensing law should be mandatory or permissive, as well as to define each licensed profession or occupation and to establish the qualifications and the manner of selection of board members—in short, to determine all aspects of the licensing plan, subject only to constitutional limitations.

The nursing practice acts contain definitions of professional nursing practice that are not cast in identical language. In many states, the definition contained in the Model Act prepared by the ANA has been adopted with little or no modification; in other states the language of the definition appears to be considerably different. Such semantic differences do not necessarily give rise to any discernible practical differences from state to state in what constitutes the practice of professional nursing. The definition in the ANA Model Act provides:

The term "practice of professional nursing" means the performance, for compensation, of any acts in the observation, care, and counsel of the ill, injured, or infirm, or in the maintenance of health or prevention of illness of others, or in the supervision and teaching of other personnel, or the administration of medications and treatments as prescribed by a licensed physician or a licensed dentist; requiring substantial specialized judgment and skill and based on knowledge and application of the principles of biological, physical, and social science. The foregoing shall not be deemed to include acts of diagnosis or prescription of therapeutic or corrective measures.

As can be noted from the language of the model definition, the definition of professional nursing is conceptual in approach; it is not a listing of specific techniques and procedures that professional nurses may perform. In some states there is additional legislation that clarifies, and sometimes extends, the definition of professional nursing stated in the nursing practice act. In addition to legislation, in many states the opinions of the state attorney-general, the rules and regulations of the state licensing board and many court decisions enumerate, describe or recognize specific procedures that fall within the scope of professional nursing. Legislation, as well as the other sources mentioned, emanate from governmental authority. There are also joint statements of state medical, nursing and hospital organizations that claim to indicate the proper scope of professional nursing practice. These statements, although they come from nongovernmental sources, may have considerable weight in legal proceedings concerned with issues involving the scope of professional nursing.

Illustrative of the materials that further define the scope of professional nursing practice in terms of the law are an Arizona statutory provision that specifically allows professional nurses to administer anesthesia;[2] an opinion of the New York Attorney-General stating that professional nurses may

[2] Ariz. Rev. Stat. Ann. §32-1661 (1956).

administer intravenous therapy;[3] a similar resolution of the New Jersey Board of Nursing regarding the same question;[4] and a joint statement of the Hawaii Nurses' Association, the Hawaii Medical Association and the Hospital Association of Hawaii, that professional nurses may perform closed-chest cardiopulmonary resuscitation in described circumstances.[5] Other rulings may declare specified activities to be beyond, rather than within, the area of practice of the professional nurse.[6] Judicial decisions in liability cases involving nursing activities sometimes provide guidelines describing or defining professional nursing practice.

The operational definition of professional nursing in a particular state is the synthesis of legislation, administrative determinations and judicial decisions. This legally recognized definition of the professional nurse can best be understood in relation to the areas of practice permitted other practitioners in the health professions and occupations, rather than as an area of activity that stands apart from other health care occupations. Under the licensing laws for physicians — the medical practice acts — a physician is permitted to provide all services and to accept all responsibilities in the care of individuals who are sick, injured, or in need of preventive health or health maintenance services. This means that, by law, the physician, and only the physician, has an unlimited license. When compared with the practice of the professional nurse, the elements that constitute the unique area of practice of the physician are diagnosis and prescribing or ordering therapeutic measures. Many statutory definitions of professional nursing specifically state that a nurse may not diagnose, nor prescribe or order therapeutic measures.

In those states with mandatory nursing practice acts, practical nurses, aides and the various auxiliary health workers all have less extensive licensed areas of practice than the professional nurse. Conceptually and practically, professional nurses may make decisions and engage in tasks that are beyond the legally recognized area of practice of these other categories of personnel within the nursing service. This reflects differences in the content of educational programs and in qualification examinations.

The area of practice of the professional nurse can also be viewed in relation to certain occupational and professional specialists within the health field. Technicians, therapists and other occupational groups have completed educational programs of equivalent or greater length than, and different from, the educational program for the professional nurse, as prerequisites for entering their specialities and obtaining their licenses. For example, the physical therapist, based on the definition of physical therapy in licensing legislation for physical therapists, can make certain decisions

---

[3] (1961) Ops. N.Y. Attorney Gen. 25.

[4] Resolution of New Jersey Board of Nursing, February 18, 1960.

[5] Joint Statement of Hawaii Medical Association, Hawaii Nurses' Association and Hospital Association of Hawaii, April 5, 1968.

[6] *E.g.,* Ruling of Massachusetts Board of Registration in Nursing, December 23, 1964, *re:* Insertion of Levine Tubes.

and engage in certain activities that are outside the scope of professional nursing. In a state with a mandatory licensing law for physical therapists, a professional nurse who provides some therapeutic measures and makes decisions related to them could be viewed as violating the physical therapy licensing law. Of course, there are procedures and decisions within professional nursing that are not within the area of practice of the physical therapist. Illustrative of these are many techniques for the administration of medication and judgments concerning reactions to therapeutic agents. There is also an area of practice shared by both the professional nurse and the physical therapist; an area of activity encompassed by the definitions of both professions.

It is necessary to consider these matters of scope of practice because they can and do influence the outcome of litigation on negligence of a professional nurse, as well as lay the basis for the imposition of sanctions on a professional nurse for engaging in practices not permitted by her license.

A court decision illustrative of the way in which the legal definition of a professional or an occupation may affect liability for negligence is the Washington case of *Barber v. Reinking*.[7] The Barber case concerned a licensed practical nurse working in a physician's office who was in the midst of administering an intramuscular injection to a child when the child moved suddenly and the needle was broken off in his right buttock. Surgical removal of the needle was attempted unsuccessfully in the office and not until approximately 9 months later was the needle finally located and removed. A suit alleging negligence was brought on behalf of the youngster against both the practical nurse and the physician. The jury decided in favor of the defendants—the physician and the practical nurse. The plaintiff appealed, claiming that the judge at the trial should have instructed the jury that, under the state's nursing practice legislation, a practical nurse was prohibited from giving inoculations. The plaintiff supported the assertion by a reference to specific language in the mandatory licensing law for professional nurses of the state of Washington, which stated that a licensed professional nurse could perform certain procedures including "...administer medications, treatments, tests and inoculations, whether or not the severing or penetrating of tissues in involved and whether or not a degree of independent judgment and skill is required...." The law also stated that these could not be done by "any person not so licensed."

The countering argument on behalf of the practical nurse was that the licensing law for practical nurses, in effect at the time, provided that they could "administer medications" and that "administer medications" included inoculations within its ambit.

The appellate court agreed with the plaintiff and held that the phrase "administer medications" in the licensing law for practical nurses did not encompass inoculations, because of the explicit language of the licensing act for professional nurses, and that, therefore, practical nurses could not

[7] 411 P.2d 861 (1966).

legally give inoculations. The court went on to say that the standard of performance to which an unlicensed person is held in performing an activity that falls within the area of practice covered by mandatory licensure is that degree of skill and care ordinarily demonstrated by the trained and skilled members of the profession. Thus, one who undertakes to perform the services of a licensed professional nurse must have the knowledge and skill possessed by licensed professional nurses, and the lack of a license permits the jury to infer that the unlicensed person does not possess the required knowledge and skill to perform the task.

Not all courts adopt the approach of the Washington court, which permits an inference of negligence in such circumstances. However, professional nurses should be aware of such a liability potential. A professional nurse who performs a task or engages in an activity beyond her legally recognized scope of practice, may find that her action, if injury is sustained by the patient, will give rise to an inference of negligence, and that her performance will be measured against the standard for its performance by a competent physician.

PRINCIPLES OF LIABILITY RELATED TO PROFESSIONAL PERFORMANCE

For liability to be imposed for negligence, 4 elements must be present. First, there must be *a duty owed* to the injured party – a duty to refrain from creating unreasonable risks of harm. In some areas of human activity there may be a substantial question of whether a particular individual, alleged to be negligent, actually owed a duty toward the person who sustained injury. However, as a practical matter, in every instance in which nurses are performing tasks and procedures and accepting responsibility for individuals entrusted to their care, a duty exists.

Second, there must be a *breach of duty* – a failure to meet the standard recognized by law for protection from unreasonable risks of harm. In the ordinary activities of life, such as operating a motor vehicle, the test applied to determine if the duty has been met is whether the individual alleged to have been negligent met the standard of care that would be exercised in the same or a similar situation by a hypothetical, reasonable and prudent person. However, the test is somewhat different when the person is engaged in the performance of professional activities. Here, the individual alleged to have been negligent is measured against the standard of performance that competent professionals in his field achieve in carrying out the particular procedure or activity that resulted in the harm. The word "malpractice" is often used to describe negligence of a professional nature.

The third element is *harm*. Even if an individual is negligent, liability may be imposed only if harm to person or property has resulted. The fourth element is *causation* – a causal relationship between the failure to meet the prescribed standard and the harm that has been suffered must be proven. While in many cases there is no serious question of the existence of a causal relationship between the negligence and the harm, there have been a number of cases involving patient care situations in which causation has not been shown. For example, in some cases involving patients who have become infected in hospitals, although poor practice on the part of personnel caring for the patient has been clearly established, the evidence has failed to indicate that the negligence was the cause of the patient's infection.

Breach of duty—the failure to meet the standard of care—is the element of the 4 described above that is of greatest importance to the practicing professional nurse. In the typical liability case, in which a nurse is alleged to have been negligent, it is necessary for the injured person to establish at the trial the standard of practice of competent professional nurses and the deviation from this standard by the individual nurse accused of negligence. The members of the jury are not expected to know the standard of competent nursing practice from their own personal experience; therefore, it is necessary to introduce evidence—testimony of professional nurses and others, often physicians—to establish the standard of competent nursing practice in the particular situation.

A judicial decision that exemplifies how conduct is measured against the standard of competent nursing practice is *Norton v. Argonaut Insurance Co.*[8] The nurse had administered 3 cc. of an injectable form of Lanoxin, which was approximately 5 times the strength of 3 cc. of the elixir form, to a 3-month-old infant who died soon after the medication was administered. The attending physician had written on the order sheet, "Give 3.0 cc. Lanoxin today for 1 dose only." The order as written indicated neither the form of the medication nor the route of administration.

Before administering the medication, the nurse, because of her concern about the order, asked physicians present on the unit whether the dose was too large, but she did not seek clarification of the order from the physician who prescribed it. The physicians to whom her inquiries were addressed assumed she was referring to the elixir form because she did not specifically inquire about the dosage in the injectable form.

The court in its opinion stated:

For obvious reasons we believe it the duty of a nurse when in doubt about an order for medication to make absolutely certain what the doctor intended both as to dosage and route. In the case at bar the evidence leaves not the slightest doubt that whereas nurses in the locality do at times consult any available physician, it appears equally certain that all of the nurses who testified herein agree that the better practice (and the one which they follow) is to consult the prescribing physician when in doubt about an order for medication. With regard to nurses consulting any available physician when in doubt about an order for medication, the testimony of [both physicians] indicates clearly that in their experience such inquiries are generally restricted solely to interpretation of the doctor's handwriting and are not usually related to dosage or route. Having elected to deviate from the general and better

---

[8] 144 So.2d 249 (1962).

practice of consulting the physician who ordered the medication in question, [the nurse] was under the duty and obligation of making herself understood beyond the possibility of error. This she did not do. . . .

There is an almost infinite number of occurrences, in the provision of nursing care to patients, that can lead to the imposition of liability. Nurses have been considered negligent in situations where they failed to summon a physician when there was serious deterioration in the patient's condition;[9] where they failed to observe at frequent intervals the deterioration of the patient's condition;[10] where they neglected to review carefully the patient's record regarding medication;[11] where they had been inattentive while assisting patients in getting into or out of beds and wheelchairs; and in a host of other contexts.

A nurse who keeps in mind the concept of the standard of care as she goes about the performance of her professional duties may find it helpful to her in difficult situations. Quite frequently a professional nurse, who has some doubt as to whether the nursing care method that she is about to employ is the correct one, can clarify the situation for herself by halting for a moment and asking herself: "If I were called as an expert witness to describe the standard of performance of a competent nurse – the standard of good nursing practice – in this situation, would I testify that the course I am about to follow is the one ordinarily followed by competent nurses?" If the answer to that question is "No," then the nurse has good reasons to believe that, if she were to proceed as she had planned, she would be creating an unreasonable risk of harm to the patient. By seeking to be objective, the nurse may be able to obtain greater insight into the particular situation, and recognize the relative risks of different courses of action.

Nurse Supervisors

A professional nurse, whether or not she has a supervisory title, often has supervisory responsibility for personnel providing nursing services to patients. If, in the performance of her supervisory responsibilities, the professional nurse deviates from the standard of good nursing practice and harm is suffered by a patient as a result, a basis for imposing liability is present.

At this point it is necessary to explain *respondeat superior*, a legal doctrine under which a master is liable for harm suffered because of the negligence of his servant, occurring within the scope of the servant's employment. Almost always, a nurse employed by an institution or agency is a "servant," and her employer a "master," for purposes of *respondeat superior*. Several rationales have been offered for imposing liability on an employer for harm resulting from negligence of an employee. To a large extent they are based on the concept that, since the employee is advancing

[9] *Goff v. Doctors General Hospital*, 333 P.2d 29 (1958).
[10] *Duling v. Bluefield Sanitarium, Inc.*, 142 S.E.2d 754 (1965).
[11] *Larrimore v. Homeopathic Hospital*, 181 A.2d 573 (1962).

the work of the employer, the employer should assume the burden for the harm incurred by others in the course of the employee's efforts. In almost every instance in which a nurse, employed by a hospital, agency or institution, is negligent, her employer can be held liable as well.[12] The nurse, however, is not relieved of her personal liability because the hospital can be or is liable under the doctrine of *respondeat superior*.

A professional nurse serving as a supervisor is not, however, the master or employer of the personnel who work under her supervision or at her direction. Therefore, a nurse who has supervisory responsibility over other nursing service personnel cannot be held liable merely because 1 of the persons to whom she assigned or delegated duties was negligent and caused harm to a patient. The supervisor is liable only for her personal negligence in performing her supervisory duties. If a nursing supervisor assigns a task to a professional nurse, a practical nurse, an aide or some other person whom she knows or has reason to believe is not competent to perform the particular task, and injury is suffered by a patient because of the incompetent or negligent performance of the task, then the supervisor could be held personally liable for her negligence as a supervisor. The standard of care applied in determining whether a supervisor has performed her supervisory duties in a competent manner is usually based on testimony regarding the level of performance of a competent, professional nurse exercising supervisory responsibility in the same or a similar situation. The employer would be liable under the doctrine of *respondeat superior* because both the supervisor and the individual who performed the task in a negligent fashion were its employees.

To a considerable extent, a supervisor may rely upon the fact that a subordinate is licensed or certified as an indication of the subordinate's capabilities for performing tasks within the scope of his license or certificate. However, where the supervisor has observed, or should have observed, that the particular individual lacks competence in certain areas of activity, it ordinarily would be deemed a departure from the standard of competent nursing practice to continue to assign those tasks to that person.

There have been very few cases fixing upon the liability of the supervisor. This may be ascribed to the fact that the injured person, where the supervisor is negligent, would have the basis for successful suits against both the individual who had been negligent in performing the procedure and the employer. Therefore, suit against the supervisor, too, may be superfluous or, at least, not essential, in the view of the patient's attorney. It is

---

[12] In several states, charitable institutions, such as voluntary, nonprofit hospitals, are not subject to liability because of the doctrine of *charitable immunity*. A considerable number of states grant immunity to governmental institutions—those institutions operated by the state, counties and other units of government. Where these immunity doctrines are in force, the institutions to which they apply are not liable under *respondeat superior*. The immunity doctrines do not provide immunity from liability to individual employees of such institutions, such as professional nurses, who have been negligent; they confer immunity upon the institutions only.

unlikely that complete perfection in the performance of supervisory responsibilities by professional nurses is the reason for the relative dearth of such litigation.

Students of Nursing

The student of professional nursing is entrusted, as part of her educational program, with responsibility for providing nursing care to patients. When a nursing student is serving at a hospital or other institution that provides nursing care to patients, she may be held liable for her personal negligence in carrying out nursing responsibilities. The fact that she is a student and is engaging in the nursing service as part of her education does not relieve her of the risks of liability, and the courts have held that a nursing student is expected to meet the standard of a competent professional nurse in the performance of professional nursing duties.[13] Thus, in determining whether a nursing student has been negligent in carrying out a particular task or responsibility, she is measured against the standard of good nursing practice—the standard of the competent professional nurse. The rationale for this position is that the patient has the right to expect and to receive competently performed nursing services, even if the care is provided by students of nursing as part of their clinical experience. Viewing the situation from the patient's expectations, it would be unfair to deprive him of the opportunity to recover damages for the injury he sustained because the institution in which he was a patient has assumed the role of providing a clinical setting in which students may become proficient, and permits students, instead of professional nurses, to minister to patients.

The supervisor of nursing students, whether a specifically designated clinical instructor or the professional nurse in charge of the unit to which students have been assigned, can be liable on the bases described earlier for the supervisory nurse. If a patient's injury is the result of a student's performance of a procedure that the student had not as yet demonstrated the capability to perform in a manner consistent with the standard of competent professional nurses, then the nurse who made the assignment would probably be deemed to have departed from the standard of nursing practice of a competent instructor. To a considerable extent, the risks of injury to patients from the performance of duties by nursing students can be minimized by the introduction of additional supervision beyond that provided when the task and procedure is being carried out by a graduate nurse. Thus, when a nursing student is to perform a procedure upon a patient, without her proficiency having been ascertained, a qualified nurse, able to intervene or assist if necessary, should be close at hand.

---

[13] *Nickley v. Skemp,* 239 N.W. 426 (1931). The same approach is taken in cases involving students of other health professions; see *Christensen v. Des Moines Still College,* 82 N.W.2d 741 (1957), for a case concerning the performance of a procedure by a student of osteopathy.

The Nurse Who Works Alone

The legal rules and principles governing the activities and performance of professional nurses who are employed in contexts other than the hospital are the same as those governing nurses in the hospital. However, the application of the rules and principles tends to vary because of the special considerations stemming from the working situation. The phrase, "the nurse who works alone," is sometimes used to describe the professional nurse employed in an occupational health facility or by a public health agency.

In a properly organized work environment, the professional nurse provides nursing care in accordance with guidelines and procedures established by the agency or organization, based on principles of correct medical and nursing practice. The professional nurse in the occupational health facility, in addition to endeavors related to preventive health and health maintenance programs, treats employees who receive injuries or become ill while working. Often, close medical supervision of the occupational health facility is lacking, and a type of judgmental ability may be required of the occupational health nurse that a professional nurse in the hospital encounters less frequently, if at all.

In a technical sense, a professional nurse in such an establishment as an occupational health facility may not exceed her legally recognized scope of practice. She may not diagnose or order therapy for patients—the area of practice reserved by law to physicians. The key issue in this context is the nature of the decisions that the occupational health nurse may make; decisions such as whether the patient's condition demands immediate treatment by her, whether she should await specific instructions from the physician, or whether perhaps his physical presence on the scene is necessary. On some occasions the physician's decision cannot be obtained with great promptness, although his intervention is required by precepts of good practice, and some care must be furnished immediately by the nurse, based upon her assessment of patient need.

The extent to which orders and guidelines have been established for the situations that can be anticipated in this kind of work is extremely important. In many establishments, relatively specific orders setting forth the procedures to be followed in particular situations are available. Nursing practice conforming with these medically-established guidelines would raise neither the spectre of violation of the medical practice act nor liability for negligence, as long as the procedures were carried out in competent fashion, even without a contemporaneous medical order. The courts recognize that a professional nurse in an occupational health facility is trained, although not to the level of a physician, to recognize symptoms of disease and injury, and to decide whether it is a situation which is within her authority to treat on a first aid basis or whether it is one that requires a physician's personal assessment first.[14] The nurse's choice of treatment is based upon information provided by the patient and her own inspection of the patient. The

[14] See *Vesel v. Jardine Mining Co.*, 100 P.2d 75 (1940).

choice must be made in conformity with the medically-established guidelines for the facility.

The nature of the working environment of the public health nurse, although similar to that of the occupational health nurse in many aspects, less frequently involves care of patients in acute situations. The issues related to the practice of the public health nurse that raise legal problems often arise from the need to determine: (1) the procedures she is legally permitted to perform without specific physician direction and (2) the extent to which she may assign or delegate certain kinds of tasks to auxiliary personnel. In deciding questions of liability for negligence when harm has been suffered because of procedures performed by her personally, the nurse in public health would be measured against the standard of performance of a competent nurse in carrying out these procedures. When the harm results from the activities of auxiliary nursing personnel, the public health nurse is measured against the standard of competent nursing practice in making assignments and allocations of duties to such personnel.

The Nurse in Private Practice

The nurse in private practice (often referred to as a private duty nurse) is considered an independent contractor whose services are purchased by a specific patient. The indicia of private practice status are that the nurse is hired by, and receives her remuneration from, the patient or the patient's representative. The nurse in private practice, like any other individual, is liable for the harm caused by her negligence. Nurses in private practice provide nursing care to patients in their homes, in hospitals and in other patient care institutions. Ordinarily, when the private duty nurse is providing care to a patient in an institution, she is not deemed an employee of the institution while carrying out duties for her patient, but maintains the status of an independent contractor.

The 2 major issues that have arisen recently with respect to nurses in private practice have concerned: (1) the degree to which she may be recognized as an employee or servant of the hospital for liability purposes, even though she is ostensibly serving in private practice status; and (2) the circumstances under which a hospital may bar a particular nurse from practice within its precincts.

Courts, in several cases, have indicated that because a private duty nurse was procured for the patient through the efforts of hospital personnel, because the hospital was the conduit for payment, or because the nature of the care provided by the private duty nurse to the patient should have been furnished by the hospital's employees, liability may be imposed on the hospital under the doctrine of *respondeat superior* for harm suffered as the result of the negligence of nurses who were engaged in private practice.[15] As a practical matter, whether or not the hospital will be liable for negligence

---

[15] See *Emory University v. Shadburn*, 171 S.E. 192 (1933), *affirmed* 180 S.E. 137 (1935), and *Hawkins v. Laughlin*, 236 S.W.2d 375 (1951).

of the nurse in private practice is of minor importance to the nurses so engaged, because the nurse will remain liable for her own negligence, even if in a particular case the hospital may be held liable under *respondeat superior.*

A hospital may exclude a private duty nurse from practicing within the hospital. In several cases, after being denied the privilege of practicing in specific hospitals, private duty nurses have sought court orders to prohibit the hospitals from barring them from practice. The courts have held that the hospitals had the right to exclude the nurses in private practice from serving patients within their institutions, unless the determination was an abuse of discretion by the hospital administration.[16] Such a result is consistent with the decisions relating to medical staff privileges for physicians. A hospital is legally permitted to establish and enforce reasonable rules and standards necessary to maintain good quality service, although they may exclude some physicians and nurses in private practice. The fact that a professional nurse possesses a valid license to practice does not necessarily entitle her to engage in private practice in a particular patient care institution.

Impact of New Technology Upon Liability Matters

Changes in nursing practice resulting from the development of new therapeutic techniques, the utilization of new kinds of equipment and the development of machines that appear to undertake responsibilities formerly viewed as part of professional nursing, have caused concern to nurses for legal and other reasons. However, the effect of automation upon the legal responsibilities of professional nurses is less extensive than a cursory review of changes would lead many to believe.

Some professional nurses are already utilizing devices and machines that automatically record and report information about their patients' conditions and, in some instances, carry out therapeutic measures with far less manual intervention by the professional nurse than was required formerly. The trend toward increased use of sophisticated equipment is very evident. However, many of the judgmental aspects and decisions of professional nursing cannot be given over to electronic and mechanical devices, at this time. As more extensive education and training of humans becomes necessary in order to perform certain tasks and to make decisions, the more difficult, and the less likely, is the development of equipment that can undertake such responsibilities. Devices are now available to obtain a variety of objective facts, such as temperature and pulse rate, directly from the patient. Observations that are more subjective in nature, such as changes in color, degree of blueness around the lips, increasing incoherence, odor and the information obtained by touch, do not at present lend themselves to instrumental measurement and require human intervention.

---

[16] See *Robinson v. Cooper Hospital,* unreported case, Super Ct., Camden County, N.J., No. C-2814-59 (1962).

Even with respect to the most advanced instrumentation — cardiac monitors, pacemakers, defibrillators, and so forth — the responsibilities of the personnel monitoring and using such equipment are not qualitatively different from the responsibilities that attend care without the use of such sophisticated devices. With respect to the scope of practice in this context, the nature and degree of discretion left to the professional nurse determines whether or not she is impinging upon medical practice. If the nurse is making decisions based essentially on objective manifestations of the patient, whether or not a sophisticated device is employed as an intermediary, and she is providing therapeutic measures in accordance with guidelines or plans established by physicians in advance, which are to be followed in such described situations, then the professional nurse is not intruding upon the area of medical practice.

The nurse runs the risk of liability for harm suffered by a patient when she fails to recognize manifestations of the patient indicated by recording and reporting devices attached to the patient, or fails to adhere to the rules established by the responsible physician regarding the appropriate therapeutic measure in the specific case. A professional nurse would ordinarily not be liable for action taken pursuant to incorrect readings obtained because of equipment malfunction, unless the readings were such as to indicate to a competent nurse that malfunction was taking place, and that the data being provided was incorrect.

Taking the long view, the technology of patient care has been in a continual process of change, although the rate of change may now be accelerated. Professional nurses have had to adapt before to new techniques and to master new kinds of equipment. In determining whether liability for negligence will be imposed in new contexts, the question will continue to be: Did the professional nurse depart from the standard of competent nursing practice with regard to the performance of the task or in her decision-making respecting the particular patient? The nurse will not be liable merely because harm has been suffered, but only because of the departure from the standard of the competent professional nurse.

ADDITIONAL MATTERS

This section is devoted to a discussion of 3 subjects, closely related to the activities and responsibilities of professional nurses, that indicate just a small portion of the variety of additional matters with which nurses should have some familiarity. These are child abuse laws, Good Samaritan laws and the principles of law related to the confidentiality of information acquired in the course of professional practice.

Child abuse laws impose a legal obligation to report instances of apparent child abuse to either law enforcement authorities, or public or voluntary agencies with responsibilities for the care of children. The laws vary considerably from state to state regarding the conduct that constitutes child abuse, the categories of persons and institutions required to make reports and to whom the reports are to be made. Almost every state has enacted a child abuse law and professional nurses are subject to the duty to report under practically all such laws. Along with the obligation to report, the law also provides a grant of immunity, to persons who render reports according to law, from any liability that might arise from an incorrect report, as long as the incorrect report was not inspired by malice.

Good Samaritan legislation is the term applied to the laws that have been enacted in almost every state to provide immunity from liability for harm arising out of the provision of emergency attention. Physicians, according to all Good Samaritan laws, and nurses, pursuant to many of them, are granted this immunity. These laws vary from state to state, not only with regard to the categories of persons provided with immunity, but also as to the language that describes the extent of immunity provided and the description of the situations in which the laws apply. The ostensible rationale for the enactment of Good Samaritan laws is to free the potential "Good Samaritan" from fear of liability for harm resulting from attention given to a person in an emergency and, thereby, encourage the furnishing of assistance. Immunity is not extended under most laws where injury is suffered by the individual in distress as the result of grossly negligent or willfully injurious conduct on the part of the person rendering the assistance. The laws do not apply to emergency care rendered in institutions.

It should be noted, in any discussion of Good Samaritan laws, that there is no body of data indicating that, prior to the enactment of such legislation, there was a considerable amount of litigation brought by injured persons against "Good Samaritans" for negligently rendered assistance in emergencies. There is also no data currently indicating that the enactment of the legislation, by freeing individuals from the risk of liability for negligence in the provision of emergency attention, has induced those persons to render assistance in emergencies who would not have been willing to furnish it without the existence of such laws.

Confidentiality, with regard to information obtained in performance of professional activities is an ethical principle recognized by many professions, including professional nursing. The nurse, according to the ethical code of the ANA, is not to make unwarranted disclosure of information learned through the care of her patients.

With regard to disclosure in court as a witness, only a handful of states recognize a privileged communication doctrine for testimony by a nurse, although more than half the states recognize it for testimony by physicians. According to the privileged communication doctrine, the patient or his representative, under certain conditions, may successfully object to the introduction at trial of testimony or other evidence regarding the patient's condition that was acquired within the confidential medical relationship.

Disclosure out of court of personal matter concerning a patient, without the patient's consent, to persons not involved in the patient's care, can provide the basis for liability for the nurse disclosing such matter. Such a disclosure may constitute, depending on its context, defamation or an invasion of the patient's privacy. In some situations, an out-of-court disclosure of confidential information may be privileged, because of the legitimate interest in the matter of the person to whom the disclosure is made and the responsibilities of the informant. However, the knowledge that liability could conceivably be imposed for improper disclosure should make the professional nurse acutely sensitive of her responsibility to exercise discretion when divulging information about patients to persons other than those engaged with her in the care of the patient. The law, in regard to issues relating to confidentiality and disclosure, varies from state to state and is extremely complex.

CONCLUSION

This chapter has only touched upon some of the large variety of legal matters with which the professional nurse must become acquainted in order both to meet her obligation to her patients and to protect herself from risks of legal difficulty. A professional nurse should keep informed about developments in the laws relating to the practice of nursing and the legal responsibilities of nurses, to the same extent that she maintains familiarity with developments in other aspects of professional nursing. The professional nurse can become familiar with the national and state legislation affecting the profession of nursing and the practice of professional nursing. There are many publications available which can assist the nurse considerably in meeting her needs for information on developments pertaining to her professional responsibilities.

A professional nurse who requires legal services for personal and work-related reasons should seek out a qualified attorney. In much the same way that a sick or injured person who treats himself, rather than seeking the assistance of a physician, increases the risks to himself, an individual involved in a situation dependent upon understanding of the law, who fails to secure the professional assistance of an attorney, must accept the risk of increasing his difficulty.

PROBLEMS

An attorney with experience in dealing with legal problems of hospitals and patient care institutions, or in litigating malpractice cases, would be ideally suited to lead the discussion of the chapter's content and the material described below. These problems are suggestions to the instructor.

1. Obtain copies of the definitions of medical practice and professional

nursing in the state licensing legislation, as well as other available items, such as opinions of the state attorney-general, regulations or rulings of the state boards, and joint statements of health organizations in the state, regarding nursing practice and specific procedures. Use this material to help develop the current functional scope of professional nursing practice in your state. (See the article by N. Hershey, "Scope of Nursing Practice," *American Journal of Nursing,* **66:**117-120, Jan. 1966.)

2. Obtain copies of the decision in *Goff v. Doctors General Hospital,* 333 P.2d 29 (1958), and discuss the nature of the standard of care, relative to the situation confronting the nurses described in the court's opinion.

3. Obtain copies of the Good Samaritan and child abuse laws of your state. Determine the nature of the reporting responsibility imposed upon the professional nurse under the child abuse law, and the extent to which she is insulated from liability for rendering the required report. Discuss and analyze the Good Samaritan law in terms of the persons provided immunity, the extent to which immunity is provided and the situations to which the law applies.

4. Obtain a copy of the decision in *Crowe v. Provost,* 374 S.W.2d 645 (1963). Use the facts of this case as a basis for discussing the range of responsibility of, and the standard of care applicable to, a nurse serving in a physician's office. (See the article by N. Hershey, "The Office Nurse," *American Journal of Nursing,* **65:**108-110, May, 1965.)

5. Obtain copies of the regulations for hospitals issued by your state hospital licensing agency. Survey the regulations to determine those that specifically or implicitly describe professional nursing responsibilities and establish standards of good nursing practice. Discuss the extent to which the nursing students have seen them implemented (and ignored) during their clinical affiliations.

6. Nurses are often called to the courts as witnesses. (a) What is meant by *adversary system?* (b) What are the *rules of evidence?* (c) What is the role of the *expert witness?*

SUGGESTED REFERENCES*

NURSING AND LAW

Bernzweig, E. P. *Nurse's Liability for Malpractice.* New York, McGraw-Hill, 1969.
* Creighton, H. *Law Every Nurse Should Know.* Philadelphia, Saunders, 1957.
Hayt, E., *et al. Law of Hospital and Nurse.* New York, Hospital Textbook, 1958.
Hershey, N. "The Law and the Nurse." A series of articles appearing in the *American Journal of Nursing.* (Monthly from Feb. 1962 until Jan. 1964, and bi-monthly since then.)
* Lesnik, M. J., and Anderson, B. E. *Nursing Practice and the Law.* Philadelphia, Lippincott, 1962.

* In each chapter all citations are footnoted and are not included here. All starred references are recommended for additional reading.

Medical Society of the State of New York, *et al. Joint Position Statements of the Medical Society of New York, New York State Nurses Association and Hospital Association of New York State.* New York, New York State Nurses Association, 1965.

Sarner, H. *Nurse and the Law.* Philadelphia, Saunders, 1968.

* Willeg, S. "Legal Considerations Regarding Drugs." *American Journal of Nursing,* **64:**126-131, June 1964.

LAW CONCERNING HOSPITALS AND PHYSICIANS

American Medical Association. *Citation.* A bi-weekly newsletter prepared by the Law Division of the AMA, Chicago, The Association.

Bernzweig, E. P. *Legal Aspects of PHS Medical Care.* Washington, D.C., Government Printing Office, 1966.

Health Law Center Division. *Hospital Law Manual.* Pittsburgh, Aspen Systems Corporation, 1959. Supplemented quarterly.

_____. *Problems in Hospital Law.* Pittsburgh, Aspen Systems Corporation, 1968.

* Horty, J. "Modern Hospital Law." A series of articles appearing in *The Modern Hospital.* Monthly since Jan. 1962.

Shartel, B. and Plant, M. L. *The Law of Medical Practice.* Springfield, Ill., Thomas, 1959.

CHAPTER

7

Relationships
and
Personal Growth

The ruling spirit in a profession is the desire to render a specialized helping service. In nursing, because of the nature of the work, you will have one of the greatest opportunities to attain this objective. As a professional person the spirit of service shall motivate your efforts rather than only the desire for financial gain. To serve well, it is essential to maintain good human relationships.

Your association with individual people and groups will vary somewhat according to the particular field of nursing you enter, but you will always find it necessary to make adjustments. Sometimes you may have to give up your own wishes graciously and adapt yourself and your ideas. It is possible for you to work wisely with others to change circumstances for the benefit of all concerned. Much of your success as a nurse, a citizen and a person depends on the kind of adjustment that you make to people and to circumstances, as well as on the way others will adjust to you.

Regardless of what field you enter—hospital, occupational health, public health nursing, private practice, office nursing, nursing education, or any other—you may become so engrossed in your work that you forget the existence outside the profession of certain contacts that are essential to the satisfactory fulfillment of spiritual, physical, mental and social needs. Your problem, then, is to make a "design for living" which will include the continuance of worth-while relationships with church, home, school, community, friends and patients, as well as with professional colleagues.

The best time to lay the foundation for desirable relationships, as you know, is during your student days. This time is a period for learning, for personal growth, and for knowing self and forming self for the type of nurse that you want to be. Have you tried to develop good relations with your fellow students, the members of the administrative and instructional staffs, and the other health personnel with whom you have had contact? Have you contributed your best toward making the social life of the school desirable in every way? Are you a good school-citizen, bearing your fair share (or even a little more) of the burden of student organizations and other school programs?

Of course you will want to succeed in carrying out your nursing responsibilities. But, as a nurse, your general influence can be very important, because people will look to you to make constructive contributions to your profession and to the community in which you live. Therefore, you have a 2-fold reason to plan every phase of your life with the aim of deriving from it the greatest possible benefit for yourself and others, not only for the present, but also for the future.

This chapter is a review of some of the major essentials in establishing and maintaining sound professional and personal relationships.

PROFESSIONAL RELATIONSHIPS

Relationship With the Patient and His Family

No 2 persons are exactly alike, and in any field of nursing you will find that you need to be prepared to understand, appreciate and adjust yourself to persons who differ in racial characteristics, cultural background and personality. It will be necessary to familiarize yourself with the likes and the dislikes of patients and to adapt yourself to them while assisting each patient to make the adaptations necessary for his welfare. You will find it necessary to accustom yourself to differing viewpoints. If you are able to do these things, you will inspire that confidence in yourself as a nurse and a person without which it is difficult to achieve success.

What patients think of you is important. One who is ill is particularly susceptible to suggestions; you may have much to do with influencing for good the thoughts, the attitudes and the actions of those with whom you come in contact. You also will be in a position to influence their families and friends. With this function of guidance in mind, it is all the more important for you to watch carefully your own attitudes and actions.

Attitudes, feelings, and what a patient thinks, says, or does at any time are not nearly so meaningful in helping the nurse to understand the patient as are the things which cause him to think, behave and speak as he does. To understand the patient and his behavior at the moment, it is important to try to learn the past experiences, the present pressures and the motives that cause his present behavior. So viewed and understood, behavior that may be displeasing can be accepted and dealt with better. Making a patient feel welcome is often all that is needed to gain his confidence and to put him at ease.

Study each patient and learn what he is like. This is the first principle to apply if you are to give him real help. Studying him means learning something about his home environment, social background, education, occupation, religion, likes, dislikes and interests. This will lead you to treat him as a personality and to show him that you consider him as such, with human rights and privileges, and not as "just another case" who is known perhaps only by a case or a room number. It is important that you be friendly, cheerful and pleasant in all your relations, but it is equally important, as you know, not to be familiar. It is genuine feeling that counts, not merely the exterior manner of friendliness toward the patient and his family.

General health education, explaining procedures used in the patient's care and answering his and his family's questions honestly and wisely are daily responsibilites of the nurse. Often the difference between a cooperative and an uncooperative patient, or between the effectiveness or ineffectiveness of a treatment, is dependent upon whether the nurse has explained what is about to be done and why. It has also been found that treatment can be made more effective by letting the patient participate in certain aspects of his care or treatment. For example, a study reported by Tryon shows that when the nurse attempts to find out how the patient feels about a procedure and encourages the patient to participate in its administration, he appears to accept the treatment better and the outcome is more effective.[1]

As you know, the patient's state of mind or spirit is often of prime importance in the recovery of physical health. He may require information about his condition, or reassurance regarding it, and you should neither alarm him unnecessarily nor reassure him falsely. For example, an emotional, high-strung, fearful patient may need careful and tactful preparation for surgery or for certain treatments. The nurse can do much for the patient by her awareness of his needs and by her thoughtful explanations and answers to his questions. By encouraging the patient to express his questions and by listening to him, the nurse can often find out what his real concerns are and base her help on relieving these, instead of giving ineffective reassurance.

Occasionally, a nurse is called on to provide for the religious care of a patient who is very ill. The nurse need not hesitate to call a clergyman. Often he may give comfort and solace which will improve the patient not only spiritually but also mentally and physically. It is important to know what is required by the different religious denominations in case of death or the nearness of death.

Sometimes death comes suddenly and unexpectedly. Sometimes a patient refuses to see a clergyman. What a great privilege it is under such cir-

---

[1] P. A. Tryon and R. C. Leonard, "The Effect of the Patient's Participation on the Outcome of a Nursing Procedure." *Nursing Forum,* **3(2):**79-89, 1964.

cumstances — and a great challenge — for the nurse to help the patient die at peace with himself and God! How important it is that the nurse herself shall have thought through the great questions of life and death in order that she may help others in this time of need!

If the patient dies at home, you are expected to take charge until the undertaker arrives, to comfort the bereaved family and even, if necessary, to make the funeral arrangements. All these matters should be arranged in an understanding, sympathetic, and gracious manner. You may need to take over temporary management quietly but firmly. See that the family eats properly and help them in every way possible to accept the inevitable situation. You are the key person in this situation and have an important responsibility to discharge. However, do not keep the members of the family from performing services if that is their desire. Making arrangements for the funeral gives them a feeling of usefulness and allays grief somewhat at this time.

Pleasant relationships must be established not only with patients but also with their families and friends and with work personnel wherever care is being provided. If you are nursing in a hospital or extended care facility, you may not be thrown into such close and constant touch with the patient's family and friends as you will be if you are nursing in a patient's home. Nevertheless, the relationships with the families and the friends of patients should be as carefully considered in the hospital as in the home. Families and friends, under strain, are likely to be critical. They probably will make impossible suggestions and ask endless questions, but you can avoid much friction if, instead of resenting this interference, you deal with them kindly though firmly, thus inspiring in them the same confidence that you wish the patient to have in you. Again, as with the patient, attempt to learn what the real concerns and fears of the family are by careful listening — and then help them deal with these. This will go far to relieve tense situations. Remember that patients and families have rights, too, and need to be able to participate in their own care to the extent that they can, as well as to feel that they are being treated with understanding and respect.

Maids, waiters, elevator boys and janitors in homes, hospitals, or other institutions in which you work are more influenced by you than you realize. Since you may be setting standards of conduct for many of them, try to realize how you are doing this. Good education is manifested largely by courteous conduct to those who serve you. We all need to learn to recognize the dignity of each individual person, valuable in himself and in his particular sphere of activity, and treat each one accordingly. If you do this, you will acquire a pleasing and useful art and also develop an important phase of a sound philosophy of life.

Relationship With Colleagues

In your relationships with members of your own profession, you will associate with 2 general groups: those to whom you are responsible, and your coworkers. Loyalty is all-important. This includes a willingness to make some sacrifices for the good of all and to cooperate with your colleagues. To make this possible, good nature and even good temperament, tolerance, cheerfulness, unselfishness and understanding must be cultivated, and such traits as envy, jealousy, rivalry and distrust must be weeded out. If present, these traits will make you less amenable to the constructive criticism of coworkers and officers of administration, less capable of cooperation and therefore less efficient.

In your association with those to whom you are responsible and who are directing you in your work, you can manifest your interest by attempting to understand and follow their directions and by accepting and profiting from their evaluation of you and your performance. Equally important is your willingness and ability to adjust yourself quickly to the routines of the organization where you work. If you accept, without faultfinding, its policies and practices as well as the facilities which it offers, you are bound to fit well into the situation. If policies and practices need to be changed, make suggestions for their revision through the appropriate administrative channels. Continuous faultfinding and griping are merely the lazy man's way of "getting around" thinking constructively to solve a difficult situation. Until you have earned your right to make such suggestions by demonstrating your competence and developing an understanding of the underlying problems and their appropriate solution, your evaluation should be reserved. A very important principle to remember, if you hope to establish good working relationships, is to go directly to those in charge or to those that generally work with the type of problem that concerns you, such as a staff committee on nursing practice or one on personnel policies, rather than gossip about it or make disparaging remarks to others.

Knowing the total scheme of an organization and where you fit therein will lessen the danger of establishing and maintaining poor cooperative relationships. If you know your place in an organization, you will be less likely to take your problems or recommendations to the wrong group or person.

In your relations with your colleagues, remember that each person has obligations and responsibilities as well as privileges and rights. If you keep this in mind, you will have little difficulty in establishing a spirit of good will and in gaining the favorable opinion of your associates. However, if you are not careful of the rights of others, you may find yourself always forwarding your own vested interests to the exclusion of those of others. For example, habitual laxness in little things, such as tardiness in attending meetings or thoughtlessness of others, may have unfortunate consequences. Likewise, constant criticism of the work of your colleagues will break down respect for you and for the profession which you represent. Those who are continuously looking at and evaluating their own methods are less likely to criticize others.

You also will associate with other members of your chosen field in professional organizations. Since these are treated at length in Part Four, it suffices here merely to mention that the same qualities of loyalty and consideration required in your relationship to other nurses while at work are the qualities that should be manifested in your association with the members of your professional organizations.

Relationship With the Medical Profession[2]

A basic principle is that the patient's confidence in the physician and the nurse promotes recovery. The physician and the nurse are partners in developing this confidence about the medical and nursing care received by the patient. For instance, if a patient or his family complains about the physician's apparent neglect, incompetence, or lack of interest, you can explain the situation if a reassuring explanation is possible; if it is not, you probably can relieve their anxiety by promising to discuss the matter with the physician and then doing so. Sympathizing with them in their anxiety or even taking part with them against the physician, yet neither telling the physician about the situation nor attempting to solve the difficulty, will not remove the problem.

The physician expects you to be conscientious in carrying out his instructions for the proper care of the patient. It is well to familiarize yourself with the varying methods of different physicians, as this knowledge will be of great value in maintaining smooth relationships. Nurses and physicians have a common interest in the prevention and care of disease and health restoration. They need the assistance and the cooperation of each other.

What Should You Do if Convinced of the Physician's Incompetence? In any discussion of the problems that come up in the relationship of the nurse to the physician, the question immediately arises as to the proper action to take if you should become convinced of inefficiency or malpractice on his part. No one formula will serve on all occasions, but in any event it is obvious that considerable tact and judgment must be employed. No nurse should openly defame or criticize a physician. If you are employed in a hospital, report the problem to the proper authority (that is, to the director of nursing service), who can help you evaluate the situation and, if indicated, will report the incident to the administrator of the hospital. In making such a report it is important to give the reasons which have convinced you that the physician is carrying on a dishonorable practice. If you are a nurse in public health, you would report such a situation to your supervisor, who in turn would take up the matter with the proper authority in the organization.

With the increasing professional responsibility that the nurse carries for patient care in clinics, extended care facilities and community health agencies, the relationship of her work to that of the physician is changing. In these work situations, because the nurse frequently carries the chief

[2] See also the discussion in Chapter 4, "Responsibility for Nursing Practice," concerning the patient-nurse-physician relationship.

burden of responsibility for the service provided, it becomes even more important that her relationship to the physician is a sharing one; that is, the nurse needs to have an awareness of the aims of medical care, as well as of the needs of the patients and their families, and must work collaboratively with the physicians involved in achieving these aims. These collaborative skills can be developed by the nurse who has a broad educational background and a real interest in providing the very best nursing care possible.

Relationship With Allied Professions

It is necessary to cooperate with all members of the health team: physicians, all personnel in hospitals, other health agencies and clergy. In most instances the nurse, by circumstance, is the coordinator of the health team, although the physician is the team leader.

Characteristics that destroy or hinder the establishment of good relationships are hot temper, sensitiveness and touchiness, and resentment or holding resentment. Characteristics that help to develop or maintain good relationships are a sense of fairness, a spirit of acceptance, a sense of humor, insight into and understanding of human nature, self-control, respect for the individuality of the people with whom one is working and awareness of self and therefore of others.

Good relations are maintained when people feel that you are perfectly fair; that you are just; that you are not eager to vindicate yourself, even at the expense of fairness; and that you are absolutely honest, even at the cost of apologies or explanations.

We all have to put up with much in this life. We need to tolerate the failings, and even the stupidities and sometimes the virtues, of those with whom we work. A sense of humor is so necessary that it often has been called the "saving sense." We need to be able to put ourselves in the place of others frequently; that is, we need to have an insight into their difficulties. Without empathy and insight we cannot maintain good relationships. Nor can we do it unless we can make each one with whom we associate feel his power and try to bring out the good in him.

When you are working in a hospital, a neighborhood clinic, an extended care facility, or another type of community organization, you will wish to establish good relationships with the social workers, the dietitians and all who are working in the interest of the patient.

If you are a nurse in public health you will associate daily with teachers, social workers and representatives of official and non-official welfare and health agencies. In the course of her work, the nurse in public health has contacts with such agencies as family and child welfare organizations, nursery schools, juvenile courts, relief agencies and civic organizations. A close working relationship with these groups brings about more effective service, preventing duplications and gaps.

One of the ways in which you can develop closer working relationships with members of other professions is by actually knowing them and by knowing what they look like. Therefore, you might try to make a special effort to attend meetings in which the various professions are represented. Inviting members of other professions to certain of your meetings will help also in maintaining good relationships with other disciplines. You also can visit your councils of social agencies if you are in an urban community, or the local department of public welfare, if you are in a rural community, in order to find out what agencies operate in your community, the nature of their activities, and to become personally acquainted with the individuals employed.

Relationship With the Community

It may be well for you to consider your relationship to the community both as an individual citizen and as a member of the nursing profession.

What services do you owe to your community? The fundamental services, of course, regardless of your particular nursing field, are preventing disease, promoting health and caring for the sick. As a nurse, you are a prime factor in making the public health-conscious. Education in health is all-important in the contemporary scheme of affairs, and you are in a position to teach health by precept and by example. The nurse in public health spreads this doctrine in her daily work, but you need not enter the field of public health to serve your community in this way. Through all your professional, civic and social relationships, you have the opportunity to teach health and to build up the social standards and values so necessary for the advancement of health.

Whatever your field of nursing, you are in a position to influence social welfare criteria, because nursing deals primarily with human relationships, and it provides an excellent opportunity to aid in the development of high moral and social norms. Toward this end you work with other socially minded persons to overcome unfortunate social conditions through legislation or other means. Bad social situations may be relieved by helping key persons involved to become aware of the underlying causative factors and by offering a feasible plan, based on a study of the situation, to improve conditions. To accomplish both of these objectives, it is important that those in the situation can take part in the planning, the thinking, and the action.

This matter of establishing good community relationships is more difficult if you are settling in a new and strange locality. Your prestige as a neighbor may be enhanced because you are a nurse, but for that very reason the community may be most observant of you. From the moment of your arrival, you will have to show by your appearance, your manner, your speech and your conduct that you are worthy of your profession. The impression you make will fashion not only the community's opinion of you and of your profession, but also its reception of the program you hope to inaugurate. Therefore, your every action, whether in professional or in social relationships, must be performed with this in mind. You have a responsibility for maintaining the social status of the nursing profession and for establishing a status enabling you to carry out effectively what the public expects of you: prevention of disease, promotion of health and recovery from sickness. In a new community it is good practice in the first year to take advantage of the social or the professional groups to which you are eligible—including civic or political groups, as well as your local nursing association—and thus explore the available sources for acquaintanceship. Another year it may seem more suitable perhaps to limit memberships to those groups that yield most pleasure and profit.

PERSONAL QUALITIES AND GROWTH

Interdependence of many elements form the personality of an individual. Many of these elements are discussed in this chapter. Although they are discussed separately, it should be recognized that they actually cannot be separated so readily when looking at the total person.

Poise

Under the general heading of poise may be considered many of those personal attributes necessary to you in your professional and social life. Health, mental and physical, is a prerequisite because of the bearing it has on your appearance, your personality, your endurance, and the quality of your work. Other important qualities affecting poise are self-acceptance, acceptance of others, and the right kind of pride. A knowledge of etiquette, a gracious manner and a mastery of social usages are also important, as is culture, in the deepest sense of that word.

How are you to continue to mold yourself into a person of whom you and your profession can be proud—one who can take her place competently and effectively in professional or social activities? It would be wise to begin with a sort of self-survey, studying yourself to know what traits of appearance and personality you now possess, which ones you need to acquire, and which ones you want to overcome.

Physical, Mental, and Spiritual Health

In any consideration of appearance or personality, health plays a leading role, for without it neither appearance nor personality can be at its best. The importance of abounding health for professional achievement and successful social relationships is self-evident and indisputable. Poor health, as you well know, makes its presence felt, and, what is more, it usually is seen in one's looks, skin, hair, posture, and especially in one's attitude toward life, self and others. Good health, on the other hand, makes itself equally apparent. Since good health is so often a matter of care, it is well to take the utmost precaution with regard to this precious attribute in order that you may reap all the benefits attendant on it and avoid anything that might contribute to ill health, through willful excess or negligence.

Much of your life will be spent in securing and maintaining sound human relationships, professional as well as social, and there are no relationships that do not suffer when one is affected by ill health. While you are teaching others that rest and sleep, proper food, correct posture, annual physical examinations, proper clothing, and sufficient exercise are not only important but necessary, you also need to try to "practice what you preach."

The health of the mind is as important as the health of the body, and for somewhat the same reasons. Mental and physical health are interdependent, the one affecting the other. Faulty adjustment to the problems of life is the main cause of mental ill health, so continued good health may be expected if the adjustments made are sound. This will be possible if you recognize a problem when it confronts you, consider it calmly and carefully, then make the necessary adjustments. Fortunately, the maintenance of mental health is, for the most part, within your own control if you keep your interests alive, varied and growing, if you multiply your social associates, if you know yourself and how you relate to others and if you know when, where and how to secure counsel when your problems become too great for you to solve alone.

Interests play a large part in the control of mental health. The sources about which they naturally revolve are your family, your friends, your community, your health, your education, your career, your recreation, and your religion, which, in the last analysis, is the integrating center to aid you in living a balanced life.

The nurse who is truly religious will understand the need of doing what she can to help to cure spiritual illness as well as to maintain her own state of spiritual health. A favorite prayer is, "God grant me the serenity to accept things I cannot change, courage to change things I can, and wisdom to know the difference."[3] Another favorite prayer is:

Teach me, my Lord, to be sweet and gentle in all the events of life —
in disappointments,
in the thoughtlessness of others,
in the insincerity of those I trusted,
in the unfaithfulness of those on whom I relied.
Let me put myself aside,
to think of the happiness of others,
to hide my little pains and heartaches, so that I may be the only one to suffer from them.
Teach me to profit by the suffering that comes across my path.
Let me so use it that it may mellow me, not harden nor embitter me,
that it may make me patient, not irritable,
that it may make me broad in my forgiveness, not narrow, haughty and overbearing.

[3] Sister Mary Berenice Beck, *Handmaid of the Divine Physician*, Milwaukee, Bruce, 1952, p. 35.

*May no one be less good for having come within my influence. No one less pure,
less true, less kind, less noble for having been a fellow-traveler in our journey
toward Eternal Life.*

*As I go my rounds from one distraction to another, let me whisper from time to time
a word of love to Thee. May my life be lived in the supernatural, full of power
for good, and strong in its purpose of sanctity.*

Closely related to your religious and other interests are your emotional responses to the persons with whom you work and the activities that you carry on. The proper utilization of emotions is essential for mental health. Friendliness, elation, gratitude, admiration, courage, pride and happiness are emotions which, on the whole, when used properly, create or maintain good mental health. Depression, boredom, hate, jealousy, fear, shame, remorse and unhappiness, if recognized in relation to the particular situation where these occur, may help you to understand the reality of the situation and influence you to do something to improve it. When these latter emotions become chronic, they cause much misery in life and frequently prevent the experience of more desirable emotions. Being negative qualities, they lead to nothing worth while or constructive. To give 2 examples of the bad effects of these emotions: persistent depression suppresses inclinations to reach desirable ends, and jealousy makes its possessor narrow and selfish. On the other hand, anger, for example, can be put to a constructive end at times and may arouse the angered person to improve a poor situation. Or, as another example, fear of an accident may cause a person to take preventive measures.

Health — physical, mental and spiritual — is not only essential for your feeling of physical well-being, your contentment and your professional achievement, but it is also basic to the success of your social relationships, for it has a great influence on you. Personality is evidenced by the way that you influence others and get along with them. It is the combination of many elements, including every trait discussed thus far: what you do and how you do things, the kind of thinking you do, the decisions you make, your emotional control, your personal appearance, your dress, manner, voice, language, conversation, interests, and all the long list of traits usually considered essential to success.

You conduct yourself so that others will be pleased; they will listen to what you have to say, enjoy being with you, seek you as a leader as well as a follower, invite you to join their societies, ask you for personal and professional advice, and believe in you as a friend and a professional colleague.

Personal Appearance

Today everyone has access to TV programs, literature and instruction on all aspects of personal appearance. It hardly seems necessary to mention it. However, a brief discussion on this vital quality is included for the purpose of emphasis.

There are few requirements of more immediate importance in your daily contact with others than a pleasing appearance, one which reflects your inner self and indicates your possession of the qualities mentioned above. First impressions count for so much that none of us can afford ever to present an appearance that will make those with whom we associate think of us as other than we would like. Your appearance depends to a great extent on the state of your health (as pointed out in the preceding section), on strength, on endurance, on being rested, on cleanliness and on attention to small details. Health and cleanliness give you good hair, good teeth, good skin and good posture. You can build on these by studying yourself, thus discovering your good features and making the most of them.

Your vitality, vivaciousness, readiness for action, interest in others and in your own work, and fertility of ideas, accompanying a good healthy appearance, go far toward making you attractive. Sometimes the most attractive persons are those who, while not beautiful, are well-groomed, expressive and vital.

Good posture is not only necessary to a pleasing appearance, but it is also an aid to good health. Quite aside from posture's important bearing on health, you know from personal observation how poor posture detracts from an otherwise pleasing appearance, while good posture can make of an otherwise average individual a striking figure.

Art of Conversation

In nursing, your relationships with your professional and social associates need to be pleasant ones. For this purpose the art of conversation is an important asset.

Conversational ability is a necessary attribute in your social life, so that you may be at ease with a dinner partner or with a group where it may be necessary for you to keep the talk going, and also in professional life where you will use it constantly to convey your ideas and thoughts.

Every day you spend a great deal of time talking with others. Anything that claims so much attention must be made worth while, and therefore it should be done well. Furthermore, conversation is the ordinary means of communication between people. The ability to make friends and to be successful in your dealings with others depends in a large measure on your success as a conversationalist. This does not mean that you must be a scintillating talker capable of impressing your listeners with how much you know. It does mean learning to express your ideas logically. It is equally important to be a good listener. A good conversationalist is one who keeps others talking, not one who monopolizes the conversation.

Everyone has conversational ability to a certain degree, but, like all natural aptitudes, it varies in different people. However, perfection is gained through personal effort, which includes persistent observance and constant application of the rules of good conversation. These are not hard-and-fast rules to be memorized and then observed rigorously. Instead, like all rules of behavior, they should be absorbed, so that they will become so familiar that you apply them instinctively and inconspicuously.

Thoughtfulness of others is the fundamental principle. Remember that everyone has some special interests which he likes to talk about. Give him the opportunity, and the conversation is launched. To keep it going, be interested in what he has to say and show this interest. A conversation is not a monologue but rather an exchange of thoughts. It resembles a game of tennis in which the phrase or the sentence is the ball served, returned, and moved back and forth. Therefore, be ready to contribute your share toward keeping the game going.

Here, too, is where a broad range of interests comes into play. The nurse must be able to converse on a variety of subjects, most of which are outside the realm of nursing, if she is to meet the needs of her patients and to communicate successfully with her family and friends.

Most people are interested in their jobs, their families, their hobbies and current events. Since there is no 1 topic of conversation suitable for every occasion, prepare yourself to talk on a variety of subjects. Once started, a conversation usually keeps going of its own accord. One thought leads to another, and the original topic is sometimes forgotten. Unless you are trying to decide on something, or have a special reason for pursuing one particular subject, such digressions are desirable, for they keep the talk alive and the interest fresh. If you want to keep the thought going, avoid making positive declarations that seem to settle a question irrevocably and preclude further discussion.

Knowing when to talk is fully as important as knowing what to say. Do your share, but do not monopolize the conversation. Often you will find that your share consists in being an appreciative audience while someone else talks. ˙

Analyze some tiresome conversations you have heard, and you probably will find 1 or more of the following defects: boasting, gossiping, incessant shop-talking, especially in the presence of patients and non-nurse friends, including minute details, correcting others and talking too much. There are also many other faults.

If you keep in mind that thoughtfulness and consideration of others are the bases of good conversation, you will not go far wrong. Here, as elsewhere in life, the more that you can forget yourself in thinking of others, the more successful you will be.

How can you possibly master the art of conversation without an adequate vocabulary? Those who always have the right word for the right thought and can use the word in a correct phrase have an invaluable gift. You are expected to make reports, to explain, to cheer and possibly to amuse. For all this you need a knowledge of words. To express yourself and to understand others you must have an adequate vocabulary. As you know, you are a teacher as well as a nurse. As a nurse you teach the proper care in sickness and the prevention of illness. You cannot accomplish this function unless you can present your thoughts logically and in the proper terms.

A short period given each day to the study of words will be of value for the later use you will make of it, and it will be interesting in itself. Anyone who has devoted spare moments to words—their derivation and their connotation—has found it a fascinating pastime. Without a good choice of words you are helpless, no matter how great may be your talents and your thoughts, for without words these must remain inarticulate. Make a point of checking on pronunciation, as the same word goes through a series of changes in pronunciation and shades of meaning in the course of years. Words, like clothes and methods, become dated and pass out of general use. In many cases, the general or the orientation tests which you have taken include some measure of your reading and speaking vocabulary. By inquiring of your teachers or counselors you may learn more about this skill and whether you are one of those who need to make special efforts for improvement.

Art of Gracious Manners

Gracious manners are sometimes referred to as "social usage." Social usage is based on consideration for the comfort and the happiness of others. A bare knowledge of the rules of etiquette will mean nothing unless you have the deep-laid qualities of courtesy, unselfishness and self-control. Possession of these qualities and application of the rules of etiquette make personal contacts smoother, and the life of the nurse is made up of one such contact after another.

The knowledge of social customs and a courteous manner will be of invaluable assistance to you in your professional activities and social life and even may be the means of securing positions for you. If a well-mannered nurse and another nurse who is equally capable but less charming in manner apply for the same position, the former is almost certain to be chosen.

Use of Tact. Tact is the art of being sensitive to people and situations. Tact is a prime requisite in one who has perfected the art of conversation, for tact tells you of what to speak, to whom to address yourself and when silence is best. Tact reaches out beyond conversation and beyond individuals to situations. Its presence, in no matter how difficult a situation, makes one sure that things will work out in the end. The nurse, whose profession requires her to see individuals and their families at periods of crisis in their lives, needs more tact than most other workers.

Tact is a combination of alertness, sympathy and resourcefulness. It puts others at their ease and relieves strained situations. Tact must be unobtrusive, however, or else it does not deserve the name. As is true of any phase of good manners, so it is true of real tact: it comes from the heart. It cannot be only on the surface, or it will fail when the real test presents itself. Tact relies on patience and charity and on an optimistic outlook that allows you full control of your temper. No one who blurts out something in anger for which he is sorry later can be said to possess true tact.

Tact should prevent inadvertent slips of the tongue, since the ignorance, the impatience and the absent-mindedness that are the chief causes of these errors, are not resorted to by the tactful person. However, if an embarrassing mistake should be made, tact immediately comes to your aid in relieving the situation. At times it is possible to laugh away the slip by turning the joke on yourself. If this is not possible, then the simplest and best action to take is that of making a sincere, but simple, apology. Long explanations usually serve only to make the matter worse.

Culture as a Personal Asset. We frequently hear patients say that they desire a "cultured nurse." The word "cultured" sometimes is misinterpreted. Some use it to describe someone who has managed to accumulate many scraps of information about many things and then proceeds to show others at all times how well informed he is. This is not culture. Culture goes deeper. Culture is a basic quality that coordinates all other personal traits. It is a normal, natural refinement that has nothing to do with wealth. It is a deep-seated characteristic, not something superficial to be used and laid aside at will. Real culture withstands strain and all social tests. It leaves a person humble and understanding even after glamorous or difficult experiences. It involves ideals and sensitivity to beauty and to human nature. It is an integral part of a person's life and personality. One definition of culture is, "the ability and the habit of feeling at ease in the presence of anyone and of making anyone feel at ease in your presence." A cultured woman is an educated woman and one whose values in life are truth, goodness and beauty.

Leisure Activities

An important problem for all of us is how to plan the use of leisure time. The wise use of leisure not only brings relaxation, recreation, or self-improvement, but it is reflected in the performance of workaday tasks. If you devote your spare hours to the most worth-while activities, you will bring to your work a refreshed point of view and an increased capacity for daily tasks.

Over and above the effect your leisure-time activities have on you as a person are those they have on your profession. The manner in which you conduct yourself in your leisure time, the friends that you make, and the accomplishments that you acquire may help or hinder the progress of the nursing profession.

Not all leisure activities need be connected with your work. It is wise to form friendships with interesting people outside of the nursing profession. The more varied the range of your interests and the more extensive your circle of nonprofessional friends, the more easily you will be able to avoid "shop talk," which seems to be some nurses' only topic of conversation. This does not mean, of course that you should not be active in your professional organizations or have close friends among your nursing associates, but merely that you also should seek other friends if you expect to be a well-rounded professional person.

There are many organizations which will be only too glad to welcome you and offer you the activities and the contacts which you seek. You will find interesting and congenial companions through participation in programs offered by church groups and local clubs such as study clubs, women's clubs, and lecture and literary societies. To satisfy more specialized interests you will find, in every community, dramatic groups and choral clubs. Other clubs of national scope with large memberships are the Business and Professional Women's Club, the Rotary Club, the League of Women Voters, the American Association of University Women, the American Association of Retired Persons, the National Retired Teachers Association, the National Association of Retired Civil Service Employees and, for nurse veterans, the American Legion. In such organizations you can participate in activities which will contribute to recreational growth and development. Most of them offer cultural programs and adult courses, providing for growth and development. One point worth remembering is that it is unwise to take on too many obligations and activities. Careful selection is important. Nurses sometimes find themselves so tied up with general club activities that they do not have time for their own professional organization meetings and for casual activities.

Aside from group activities, there are many ways in which you may enjoy leisure hours alone. Music, handicrafts and reading newspapers and other literature are old standbys. Reading is made even more interesting if it is done with a purpose. Your special interest may take the form of a home-study course in some subject that always has been of particular interest to you, or it may be in pursuance of a hobby. Hobbies are invaluable, and there is sure to be one or several which will fascinate you. Your fancy may run to writing, sewing, raising flowers, or cooking, or it may incline you toward amateur astronomy, stamp or shell collecting, photography, antique hunting or raising tropical fish. You can enjoy some of these hobbies no matter where you live, how small the space or how limited your time and money.

In considering the use of leisure time, an item that cannot be overlooked is further education. It would be wise to use part of your leisure in attending school.[4]

LIVING A WELL-BALANCED LIFE

The opportunity to live a well-balanced life is important if you expect to do your best.

To maintain balanced living as a nurse, a citizen, and a fully developed person you need to establish fine social and professional relationships. To

[4] See Chapter 16, "Continued Education for Nurses."

do this it is presupposed that you have a good understanding of your own functions, an appreciation of the responsibilities of others as they relate to yours and a knowledge of the psychology of living well.

Poise is essential for maintaining fine human relationships. It is determined by physical and mental health, personal appearance, conversation, self-acceptance, sensitivity to people and situations, good manners and, above all, ethical ideals and practices. Other factors which influence social and professional associations and relationships are living conditions and leisure-time activities.

As a final consideration, you might reflect on those traits which are going to aid you to make the most of your opportunities. If you cultivate the art of conversation, if you are tactful and thoughtful toward others, if you know and practice the rules of etiquette and if you acquire the all-important quality of social poise, you will be doing much toward assuring a successful and a beneficial life for the present and the future.

PROBLEMS

1. (a) Differentiate ethics and etiquette. (b) What considerations should nurses observe relative to smoking and drinking? (c) Outline how you think the problem of drug use by students should be handled.

2. Plan a symposium on "Interrelationships in Nursing," using the following or similar topics: (a) Suggestions for Improving Relationships with the Medical Profession; (b) Essentials to Consider in Maintaining Cooperative Relationships with Other Helping Professions in the Field of Health; (c) Considerations in Establishing Good Community Relationships; (d) Factors that Promote Sound Relationships with Nurse Colleagues; (e) Practices Useful for Maintaining Workable and Pleasant Relationships with Patients and Their Families.

3. (a) What constitutes "shop talk"? (b) Suggest some ways in which "talking shop" may be overcome in a group of nurses. (c) What is the difference between "talking shop" and carrying on an intelligent professional conversation? (d) Give illustrations of when appropriate conversations on a professional topic can be of the very best type of conversation.

4. How does your mode of living influence your professional and social contacts?

5. The nurse may sometimes find herself in a tight spot when she is asked about a diagnosis or prognosis. (a) How much of the "facts" may she reveal (b) Should a patient or relatives be told the diagnosis of terminal cancer by the nurse?

6. (a) What is your recreational plan for this year? (b) for next summer?

7. What advantages would you derive from membership in (a) the Young Democrat's Club or the Young Republican's Club? (b) Make a list of professional, social and civic clubs for both men and women that are available in your community in which you might participate now and after graduation.

8. (a) How does fatigue affect your social and professional relationships? (b) What can be done to overcome fatigue?

9. Discuss with your fellow-students the questions that you believe should be included in a self-survey to determine how you rate as an all-round person, citizen and potential professional worker.

10. What suggestions do you have for maintaining good communication and cooperative relationships between the patient, the nurse, the physician and other members of the helping professions in the health field?

SUGGESTED REFERENCES*

COMMUNICATIONS: GENERAL

* Craytor, J. K. "Talking With Persons Who Have Cancer." *American Journal of Nursing*, **69**:744-748, Apr. 1969.
* Lambertsen, E. C. "Let Others Extend Eyes and Ears of the Nurse." *Modern Hospital*, **109**:140, Nov. 1967.
Lockerby, F. K. *Communication for Nurses*. St. Louis, Mosby, 1968.
Slavens, M. K. "Language: Communications in Interpersonal Relationships." *AORN Journal*, **7**:74-77, Jan. 1968.
Spiegel, A. D. "Questions of Hospital Patients—Unasked and Unanswered." *Postgraduate Medicine*, **43**:215-218, Feb. 1968.
* Strikwerda, G. G. "Are You Really Listening?" *American Association of Industrial Nurses Journal*, **15**:11-12, Dec. 1967.
* Theis, C., *et al.* "Three Factors that Affect Practice: Communication, Assignments, Attitudes." *American Journal of Nursing*, **68**:1478-1482, July 1968.

NURSE-PATIENT-PHYSICIAN RELATIONSHIPS

Alman, B. "Patients Participate in Nursing Care Conferences." *American Journal of Nursing*, **67**:2331-2334, Nov. 1967.
* Armiger, Sister Bernadette. "Reprise and Dialogue." *Nursing Outlook*, **16**:26-28, Oct. 1968.
Bergman, A. "A Shared Experience." *International Nursing Review*, **14**:39-42, Sept./Oct. 1967.
Berkowitz, P. and Berkowitz, N. S. "The Jewish Patient in the Hospital." *American Journal of Nursing*, **67**:2335-2337, Nov. 1967.
* Cerdes, L. "The Confused and Delirious Patient." *American Journal of Nursing*, **68**:1228-1233, June 1968.
* De Jean, S. "Empathy: A Necessary Ingredient of Care." *American Journal of Nursing*, **68**:559-560, Mar. 1968.
* Ewell, C. M. Jr. "What Patients Really Think About Nursing Care." *Modern Hospital*, **109**:106-108, Dec. 1967.
Fletcher, G. P. "Legal Aspects of the Decision Not to Prolong Life." *Journal of the American Medical Association*, **203**:65-68, Jan. 1968.
Francis, G. M. *Promoting Psychological Comfort*. Dubuque, Wm. C. Brown, 1968.
Frenay, Sister Agnes Clare, "Helping Students Work with the Aging." *Nursing Outlook*, **16**:44-46, July 1968.
Glaser, B. G. and Straus, A. L. *Time for Dying*. Chicago, Aldine, 1968.

---

* In each chapter all citations are footnoted and are not included here. All starred references are recommended for additional reading.

* Goldsborough, J. "Involvement." *American Journal of Nursing*, **69**:66-68, Jan. 1969.

Gould, G. T. "The Nurse-Patient Relationship: A Monologue." *Nursing Clinics of North America*, **3**:129-134, Mar. 1968.

Gozzi, E. K., *et al.* Gaps in Doctor-Patient Communication: Implications for Nursing Practice." *American Journal of Nursing*, **69**:519-533, Mar. 1969.

Hallan, M. B. "Attitudes Toward the Unwed Mother." *Nursing Clinics of North America*, **2**:775-784, Dec. 1967.

* Hershey, N. "Questions of Life or Death." *American Journal of Nursing*, **68**:1910-1912, Sept. 1968.

Hyams, D. E. "A Realistic Look at Geriatrics." *Nursing Times*, Part 1, **63**:1447-1449, Nov. 3, 1967; Part 2, **63**:1507-1509, Nov. 10, 1967.

* Kalkman, M. E. "Recognizing Emotional Problems." *American Journal of Nursing*, **68**:536-539, Mar. 1968.

* Kneisl, C. R. "Thoughtful Care for the Dying." *American Journal of Nursing*, **68**:550-553, Mar. 1968.

* Kramer, C. H. "How to Become a Better [Nurse] to Your Aged Patients." *Geriatric Nursing*, **3**:14-16, Oct. 1967.

* Laney, M. L. "Hope As a Healer." *Nursing Outlook*, **17**:45-46, Jan. 1969.

Leininger, M. M. "Nursing Care of Patients from Another Culture." *Nursing Clinics of North America*, **2**:745-762, Dec. 1967.

* Levine, M. E. "The Pursuit of Wholeness." *American Journal of Nursing*, **69**:93-98, Jan. 1969.

Martucci, M. E. "Individual Conferences as a Means of Resolving Stressful Situations." *Journal of Psychiatric Nursing*, **6**:27-34, Feb. 1968.

* Mead, M. "The Right to Die." *Nursing Outlook*, **16**:20-21, Oct. 1968. (Read with article by Sister Bernadette Armiger.)

"Morale Boosting in Cystic Fibrosis." *American Journal of Nursing*, **69**:322-323, Feb. 1969.

Moses, D. V. "The Older Patient in the General Hospital." *Nursing Clinics of North America*, **2**:705-714, Dec. 1967.

Patrick, M. L. "Care of the Confused Elderly Patient." *American Journal of Nursing*, **67**:2536-2539, Dec. 1967.

Phillips, B. D. "Terminating a Nurse-Patient Relationship." *American Journal of Nursing*, **68**:1941-1942, Sept. 1968.

* Quint, J. C. "Awareness of Death and the Nurse's Composure." *Nursing Research*, **15**:52-55, Winter 1966.

Roch, S. "The Care of the Dying." *Nursing Times*, **64**:157-160, Oct. 11, 1968.

Saunders, C. M. "The Care of the Dying." *Gerontologia Clinica*, **9**:385-392, 1967.

Sharp, D. "Lessons from a Dying Patient." *American Journal of Nursing*, **68**:1517-1520, July 1968.

Shephard, M. W. "This I Believe About Questioning the Right to Die." *Nursing Outlook*, **16**:22-25, Oct. 1968.

* Smith, D. W. "Patienthood and its Threat to Privacy." *American Journal of Nursing*, **69**:508-513, Mar. 1969.

* Spradlin, W. W. "Family Roles of the Elderly as a Focus in Teaching Comprehensive Medicine." *Journal of Medical Education*, **42**:1045-1048, Nov. 1967.

Thomas, M. D. "Anger in Nurse-Patient Reactions." *Nursing Clinics of North America*, **2**:737-745, Dec. 1967.

* Ujhely, G. B. "What is Realistic Emotional Support?" *American Journal of Nursing*, **68**:758-762, Apr. 1968.

_____. *Determinants of the Nurse-Patient Relationship.* New York, Springer, 1968.

Verhonick, P. J. "I Came, I Saw, I Responded: Nursing Observation and Action Survey." *Nursing Research*, **17**:38-44, Jan./Feb. 1968.

* Verwoerdt, A., *et al.* "Communications with Fatally Ill Patients: Tacit or Explicit?" *American Journal of Nursing,* **67:**2307-2309, Nov. 1967.
* Watson, M. J. "Death a Necessary Concern for Nurses." *Nursing Outlook,* **16:**47-48, Feb. 1968. See also references at end of this article.
Weinstock, C., *et al.* "Problems in Communication to Nurses Among Residents of a Racially Heterogeneous Nursing Home." *Gerontologist,* **8:**72-75, Summer 1968.
* Wygant, W. E. Jr. "Dying, But Not Alone." *American Journal of Nursing,* **67:**574-577, Mar. 1967.

See also references in Chapter 2 on "Aging."

PROFESSIONAL RELATIONSHIPS

Berkowitz, N. H. and Malone, M. F. "Interprofessional Conflict." *Nursing Forum,* **7**(1):50-71, 1968.
Dalrymple, S. Z., *et al.* "Implications of a Study in Nurse-Physician Relationship." *Nursing Forum,* **7:**21-27, Winter 1968.
Hall, B. L. "Human Relations in the Hospital Setting." *Nursing Outlook,* **16:**43-45, Mar. 1968.
Hutchinson, D. T. "The Supportive Role of the Nurse in Relation to Health Service Workers." *Nursing Clinics of North America,* **3:**153-163, Mar. 1968.
Kramer, C. H., *et al.* "How to Achieve a Good Relationship Between the Nurse and the Physician." *Geriatric Nursing,* **4:**22-23, May 1968.
* _____. "Ten Ways to Improve Staff Relationships." *Geriatric Nursing,* **3:**19-23, Nov. 1967.
* Lambertsen, E. C. "Let's Stop War Between Nurses and Administrators." *Modern Hospital,* **109:**130, Sept. 1967.
O'Connell, P. E. "Communication in the Public Health Team." *District Nursing,* **10:**142-144, Oct. 1967.
Peoples, E. H. "Social-Psychological Obstacles to Effective Team Practice." *Nursing Forum,* **7:**28-37, Winter 1968.
* Peplau, H. "Interpersonal Relationships and the Work of the Industrial Nurse." *American Association of Industrial Nurses Journal,* **15:**7-12, Nov. 1968.
Pratt, H. "The Doctor's View of the Changing Nurse-Physician Relationship." *Journal of Medical Education,* **40:**767-771, Aug. 1965.
Rutherford, M., *et al.* "Observer Effects and Hospital Interaction." *Nursing Research,* **17:**65-68, Jan./Feb. 1968.
Schlotfeldt, R. M. "The Nurse's View of the Changing Nurse-Physician Relationship." *Journal of Medical Education,* **40:**772-777, Aug. 1965.
Selmanoff, E. D. "Strains in the Nurse-Doctor Relationship." *Nursing Clinics of North America,* **3:**117-127, Mar. 1968.
Stein, L. L. "The Doctor-Nurse Game." *American Journal of Nursing,* **68:**101-105, Jan. 1968.
Strauss, A. "The Intensive Care Unit: Its Characteristics and Social Relationships." *Nursing Clinics of North America,* **3:**7-15, Mar. 1968.
Sward, K. M. "The Nurse as a Practitioner and Colleague." *Journal of the American College Health Association,* **16:**324-329, Apr. 1968.
Weiss, E. D. "The Role of Nursing Service and Administration in Staff Development." *AORN Journal,* **7:**71-72, Mar. 1968.

WELL ADJUSTED LIVING

Allport, G. W. *Pattern and Growth in Personality.* New York, Holt, 1961.
* American Bankers Association. Savings and Mortgage Division. *Personal Money Management.* New York, The Association, 1967, pp. 23-29.

* Hayes, Rev. E. J., *et al. Moral Principles of Nursing.* New York, Macmillan, 1964.

* Kelly, H. S., *et al.* "Interpersonal Relationship Skills." *Perspectives of Psychiatric Care,* **6:**110-115, 1968.

Kemp, E., *et al.* "Nurses Attitudes: Fact or Fallacy?" *Canadian Nurse,* **64:**51-54, Feb. 1968.

Kramer, C. H. "Self-Inventory for Growth." *Geriatric Nursing,* **4:**14-17, Mar. 1968.

* National Recreation Center. *Adventures in Arts and Crafts: A Bibliography.* 8 West 8th Street, New York, N. Y., The Center, n.d. Many excellent materials on leisure and hobbies can be obtained from the Center.

* _____. *Your Hobbies: A Bibliography.* New York, The Center, n.d.

Stauffacher, J. C., *et al.* "The Prediction of Subsequent Professional Activity of Nursing Students by the Edwards Personal Preference Schedule." *Nursing Research,* **17:**256-260, May/June 1968.

Thurston, J. R., *et al.* "The Relationship of Personality and Achievement in Nursing Education." *Nursing Research,* **17:**265-268, May/June 1968.

* "21 Ways to Improve Your Conversation." *Christopher News Notes.* New York, The Christopher Association, May 1964.

Vanderbilt, A. *Amy Vanderbilt's New Complete Book of Etiquette.* New York, Doubleday, 1963.

Voeks, V. *On Becoming an Educated Person.* Philadelphia, Saunders, 1964.

Wright, M. *The Art of Conversation and How to Apply Its Technique.* New York, McGraw-Hill, 1936.

See also current issues of various fashion magazines.

PART 3

Choosing, Preparing for and Succeeding in a Field of Nursing

PREVIEW

The typical student who is about to graduate from a nursing school is concerned with choosing a field of work and succeeding in it.

This part of the book, consisting of 10 chapters, deals with this subject. The first chapter is a survey of the occupational opportunities for nurses, both inside and outside the profession. Chapter 8 also includes a brief overview of some contemporary occupational trends. The next 3 chapters (9, 10 and 11) present a brief review of the major fields of work for nurses and of nursing positions important in society. Although nursing education is described separately as an occupational field, it should be remembered that all nurses, whatever their field of work, carry some type of teaching responsibility, even though their career is not in teaching. Chapter 12 describes the functions of nurses in a national disaster or emergency program. Chapter 13 emphasizes your need to analyze yourself so that you may make a wise occupational choice. It also includes suggestions for an occupational study of one or two types of work in which you may be interested. The next chapter (14) presents some of the answers to the principal questions that will arise when you are faced with the problems of obtaining, filling and resigning from a position. It deals with such phases as the means of locating the kind of work you desire and the ways of employing the best practices for obtaining it. It also points out some reasons why people succeed in work or fail. The difference between holding a job and filling it is emphasized, and the general procedure to follow in resigning from a position is discussed. Chapter 15 takes a look at ways in which you can plan to attain your future financial security goals. Chapter 16 outlines some of the factors that you will need to consider when planning for continued education for your future professional and personal growth. It points up the kinds of educational programs available and places emphasis on the need for continued education for professional growth. The final chapter (17), dealing with your leadership role, is presented with the hope that it will help you to analyze and grow comfortable with this important function given to you by society and your fellow workers.

When you realize the importance of a wise solution of the problems raised in this part, you will have little difficulty in making good professional adjustments; and you will fully understand and appreciate the nature of your profession, your professional responsibilities and how to succeed in the work of your choice.

CHAPTER

8

General Survey of Occupational Opportunities for Nurses

Formerly the nurse found it very simple to select a field of nursing. This is not so simple today, for great changes have taken place in nursing. Some types of nursing have declined in importance because of lessened demand, while others have increased in importance because of greater demand and personal satisfactions; modern developments have opened new fields. This chapter reviews the types of work in which nurses may be employed and points out some occupational trends.

HISTORICAL ASPECTS

The whole field of nursing was divided formerly into 3 main areas: private practice, visiting nursing, which often was called district nursing and is now part of nursing in public health, and institutional nursing. Private practice is probably the oldest of the 3 if the nursing coincident with early family life is considered; visiting nursing may be the next oldest, and what is commonly called institutional nursing, hospital and other institutional nursing as we know it today, is probably the youngest.[1]

[1] L. L. Dock and I. M. Stewart, *A Short History of Nursing from the Earliest Times to the Present Day,* New York, Putnam, 1938, p. 299.

Development and Growth of Private Practice in Nursing

There have been various types of workers in private practice, including the slave, the servant, the hireling and the mother. At least some part of nursing has been done by many different groups: male and female, religious and secular, ethical and unethical. Early private practice was done in the home, but later it spread to hospitals, where it was called special duty. In some instances the fees went, not to the nurses themselves but, as in the case of religious communities, directly to the motherhouse or the community. Today this phase of nursing service is called private practice, or private duty, and the fees go to the nurse herself. The nurse in private practice may do group nursing in the hospital or hourly nursing in the home, and sometimes she is asked to do relief general staff nursing in the hospital.

Since no special training for private practice was required beyond preservice education in a hospital school of nursing, it was an easy field to enter. Also, there was a great demand for nurses in private practice among wealthy patients who wanted special service and individual care. The private physician increased the demand by requiring private duty nurses for paying patients. Another reason these nurses in private practice increased in number was that hospitals could not be staffed adequately with students who were there to secure an education, and consequently there was a demand for more nurses in private duty nursing. Furthermore, the social philosophy of this country influenced the demand for this type of nursing service.

Some Factors That Have Changed Private Practice in Nursing

Nurses in private practice had little choice of work opportunities in the early part of this century. Now nurses can choose from among a number of opportunities.

The 8-hour day, requiring 3 nurses around the clock, has placed the use of nurses in private practice beyond the pocketbooks of a large segment of the population, unless the patient carries insurance to cover this. Furthermore, since the nurse is an independent contractor, there are certain other disadvantages. These are discussed more fully in Chapter 9.

Private practice in nursing is taking on new aspects. Patients who have undergone radical surgery, as in cardiac and pulmonary procedures, require expert nursing care. Here and there such expert nurses are found. One hospital mans its postsurgery-anesthesia recovery room with private nurses, and the patients share the costs.

The nurse in private practice who does not keep up to date will be an anachronism, because diagnostic and treatment procedures have changed and continue to change rapidly. These advances increase the need for expertness to practice in special areas of patient care. For example, the understanding and use of new drugs and new technological equipment – monitoring devices, artificial kidneys and others—makes continuing education for the nurse in private practice as essential for her as for all nurses. In order to assist with this need, some hospitals today open their inservice staff education programs to nurses in private practice in their institutions.

The number of registered nurses in private practice has been declining gradually over the past few years. In 1966 there were 57,193 in active practice in contrast with 70,200 in 1960 and 74,000 in 1954. Nurses in private practice represented 9.7 per cent of all employed nurses in 1966; in 1962 this percentage was 12.1. The extent to which private nursing care is included in health and insurance plans, the utilization of private practice nurses in recovery rooms and in intensive treatment areas in hospitals, and the growth of practical nurses in private practice will influence the future demand for private nursing among registered nurses. Also, the rise in general staff nursing, which began in the 1930's and has continued to expand since that time, has created a lesser need for the private nurse.

A factor that keeps many nurses in private practice is the control it allows over the time when one will work. Married nurses, with homes and children to care for and with cars and other items to pay for, find private practice a means to an end and more convenient. Also, private nursing is practiced by nurses going to school who are free to work only at certain hours.

Private practice remains a most gratifying field for expert nurses because they are able to provide nursing care of high quality.

Origin of Public Health Nursing

Public health nursing, first called *visiting nursing* and later called *nursing in public health,* began as a free service given in loving kindness. It can be traced to women in the early Christian era. Later, sisterhoods became interested in it, but now, in the 20th century, it has become a part of the important and broadening field of public health. The advent of Medicare and Medicaid have greatly expanded the work of the public health nursing agencies and enlarged the opportunities in this field for the young graduate. The focus on nursing of the sick at home, on use of neighborhood clinics and on the growing use of extended care facilities, together with the changing and expanding role of the nurses in public health, makes community nursing an exciting field. Development of expertness and continuing education will be important for these nurses, too, in order that they can function effectively in a field that will be developing and growing in many ways during the next decade. There is a growing trend to call this field of nursing *community health nursing,* and the mental health nurse in this field is now called the *community mental health nurse.* Many nurses find public health nursing a particularly satisfying kind of work because of the opportunity to work with families, as well as with patients, and the challenge of community health work.

Institutional Nursing

The term *institutional nursing* had been used until recent years to designate nursing carried on not only in hospitals, but also in such places as nursing homes and other extended care facilities, and a variety of other types of institutions where nurses may be found working, such as those for the mentally retarded.

By far the largest group of nurses employed in institutions is the general duty or staff nurses. Prior to 1930, much of the nursing done in hospitals was carried out by nursing students. During the 1930's, known as the "Depression Years," many nurses who would have turned to private practice turned to hospital general staff nursing instead. General staff nursing offered them more regular employment as well as the benefits other persons enjoyed, such as vacation time, holidays, sick leave and other benefits. Following the 1930's, the growth in hospital services opened many new opportunities for general staff nursing, both in the hospitals and in outpatient departments. Today, the opportunities for general staff nursing far exceed the number of nurses available.

Present-day Occupational Areas Other Than Private Practice, Public Health and Institutional

In addition to these kinds of nursing, nurses work in the areas of nursing education, consultation and research. However, how nursing is classified occupationally depends on whether it is done by services which nurses carry on — nursing service or education — or by the functions involved — clinical nursing, administration, supervision, curriculum development and improvement, teaching, consultation or research or some combinations of these.

It is of interest that in the early part of the century relatively few nurses were employed in administration, supervision, consultation or research. But development of these areas in both nursing service and nursing education was inevitable as nursing service grew more complex and as the medical, health and social sciences made unprecedented rapid progress. A response to this growing complexity is the recent emergence of the clinical specialist in nursing.

Within the area of nursing service in recent years, occupational health nursing, school nursing and office nursing have expanded rapidly. Although in 1966 the largest proportion of employed nurses worked in hospitals and related institutions (387,847) and the second largest group continued to be in private practice (57,193), the third largest group were office nurses (47,628). Occupational health nurses (18,155) were exceeded by the public health nursing group (26,001) and the growing numbers of school nurses (20,348).

OCCUPATIONAL TRENDS[2]

Do We Have the Same Occupational Opportunities in Nursing Today That We Had 20, 10, or Even 5 Years Ago?

Some nursing positions retain the same title, but there have been changes in function and in organization of areas and work.

Each year the ANA's *Facts About Nursing* includes information about the distribution of nurses in the various fields of work and about trends of employment in nursing. We suggest that you study these figures annually and compare them with those presented in previous years.

The gap between the expanding population that requires nursing care and the number of nursing personnel to provide such care has been and is a major problem. After World War II there was a shortage of nurses. This shortage still exists. It is not due to a decrease in the number of available nurses. Actually there are more nurses employed now (1970) than ever before. Nursing is the largest of the health professions. The shortage of nurses is due to the increased demands for nursing services because of the expansion of hospitals, extended care facilities and other community health services, the introduction of Medicare and Medicaid, advances in health sciences, lack of qualified nurses and poor distribution of available nurses, and to the complexity of the whole health treatment situation.

An important factor in the supply of and demand for nurses is the increase in population over the past 50 years, and the population continues to expand with increased momentum. Furthermore, because of improved social and health conditions, the proportion of population in the older age group is growing. It is reported that "by 1990 there will be 27 million Americans, and 1 in every 10 will be aged 65 or over. Of that number 10 million will be at least 75. In 1900, by contrast, only 3 million—or 1 in every 25—were over 65 and only 900,000 over 75."[3] In 1968 there were 659,000 nurses in employment, or 331 per 100,000 population. In fact, registered nurses increased by 3 per cent between 1967 and 1968 while the population increased by only 1.1 per cent. However, more nurses by count is not the equivalent of nurse power per population. One must remember that nurses are not necessarily evenly distributed; for example, in 1966 there were 536 registered nurses in practice per 100,000 population in Connecticut but only 133 in Arkansas. You may be interested in studying the situation in your own state.

The largest group of nurses employed in 1966 was in the hospitals in this country; it was estimated that 360,969 registered nurses were employed in 5,342 hospitals. At the same time, it was estimated that a 22 per cent increase would be necessary for optimum care.

[2] Figures in this and the preceding section have been taken from the annual statistical summary—*Facts About Nursing*—published by the American Nurses' Association.

[3] "Meeting the Needs of the Aging," *Nursing Outlook*, **16**:49, Sept. 1968.

TABLE 8-1. REGISTERED NURSES EMPLOYED IN NURSING IN USA, BY FIELD OF EMPLOYMENT

Field of Nursing	1962[1]	1966[2]
Totals	532,118	593,694
Hospital or other Institution	335,404	387,847
School of Nursing	16,294	20,818
Private Duty Nurses	64,155	57,193
Public Health Nurses	23,983	26,001
School Nurses	16,704	20,348
Industrial Nurses	17,569	18,155
Office Nurses	43,558	47,628
Other Specified Field	2,496	1,885
Field not Reported	11,955	13,819

[1] Source: American Nurses' Association, *Facts About Nursing: A Statistical Summary,* New York, The Association, 1965, p. 18.
[2] Source: *Ibid.,* 1968 edition, p. 25.

It is interesting to note that it has been estimated that approximately 31,000 registered nurses were employed in nursing homes in 1967. There were 20,031 long-term care facilities in 1967, a great majority of which were proprietary institutions.

The ratio of nurses and auxiliary nursing personnel to the number of patients seems to vary greatly in the different types of hospitals. In 1966 there were 2.4 registered nurses per practical nurse employed in hospitals but the number of other auxiliary nursing personnel (aides, orderlies and attendants) exceeded the number of registered nurses. The determination of appropriate ratios of nursing personnel to patients is one of the major problems in nursing. The important fact is that the need for nursing personnel in hospitals continues to be great. The Report of the Surgeon General's Consultant Group on Nursing (1963) recommended a general ratio of 50 per cent of direct patient care in general hospitals be given by professional nurses and 30 per cent by practical nurses.

The number of nurses employed for public health work in 1966 in the USA, Puerto Rico, and the Virgin Islands was 41,254. Of this number, 3,370 were employed part time.

The largest increase in recent years is due, in part, to the gain in the number of nurses employed by local boards of education, the second largest employers of public health nurses. The need for more nurses in public health continues. It has been recommended that by 1970, we will need 86,000 nurses in public health work, at least half of whom will need to be qualified public health nurses.

The number of nurses employed in health services in industry was 18,155 in 1966. This represented a slight increase over 1962. Occupational health nurses are usually employed in the larger companies, those with several hundred workers and having a full-time health service.

It is of interest to note the continuing increase in the number of office nurses employed. Frequently, 2 or more physicians share the services of a nurse. Office nursing, in 1966, continued to be the 3rd largest employment field in nursing.

In 1967, the Army, the Navy and the Air Force Nurse Corps had a combined force of 10,969, as compared to 8,985 in 1962. In general, all of the Corps have been increasing the number of nurses. The figures reported fluctuate, depending on troop ceilings. Any national emergency could change this picture.

According to Table 8-1, there was an increase of 4,524 nurses employed in nursing education programs from 1962 to 1966. Estimates made by the NLN as of January 1968 indicated that there were 22,478 nurses employed in these programs, 17,607 in initial and graduate programs for registered nurses and 4,866 in those for practical nurses. Despite the fact that there had been an increase in total numbers employed, there was an estimated vacancy of 1,516 budgeted positions in the schools reporting. During the period 1966 to 1968 there was an increase in numbers of all types of programs (except diploma programs, which declined) and an increase in numbers of faculty needed. There continues to be a critical need for well-prepared faculty in schools of nursing.

In Table 8-1 the category "other" includes nurses employed in national and state nurses associations and in other organizations of this nature. Many new opportunities for nurses prepared in consultation, research and other special fields are opening up in these areas.

The opportunities today for the nurse with a good personality and desirable qualifications, who has continued to study and has let each new experience add to her education, are increasing greatly. Opportunities exist, not only in the USA, but throughout the world.

Some Economic Influences That Have Affected Nursing in Recent Years

The changes that are taking place in nursing's occupational opportunities are due to economic influences, social and political developments, scientific advances, changing concepts such as those relating to occupational and team relationships, and other influences within the health professions and nursing itself.

First of all, the prosperity after World War II encouraged expansive government and private enterprise. There was greater personal spending, and health services got their share of money from all of these sources. Many hospitals were built, or additions were added, through the use of funds of the *Hill-Burton Act* and the distribution of funds by the Ford Foundation and other groups. There has been an increased sale of health and medical insurance and of Blue Cross. Medicare and Medicaid programs have had a tremendous impact on the increase of hospital and extended care facilities. Consequently, larger and larger nursing staffs, as well as nurses technically and educationally prepared to function in an ever more complex situation, have been required, but the demand for nursing services has not been readily met.

There are a number of factors involved in the continuing high birth rate. This increase in birth rate brings with it problems of nursing care both in hospitals and in public health agencies. The Children's Bureau of the U.S. Department of Health, Education, and Welfare has been very active in its efforts to improve conditions in maternal and infant care, as have many other groups and individuals. It is still too soon to estimate the effect of groups interested in population control.

As mentioned elsewhere, a major problem after World War II was that of the increasing shortage of nursing personnel and the consequences of this shortage upon the quality of nursing and medical care. *A Program for the Nursing Profession,* published in 1948, dealt with the shortage problem in nursing.[4] Recommendations in this report were a factor in introducing team nursing to secure more economic and better use of the practical nurse and the nursing aide, with the registered nurse serving as team leader. The introduction of intensive care units, including recovery care rooms, coronary care units and the more recent extended care units, have greatly expanded the functions and responsibilities of the nurse. The effects of specialization in nursing are also beginning to be felt.

Auxiliary nursing personnel came into the hospital as a necessity, primarily for 4 reasons: (1) because registered nurses were withdrawn in large numbers from civilian services for military services; (2) because of the increasing withdrawal of student service; (3) because of the great increase in hospital population, which has outstripped the supply of registered nurses; (4) because the shortage of skilled workers in all fields has helped to establish a principle that skill must be utilized wisely; and (5) because it is economically impractical to pay a highly skilled person's salary for work that requires much less skill. Thus, personnel who are not nurses are being used for those activities that are essential but do not require professional skill and for certain ward management positions, in order to free nurses for nursing functions. Industry established this principle and practice as a necessity during World War II when skilled manpower was at a premium. The use of these various auxiliary nursing personnel place additional responsibility on the registered nurse for teaching, directing and supervising their work.

The work of the general staff nurse has undergone and continues to undergo change. As more hospitals introduce team nursing, the general staff nurse appointed by the head nurse as the team leader carries, with the

---

[4] Committee on Functions of Nursing, *A Program for the Nursing Profession,* New York, Macmillan, 1948, pp. ii-iii.

other members of the team, the major responsibility of planning the nursing care required by a group of patients assigned to the team. As the team leader, the general staff nurse directs and supervises the other members of the team in carrying out the nursing care plan, in participating in the provision of nursing care, and in providing the means whereby the team continuously can evaluate and revise the plan to meet the needs of patients. The team may consist of different personnel in different hospitals.

The advent of the 8-hour day for nurses in hospitals and in private practice has been a major economic influence. It has called for more nurses. It also has caused a strain on the patient's pocketbook, tending to change the habits of patients using private practice nurses. There are other effects of the introduction of the 8-hour day you will think of. If shorter work weeks become the vogue, there will no doubt be movement toward shorter work weeks for registered nurses and auxiliary nursing personnel.

In a 1967 article, Dr. Ginsberg has reviewed the nursing accomplishments made since 1948. In his opinion, the response of nursing to demand has not been bad. The nurse-population ratio has gone up. He does not agree that there is a nursing shortage, but believes rather that the consumer can afford and wants more health services, including nursing services. He does not believe that nursing has made much progress in improving the utilization of nursing personnel, and recommends that groups of hospitals do cooperative research with the purpose of determining the effects of different patterns of utilization.[5]

It was mentioned earlier that there are not enough well-prepared nurses to take the newer positions created by demands, and that there has been an unequal distribution of nurses, especially in the rural areas, even though efforts were made by special national and Federal nursing agencies to equalize distribution before, during and since the Korean War, and during the war in Vietnam.

One of the most significant changes occurring in the nursing situation has been the dramatic rise in the use of part-time nurses. According to a survey carried out jointly by the Division of Nursing of the U.S. Public Health Service and the American Hospital Association in 1961 (the latest figures available in 1970), and covering nonfederal and allied special hospitals in the continental USA, the number of nurses employed part time rose from 17,188 in 1948 to 77,359 in 1962. It was estimated that there was about 1 part-time nurse to every 2 full-time nurses and that this ratio was very likely to become higher.

Major reasons given by nurses for working part time were: (1) to supplement income, 51.7 per cent, and (2) to maintain professional skills, 39.7 per cent. Most of the part-time nurses were married and could work only part time because of family responsibilities.[6] The proportion of employed nurses

---

[5] E. Ginsberg, "Nursing and Manpower Realities," *Nursing Outlook,* **15**:26-29, Nov. 1967.
[6] A. Testoff, *et al.,* "The Part-time Nurse," *American Journal of Nursing,* **64**:88-89, Jan. 1964.

who are married has increased over the years. In 1966, according to the ANA inventory, 63.5 per cent of employed registered nurses were married as compared to 22.4 per cent who were single, thus making nursing a field of work predominantly composed of married women. While the number of men in nursing continues to remain proportionately small, the percentage of male nurses increased from .9 in 1962, when the previous inventory was made, to 1.1 in 1966. Office nursing remains the field with the largest proportion of married nurses. Up until this last inventory (1966), schools of nursing was the one place over the years where single nurses were in a majority; this is now changed, and a majority of nurses in all fields are married.

One of the major factors affecting the increasing need for nurses is the rapid expansion in the use of nursing homes. As pointed out elsewhere, in 1967 it was estimated that there were 31,000 nurses employed in this type of facility. It is urgent that registered nurses assume the leadership positions in these increasingly important nursing care institutions.

Another factor affecting the need for more registered nurses is the trend toward providing care for psychiatric patients in general hospitals, day and night hospitals, half-way hospitals, community clinics, and at home or in foster homes. This trend will require that the number of nurses with advanced preparation in psychiatric nursing be doubled. This field is wide open as a dramatic and rewarding type of service for nurses.

The changes in nursing activities, such as those resulting from the use of new equipment, ranging all the way from disposables through electronic processing equipment, the use of tranquilizers for the mentally ill, and the taking on of functions that were once physicians', are all factors influencing changes in the nurses' work and its organization in the different fields.

The economic security program of the American Nurses' Association has been a determined effort to improve the income and work conditions of nurses. The results of this program have significant implications for nurses. They are discussed in Chapter 15.

Finally, a factor to recognize is the growing understanding of the public that "keeping people well" is more economical than "treating disease." This has made nurses conscious of their health education responsibilities.

What Are Some of the Social Developments That Have Affected Occupational Opportunities in Nursing?

The public-health movement with its emphasis on mental health, social hygiene, accident prevention, school health, health education (including nutrition education), parent education, child health, geriatrics, and control of such communicable and chronic diseases as tuberculosis, cancer, stroke and heart disease, has introduced new administrative, consultative and teaching positions as well as new opportunities in the field of public health.

The continued interest in child welfare has brought many opportunities in child-guidance work, parent education, camp nursing and health supervision in homes of dependent children. Considerable emphasis is on care and supervision of the handicapped child, including the mental retardate.

At the same time that urbanization and the increasing growth of suburbs have added to the complexity of health problems, the problems of rural health continue. Many families living in rural communities and sparsely settled areas of our country are still without medical and nursing facilities. The hospital construction program under the Hill-Burton Act has provided facilities in some rural areas, but facilities without plans for adequate staffing do not meet the need. Greater attention must be given to attracting nurses in greater numbers to these rural areas. It is interesting to note that congressmen are suggesting that more funds also need to be used for improving hospital facilities in urban areas. In addition to increased facilities, many communities have had increased health and hospital insurance coverage and a growth of organized home-care plans. These, too, have created further demands for nursing personnel. Medicare and Medicaid have brought renewed emphasis on extended care facilities, home care of the sick and disabled and the use of home health aides and homemakers.

Occupational health nursing has taken on a new and important significance. Nursing in industrial centers, which sprang up mushroomlike during and after World War II, has continued to be a vitally important health service. Occupational health nursing, probably has received its greatest impetus because management has found that lost man-hours decline when a good health program exists.

A tremendous expansion of community health centers, clinics and outpatient departments has taken place. This expansion has increased greatly the number of positions for nurses in both hospital outpatient departments and the clinics of health organizations.

Because of the size and the complexity of the problem of care of the mentally ill in institutions, in day hospitals, in outpatient services and in their own homes, well-prepared nurses are badly needed to work in this field. Owing to the newer forms of therapy, more patients are being discharged from mental institutions to care in the community, thus presenting another challenge to the nurse in public health to whom the patient and his family are referred. This field, as pointed up elsewhere, is and will continue to be extremely important.

As all nations have turned their attention to the conservation of health and life and to the care of the chronically ill, of people of advanced years and of the crippled, as well as to rehabilitation programs for the handicapped and the addict, health programs have widened in scope and increased in importance, requiring the services of many nurses. This is true not only of our country, but also of others, which still lack nurses as well as other health personnel and necessary resources.

What Occupational Opportunities Have Been Brought into the Field of Nursing Through Political Developments?

World War I not only influenced the profession of nursing by movements such as the emphasis on rating, surveys and research, but also brought in new work opportunities, especially with the Veterans Administration and other government nursing services. These opportunities were increased even more by World War II, which tremendously affected occupational opportunities in the profession. The military services expanded enormously; besides the usual opportunities – general staff nurse, head nurse, supervisor and chief nurse – the advent of students of nursing in the Federal nursing services, with their need for supervision and continued education, brought in the nurse educator as instructor or consultant. Opportunities in the other Federal nursing services also increased both in numbers required and in types of services. The Korean and Vietnam Wars increased international activities of nurses in the armed services, of missionary nurses, and of nurses assigned for a variety of nursing work by various agencies of the Federal Government in foreign countries. Opportunities for nurses to serve in the Peace Corps, on the Ship Hope and in similar health services are other developments. These are discussed in Chapter 25.

The poor physical condition of so many of our men who were examined for military service during World War I was a shock to the nation. Probably this, as much as any other factor, stimulated government spending on health services. This created many occupational opportunities for nurses. The development of rehabilitation as an important part of medical and nursing care came about primarily as a result of the needs of disabled veterans of World War II. Rehabilitation has since grown into an important part of the care of all disabled and has created additional demands for nurses skilled in rehabilitative procedures.

Some legislative acts and political reorganization movements have created certain positions for nurses and made others less important. Some of the most important positions during recent years were those sponsored because of the *Social Security Act,* the *Bolton Act,* the *Mental Health Act,* the *Tuberculosis Control Act,* the *Hospital Survey and Construction Act,* the *Vocational Rehabilitation Act* of 1965, the *Health Insurance for the Aged Act* (popularly known as Medicare), the *Comprehensive Health Planning Act* of 1966, the *Heart Disease, Cancer, and Stroke Amendments* of 1965 *(Public Law 89-239),* which authorized the Regional Medical Programs, and *Public Law 90-574* of 1968, which extended and amended the original Regional Medical Programs. Government reorganization created significant changes, beginning in 1953.

Other important influences resulting directly or indirectly from political developments are:

Expansion of the Army, the Navy, the Air Force Nurse Corps and the nursing units in the Public Health Service.

Acceptance of men nurses in the armed forces through the bill which gave them commissions. The commissioning of men in nursing is considered, by many, to be a milestone in the progress of American nursing.

Increase in the number of nurses prepared for positions in teaching, administration and supervision in nursing service and nursing education and for beginning nursing positions in public health through traineeships provided under the *Health Amendments Act* of 1956 *(Public Law 911)* and *Public Law 105* of 1959, the *Nurse Training Act* of 1964 *(Public Law 88-581)* and the *Manpower Health Act (Public Law 90-490)*, which continues the *Nurse Training Act.*

Increase of obligations of nurses in many foreign countries since the USA has become an important world power. War and its aftermath have created vast problems of health and rehabilitation in Europe and Asia. People in those countries have looked to the USA as well as other countries for medical and nursing services in order to rebuild the minimum conditions for living a useful and a healthy life. Nurses have been sent into other countries to help to reconstruct or to start new nursing service and nursing education programs and to serve as consultants in all nursing service areas. One of the greatest barriers for American nurses in taking advantage of international opportunities is language. Another problem grew out of the attempts by nurses from the USA to reconstruct foreign education and nursing service programs according to our patterns, without taking into consideration the differences in educational and health systems and cultural attitudes of other countries. These are problems for nurse educators to consider in curriculum planning.

Increased social and health legislation. Each time a legislative measure (Federal or state) is enacted for the improvement of the health of the nation or the state (and many have been enacted since 1935), implicit in such enactment is the need for more nursing personnel. For example, Medicare, Medicaid, the Regional Medical Programs and the Comprehensive Health Planning Act have had a great impact on health care services and facilities and have placed new demands and responsibilities on nurses. Also as a result of this health legislation, as well as of the position taken on nursing education in 1965 by the ANA, many state nurses associations, in cooperation with other groups, are examining their nursing needs and resources, with a view toward better planning for nursing service and education and better utilization of the nursing and educational resources available.

How Has Scientific Advance Affected Work Opportunities in Nursing?

The effects of scientific advance and discoveries have been numerous. New treatments have brought in new nursing procedures, practices and approaches to nursing, and have produced a variety of occupational opportunities. Clinical laboratory research and other research, especially medical, has made the care of patients generally more scientific. For example, advances in cardiac surgery have created a need for nurses highly skilled in the care of these patients. Other newer methods of treatments requiring highly skilled nurses include: organ transplants, long-term hemodialysis, hyperbaric therapy, radical surgery for cancer, and others. Nurse research workers in nursing organizations and Federal agencies are becoming more numerous and important. You will want to watch with interest the nursing research being undertaken by the Clinical Centers of the U. S. Department of Health, Education, and Welfare at Bethesda, Md.; by nurses in the Walter Reed Army Institute of Research in Washington, D.C.; by the Nursing Research Division of the Naval Medical Research Institute in Bethesda, Md.; by the Institute of Research and Service in Nursing Education at Teachers College, Columbia University, New York; and by other universities, such as Johns Hopkins.

Opportunities for nurses in research have greatly increased and continue to increase. They range from that of the young staff nurse who assists in the collection of data, the research nurse on the research team, the nurse carrying major responsibility for a piece of original research, to the nurse who directs a major research project. It is interesting to note that in 1969, there were 6 graduate programs in nursing offering a doctorate in nursing. Some of the nurses in these programs will be the nurse researchers of the future. However, all professional nurses need an orientation to research methods, in order to assist with research projects and to evaluate and implement research findings.

Interest in preparation of the nurse-scientist is growing also. In 1961 funds were first made available through the Public Health Service for the development of university programs to prepare nurse-scientists. By 1969, awards had been made to 10 universities (2 were terminated in 1966). The purpose in giving these awards is to expand predoctoral programs and to pay stipends to nurses who have been chosen by the universities as candidates for a doctor degree.[7] The program combines study in nursing with a major in one of the behavioral or biologic sciences within the university.

Clinical specialists, to aid general nurses and supervisors, are growing in number in nursing service agencies as a result of advances in diagnostic and treatment procedures. Public health agencies have demonstrated, for a long time, the value of the expert practitioner in nursing as a consultant to help the general nurse keep abreast of new knowledge and know-how. This kind of service is opening up in hospitals and will offer great opportunities to more and better prepared nurses.

Advances in science leading to explorations in space have opened up new roles and functions for nurses. Nurses will play a part in maintaining healthful conditions for those participating in these experiments in outer space.

[7] E. M. Vreeland. "Nursing Research Programs of the Public Health Service." *Nursing Research,* 13:156, Spring 1964.

One of the conflicting factors in our scientific period is the group of allied professional workers who want the oldtime R.N., the bedside nurse of the 30's, with the scientific know-how of the 70's. Others contend that advances in health care have created the demand for a modern approach to nursing care. Many others believe we need to examine current patterns of nursing service to see how we can make it possible for nurses "to nurse." The speed with which major changes in health care have come about has created dislocations which may take time to correct. However, as a result of recent legislation and the efforts of organized nursing to promote the type of nursing education and service required, there has been renewed emphasis on planning in terms of health care needs.

These are only a few of the influences in this realm; no doubt you will think of many others.

How Have Changing Concepts and Other Influences Within the Profession Affected Opportunities for The Nurse?

Greater development of university programs in nursing, undergraduate and graduate, has brought opportunities for the nurse prepared for expert clinical practice, educational administration, curriculum development and improvement, teaching, supervision, consultation and research. The development of educational programs for the preparation of technical and practical nurses and inservice and continuing education programs are providing increasing opportunities for nurse educators. University and college education programs in nursing call for field coordinators and teachers who act as liaison between the educational institution and the participating agencies used for practice in nursing.

The continued emphasis on curriculum development and improvement, and on educational administration and the utilization by educational programs of hitherto unused clinical facilities of Federal services have increased opportunities for all kinds of educational positions, such as field supervisors, teachers and consultants.

The reorganization of the national nursing organizations has brought in new opportunities, such as director of headquarters or executive secretary, director of studies, field representative, director of public relations, consultant in nursing, counselor and editor. These are some of the positions, but there are other important ones in national as well as in state nurses organizations.

An important development within the nursing profession which has influenced the occupational opportunities for nurses was the organization in May 1945 of the American Nurses' Association Professional Credentials and Personnel Service. This service helps nurses to find positions for which they are best qualified and in which they can make their greatest contribution. A square peg in a round hole usually means loss of time, money and happiness, and such losses ought to be reduced to a minimum. Besides seeking professional counsel, study your own abilities and potentialities as objectively as you can and try to do the kind of work for which you are best fitted. This is discussed more fully in other chapters in this book.

SCOPE OF NURSING AS AN OCCUPATION

As has been emphasized in the foregoing pages, the major employers of nurses are hospitals and related institutions, nursing education institutions, public health agencies, boards of education, industry and private individuals (physicians and patients). Within these employing agencies are many diverse job opportunities enabling you to satisfy your interests and use your abilities as you progress in experience and continuing education.

The following classification of positions according to type of work gives a general idea of the scope of nursing.

POSITIONS IN NURSING SERVICES

Hospitals and Similar Health Facilities

Positions Usually Restricted to Nurses

Director of nursing service
Associate director of nursing service
Assistant director or assistant to director of nursing service (administrative or educational)
Director of nursing service personnel division
Director or instructor for inservice educational program or on-the-job training program
Coordinator of patient education
Consultant in nursing service or clinical nursing specialty
Supervisor in a clinical division of nursing service, such as medical,
pediatric, maternity, psychiatric, intensive care unit, coronary care unit, self-care unit, operating or outpatient (day or night)[8]
Head nurse or assistant of a unit of a clinical division of the nursing service department[9]
Nursing team leader
General duty or staff nurse
Private practice nurse (work with single patient or on a group basis)
Visitor or consultant for state hospital or nursing homes licensing boards

Positions in Which Nurses Are Sometimes Employed[10]

Assistant to surgeon, such as office nurse or scrub nurse in operating room
Clinical laboratory technician
Clinical psychologist
Dental assistant

[8] If this position is combined with an educational one, there should be also a title to indicate the educational function, such as "instructor of obstetric nursing" or "instructor of medical and surgical nursing." This same principle applies to other positions requiring dual functions.
[9] The title to indicate the educational function of the head nurse may be "assistant instructor" of psychiatric nursing, medical and surgical nursing or some other nursing course.
[10] It will be recognized that many of these positions are not nursing positions and do not require nursing preparation. The fact that they are listed does not mean that they are recommended. It is hoped that nurses will go into and remain in positions in nursing, rather than in those which are not nursing.

Dental hygienist
Diathermist
Dietitian
Director of nursing home
Director of nursing research
Director of volunteer service
Electrotherapist
Group therapist
Historian in hospital
Hospital admitting officer or clerk
Hospital consultant
Hospital secretary
Hospital or medical social worker
Hospital statistician
Hospital administrator or assistant
Hospital personnel manager
Housekeeper in hospital or nurses' residence
Hydrotherapist

Instructor of patients in a rehabilitation sheltered shop
Librarian in hospital
Manager of nurses' residence
Masseuse
Mechanotherapist
Methods analyst
Nurse anesthetist
Nurse epidemiologist
Occupational therapist
Patient-care, or home-care, coordinator
Pharmacist
Physiotherapist
Record clerk or curator
Research assistant
Social director or hostess in nurses' residence
X-ray technician

Other Institutions and Agencies

Health supervisor or resident infirmary nurse in a boarding school, a college, a university or a normal school
Resident nurse in a prison, a reformatory or an almshouse
Supervisor of health service in a department store

Administrator of an orphanage, a home for the aged, or a convalescent home for children or adults
Administrator of first aid in a department store
Resident nurse in a hotel (may have charge of a hospital department or first aid room)

POSITIONS AVAILABLE IN COMMUNITY HEALTH PROGRAMS

Positions Usually Restricted to Nurses

Director of a nursing service in a public health agency, generalized or specialized[11]
Associate or assistant director in such agency (administrative or educational)[12]

Supervisor
a. General service
b. Field service
c. Area service
d. Special service (see list under staff nurse)[13]

[11] A community nursing service is private if supported by private contributions, official if supported by taxes, a combination of private and official if its funds are derived from both sources. Examples of private services are visiting nurse associations. Examples of official agencies are the Public Health Service of the U. S. Department of Health, Education, and Welfare, state, county, city and town departments of health, and services under village or township boards, as well as under departments or boards of education in any government unit.

[12] There seems to be a tendency to eliminate the position of educational director and to delegate the main responsibility for the educational program to an associate or assistant director.

[13] Generalized services are preferred to specialized.

Positions Usually Restricted to Nurses (Continued)

Assistant supervisor

Staff nurse rendering general service or special service, such as school nursing, camp nursing, occupational health nursing, midwifery, maternity nursing and child health, orthopedic nursing, psychiatric nursing, tuberculosis nursing, venereal disease nursing and other clinical nursing

Community nurse, i.e., a nurse working alone in a small town

Rural or urban nurse

Consultant in various nursing specialties to official or private agencies, such as the Public Health Service and the Children's Bureau of the U. S. Department of Health, Education, and Welfare, or other government units such as state boards of health, or a community organization such as a council of social agencies.[14]

Infant welfare nurse

Preschool nurse – day care nursery nurse

School nurse

Nurse teacher in school system

Health supervisor in private or public schools, camps and similar places

Obstetric, infant or child health nurse

Midwife

Occupational health nurse in administrative, supervisory or staff position, such as in factory, bank, theater, store, office building and many industries[15]

Tuberculosis nurse

Nurse for cancer service

Cardiac nurse

Positions in Which Nurses Are Sometimes Employed*

Administrator of an organization such as a community health center or a day nursery

Camp counselor

Director of or teacher in a nursery school

Medical, psychiatric or family social worker

Mental health supervisor

Missionary worker, home or foreign

Nutritionist

Recreation director

Playground supervisor

Quarantine officer

Sanitary inspector or investigator

Social hygiene consultant

Specialist in parent education

Specialist in child guidance

Health educator, as in normal school, college or public school system

Prevention-of-blindness worker

---

[14] Consultants may carry special responsibilities for industrial nursing, midwifery and maternity nursing, orthopedic nursing and physical therapy, public health nursing, trachoma nursing, tuberculosis nursing, polio nursing, venereal disease nursing, pediatric nursing, cancer nursing, mental health, education and others.

[15] Several areas of nursing service seem to claim the industrial or occupational health nurse, but she is finding a separate niche.

* For most of these positions being a nurse is not important. Other professional skills are needed.

POSITIONS OPEN TO NURSES IN PRIVATE PRACTICE

General nursing

Nurse in specialties such as obstetric nursing, nursing of children, medical nursing-surgical nursing including heart and cancer nursing, geriatric nursing, communicable disease nursing, psychiatric nursing, neurologic nursing, tuberculosis nursing, orthopedic nursing, gynecologic nursing, genitourinary disease nursing and nutritional disease nursing. (Usually nurses in the field of private practice care for any type of patient.)

Special nurse in the home, the hospital, the hotel or the sanatorium, or nurse acting as supervisor of family when traveling, or traveling companion to a patient

Hourly nurse (nursing in the home for 4 hours or less)

General duty or staff nurse in a hospital

Group nurse in a hospital

POSITIONS IN AND ASSOCIATED WITH NURSING EDUCATION

Positions Usually Restricted to Nurses

Dean or director of a nursing school or a division of nursing in a university or a college

Associate or assistant dean or director of a nursing school or a division of nursing in a university or a college

Assistant to the dean or director of a nursing school or a division of nursing in a university or a college (administrative or instructional)

Director of a nursing school in a hospital[16]

Director of a specialty program in nursing at the graduate level in a university or college[17]

Associate or assistant director of a nursing school in a hospital

Assistant to the director of a nursing school in a hospital (administrative or educational; the latter sometimes called educational director or instructional leader)

Director of other types of educational programs in nursing, such as technical or practical nurse, nursing aide or attendant

Director or coordinator of curriculum or instructional leader for various types of educational programs in nursing: professional, technical or practical nurse

Teacher in various types of educational programs in nursing: preservice, graduate, and inservice. (This includes all types: social science[18]; physical and biologic science; fundamental or general nursing; nursing in special fields, such as medical and surgical, pediatric, maternity, psychiatric and mental health, cancer, orthopedic, geriatric, and others; other functional areas, such as administra-

[16] Sometimes, the director of a hospital nursing school also may be the director of a nursing service in a hospital. This may apply to her associate and assistant also.

[17] Sometimes the director of a specialty program has a joint appointment in the hospital nursing service providing the clinical field for the students.

[18] Very few nurses teach in the area of social science or social studies, because the social science teachers in general education generally are utilized for such teaching.

Positions Usually Restricted to Nurses (continued)

tion, supervision, curriculum and teaching, consultation and research, as these relate to all phases of nursing service and nursing education. Those qualified on faculties of universities and colleges hold the appropriate professorial rank.)

Coordinator or supervisor of field work for any of the educational programs in nursing

Itinerant or visiting teacher

Executive secretary, state supervisor, educational director or visitor for a state board of nursing

See also some of the positions listed under "Positions Available in Nursing and Allied Organizations" in the next section

Positions in Which Nurses Are Sometimes Employed

Director of research program

Counselor or director of student-life services

Director of or house mother in student residence

Secretary or clerk in school office

Social director or hostess in student residence

POSITIONS AVAILABLE IN NURSING AND ALLIED ORGANIZATIONS

Positions Usually Restricted to Nurses

Top administrators

Director of special divisions at headquarters office, such as hospital nursing, public health nursing or nursing education

Editor of official nursing magazine

Field worker in different areas of nursing service or nursing education

Counselor or registrar of a professional placement service, a professional registry, a regional or a national or a community-nursing council

Consultant or specialist in nursing service (hospital or public health), nursing education, special nursing field, legislation and other

Positions in Which Nurses Are Sometimes Employed

Specialist in:
  Labor-management relations
  Test construction
  Community organization
  Public relations
  Writing
  Editing
  Research
  Statistics
  Personnel and placement
  Business administration

Executive secretary or field secretary of a health or a social organization, such as
  Heart Association
  Cancer Society
  Red Cross Chapter
  Tuberculosis Association
  Community Chest
  Family Welfare Association
  Council of Social Agencies
  Medicare Agencies

MISCELLANEOUS POSITIONS NOT PREVIOUSLY LISTED

Positions Usually Restricted to Nurses

Camp nurse
Flight nurse
Missile nurse
Missionary nurse
Parachute nurse
Physician's office nurse

Space nurse
Teacher of home nursing, first aid or child care (as under American Red Cross)
Transport nurse: airline, ship or train

Positions in Which Nurses Are Sometimes Employed

Airline hostess
Anatomic artist
Assistant to mortician
Author of nursing textbook or other publication
Camp counselor
Dean of women or adviser of girls
Demonstrator of appliances, instruments or food
Editor of a periodical
Feature writer on nursing subjects
Ghost writer
Health education instructor
Kindergarten worker
Lecturer

Lobbyist
Manager of nurses' clubhouse or hotel
Oral hygienist
Personnel or guidance worker
Physical education instructor
Police matron
Probation officer
Promotional educational worker
Publicity specialist
Traveler's-aid counselor
Vocational guidance counselor
Worker with juvenile delinquents
Writer for magazine

WHERE NURSES WORK

Positions may be classified according to the agency or auspices under which the nurse works or through which she secures work:

Private patients cared for at home, in hospitals or in other institutions, and nurse employed through professional nurses registries, or by physician or patient
Private or nonofficial agencies, organizations or institutions
  Hospitals, proprietary and nonprofit, general or special
  Dispensaries, infirmaries, convalescent homes, and foundations
  Nonofficial public health nursing organizations
  International, national, state and local nurses associations
  Religious and missionary associations
  Insurance companies
  Industrial organizations
    (1) in an employee health service, or
    (2) to promote the use of a product, for example, hospital equipment

Foundations
Regional medical planning organizations
Business organizations, such as management consultant firms
Transportation agencies
Nursing Service of the American National Red Cross
Official agencies, organizations or institutions
International Organizations, such as the World Health Organization
Federal and allied government nursing services
U. S. Army Nurse Corps
U. S. Navy Nurse Corps
U. S. Air Force Nurse Corps
Public Health Service of the U. S. Department of Health, Education, and Welfare in various divisions and offices
Veterans Administration Nursing Service
Children's Bureau, U. S. Department of Health, Education, and Welfare
U. S. Office of Civil and Defense Mobilization
U. S. Civil Service Commission, Medical Division
Manpower programs
OEO Health project agencies
Missile Base
State, county, township and municipal departments and private agencies which are responsible for health or educational work in nursing
Boards of health
Psychiatric and other types of special hospitals
Infirmaries of state institutions for the deaf and the blind
Boards of education
Any health organization or service supported by the state, county, township, or village funds, such as narcotic farms and sanatoria for tuberculosis patients
Combination of official and nonofficial agencies, organizations or institutions
Professional and other health or related organizations
Educational institutions
Colleges and universities
Associated field centers, such as hospitals and related institutions, public health and other community agencies

OCCUPATIONAL OPPORTUNITIES FOR MEN IN NURSING

Men in nursing in the USA represent a total of 1.1 per cent of the number of employed registered nurses. Ever since the first school for men nurses was opened in New York City in 1888 (the Mills School of Nursing for Men) they have had increasing opportunity for service in this field. The number of men who have elected to come into nursing may in part be a reflection of the feeling that it is a predominantly female occupation and of the fact that nursing education for so long has been mainly outside of educational institutions, such as colleges and universities.

Today the picture is changing, and one finds a gradually growing number of men in nursing. In the 1966 inventory of the ANA 6,590 employed men nurses were found, as compared to 3,630 in the 1956 to 1958 inventory. An additional 2,044 were enrolled in schools of nursing during the academic year 1965-1966. As young men become more aware of the opportunities for them in nursing, and as nursing education programs in both junior (or community) and senior colleges become more readily available to them, an increasing number of men can be expected to come into nursing. The Surgeon General's Consultant Group on Nursing urged that action be taken to attract more men to nursing and commented that, "Men in nursing are making outstanding contributions as leaders and teachers."[19]

Traditional Occupational Opportunities for Men Nurses

It is said by some nurses that men nurses are able in some instances to give better nursing care to men patients because they understand them and can perform the required nursing procedures without embarrassment to themselves or the patients. It also has been implied that because of the lack of men nurses, some men patients receive, from relatively untrained personnel, nursing care and treatments that should be given by professional personnel. For example, a urologist has said recently that approximately 70 per cent of the bladder infections he saw in males "came from being catheterized by orderlies." Some men patients have said that they feel freer in discussing their conditions with a man nurse and consequently they react better to the guidance of a man nurse. On the other hand, men nurses generally prefer to think that their practice is not limited to the nursing care of men, but that they are prepared to function in all fields as a *nurse*.

World War II and the Korean and Vietnam Wars drew many registered men nurses from hospitals into the armed forces or occupational health nursing. Those in military service were not inducted as nurses but took their chances along with other service men. To change the regulations of the armed forces to include men nurses presented some administrative problems that were not easily solved. However, these problems were finally resolved. In 1955, the bill (H.R. 2559) presented by Representative Frances Payne Bolton successfully passed the House and the Senate and was signed by President Eisenhower on August 9 of that year. A 25-year-old man, Edward L. T. Lyon, was the first man to receive his commission under the terms of the new legislation. LeRoy Craig was one of the pioneers in the drive to se-

[19] U. S. Department of Health, Education, and Welfare. Public Health Service, *Toward Quality in Nursing: Needs and Goals*, Report of the Surgeon General's Consultant Group on Nursing, Washington, D.C., Government Printing Office, February 1963, p. 29.

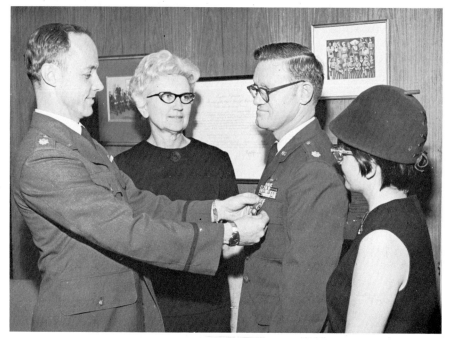

Fig. 8-1. Major George E. Farrell II, graduate student in the University of Colorado School of Nursing, receives the Bronze Star for his service under fire in South Vietnam. Left to right: Maj. Frank H. Brunstetter, liaison officer for Air Force officers studying at the CU Medical Center; Dr. Kathryn M. Smith, dean of the nursing school; Major Farrell and his wife. (University of Colorado Medical Center)

cure the legislation. Mr. Craig made the following comment about this legislation: "Commissioning of the man nurse . . . will [create] a long stride in democracy, understanding, and planning [in nursing]. The real challenge facing nursing is how to expedite our present plans toward sounder relationships of all concerned with nursing and education for adequate nursing service."[20] Figure 8-1 shows a picture of Major George E. Farrell receiving the Bronze Star for his service under fire during air-evacuation duty in South Vietnam. He served as a flight nurse and as assistant chief nurse of the 903rd Aeromedical Evacuation Squadron at Tan Son Nhut in South Vietnam from July 1967 to July 1968.

Educational positions in nursing schools have been available to men nurses, as well as administrative and supervisory positions in the nursing services of hospitals. In public health agencies, opportunities have also been available. The Veterans Administration and state hospital systems have increasing opportunities for men nurses. These are opportunities for men who qualify to make a decent living for their families. Nursing services of American companies in foreign lands also offer positions for men.

[20] From letter dated April 18, 1958, addressed to one of the authors.

Emerging Occupational Opportunities for Men Nurses

The 3 fields of nursing where the majority of men nurses are found today are hospitals and other institutions, 79.8 per cent; private practice, 6.6 per cent; and industry, 4.4 per cent. In contrast, the majority of women are in hospitals and other institutions, 65.2 per cent; private practice, 9.7 per cent; and office nursing 8.1 per cent. Men are to be found in all fields of nursing employment, and the majority—as in the case of women—are employed as general staff nurses; but a larger percentage of men are in head nurse, supervisory and administrative positions. However, in making these comparisons, it must be remembered that the numbers of women in nursing are much greater.[21]

Mannino found that a large majority of the men nurses surveyed were working in nursing, 48.9 per cent. Of the remaining, 31.3 per cent were in related health fields. A large number of men nurses continue to become nurse anesthetists. Other health related fields in which men were to be found working were: physicians, medical detailers, hospital administrators, physical therapists, pharmacists and directors of laboratories.[22]

Today the man nurse is accepted in all areas of specialization, and his basic educational preparation is the same as for women nurses. An increasing number of men nurses receive baccalaureate and higher degrees.

What Are Some of the Persisting Problems in Relation to Nursing by Men?

1. There still seems to be some difference of opinion among men in nursing about where men should work and how they should be prepared for nursing. For example, one man in nursing said this:

The question of training in obstetrics has been debated pro and con for many years. In order to have a broad spectrum of the whole nursing field, an adequate knowledge of obstetrics is essential. While it is doubtful that men would choose obstetrics as a specialty, they should certainly be familiar with all problems and procedures involved. For men in nursing administration, a good background in obstetrics would certainly be essential. The usefulness of men in pediatric wards has been demonstrated many times.

A comment from another man nurse was:

Men nurses—and as a matter of fact all nurses—need training in obstetrics not to become practitioners but for a better understanding of human growth and development.

Another comment made by a man nurse is:

All pediatric units should have some men nurses on their staffs. The sick child from a good home has equally strong needs for both a mother and a father. The

---

[21] American Nurses' Association, *Facts About Nursing: A Statistical Summary*, New York, The Association, 1968, pp. 8-9, 21.

[22] Mannino, S. F., "The Professional Man Nurse: Why He Chose Nursing and Other Characteristics of Men in Nursing," *Nursing Research*, 12:185-187, Summer 1963.

child's anxiety from illness and the strange surroundings in the hospital may be lessened if there is a good father figure to whom he may relate. As a director of nursing service I would not hesitate to place a well-prepared man as supervisor on an obstetric or a gynecologic unit.

According to one man who is a director of nursing service and an assistant professor of nursing:

The goals for men in nursing should be for equal opportunity, not selective priorities. The best applicant should be selected for positions in nursing whether this be a man or a woman. Men in nursing are more apt to remain in the profession. Theirs is a career choice and their careers are uninterrupted; for example, marriage, babies and family responsibilities generally do not interfere with their careers in nursing. It is believed that nursing can be a rewarding career for men, both financially and in satisfactions. The recruitment of men into nursing should be given the highest priority.

One man commented on the curriculum problem relating to obstetric nursing in this way:

I would agree that at one time this was a real problem, but accrediting and approving groups have settled this problem to a large extent.

Another man in nursing has sent this comment:

In most nursing situations it seems that men and women nurses have equal ability and contributions to make at all levels from the director to staff nurse and concerning the care of patients of either sex. I believe in the present-day concept in nursing education that a sick woman has the same problems as a sick man and vice versa. Many of the challenges confronting nurses are based on old misconceptions regarding what we can do for a patient.
A sick man has the same feeling as a sick women. Men nurses assigned to units of a psychiatric hospital where women are cared for have demonstrated the value of their presence in meeting the psychological and emotional needs of women patients. Likewise, women nurses are valuable on the services for men patients in psychiatric hospitals.

Do you know what stand the state board of nursing in your state takes toward this question of where men can work in order to facilitate interstate licensure?

2. It appears that one of the major problems is the development of a plan for recruitment of men for nursing. There has been some attention given to this by the nursing organizations and, as stated before, the Surgeon General's Consultant Group in Nursing urged more attention be given this problem. The concerted and vigorous efforts of all groups, including men nurses, will be needed. What is being done in your state to recruit men into nursing?

3. Related to the second problem has been the dearth of career publicity which has resulted in a lack of well-qualified men applicants for admission to nursing schools. The NLN has published career pamphlets to overcome, this lack, in part.

4. Some men believe that a major problem revolves around the acceptance of the qualified man in nursing by the medical profession. It is said that physicians confuse men nurses with untrained attendants and do

not give them proper recognition. Other men do not feel this has been a problem.

5. Recognition by the public of the difference between the prepared and registered man nurse from the orderly and man aide also seems to be a big stumbling block for the well-prepared men in nursing. It is believed that this problem can be solved only through appropriate educational efforts.

Encouraging Developments in Relation to Men in Nursing

Some of the more encouraging developments in relation to men in nursing are:

1. Passage of the bill which commissioned men nurses in the armed forces in 1955.

2. The appointment of men nurses as chief nurses and in other nurse positions in the Veterans Administration.

3. The appointment of well-prepared men nurses to instructional staffs in both preservice programs for nursing and graduate programs for nurses, and to state boards of nursing.

4. The appointment of men nurses as deans of nursing schools in baccalaureate and associate degree programs.

5. The election of a man to serve on the first Board of Directors of the National League for Nursing.

6. The appointment of a man nurse on the Board of the American Journal of Nursing Company, and of another to the position of publishing director of the Company.

7. The appointment of men in increasing numbers as consultants in mental health and psychiatric nursing in states and by the NLN. Some of the states in which men have been employed as consultants are: Maryland, Michigan, New Jersey, Oklahoma, Pennsylvania and Virginia. Men nurses have also been employed on the professional staff of the ANA and the NLN.

8. The election of a man to the ANA Board of Directors in 1958.

9. Men have been elected as state nurse association presidents, for example, in Vermont, Michigan and Pennsylvania.

10. The effort of the nursing profession to improve economic conditions for men nurses, which, in the past, have been deplorable.

OCCUPATIONAL OPPORTUNITIES FOR NURSES IN MISSIONARY WORK

Objectives of Missionary Nursing

One of the objectives of missionary nursing is to help the people in developing sections of the world to understand the dignity of the human being through the kindly example it gives in ministering to the needs of man's threefold nature—physical, mental and spiritual. It is especially missionary nurses' aim in many countries to work with and for the women in order to gain for them the dignity and respect God meant them to possess.

To work with these people and gain their confidence requires that one recognize the fact that differences in custom and tradition do not necessarily indicate inferiority; on the contrary, at times they may signify a higher and more spiritual philosophy of life. By a sincere attempt to understand the culture of the people, it is the hope of missionary nurses that such enlightenment and tolerance will serve to unify and strengthen intergroup relations among the various peoples of the world and eventually draw all into the light and the kingdom of God.

To establish good standards of nursing, to conduct nursing schools for local youth, and to raise the general level of health, sanitation and habits of living to standards of ordinary safety, comfort and decency are also objectives. Another objective is to train and educate the young people for positions of leadership in nursing in their countries for the time when they may have to carry this responsibility. In the past some nurses in missions have worked long and hard themselves, but they have kept the people of the country out of responsible positions. Nursing in the mission field is a cooperative venture. Sometimes, but not always, in top positions it is more difficult to help others to develop in responsible positions than to give orders. However, one of the goals of missionary nursing is to give guidance and to develop responsibility in those who show promise of leadership.

Helping the local women to achieve status and dignity and the local nurses to achieve professional status may be difficult. However, many missionary nurses can help to raise professional standards by helping the nurses to develop nurses-association activities and the needed laws for securing appropriate legal recognition of nursing personnel.

Another objective closely allied with that last mentioned is for the missionary nurse to act as a consultant to nurses who are beginning to assume positions of leadership and responsibility in the health field. In the past, it was often necessary for the missionary nurse to assume and maintain a leadership role and to carry the greater responsibility in the mission hospitals, schools of nursing and other community health agencies. Now, with increasing feelings of nationalization, changes in this regard are taking place. The nursing practice act in some countries specifies that only a citizen of that country may be the educational administrator of a school. This is done in the Philippines, for example. In other countries, nurses from the USA may not be granted reciprocity.

It is very important that missionary nurses respect the people they work with and their need to feel proud of their own abilities and accomplishments.

Types of Work Done by Missionary Nurses

In general, missionary nurses engage in much the same kinds of work as nonmissionaries: they work in hospitals and dispensaries, visit the sick in their homes, open and conduct nursing schools where local qualified youth are trained so that eventually they may do all the nursing for their own people. Missionary nurses also assist in establishing and maintaining health standards, and start nursing organizations when the situation warrants this progressive measure. As one nurse put it:

It's using everything a nurse has ever learned in a school of nursing and everything that she has read in nursing journals. It's forcing fluids on a child dying from diarrhea. It's delivering babies, preparing diets, and assisting the doctor. It's watching and working day and night to bring a critically ill patient through. It's sympathizing with patients' relatives.[23]

As soon as possible, missionary nurses usually begin training local "helpers" for nursing. Eventually this seems to lead to the development of nursing schools operated under gradually better standards. In nursing education, therefore, there are ever-increasing and challenging opportunities for nurses in the mission field.

Few countries in which missions have been established have enough nurses in public health; they are vitally needed. Nurses with preparation for public health work are faced with the dilemma of whether they should do actual field work themselves or concentrate on the training of local youth and nurses for nursing in public health. Public health nurses are usually involved in social action. They work with groups in the community to identify problems and provide possible solutions, and present these to the appropriate authorities for approval and initiation.

Nurses also are asked to work on social welfare committees or to serve as consultants to professional nursing groups, both government and voluntary. A number of missionary nurses are serving as consultants to personnel in hospitals and schools of nursing.

There is a great need for nurses specially prepared in administration, teaching and consultation in both nursing service and nursing education—all fields. Maternity nurses and nurse midwives are greatly in demand.

Conditions of Mission Life

Conditions of mission life vary widely with the climate, the language, the cultural differences to which one must adapt, the country, the particular part of the country, the degree of development of the people, the age of the mission, whether just beginning or long established, and the general economic, political and social condition of the immediate community. Life is doubtless very hard and lonely on some missions; interesting, lively, and even fascinating on others; fairly easy and comfortable, not too unlike home conditions, on still others. It probably takes heroic strength to live in some mission situations and comparatively none to live in others. We may be sure the mission field offers great compensations for those who work solidly and well, imbued with the true spirit. There are undoubtedly nurses who, with a special calling for this type of work, are happiest when doing it.

[23] M. R. Maxwell, "Missionary Nursing," *Nursing Outlook*, 11:895, Dec. 1963.

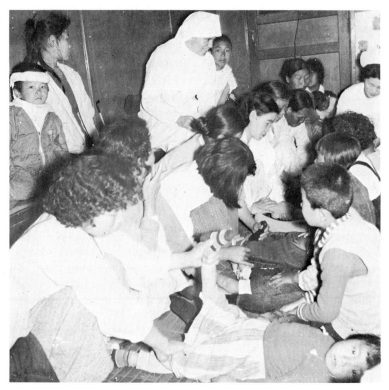

Fig. 8-2. Physiotherapy room in the clinic at Pusan, Korea. Maryknoll Sister is instructing mothers in exercises for children in plaster casts. Notice the crowded conditions current in mission clinics and also the intelligent use of local personnel. (Maryknoll Sisters)

To illustrate the spirit of service on a mission, as viewed by one nurse who perhaps expresses the sentiment of many others in mission service, here is an abstract from a letter received from a nurse who returned from a mission field:

It is often a matter of comment that . . . those who have once been working in the foreign mission field simply cannot resign themselves to the drab life "at home." There is a thrill to it, especially to the knowledge that one is relieving the sufferings of the poorest of the poor. While I speak from the point of view of a [nun], I know very well that lay people have the same enthusiastic love for the foreign mission field. I traveled with Protestant clergymen and their wives. All share in the same enthusiasm. . . .

If hundreds [of missionaries] can respond to the missionary urge and live happily in foreign lands on a small salary, enduring many privations, it is because the work is satisfying. The salary is, relatively speaking, small — but labor is cheap.

Some bring forward the element of loneliness. Nowhere else in the world does one form such friendships as in a foreign mission. Usually religious and national boundaries do not exist. Every missionary will help every other one. . . . Hospitality is freely given among the missionaries and money for the same accepted only under protest, even though badly needed.

You will be interested in what another missionary nurse wrote after reading the preceding letter. She said:

I like this letter. It is a good description of what missionary work may be, but it especially indicates what it feels like. I would have liked her to have mentioned also that, although we have failures and disappointments of great concern to us, there is the satisfaction of watching the amazing development of individual nurses as well as the nursing profession in these developing countries. There is also a personal satisfaction in being able to share in these developments when, at the same time, there is no one else to do it — a sense of accomplishment that I doubt can be equaled elsewhere. In fact we are, at times, almost forced to do things we did not think we were capable of.

Figures 8-2 and 8-3 show examples of the kind of activities carried on by missionary groups from different religious denominations.

What Should Motivate the Missionary Nurse?

The missionary nurse needs to be imbued with a deeply religious spirit and devotion to the service of mankind. She must have a very real love of the people to whom she ministers. On the missions, more than in any other field of social work, it is necessary to follow the precept of St. Vincent de Paul to love the poor very much so that they can forgive one for the bread given them. This is especially true in the Orient where the concept of "losing face" is so strong.

What Nurses Should Enter the Mission Field?

Only those nurses should enter the mission field who, besides possessing good sense, infinite patience, good health, and the qualifications of good

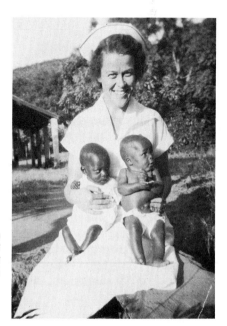

Fig. 8-3. Jack and Jill, premature orphan twins would have died if this Seventh-day Adventist missionary nurse (Anna May Vaughan) had not gone to Mwami Mission in Zambia. (Loma Linda University)

nurses, are both able and willing to lead exemplary lives as models for those whom they are trying to lead to God, and to show fortitude in their tolerance of privations and different cultural patterns and behavior. A most important quality for the nurse to possess is a sense of humor. To be able to detect the incongruities of life, to be able to laugh—even at oneself—is a great asset in weathering the problems of missionary life.

Generally missionary nurses have limited supervision of local doctors and complete supervision of nurses, so they should have initiative, unusually good judgment, and ability to carry much responsibility and to meet emergencies adequately. They must be able to improvise when necessary equipment is lacking and to get along with old-fashioned equipment and supplies. On the other hand, not all missionary nurses have these problems. Some may find themselves in a well-equipped hospital or agency where medical and nursing care are very advanced. While the missionary nurse should be of leadership caliber, she must also be willing to assume the role of coworker and follower. In this role she has many opportunities to help others grow into positions of leadership.

It is essential that the missionary nurse have a good knowledge of the language and the culture of the people that she will be working with. It is becoming increasingly important for her to have completed work for her baccalaureate degree, and often an advanced degree is desirable. Advanced courses in tropical public health, tropical nutrition, health education, anthropology and international relations will be helpful as background. Preparation in midwifery may be important in some instances. Some religious groups themselves provide excellent programs for the preparation of their nurse missionaries for work in the foreign field.

Admission and Term of
Assignment in Mission Work

The best way to learn the requirements for missionary nurses in your particular religious group is to obtain the name and address of one or more persons in charge of such work and write to or interview them, asking for all available information. It may be well to compare different kinds of mission work and different groups engaged in it, so that you may make a wise choice. Get as much information as possible, from a circular or a book, regarding the life of the missionary nurse, her work, her particular obligations and responsibilities, and the kind of life she will be expected to lead. Foresee the situation as clearly as you can and decide whether you will be willing and able to live in it.

In the USA the Catholic Mission Board and more than 100 Protestant mission boards operate medical missions in other countries. It may be that your church publishes a list of such mission societies or communities from which you can get names and addresses of several in which you may be interested. *The Official Catholic Directory,* revised annually, includes the name and the address of every Catholic religious community in this country, with a brief description of the community's work, institutions and location. The national mission boards of a number of denominations publish similar directories. One general source of information on Protestant medical missions is the Christian Medical Council for Overseas Work, 156 Fifth Avenue, New York, N.Y. 10010. Articles and books on nursing in the mission field are published from time to time. You will find some listed at the end of this chapter.

The term of a missionary nurse can be anywhere from 2 to 6 years, depending on the policy of the mission organization, the country to which she is assigned and the type of assignment. At the end of the term, the nurse usually returns home for rest, speaking engagements and further study. A nurse who is interested in missionary work can gain much valuable information as to the needs and nature of the work in a particular country or area by interviewing a nurse who is on furlough. The names and addresses of nurses on furlough can usually be secured from the headquarters of each denomination.

NEED FOR KEEPING INFORMED ABOUT OCCUPATIONAL CHANGES

Today more than at any time in history the entire world needs nurses, both men and women nurses, who are competent and who can carry responsibility. Nurses have a very special and important part to play in the programs of communicable disease control (including tuberculosis, leprosy and syphilis), maternal and child health, cancer control, control of occupational diseases, prevention of blindness, care of crippled patients, promotion of mental health, civil defense and in geriatric and rehabilitation programs.

Health problems are universal, and the contribution of nurses in health programs at home and in all countries of the world is tremendous. Here is a real opportunity for all nurses to use their influence to bring about international peace.

Keep in touch with world as well as local changes, because they affect nursing as a whole and occupational opportunities in particular, and because this knowledge is very helpful in sensing which positions are declining and which are increasing in relative importance.

Nurses are needed, both men and women nurses. Opportunities definitely are increasing. Those who plan soundly and who qualify spiritually, intellectually, personally, socially and technically are wanted in all nursing fields.

Chapters 9, 10 and 11 discuss in detail the qualifications and the preparation for nursing in different fields of work.

PROBLEMS

General

1. (a) What is the proportion of practical nurses to professional nurses for each 10-year period since 1920? (b) What is the present proportion of aides to registered nurses? (c) What is the present proportion of aides to practical nurses? (d) Is the ratio increasing or decreasing? (e) What are the implications for nursing of the trend in this situation?

2. (a) Study the supply and demand of nurses in your state. (b) Keeping in mind the goals recommended in the report, *Toward Quality in Nursing: Needs and Goals*, what are the prospects in your state?

3. (a) Ask some of the leaders in nursing in your community what they believe are the emerging opportunities for employment in nursing. (b) On the basis of your survey see what additional suggestions and classifications you can make about the opportunities in nursing that are presented in this chapter.

4. Study each issue of the *American Journal of Nursing, Nursing Outlook, Nursing Research* and the *International Nursing Review* for the last year and determine what were the special occupational demands for nurses.

Men in Nursing

1. Discuss the idea expressed in the following comment made by a man in nursing: "I was graduated from nursing and began as a clinical instructor at . . . in 1936. It was felt then that it would be a good idea to have a 'mother' and 'father' image on each of the large pediatric units of the hospital. The head nurse on the boy's pediatric surgery was a woman nurse and I was the clinical instructor. We conducted no controlled experiment. We believed, however, that on the units where a man and woman were jointly in charge, the children responded better. . . ."

2. (a) What men are serving on boards, committees, and other groups in the national nursing organizations? (b) What contribution have men nurses made to nursing in your locality? (c) What men nurses are serving on the state board of nursing, committees and other groups of the nursing organizations in your state and local community?

3. Identify the following men in nursing and describe their contributions to the profession: Luther Christman; Philip Day; Richard O. Hakes; Clifford H. Jordan; Sandy F. Manino; John H. Wick; Edward O. Wray.

4. (a) How can the scope of the recruitment program for students of nursing be broadened so as to reach potential men candidates? (b) Do you think recruitment should start with students in the elementary schools?

Nurses in Missionary Work

1. (a) In working for and with people from other countries of the world, what should be our own attitude toward their health practices? (b) What are

some factors one should understand before evaluating people of another culture?

2. (a) Correspond with a nurse in the mission field in a foreign country. (b) Learn from her all you can about the country, its people, its nursing and health programs, how she works with government and voluntary nursing and allied groups, and what she does and does not like about her work. (c) Learn what the government regulations about nursing are, and what is the attitude of the people in government toward nursing in the country. (d) Decide whether you would be interested in missionary nursing.

3. (a) Try to keep informed about world affairs, especially in Asia, South America and Africa. (b) Talk to some missionaries and learn what they think are the differences between working as a missionary nurse in these 3 parts of the world.

4. If you were planning to do missionary work in the Far East, what do you think might be the major problems you would face there? In Africa? In South America?

SUGGESTED REFERENCES*

GENERAL

* American Nurses' Association. *Facts About Nursing: A Statistical Summary.* New York, The Association, Current edition.
_____. *RN's 1966 ... An Inventory of Registered Nurses.* New York, The Association, 1969.
"Challenges to Nursing in Medicare." *American Journal of Nursing,* **65**:68-75, Nov. 1965.
* Cherescavich, G. "Utilizing the Professional Nurse." *MLN Bulletin,* **15**:3-8, July 1967.
* Fischelis, M. C. and French, N. H. "Three Full-time Jobs: Nurse, Wife and Mother." *American Journal of Nursing,* **68**:76-79, Jan. 68.
* Gabrielson, R. "Impact of Medicare on Nursing." *Arizona Nurse,* **20**:4-5, Jan.-Feb. 1967.
Hess, A. "Through Government Action: Medicare Begins." *American Journal of Nursing,* **66**:1295-1297, June 1966.
Kay, E. *Nurses and What They Do.* New York, Franklin Watts, 1968.
Kramer, M. "A Look at the Facts." *Nursing Times,* **63**:851-853, June 30, 1967.
Lambertsen, E. C. "The Emerging Health Occupations." *Nursing Forum,* **7**:87-97, Winter 1968.
Lesparre, M. "Retired Nurses Return to Nursing." *Hospitals,* **40**:46-48, passem, July 1, 1966.
Mussallem, H. K. "Manpower Problems in Nursing." *Canadian Nurse,* **63**:25-26, Aug. 1967.
National League of Nursing Education. Committee on the Grading of Nursing Schools. *Nurses, Patients and Pocket-books: A Study of the Economics of Nursing.* New York, The League, 1928, pp. 35, 36, 38, 40, 42.
Platou, C. N. and Pederson, W. D. "Can More Part-time Nurses be Recruited?" *Hospitals,* **41**:77-82, Dec. 16, 1966.

* In each chapter all citations are footnoted and are not included here. All starred references are recommended for additional reading.

Pope, I. "Medicare's Impact on Hospital Nursing Service." *Nursing Outlook,* **14**:60-61, June 1966.
Scott, J. M. "Three Years with the Nurse Training Act." *American Journal of Nursing,* **67**:2107-2109, Oct. 1967.
U.S. Department of Health, Education, and Welfare. Public Health Service. *Nurse Training Act of 1964: Program Review Report.* Washington, D.C. Government Printing Office, December 1967.
See also the Guide Issue of *Hospitals,* Journal of the American Hospital Association, published in August, each year. This issue includes information on the distribution of personnel in hospitals, including nurses. See also references at end of Chapters 9, 10, and 11.

MEN IN NURSING

Campbell, K. "The Male Health Visitor." *Nursing Mirror,* **126**:35-36, Jan. 26, 1968.
* Craig, L. N. "Another Goal Achieved." *Nursing Outlook,* **4**:175-176, Mar. 1956.
Fosberg, G. C. "Men Nurses are There." *American Journal of Nursing,* **69**:310-315, Feb. 1969.
Harden, L. M. "Maternity and Men." *American Journal of Nursing,* **63**:102-104, Apr. 1963.
Haynes, I. "Commissions and Men Nurses." *American Journal of Nursing,* **56**: 775, June 1956.
Johnson, G. A. "Obstetric Nursing is for Men, Too." *American Journal of Nursing,* **66**:2714-2715, Dec. 1966.
* Mannino, S. F. "The Professional Man Nurse: Why He Chose Nursing and Other Characteristics of Men in Nursing." *Nursing Research,* **12**:185-187, Summer 1963.
"Men in Nursing." *Hospitals,* **42**:41, May 1968.
Thomas, K. "Men Nurses in Public Health Work." *Christian Nurse,* **213**:15-16, Aug. 1967.

MISSIONARY NURSING

"Expedition to Nepal." *Nursing Times,* **64**:15-17, Jan. 1968.
Fox, J. E. "Papal Volunteer in Peru." *American Journal of Nursing,* **67**:2565-2568, Dec. 1967.
Hayes, D. A. "A Typical Day in My Utopia." *Midwife and Health Visitor,* **3**:505-506, Dec. 1967.
* Long, R. F. *Nowhere a Stranger.* New York, Vantage Press, 1968.
* Maxwell, M. "Missionary Nursing." *Nursing Outlook,* **11**:895-897, Dec. 1963.
* Monteith, M. C. "International Aspects of Nursing." *Nursing Outlook,* **12**:56-58, Jan. 1964.
Sister Maria del Rey. *Safari by Jet.* New York, Scribner, 1962.

CHAPTER

9

Fields of Work in Nursing Services

The purpose of the authors in this and the next 3 chapters is to discuss briefly the main characteristics of and requirements for work in the major fields in nursing and to stimulate your interest in making a comprehensive investigation of occupational opportunities.[1] You might consider making an occupational plan based on a study of one or more types of nursing work, bearing in mind your own interests and qualifications. Chapter 13, "Choosing a Field of Nursing," will be helpful in preparing materials, especially in analyzing your potential.

We suggest that you read Chapter 16, "Continued Education for Nurses," in connection with these chapters on the various fields of work in nursing. The beginning field of work will be generally one in which you will become proficient in nursing care. As you progress in your chosen field you no doubt will begin to feel the need for additional professional preparation, "continued education," in your field of work. Chapter 16 will tell you about the routes that you can take to graduate education.

NURSES IN PRIVATE PRACTICE

Nurses who derive satisfaction from giving close, continuous and highly personal nursing care to patients will find private practice, or private duty,

[1] Earnings are discussed in Chapter 15, "Planning Economic Security."

the perfect field of endeavor. Nurses in private practice are called on to be expert clinicians as well as expert generalists in nursing. Some nurses in this field continue to use the title *private duty;* others prefer the newer term *private practice.*

The nurse in private practice is one who independently contracts with a patient or his family to give expert nursing care to the patient. She is responsible for the total nursing care of the patient during the period she is with him. She is called upon to use her knowledge and skills to the fullest extent.

The role of the nurse in private practice, like that of other registered nurses, is expanding as a result of the changes and advances in medical care. Because her work often entails care of the acutely ill, of patients in intensive care units, of those who have had organ transplants and of other surgical patients requiring the utmost in modern professional care, she is expected to be an expert clinician. Actually many nurses in private practice, because of the type of patients they are called in to care for, may become experts in a particular field. It appears possible that the clinical specialist may eventually find a place in this field of nursing in the future.

The nurse in private practice cares for patients in the hospital and in the home; she may be called upon to travel with a patient. Some private practice nurses occasionally provide relief for general staff nurses on a per diem basis; others may do temporary work, such as camp nursing, or work with the Red Cross during epidemics and catastrophes.

The nurse in private practice can gain many rewards and satisfactions by actively participating in local, state and national association activities. Not only can she gain much but she can have the satisfaction of working for improvements in her field of nursing and enjoy many pleasant relationships with coworkers.

Major Functions and Qualifications for a Nurse in Private Practice

In the past decade modern advances in medicine, surgery and technology have presented a new challenge to all nurses, especially those in private practice. Nursing care is much more complex today. It is not a matter of giving bedbaths, feeding the patient, taking temperature, pulse, and respirations, giving enemas and making the patient comfortable. True, it includes all of these, but it also demands much more.

Because the nurse in private practice has the responsibility for the total nursing care of the patient, she performs the following nursing functions:

1. Formulation of a plan of care based on the individual needs of the patient.

2. Control of the environment of the patient, whether it is the home, the hospital or elsewhere.

3. Observation of symptoms and the reactions to medications and

treatments in relation to symptoms; evaluation of progress and contribution to the rehabilitation of the patient.

4. Keeping of accurate and complete records for the benefit of the patient, the physician, the nurse and the hospital, and for legal reasons. The nurse also needs to keep adequate records of patients cared for, so that she can summarize her experience each year. Such records are of value when studying nursing in this field, and they are essential for income tax reporting.

5. Direction and instruction of the licensed practical nurse or any other person who may substitute for the nurse in the home in the absence of the nurse.

6. Conducting any procedure involving the practice of a medical act under the supervision or the direction of a licensed physician. In some places the nurse is expected to give intravenous infusions and medications, such as aminophylline. Yet many hospitals do not permit the nurse in private practice to give intravenous medications but will allow general staff nurses to give them.[2]

7. Carrying on of those procedures that are concerned with the comfort and the hygiene of the patient and of certain emergency measures.

8. Health direction, including activities of psychologic and sociologic significance as they relate to the individual patient and his family.

Some nurses in private practice are specializing in a particular field of nursing and are taking on responsibilities which require additional or advanced preparation. For example, one nurse has been employed to care for a patient who had an unusual type of cardiac operation. In this instance she not only is giving expert nursing care, but she also is serving as a member of a research team which is developing a new method in this type of surgery and a detailed program of preoperative and postoperative care.

From a review of these general functions of the nurse in private practice, you can see that nursing in this field requires knowledge, specialized skills and sound personal and social attitudes.

Important qualities for you if you are considering entering private practice are those that are possessed in some degree by all successful nurses: scientific knowledge, sound concepts of nursing care, nursing skill, emotional stability, ingenuity, high professional ideals, adaptability, wisdom, tact, tolerance, reliability, patience, gentleness, good powers of observation, courtesy and the qualities essential for leadership in proportion to your status and responsibilities. Also of importance are courage, intelligence, vision, initiative, insight, openmindedness, self-confidence, energy which comes from good health, sincerity, versatility, maturity of judgment, the ability to work with people and a genuine liking for people.

Some of the abilities which you as a nurse in private practice will need

---

[2] Some state nurses associations are developing joint statements with medical and hospital associations that serve as guides for conditions under which certain medical procedures may be carried out by nurses in private practice.

especially are ability to adjust to patients and surroundings, particularly in homes; ability to inspire confidence and to meet emergencies; ability to show genuine liking for people and to establish close interpersonal and interprofessional relationships and ability to give total nursing care. Too, it is important to have respect for the religious beliefs of patients and to be able to help them in securing and maintaining peace of mind and spirit. Patients also expect their nurses to be well read and informed so that they can carry on intelligent conversations and be able to discuss current topics.

In general, the nurse in private practice carries responsibilities for evaluation of her own work, for self-improvement and for continuing education to an even greater extent than the nurse in a field having a planned program of evaluation and education. She must, therefore, be self-directing and willing to plan for her professional improvement.

Some Advantages and Disadvantages of Private Practice

While nursing in private practice you have the chance to see life as it really is, to study human nature and to know at close range interesting people of different nationalities, cultures, religions and status. You also have the opportunity to make some real friends. People have unusual confidence in a good nurse, thus giving her the chance to use her influence, while at the same time placing on her the responsibility of giving the right kind of guidance and doing effective health teaching.

Nursing in private practice is filled with adventure for those who grasp its deepest significance, because there is always something new and unknown waiting around the corner. Sometimes travel and a chance to see the world come to the nurse in this field.

One of the chief advantages of private practice cited by some nurses is that they can plan their own time. This is an advantage particularly for the married nurse, or the nurse attending school. Many nurses in private practice have home responsibilities, such as caring for aged parents or families. Some nurses say that they stay in the field because it enables them to adjust their work and private lives satisfactorily. However, the nurse who depends on private practice for her entire income generally finds it necessary to work about 240 days a year and does not limit her work by too many exceptions, such as types of patients and hours of work.

Modern medicine and surgery have increased the demands for nurses in private practice. Physicians often insist on special nursing care as an essential for the patient who has had a tracheotomy or eye, chest, brain, organ transplant, cardiac or other major surgery, or one who has a respiratory or a heart condition. In fact, nurses in private practice are more and more being used only to care for the acutely ill patients and those requiring intensive and complex nursing. The nurse who keeps abreast of new knowledge and procedures and who feels competent to care for such patients finds nursing an exciting, stimulating experience, with an infinite variety of problems to solve and personal satisfactions to be gleaned.

One disadvantage of private practice is that the nurse must pay a higher percentage of her total social security tax. She must also plan for herself for any of the so-called "fringe benefits" such as holidays, vacation, health and hospital insurance and retirement income.

Salaries and economic security as they relate to the nurse in private practice are discussed in Chapter 15, "Planning Economic Security."

Problems in the Field of Private Practice

The following problems of nurses in private practice seem to be the most important ones as noted from a survey the authors have made.

1. The persistent fundamental problem common to all fields of nursing is the wide variation in background, education and experience of nurses. Actually some so-called professional nurses do not and cannot give as good care as licensed practical nurses who have graduated recently from good schools of practical nursing. The problem of the nurse who gives poor care is one of real concern to the private practice group; fortunately, it is being faced realistically in some localities and by the ANA.

2. One criticism that seems important to consider, especially in view of the trend to help patients to help themselves and to be rehabilitated so that they can retake their places in society, is this; some nurses create and maintain a situation in which patients become totally dependent on them. No doubt part of this is due to the nurses' feelings that they may not be earning their fees unless they wait on their patients every minute, and part may be due to their job insecurity.

3. The problem of securing enough nurses in private practice for the evening and night hours and for holiday, weekend and vacation periods is a major one from the standpoint of patients, physicians and hospitals.

4. The nurse in private practice has had the disadvantage of being more or less a lone operator. Among other factors, this has sometimes created poor personal relationships with hospital personnel, especially with general staff nurses. This situation has caused criticism and confusion for the patient and his family.

5. A disputed point by some nurses is whether or not nurses in private practice should consider themselves under the supervision of administrative personnel in the hospital. The question one might raise in this connection is: Should the administrative and legal implications be considered in this problem by the nurse? The ANA has stressed that the nurse in private practice in the hospital is responsible to hospital administration. Legal opinions have been given substantiating the responsibilities of hospitals and nurses to each other, as well as to the patient.

6. On the other hand, the nurse in private practice complains that she has difficulty in getting assistance from the head nurse when a patient is critically ill and she needs help in giving a treatment or in changing

the position of a patient. She says she sometimes goes without meals because the head nurse does not arrange for relief when a patient cannot be left alone. This attitude is reflected in the staff if the head nurse is not sympathetic in understanding the problems of the nurse and in fulfilling her own responsibility for all patients on her unit.

7. The fact that many nurses in private practice carry full home responsibilities as well as professional obligations makes active participation in professional activities difficult or impossible. Some of these nurses are unable to attend meetings, serve on committees and hold office. Also, the fact that they do attend meetings at their own expense with corresponding loss of salaries is a real problem.

8. A problem that the nurses in private practice believe they need to consider is whether the nurse who is very experienced and well qualified should receive the same fee as the newly graduated nurse. Experimentation has begun in California to qualify and pay an increased fee to the nurse with additional education and experience.

9. The problem of the nurse in private practice as an independent contractor and her need for liability insurance is a growing one.

What Is Being Done to Solve Problems of Nurses in Private Practice

Much is being done to change conditions in the field of private practice that should benefit both patients and nurses.

Nurses themselves, working in their professional organizations, both in their special sections and with other groups, are doing a great deal in trying to solve their problems, but greater participation by all nurses in private practice is essential. The private practice nurse, because of her independent status, needs her professional organization almost more than other nurses.

State nurses associations are accomplishing much in helping solve the problems of nurses in private practice. In some hospitals they are invited to participate in the inservice education programs. Some nursing organizations have sponsored institutes and short courses in medical, surgical, cancer, cardiac, geriatric, rehabilitation and other types of nursing. However, it is still true that nurses in private practice have a very difficult time planning continued educational programs. Some state nurses associations are also working very effectively for the economic security of the nurse in private practice.

Many nurse placement services or registries have been using the ANA Professional Credentials and Personnel Service forms in keeping records and references on private practice nurses. They are also providing counseling services to help the inadequate nurse to improve. If her work continues to be unsatisfactory, her name is removed from the registry list. More stress is being placed on the fact that any nurse employed through a registry is recommended by the registry. In some areas, registries require that all nurses on the roster be evaluated on a regular annual basis by the hospital supervisor. This is a written evaluation and can be used for counseling by the registrar.

NURSES IN HOSPITALS AND SIMILAR HEALTH FACILITIES

What Is Hospital Nursing?

Nursing in hospitals and related health facilities such as, extended care facilities, nursing homes, and neighborhood clinics, comprises all of the basic components of comprehensive patient care and family health. The concept of the modern hospital as a community health center where inpatient and outpatient care are continuous describes the goal of medical care in most general hospitals. The goals of bringing care to the patient and of continuity of care are emphasized by the development of extended care facilities and the increasing use of home care (both resulting from the Medicare program), and by the use of neighborhood health centers affiliated with the local hospitals (a result of the Office of Economic Opportunity programs).

The nurse participates, as a member of the health care team, in all phases of patient care: the care of the acutely ill; the convalescing; the patient requiring bed care; and the ambulatory patient. She cares for the patient in the hospital and in the outpatient department, and she plans for the nursing care needs of the patient referred for extended care or home care. She performs nursing measures that will meet the patient's physical, emotional, social and spiritual health needs while he is in the institution and helps him and his family plan for his further health care needs when he returns home. Her functions involve evaluation of patient needs for nursing and planning for and giving, or providing, the care indicated — whether this be personal care, rehabilitation measures or health instruction. Her functions include participation in the research and teaching carried on in the hospital; she is often responsible for teaching auxiliary personnel and for assisting in medical student education.

Today, the actual job of ensuring continuity of care falls, in great part, upon the nurse, who is often responsible for initiating and following through on the referral of patients to the extended care facility or the home health agency. In extended care facilities and nursing homes, the importance of the role of the nurse cannot be overemphasized. Here, where the main purpose of the institution is the provision of nursing care, she performs the range of functions we have listed.

The practice of nursing in a given hospital is influenced by the philosophy underlying the operation of the hospital, by its objectives, by its physical and environmental facilities, by the personnel selected and by its organization and administration. Hospital nursing changes as these aspects of the hospital change to meet society's needs. Hospitals grow out of the needs of people. Certain health needs, such as the care of the sick and the injured, are met by many hospitals. Each hospital sets its own functions designed to carry out the purposes listed in its articles of incorporation. The purposes may be broad, as for general hospitals to provide for the care of all kinds of patients, or they may be limited, such as "to give care to the child with crippling conditions." The primary purpose of some hospitals may not be the care of the sick. Hospitals may have other purposes, such as "to do research into the cause of disease," as in the Clinical Center, National Institutes of Health, U. S. Department of Health, Education, and Welfare in Bethesda, Md. Other hospitals may have education as their primary purpose. The hospital in the community health center has many teaching functions, such as prenatal counseling, parents' classes, and speech correction. Other hospitals, particularly those for the care of the mentally ill, may be set up for "day care" or "night care" only. Some hospitals have departments where all kinds of diagnostic testing, including psychologic, may be done for the community. Hospitals can be used, also, for the practical education of physicians, nurses, dietitians, laboratory technicians, occupational therapists, x-ray technicians, social-service personnel, hospital administrators, residents, interns, and other hospital personnel.

The work of the nurse practitioner in a given hospital is influenced by

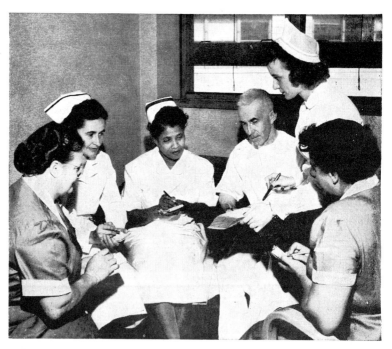

Fig. 9-1. A nurse instructor supervising the planning of nursing care by the nursing team. (Teaching Demonstration Center, Delafield Hospital, New York)

the organizational plan of the hospital departments for carrying out the purposes of the hospital, the organizational plan of the nursing service for carrying out its functions, the concept of nursing practice subscribed to – the objectives and the type of over-all planning for patient care – the kind of interdisciplinary relationships among personnel concerned with the patient, and the provision of conditions that make it possible for personnel to provide patient care. For example, the involvement of the nurse in planning on medical and hospital committees can be a factor in improving the quality of patient care.[3]

Other influences on the work of the nurse in the modern hospital grow out of various types of work divisions, new types of assignments and new relationships which must be tested and evaluated in terms of their usefulness. Because of the high cost of hospital care and the rapid pace of technological change, the emphasis today is on experimentation in staffing patterns, in types of personnel employed, in patient environment, as well as in the actual treatment afforded the patient. Changes in medical care have resulted in shorter hospital stays for patients. As a result, there are more continuous peak-load conditions and a frequent turnover of patients, which creates a demanding situation requiring stability and organizational ability on the part of the nurse.

The establishment of recovery rooms and intensive care units, as well as the automation of certain procedures, such as patient monitoring, are important influences on changing medical care. Emphasis on family-centered maternity care together with rooming-in allows the parents to participate in the care of their newborn infant. Permitting parents and relatives to participate in the care of patients is another innovation. The relocation of patients from segregated services, such as medical, surgical or communicable disease, to patient groupings based on age or degree of illness – for example, progressive patient care – are also major influences on the nurses' work. These trends in patterns of organization for care are requiring more teaching and supervision of other personnel and of patients and their relatives by the nurse. The use of floor managers and ward clerks, team nursing, group nursing and the use of clinical specialists in nursing are other influences on the work of nurses. The initiation of the position of administrative assistant to the director of nursing service permits the director to concentrate on the professional nursing aspects of her job. Finally, the availability of modern inservice education and staff development programs create a climate where good practice and sound experimentation can occur.

Types of positions available to nurses in hospitals are listed in Chapter 8, "General Survey of Occupational Opportunities for Nurses," in the section entitled "Positions in Nursing Services: Hospitals and Similar Health Facilities."

[3] A. L. Conta, *et al.,* "Professional Performance Committees," *American Journal of Nursing,* **69:**2601-2607, Dec. 1968.

Types of Hospitals and Similar Agencies Where Nurses Work

Hospitals usually are classified according to type of control, type of service offered, size and basis of accreditation.

Hospitals classified according to control are:

1. Governmental (official), including: Federal, such as those operated by the armed forces, Veterans Administration, and Public Health Service of the U. S. Department of Health, Education, and Welfare; state; county; city; and city-county

2. Nongovernmental (nonofficial), including: nonprofit groups, such as church or church affiliation, fraternal, private voluntary; and proprietary, such as individual, partnership and corporation

Hospitals classified according to type of service offered are usually divided into 2 groups:

1. According to sex or age, for example: women's, children's, babies', maternity or for men only

2. According to disease entity or condition cared for, such as: general, cancer, cardiac; eye, ear, nose, and throat; orthopedic and psychiatric

3. According to the nature of care required, such as acute hospital, extended care facility or nursing home

Hospitals are classified by size according to the number of beds available and the daily average number of patients.

Classification of Hospitals on Basis of Accreditation

The classification of hospitals on the basis of approval includes lists prepared by the following: (1) state agencies under licensing laws; (2) American Hospital Association (AHA), which lists registered hospitals meeting specified requirements; (3) American Psychiatric Association; (4) Council on Medical Education of the AMA for the approval of internships and other organizations' residency programs; (5) American College of Surgeons for approval of cancer programs; and (6) the Joint Commission on Accreditation of Hospitals.

Some people believe that the most significant approval agency for hospitals is the Joint Commission on Accreditation of Hospitals. Member organizations of the Commission are: the American Hospital Association, the AMA, the American College of Surgeons and the American College of Physicians. Major objectives of the Commission are to establish standards of hospital operation and to promote high quality of medical and hospital care in all their aspects. Evaluation is based on minimum standards consistent with safe patient care. The standards, based on principles of good practice, apply to all hospitals — large, small, or specialized. Nursing service evaluation is also a part of the total evaluation.

In 1966 the Commission also assumed responsibility for the accreditation of health care facilities other than hospitals. At that time, the American

Association of Homes for the Aging and the American Nursing Home Association became participating members of the Commission.[4]

The ANA and NLN both work toward the development and implementation of standards for nursing services. In 1965, the ANA published its *Standards for Organized Nursing Services in Hospitals and Public Health Agencies, Nursing Homes, Industry, and Clinics*, which was developed by its Committee on Nursing Service. Following the reorganization of the ANA, the ANA Commission on Nursing Services became responsible for developing standards and gaining their acceptance, for stimulating studies of the organization and management of services, for evaluating scientific and educational changes, as well as changes in health needs and practices, with their implications for nursing services and nursing manpower needs. The Commission also develops guides for the organization and management of nursing services and recommends action concerning Federal and state legislation related to health manpower and nursing services.[5]

Hospital Facilities in the USA

The number of hospital beds has increased tremendously since the turn of the century. According to the annual survey of the American Hospital Association in 1967, there were 1,671,125 beds in the 7,172 hospitals registered by them. A majority of the hospitals were community hospitals (nonfederal, short-term general and special hospitals, other than psychiatric and tuberculosis). This survey also stated that 22 per cent of the reporting hospitals reported having coronary care units, 67 per cent had postoperative recovery rooms and 8.4 per cent had a home care program. It was estimated that approximately 1,200 community hospitals (more than 20 per cent) provided hospital-based extended care services.[6]

Part of the hospital expansion is due to increased use of private, prepaid hospitalization insurance plans, an aging population beset with geriatric ailments and the introduction of Medicare and Medicaid programs. Regional planning of facilities on the basis of need, as under the Regional Medical Care programs, for example, and of the establishing of relationships between smaller hospitals in rural areas and large medical centers should help to distribute services more equitably. In this way complex services can be made available to more people, there can be better use of scarce personnel and unnecessary duplication of costly services can be avoided. Another trend of importance is the affiliation of health department clinics, hospital outpatient departments and neighborhood clinics in the interest of better continuity of

[4] Joint Commission on Accreditation of Hospitals, *Standards of Accreditation of Extended Care Facilities, Nursing Care Facilities and Resident Care Facilities*, Chicago, Joint Commission, 1968.

[5] American Nurses' Association, *Bylaws*, New York, The Association, 1968, p. 20.

[6] "The Nation's Hospitals: A Statistical Profile," *Hospitals, Journal of the American Hospital Association*, **42**(Part 2, Guide Issue):437-438, Aug. 1, 1968.

medical care. It would be an enlightening experience for you to explore other trends in hospital expansion.

In addition to hospitals, as of January 1, 1967, there were 20,031 long-term facilities in the USA and Puerto Rico with a total bed capacity of 974,277.[7] These included facilities providing skilled nursing care, those providing both personal care services and skilled nursing and those providing only personal care. The nursing home is becoming significant among the country's health-care facilities. Some of the skilled nursing care homes meeting Medicare requirements have entered into agreements with hospitals to become the extended care facilities for the hospitals. You will wish to keep informed about the changes taking place in the purposes and the character of facilities for such homes.

Nursing Positions Available in Hospitals and Similar Institutions: Essential Preparation and Qualifications

Nursing has developed in such complexity that its functions are performed by a variety of workers with different levels and length of preparation. The demands for nursing service have brought into hospitals greatly increased numbers of licensed practical nurses, auxiliary personnel trained on the job and other types of allied nursing personnel in addition to the technical and professional nursing personnel.

The main positions for nurses in hospitals related directly to nursing service or care of the patient are as staff or general duty nurse, head nurse, supervisor, clinical specialist, associate or assistant director of the nursing service, and director of the nursing service. Many hospitals also employ an assistant director or an instructor with the responsibility for inservice education and staff development.

Because nursing positions in hospitals and similar institutions include a wide variation in the range of responsibilities and activities, the educational preparation and the experience required for effective functioning in them also differ. In 1965, the ANA, in its position on nursing education, recognized the need of preparation for both technical and professional nursing practice. See Chapter 2 for trends in nursing education. Larger hospitals generally have a greater variety of positions and supervisory levels, but in small hospitals, especially in rural areas, the nurse may need to take responsibility for self-direction and self-development within her general staff practice.

The Staff Nurse. The general staff nurse is concerned directly with the nursing care of patients and in some instances is the team leader of the personnel responsible for nursing care. Her preservice preparation equips her with basic competencies in most of the clinical nursing areas. If she continues to function in a particular clinical field, she needs to keep up to date by reading current relevant literature, especially nursing journals

[7] American Nurses' Association, *Facts About Nursing: A Statistical Summary*, New York, The Association, 1968, p. 203.

such as the *American Journal of Nursing;* by active participation in her professional associations and in their program meetings; and by attending institutes and being an active participant in the inservice program in the hospital. Perhaps more than any other nurse, she must be alert to changing medical practice and the newer demands made on nurses. This means that her attitude needs to be one of willingness to accept change and that she must be able to see the broadening scope of her job. As a leader of the nursing team, she needs to develop teaching, supervisory, coordinating, collaborating and managerial skills. She needs ability in problem solving, interpersonal and interprofessional relations and teaching, as well as clinical expertness and group conference leadership.

The Head Nurse. The head nurse is responsible for the administration of a unit of approximately 24 to 50 patients within a division of a nursing service of a hospital. Some of the newly constructed hospitals are planned on the basis of 40 to 60 patients per unit with the organization of the nursing service staff into approximately 4 or more teams.

The head nurse, the supervisor and the nursing service director are all members of the professional nursing service administrative team whose joint appraisal, planning and organization of patient care set the standard for the quality of nursing care given. The head nurse needs to be an expert clinician and teacher if she is to be successful in evaluating the needs of patients, planning for their care, and guiding the work of others in the provision of the care. She also needs some understanding of the processes of administration and supervision. The head nurse, in preparing for her position, would do well to take advanced courses in the process of administration, teaching, and supervision, interpersonal relationship, public relations in hospitals, communication skills, legal aspects of nursing, general nursing or a nursing specialty, and those courses which will help her to understand people and to meet better the demands of her particular job. In addition to having a good educational preparation, the head nurse should possess personal qualifications which include a keen interest and understanding of the needs of patients and of coworkers. Like the staff nurse, it is important that she keep abreast of current literature and be active in her professional associations.

The Supervisor. The Supervisor is responsible for the administration of a division of a nursing service in a hospital, such as generalized nursing, medical and surgical nursing or maternity nursing. Another kind of divisional pattern might be on the basis of patient needs, for example: critical, long-term extensive nursing, rehabilitation, ambulatory or long-term custodial care. The supervisor could be in charge of any one of such divisions, or she could be responsible for 3 or 4 units of private patients. Regardless of the type of division, the supervisor is responsible for the direction of all personnel in the division and works directly with and through the head nurse in the division. She should be very well prepared in generalized nursing or a specialized field of nursing; have an understanding of research methods, including the ability to evaluate and use the findings of research; and have a working knowledge of the functional processes of administration, supervision and teaching. Other important areas of instruction are hospital administration, the behavioral sciences, communication skills, legal aspects of nursing and professional and social ethics. She must be an expert in such areas as staffing patterns, staff education, quality controls such as nursing audits, trends in automation and interdepartmental relations. Because the head nurse and the supervisor are key people in the administration of nursing service, they should have a thorough understanding of their relationships to each other and, also, the relationship of the units or divisions for which they are responsible to other units within the nursing service and to other hospital services, so as to promote the carrying out of interdivisional and interservice functions effectively. In addition to having an appropriate education, the supervisor, like the head nurse, should possess an interest in and an understanding of the needs of patient and of coworkers. Above all, the supervisor, as well as the head nurse, must be an expert clinician and have the ability to develop in those under her supervision the ability to give expert care.

The Clinical Specialist. A growing number of hospitals are employing clinical specialists or clinical supervisors who, by education and experience, have developed a high level of knowledge and skills in a special area of practice, such as geriatric nursing, maternal and child health nursing, or coronary care nursing. The clinical specialist is the expert practitioner responsible for improving the quality of nursing care through work with patients and by guiding the work of others giving the nursing care. According to Fagen, the clinical specialist has great potential as: (1) a role model, (2) a participant-observer, (3) an informal teacher, (4) an investigator, (5) an innovator, and (6) an evaluator-assessor. She must have the ability to evaluate research in her specialty and to assist the staff in implementing the findings of research. Her background should include an introduction to research methods, which will enable her to identify what needs research and to initiate new studies with the goal of improved practice. As more nonnurse assistants or secretaries enter the picture, there may be less need for the administrative supervisor and a greater movement toward the use of the supervisor who is a clinical specialist.[8]

The Associate Director. The associate or assistant director of a nursing service shares the administration of the service with the director and usually serves as deputy director. There is a difference between an assistant director of nursing service and an assistant to the director of nursing service. An assistant to the director is responsible only for the activities which are assigned to her by the director, and in some instances she may not be a nurse. Sometimes she is called an administrative assistant. The assignment depends on the size of the nursing service, the number of people available, and the plan of allocation of activities based on a functional analysis and distribution of the tasks involved. An assistant director may be responsible for adminis-

[8] C. M. Fagin, "The Clinical Specialist as Supervisor," *Nursing Outlook,* **15:**34-36, Jan. 1967.

trative, educational, or personnel functions or for all 3. Assistant directors may be assigned to carry responsibility for various units of the nursing service, such as maternity. The assistant should be well prepared for whatever functions are assigned: educational, administrative, personnel or other.

The Director. The director of nursing service in a hospital is responsible for the general administration of the service. As a member of the executive staff, she is responsible for interpreting nursing and the nursing service needs of patients to the hospital administrator and other department heads. She is involved in the affairs of the hospital as a whole and with its place in the community. She should have the best preparation possible. It is desirable that she complete those advanced courses which will help her to become an effective leader of people and a capable administrator in all areas of nursing service under her direction. In addition to the courses suggested for the preparation of a supervisor, community health organization and problems in administration of a hospital nursing service are recommended. Necessary are courses in budgeting, accounting, preparation and use of nursing service statistics, the writing of comprehensive and convincing reports, hospital law, and legal aspects of nursing. It should be emphasized that for the director of nursing service, understanding of administration is equally as important as understanding the principles of good nursing care. She must have the capacity to see nursing in relation to the other disciplines involved, the ability to reach out and make use of the findings of research in nursing and in related areas, the awareness of standards as set by the various official bodies, and familiarity with the sources of funds which might be available to improve nursing services. The position also requires that she be knowledgeable about both preservice and graduate education in nursing.

In addition to the hospital positions for nurses which have been described, there are several other positions of importance. These are director or coordinator of inservice education programs including on-the-job training programs, coordinator of patient education, methods analyst or nursing service research director and consultant in nursing service.

Preparation of nurses for direction and teaching in inservice programs in hospitals is discussed in the section of Chapter 10 headed "Nurses in Education. . . ." Special mention of the great demand for teachers for inservice programs in hospitals, however, is made again here for emphasis because of the great need for such workers.

A word should be said also about nursing in the outpatient department. Nursing in hospitals includes nursing of the ambulatory patient. This type of nursing is becoming increasingly important as the hospital becomes a community health center. There is a trend toward expanding the role of the nurse in outpatient and neighborhood clinics. She is assuming more responsibility for assessing patient care needs and for teaching patients and their families. Nurses who are interested in health teaching and preventive care will find outpatient department nursing a very challenging type of work, one that makes use of all of their professional skills.

So far, this discussion has centered on positions available primarily for nurses in hospitals. There is a large and growing number of allied nursing personnel employed in hospitals, such as licensed practical nurses, attendants, nursing aides, orderlies, ward clerks, secretaries and stewards. It is suggested that you refer to the latest "Guide Issue" of *Hospitals* and to the latest edition of *Facts About Nursing* to review the statistics about these groups. The role of these groups in hospitals is expanding. What the extent of the expanding role of these groups will be in the future is unpredictable. At any rate, these are implications for nurses to consider. Perfection of professional nursing skill in coordinating nursing-care services provided by various members of the nursing team is one need to consider. Another need to consider is that of determining those areas of nursing responsibility which the registered nurse should retain and not turn over to less qualified personnel.

Perhaps the group of most importance to nursing because of their expanding role are the licensed practical nurses. Licensed practical nurses, called vocational nurses in certain parts of the country, are rapidly increasing in numbers. Furthermore, as the educational programs for these nurses has been upgraded, they have been accorded more responsibilities in patient care. It is important that registered nurses know the proper functions of licensed practical nurses and learn to work effectively with this group. We suggest that you explore the whole question of the changing functions of nurses and auxiliary personnel, particularly as these relate to general staff nurses, the auxiliary nursing personnel and the necessary relationships for effective service.

Hospital nursing can be satisfying for the nurse who really wants to be with patients. In the hospital a nurse has an opportunity to learn more about patient care; first, because of the number of patients, and second, because it is essentially in hospitals that new developments in patient care are introduced. It is important, however, for the young nurse to choose carefully the hospital in which she will work. For instance, if you are interested in doing hospital nursing, you could inquire into: (1) the reputation of the hospital in the community; (2) its philosophy of patient care, and whether you will have the opportunity to give nursing care or if this responsibility has been assigned entirely to auxiliary nursing personnel; (3) its personnel policies (learn if these are in accord with the standards of the state nurses association) and (4) the kind of inservice education or staff development program it provides.

Expanding Objectives and Trends in the Modern Hospital Which Affect Nursing

The 2 major trends one hears mentioned most frequently are those of the rising cost of health care and the growing involvement of government in support of health care programs. Much effort in the next few years will go into the attempt to reorganize our system of health care in order to halt the rising spiral of costs to both government and those who use health services. Nursing, because it represents the largest group of professional workers in the health field, is a very important factor in the economics of health care. Therefore, nurses in both nursing education and nursing services will be involved in any effort to effect greater efficiency in the provision of services.

Some of the other trends which affect nursing are:

1. One of the greatest changes in hospitals has been the expansion of objectives. The main function in the past has been the care of the sick. This objective remains just as important as ever, but others are assuming more importance than they formerly did. Today the hospital is as essential for the rich as for the poor. More and more persons and families of all kinds are using prepaid hospital insurance, either through private plans or through Medicare. Not only the groups to whom service is rendered, but also the types of service, are changing rapidly. A primary objective of the hospital today is to serve as a major community health center.

2. The educational objective of the hospital is constantly increasing in importance. Hospitals are providing instruction and experience for administrative residents, nurses, social workers, dietitians, different kinds of technicians, and others. Thus, they are serving as field training centers for the educational institutions offering education to personnel in the health professions. They also provide important materials for study and research in the healing sciences. Some hospitals have as a primary or sole objective either research or education.

3. Much of the progress in hospitals has resulted from the approval and the educational programs of the American College of Surgeons, the AMA, the American Hospital Association, the Catholic Hospital Association, the American Protestant Hospital Association, and the Joint Commission on Accreditation of Hospitals. The work of the international and the national nursing organizations also has had a major influence on the nursing care of patients.

4. The work of the Commission on Hospital Care which resulted in the publication of *Hospital Care in the United States,*[9] the survey of hospital facilities state by state, the increased development of state hospital licensing, and the provision of Federal funds for the construction of public and nonprofit hospitals under the *Hospital Survey and Construction Act* all aided in the improvement of physical facilities, the quality of patient care, the distribution of services, and the operation and the interrelationship of hospitals. All these movements increased job opportunities in all of the health professions, in addition to creating new ones. They brought direct pressure to secure better and more qualified personnel in all of the health fields.

5. Other important and far-reaching changes, some good, some bad, have occurred in the last several years which have profoundly affected

[9] New York, Commonwealth Fund, 1946.

patient care in hospitals. These are: (a) fundamental changes in diseases, particularly decrease in acute and increase in chronic diseases; (b) increased emphasis on care of the aging; (c) revolutionary advance in knowledge and skill in all phases of patient care diagnosis, treatment, prevention and rehabilitation; (d) marked increase in the number of patients seeking hospital care; (e) increased number of health personnel, both in total number as well as in technical and special fields; (f) the practice, in some institutions, of using licensed practical nurses and aides for almost the whole care of patients and (g) change in the public's attitude about health. People are much more aware today of the advantages gained from good health services, both from the standpoint of the community as well as from that of the individual, and are demanding the type of services they have learned to value.

6. Patient care has changed in the last 12 or more years. More full-time physicians are employed on staffs of hospitals. More oxygen and more intravenous injection sets are used. More electrocardiograms are ordered. In addition, patient care has changed by the incorporation of rehabilitation, teaching, and the inclusion of all kinds of new medicines. Technologic advances have brought automation into many areas of the hospital. The fantastic electronic equipment recently introduced can be expected to expand greatly. New types of surgery, such as vascular and heart surgery, and various organ transplants, have added to the need for highly skilled clinical nurses—technically skilled and skilled in human relations. The whole patient-care practice in the hospital is more complex. Consequently, nursing is more complex. Some of the factors responsible, in addition to those just mentioned, are: expansion of physical medicine; increase in referrals among agencies for follow-up care and the employment of a nurse as home care coordinator to facilitate referrals and continuity of care; closer collaboration of the social service and nursing service to facilitate continuity of patient care after discharge from the hospital; inservice programs for all levels of nursing service personnel and a change in the philosophy of patient care from doing things "to" the patient, to helping the patient, to "helping him help himself" by working with him.

7. Today the health professions need to study more intensively the problems of patient care in the hospital. The physician, the hospital administrator, the nurse and persons of other health groups must begin to realize that the provision of good patient care is going to take their combined efforts. More interdisciplinary collaboration is essential. Also, more community participation in this planning needs to be encouraged.

8. The emphasis on the need for continuous investigation of patient care has influenced hospital administrators to provide methods analysts as regular members of nursing service department staffs. The research carried on by groups outside the hospital, such as the ANA, the NLN, the ANF and the Division of Nursing of the Public Health Service of the

U. S. Department of Health, Education, and Welfare, has also had a direct bearing on the improvement of hospital and nursing service practices.

A major responsibility of the nurse is to make regular appraisals of her nursing practice and to participate in and make use of appraisals made by professional groups, nursing and interdisciplinary, aimed at improved patient care. Professional standards of practice developed through organized study, such as those currently (1970) being developed by the ANA Divisions on Practice can be used in both self- and group-appraisals.

9. There has been a change in general hospitals in the relationship of the hospital census to the number of admissions and length of stay in the last 15 or more years. While, in general, it appears that the average daily census and the number of daily admissions have increased, the average length of stay of patients in hospitals has decreased, because physicians do not keep patients in hospitals for periods so long as formerly. This change causes an active turnover of patients and affects the character of the work of the nurse as well as of other personnel in the hospital.

10. A major trend in hospitals, which has implications for the preparation of all types of students of nursing and for assignment of personnel for patient care, is the introduction of new ways of grouping patients. These newer groupings grew out of an attempt to secure a maximum utilization of nursing skills. Some examples, as mentioned elsewhere, are self-care units, minimum-care units, intensive or maximum-care units, recovery rooms, extended-care units, ambulatory units, and units for long-term extensive illness and long-term custodial care.

11. Staffing patterns in nursing in hospitals are rapidly changing, but it is not easy to gain a picture of what is happening. The number of part-time staff nurses, and particularly the number of married nurses, many of whom work part time, has increased greatly; the number of administrative nurse personnel has increased; and the number of auxiliary nursing personnel has increased most of all. The number of full-time nurses employed has decreased, and so has the number of nurses in private practice. The head nurse is responsible for the direction of approximately twice the number of nursing personnel that she directed 20 years ago. There is, however, an increasing trend for personnel and payroll departments to assume responsibilities once carried by the nursing service, such as collecting credentials and hiring personnel. The length of the work week has decreased, generally from 48 to approximately 40 hours, and there has been considerable improvement in personnel policies and salaries for the registered nurse.

12. There appears to be greater recognition by nursing service, as well as nursing education personnel of the contribution of nursing services in hospitals to nursing education, preservice and graduate. Nursing service personnel seem to be more attuned to their responsibility for providing a

suitable environment for learning even though they may not always be directly responsible for the teaching of the students. Their attitude toward and acceptance of students is important if sound learning situations are to be provided for students of nursing in hospitals.

13. There is a trend to include the special services, such as psychiatric care, in departments of general hospitals. There is the trend, also, toward greater coordination of hospitals with other community health services — even to the point that some buildings are being erected to house all of these. Another trend is the development of institutions, or units, to care for patients at times other than that traditional in the general hospital; for example, "day hospitals," "night hospitals" and neighborhood clinics which attempt to bring service to the patient and his family at times and in ways acceptable and convenient to them. Neighborhood clinics have been established in poverty areas, but there is a growing belief that bringing services *to* the people may be a better way to serve everyone, not just those who cannot afford care.

14. Regionalization of health care planning is a trend that will influence the types, size and the location of hospitals and other types of health facilities. It will even affect decisions regarding specialty services in institutions — for example, whether or not each of 2 neighboring hospitals will provide for extensive heart surgery.

15. A trend or influence, which in turn will affect nursing, is the growth in professional specialization. To what extent clinical specialization in nursing is desirable or necessary is currently under debate.

It is difficult to predict how all of these dynamic changes will ultimately influence nursing. One thing is certain — there are many exciting, demanding, and enriching occupational opportunities for nurses in hospitals or related facilities.

NURSES IN PUBLIC HEALTH AGENCIES[10]

Broad social and economic changes, technological advances, and changes in medicine and in patterns of medical and health care continue to create the need for an increasing number of nurses in public health. The extension of public health services to all persons, regardless of religion, race, creed, color or economic status; the broadening of the concept of public health to include prevention and control of chronic, as well as communicable disease and the increasing enlightenment of the public about health needs have all demanded the cooperative efforts of a team of qualified health workers, such as physicians, nurses, epidemiologists, dentists, sanitary engineers, nutritionists, health educators, social workers, the consumer and others.

Effective coordination based on mutual understanding of and respect for

---

[10] *Community health nursing practice* is the broad term which embraces the work of the nurse in public health, in school health and in occupational health services. See "Division Executive Committee Defines Community Health Nursing Practice, Sets Forth Goals," in *Community Health Nursing,* the first newsletter of the ANA Division of Community Health Nursing Practice, New York, American Nurses' Association, April 1968. p. 13.

the functions of each worker is important if the public health needs of society are to be served efficiently and well. Nurses have an important part in all public health work; they comprise the largest group of public health workers. The number of nurses needed in this field of work continues to increase as programs expand.

Evolution of Philosophy Underlying Nursing in Public Health

Nursing in public health is a community service organized as a part of a community health program for the prevention and the control of disease, the care and rehabilitation of the sick and the disabled, and the promotion of healthful living. The nurse in public health provides nursing care and counsel to persons and families. She provides this service to individuals and groups in clinics, in their own homes, in schools and at work. She also participates in programs for the education of all types of nursing personnel, allied professional and technical workers, and community groups, and cooperates with others in the health professions and allied technical and citizen groups in studying, planning and carrying out the community health program.

In the USA, modern public health nursing developed in the latter part of the 19th century with the organization in many cities of voluntary agencies called "visiting nurse associations." The purpose of these agencies was to care for the sick at home on a part-time basis.

As time went on the services of nurses in public health broadened to include prevention and control of disease, health education, rehabilitation, and the promotion of healthful living, as well as care of the sick. The services of the public health nurse became an important part of official health departments. Her concern from the beginning was not only for individuals but for families, neighborhoods and communities. Although in the beginning, public health nursing efforts (like all public health effort) were directed largely toward the prevention of communicable disease, today they are aimed more at the prevention and the control of chronic illness and its effects and at the rehabilitation of individuals and families to the fullest extent possible. She is concerned not only with their physical health but also with their social and mental health as well.

In the early part of this century, nurses in public health agencies were employed to carry out such specialized functions as infant health and tuberculosis nursing. Today, whether she is serving in the clinic, the home, the school or in industry, each nurse is responsible for a generalized service to individuals and families—that is, her concern is for all the needs presented. She also serves, along with other members of the public health team, in the scientific diagnosis and treatment of the whole community as a patient.

What Nurses in Public Health Agencies Do

The nurse in public health, whether she is concerned with the prevention and the control of disease, with the care and the rehabilitation of the sick and the disabled, or with a program for the promotion of healthful living, works closely with the health officer, the physician, the nurse in the hospital, the sanitarian, the health educator, the social worker and other members of the health team. In recent years, with the advent of Medicare and the opportunity for more comprehensive care of the patient at home, the public health nurse operates within a team comprised of a registered nurse, licensed practical nurse, aide, physical therapist, speech therapist and others. Hence, she has greater responsibility for developing comprehensive plans for nursing care, for team leadership and for the supervision of auxiliary personnel. With the increasing number of auxiliary nursing personnel, she has become responsible for the teaching of licensed practical nurses and aides, as well as volunteers. She also cooperates with civic groups and leaders, church groups, the community's social agencies and similar organizations.

In the public health agencies providing nursing care of the sick at home, the nurse works closely with the physician. She interprets her service to him and explains and teaches nursing care and treatments to patients and their families. Under organized home care programs, she assists in the coordination of care to the family, serving as liaison between the hospital and the home. And with the growing number of agencies serving some of her patients and their families, the public health nurse is frequently the person who helps patients to understand and integrate the services provided and aids them in taking responsibility for determining and planning their own care.

In the child health conferences administered by public health agencies in order to prevent and control disease, the nurse assists in the provision of service for healthy mothers and children. This includes health guidance and immunization services for the protection of health. Clinics are provided for the examination, the treatment, and the health supervision of the tuberculous person and his family; for the diagnosis, the treatment, and the health supervision of persons with venereal diseases or physical handicaps such as orthopedic or cardiac conditions and for the detection of illness or defects, such as cancer and diseases of the eye. Other specialized clinics are provided wherever they are required. In all of these, nurses work with others in the epidemiologic aspects of tuberculosis, venereal disease, and other communicable diseases and such noncommunicable diseases as cancer and heart disease, through conferences with patients, families and various others in the community. For the clinic nurse, also, the nursing role is expanding to include assessment of patient needs and teaching the patient and his family.

The nurse in public health helps families to a better understanding of mental, emotional or social problems which are a handicap to the family's well-being and an obstacle to the recovery of the sick. She helps families to use other health and welfare services which the community offers through interagency referrals, through conferences with other health workers and in other ways.

Fig. 9-2. The nurse giving care in the home. (Visiting Nurse Association of Brooklyn, N. Y.)

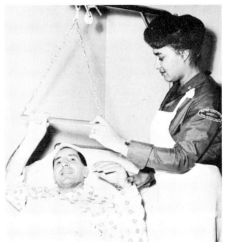

An increasing number of agencies are providing nursing care to families where there is mental illness. The use of newer drugs and treatments has facilitated the home care of many of the mentally ill. The nurse assists in preparing the family for the return of the patient and with the care and rehabilitation of the patient in the home and the community. Nurses have an important role in interpreting the needs of these patients to the community.

In the program for the promotion of healthful living, nurses in public health assist in the work of health supervision in a total health program which includes prenatal and maternity service and health service for infants, children in preschool years, school children, adolescents, adults and the aged. Consultation in nursing homes and working in rehabilitation programs

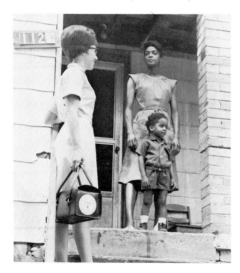

Fig. 9-3. The nurse making a visit in the interest of a child's health. (Washtenaw County Health Department and Affiliated Agencies, Michigan)

are also part of the nurse's work, as well as service in day care centers for children and adults, and in programs for the alcoholic and the addict. Nurses do health teaching in clinics, schools and offices or through visits in the field. The term *field* can mean a visit to a home, to a school or health conference, to another agency interested with the nurse in the health and the welfare of the same family, or to professional meetings or conferences concerning the health problems of families in the community.

The nurse's activities include many phases of community health work. For example, while visiting a family on a maternity service, she could bring to the mother's attention obvious accident hazards for the preschool child as well as for other members of the family. On a call to a geriatric patient, the plumbing situation may prompt her to arrange for a visit with a sanitarian in her health department. She also takes part in community action for day-care centers, boys' and girls' clubs and playgrounds. All of this is done in the interest of preventing disease before it strikes, assisting in the cure if illness comes, and improving the general health of the community as a whole. Figures 9-2, 9-3, 9-4 and 9-5 show the nurse in public health at work.

As you can see, the scope of the work of the nurse in public health agencies is as broad as are the health needs of people. The nurse who is interested in working with individuals and families in community settings outside of the hospital, in joining with other community health workers in improving community health, and in drawing on all aspects of her professional preparation in her service to individuals and families, will find this type of work both satisfying and enriching.

Positions Open to Nurses in Public Health

Public health nurses are employed by private (voluntary) agencies such as visiting nurse associations and other nonofficial health agencies, by official public health nursing agencies (tax supported), and by combination agencies where both official and nonofficial agencies work together.[11] Public agencies include city, county and state departments of health, Federal nursing services and public schools. Nursing in schools may be an integral part of the generalized public health nursing program. However, an increasing number of nurses are found working for boards of education and in colleges and universities. For this reason a discussion of the work of nurses employed in schools under boards of education is included in a later section. Public health nurses are employed as staff nurses, clinical nurse specialists, assistant supervisors, supervisors, educational directors, consultants, assistant directors and directors of public health nursing services, and as teachers in all types of educational programs for nursing. Nurses with public health backgrounds can also be found working in hospitals—with ambulatory

---

[11] Official agencies are those supported by taxes and operated by the Federal, state or local government. Nonofficial agencies are those not operated by the government; they depend on endowments, donations, campaign subscriptions, contracts and patients' fees for financial support. Sometimes, however, nonofficial agencies receive fees from tax funds.

Fig. 9-4. The nurse and the physical therapist evaluating the rehabilitation of a young patient. (Visiting Nurse Association of New Haven, Conn.)

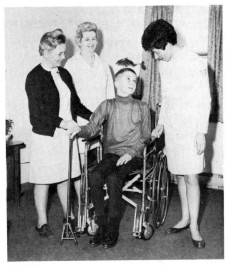

services, as coordinators or as liaison nurses responsible for the provision of patient care continuity following discharge from the hospital, and between the hospital clinic and the community nursing services. They hold positions not only in the USA, but also in other countries, where preparation and experience in public health nursing are often basic requirements to employment.

For a complete list of positions open to nurses in public health consult Chapter 8, "General Survey of Occupational Opportunities for Nurses," the section entitled "Positions Available in Community Health Programs."

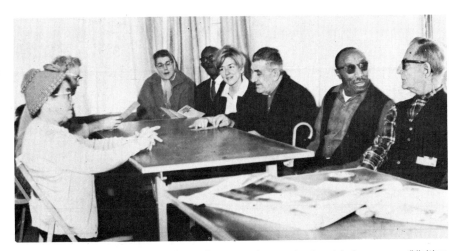

Fig. 9-5. The nurse leading a discussion group in a center for elderly persons. (Visiting Nurse Association of New Haven, Conn.)

Some Trends in Nursing in Public Health

Many of the trends which affect the nurse in hospital nursing also influence the nurse in public health, such as the spiralling cost of health care, the growing involvement of government in supporting and planning for health care, the impact of Medicare and regional planning programs, the provision of care for a growing number of the chronically ill aged in our population and changes in the populations of our cities.

The following list represents a few major trends that influence nursing in public health. You will be able to add to this list in your discussion.

1. Advances in medical care, including the use of new drugs and treatments in the care of the sick, including the mentally ill, at home

2. The trend toward shorter hospital stays, particularly for the surgical patient and the postpartum patient (This situation often requires follow-up at home)

3. The development of organized home care programs

4. Continuing emphasis on rehabilitation as a function of public health nursing

5. The acceptance of care of the sick at home as a function of official as well as voluntary public health nursing agencies

6. The increasing use of auxiliary nursing personnel, practical nurses, and the community or indigenous worker and aides in public health agencies

7. An increasing concern about the effective utilization of personnel

8. The problems of the inner, or "core," city that are demanding new and different approaches, such as working more actively with the recipients of service in planning for the delivery of health services and experimenting with new methods of providing health care

9. The influence of rapid suburbanization and urban redevelopment on extension and expansion of public health services

10. A trend toward the inclusion of public health nursing services in centers for senior citizens and housing for the aged

11. The use of homemaker services, meals on wheels, etc., to support the care of the chronically ill at home

12. The growing need for care of the aged chronically ill at home

13. A continuing increase in the number of communities where, through contractual arrangements or combinations, there is coordination of the public health nursing services of the official and voluntary agencies

14. The introduction of Medicare and Medicaid programs

15. The trend toward health insurance coverage of nursing care of the sick at home

16. Changing patterns of parent education—expectant parents classes and classes in education for childbirth

17. Growing recognition of the vital function that public health nursing

performs as one of the most important health services in communities today

18. The increase in the number of nurses in public health who have baccalaureate degrees and other higher educational preparation

19. The development of many more opportunities for public health nurses to work on interdisciplinary teams, or on assignments to special projects demonstrating and experimenting with new methods of organizing and delivering health care

NURSES IN SCHOOL HEALTH PROGRAMS

School nursing is provided under 2 different auspices in this country. In some communities the local public health nursing agency provides service in the schools as part of the generalized public health nursing program in the community. In other communities the school health program is administered by the local board of education.

The number of nurses employed by boards of education has grown steadily in the past few years. In 1966, the last year at this writing for which figures are available from the U. S. Public Health Service, 14,048 nurses were employed full time and 1,234 part time by 5,209 boards of education.[12] The following material pertains in part to the nurse serving on a specialized basis in school health — read also the preceding section, "Nurses in Public Health Agencies," for details regarding school nursing as part of a generalized public health nursing program.

How Does the Nurse Function in Schools?

The primary function of the school is education. The school health program assists the school to carry out this function by providing a health services program geared to having the students and the faculty gain in their understanding of health. Education for a better understanding of health permeates the health services program, which emphasizes health promotion, prevention of disease and disability and follow-through of any findings that indicate a need for medical care and treatment.

Responsibility for the school health program is shared by all school personnel, but major responsibility for its leadership resides in the school nurse. She works in a team relationship with a variety of other groups in the area of pupil personnel services, as well as with the total school staff. Her activities will depend in part on the size of the school or the school system in the community, the health needs of the pupils, and the other personnel available, such as guidance counselors and social workers. According to the statement of functions developed by the Committee on Practice of the

[12] American Nurses' Association, *Facts About Nursing: A Statistical Summary,* New York, The Association, 1968, p. 34.

School Nurses Branch of the Public Health Nurses Section of the ANA, her broad functions can be classified under 5 broad groupings: assessing, planning, implementing, evaluating, and study and research. Specific functions and related activities are spelled out under each of these classifications. For example, under "assessing," the nurse's functions are to identify "health needs of pupils and school personnel" and to analyze "the nurse's responsibilities in relation to the educational structure, and the relationship of the nurse to other faculty members and community groups."[13] It is suggested that you review all of the functions and activities as developed for the school nurse.

The School Nursing Committee of the American School Health Association has also defined the responsibilities of the nurse in the school health program. They classify responsibilities under (1) organization and implementation of the school health program, (2) functions directly related to pupil health, (3) coordination of the school health program, (4) evaluation, (5) functions related to the health of school personnel, and (6) professional responsibilities as a member of the teaching profession as well as of the nursing profession.[14]

The organization and the administration of the school system will affect the activities of the school nurse. In some instances she may be the only health specialist in the school. The school physician may be employed on a part-time or full-time basis. A few have administrative responsibility for school health services, but in most instances, the physician simply provides medical supervision while the principal of the school carries out, or delegates, the related administistative responsibilities. In some of the larger school systems, the health services program is part of a larger unit known as "pupil personnel services." This unit includes school personnel concerned with health and learning problems of students. Members of this team may include nurses, physicians, psychologists, guidance counselors, attendance workers, dental hygienists and school social workers.

Today opportunities are increasing for the specialized school nurse, or the "school nurse teacher" as she is sometimes called, to advance to supervisory and administrative positions. These advancement opportunities are available mainly in the larger school systems where nurse supervisors may be employed.

What Are the Qualifications for School Nursing?

If you are thinking of working as a specialized school nurse, you will need to know not only about the general qualifications for school nursing but also the specific requirements in the state in which you plan to work. Ideally,

[13] American Nurses' Association, *Functions and Qualifications for School Nurses,* New York, The Association, 1966.
[14] American School Health Association, School Nursing Committee, "The Nurse in the School Health Program," *Journal of School Health,* 37(2a):7-10, Feb. 1967.

for your first position as a school nurse you could seek to work in a school nurse program where you will have the benefits of supervision, or in a generalized public health nursing program offering school nursing.

General qualifications as recommended by the Committee on Practice of the School Nurses Branch of the Public Health Nurses Section of the ANA include graduation from a state accredited school of nursing and licensure to practice nursing. In addition, a baccalaureate degree and completion of a program of study in education, behavioral and social sciences, school health and public relations are recommended, as well as at least one year of experience in generalized public health nursing practice under supervision.[15] The School Nursing Committee of the American School Health Association recommends, in addition, that the nurse preparing for school health work should have graduate education in school nursing.[16] These qualifications are considered important because of the high degree of responsibility the school nurse carries for independent functioning and because she will be applying her nursing knowledge and skills in a setting that has education as the primary function rather than care of the sick.

In addition to the above qualifications, some states require the school nurse to have a teaching certificate. This certification will entail meeting a few additional requirements.[17]

What Are Some of the Other Qualities a School Nurse Should Possess?

Nurses working in school health programs under boards of education should possess sufficient professional maturity to be able to work cooperatively with a variety of other disciplines where she is oftentimes the only health worker. Nurses who select school nursing should be those who enjoy working with children. Further, they need to be able to work through and with others (school personnel, children, and parents) to achieve their objectives. They should be persons who can accept the education function of the school and be committed to the promotion of health through education.

NURSES IN OCCUPATIONAL HEALTH SERVICES

Professional nurses are employed in employee health services in industry and in commercial and service establishments. Even though one still occasionally hears the term, "industrial nurse," the accepted designation today is "occupational health nurse." This latter title is more in keeping with

---

[15] American Nurses' Association, *Functions and Qualifications for School Nurses*, New York, The Association, 1966.

[16] American School Health Association, School Nursing Committee, "The Nurse in the School Health Program," *Journal of School Health*, **37**(2a):20, Feb. 1967.

[17] American Nurses' Association, *A Rationale for School Nurse Certification*, New York, The Association, 1966.

modern goals of occupational health programs, which are geared to health maintenance and health promotion activities for groups of persons who are occupied or employed.

Objectives of Occupational Health Programs

Modern occupational health programs continue to be concerned about protecting employees against the hazards of the job itself and of its environment. However, the health program, which is financially supported by management, also concerns itself with suitable placement, attempting to match the person with the job according to his physical and mental capacity and emotional makeup. Two additional important objectives of the program are: (1) assurance of adequate medical care, including rehabilitation of the competent worker who is occupationally ill or injured and (2) promotion of personal health maintenance of all workers.

For further information about the occupational health program it is suggested that you read, *Scope, Objectives, and Functions of Occupational Health Programs,* published in 1960 by The Council on Occupational Health of the American Medical Association.

The Nurse in the Occupational Health Service

The occupational health nurse is a member of a team that also includes medical, safety and industrial hygiene specialists employed to conserve and promote the health and effectiveness of workers at their place of employment. Her particular responsibility as a member of this team is to apply nursing principles to develop and carry out a nursing service tailored to the environment of the particular company and the needs of its employees.[18] She is often, particularly in a one-nurse service, responsible for the administration as well as the implementation of the nursing service. When the nursing service is provided through a contractual arrangement with the community nursing service, she will be a member of the community nursing service and may be only part time in the industry, spending the rest of her time with community nursing service work.

The occupational health nurse generally works with the physician employed either full or part time by the industry. Sometimes, and in fact all too often, he is "on call" only. In small industries where the physician is employed on a part-time basis, much of the success of the program will depend on the nurse's concept of occupational health and her initiative, vision and judgment.

The scope of the nursing service will depend on the type and the size of the industry and on the specific health needs of the employees. In a small industry the nurse may be the only professional person assigned full time to the

[18] American Nurses' Association, *Functions and Qualifications for an Occupational Health Nurse in a One-Nurse Service,* New York, The Association, 1968, n.p.

health service. A large industry may have a team of health workers including a staff of nurses. When there is a nursing staff, one member is assigned to be director of nurses.

Responsibilities of the Occupational Health Nurse

The responsibilities of occupational health nurses vary depending on the size, the type and the complexity of the industry. For example, working in a health service in an automobile manufacturing industry or in a department store, or working in a health service on a construction site or at a missile base, would all pose different kinds of problems and entail different kinds of responsibilities. However, many of the basic responsibilities for the health of the workers remain the same.

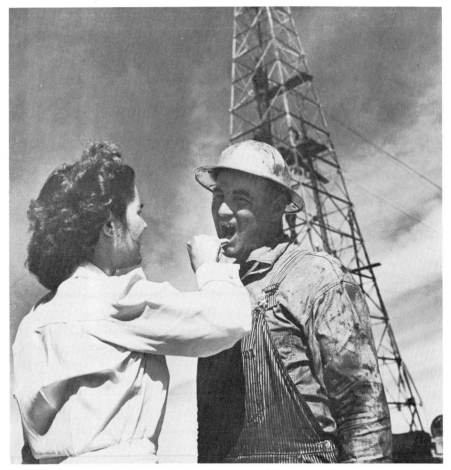

Fig. 9-6. Industrial nurse visits employee who has returned to work after sick leave. (Humble Oil Company)

The occupational health nurse, especially in a one-nurse service, will share responsibility with management and the doctor for developing, keeping up-to-date, and implementing administrative policies. These policies will define the scope and the objectives of the health service and will include written medical direction for emergency nursing care and treatment, and a list of the nurse's functions and responsibilities.

The main responsibilities of the occupational health nurse are, of course, related to the prevention of illness and accidents and to the emergency care of both occupational and nonoccupational injuries and illnesses. The nurse uses her professional nursing knowledge and skills not only to give emergency care but also to teach others, or plan for others to be taught, to perform first aid. Her responsibility for teaching will include also safety education and individual health counseling. For example, she may contribute to the plant newspaper such material on health as items about good nutrition or the prevention of colds; or she may counsel a diabetic worker about skin care. Counseling will include appropriate referrals to health and welfare services.

As in other fields of nursing, the nurse in the occupational health service is expected to keep adequate records and to make reports. She is in a unique position to interpret nursing and health care to both management and the employees of the industry. She can interpret the health program of the industry to the community and to community agencies and work cooperatively with them.

For a discussion of the unique practice of the occupational health nurse, it is suggested that you read the section on the "Distinctive Characteristics of Occupational Health Nursing" in *Selected Areas of Knowledge or Skills Basic to Effective Practice of Occupational Health Nursing,* published in 1966 by the ANA. Figures 9-6, 9-7 and 9-8 are illustrative of some activities of the occupational health nurse.

What Qualifications Are Needed to Do Occupational Health Nursing?

A nurse electing to work in occupational health should have a sincere interest in working with people and the ability to be professionally self-directing. In addition to graduation from a state accredited school of nursing and current state licensure, it is considered helpful for her to have had some supervised experience beyond graduation in such fields as public health nursing, outpatient department, or emergency clinic nursing. It is helpful, too, if she has had additional preparation in occupational health. Her first work experience in this field should be in a situation where she will have nurse supervision.

She should have the ability to work well with people and be skillful in communications, both written and verbal. Because she often works alone, she should have the ability to evaluate her own work and to provide for her own professional development. Maintaining membership in her professional

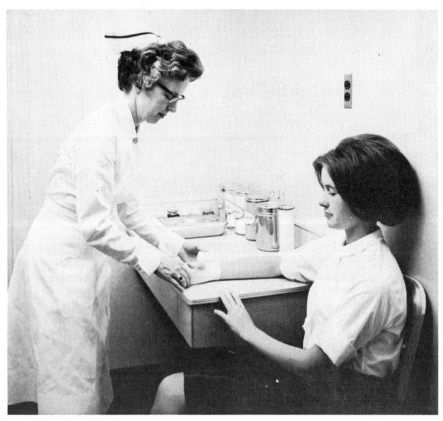

Fig. 9-7. Industrial nurse giving nursing care to a young employee with an injury. (Eastman Kodak Company)

association and subscribing regularly to professional journals will help her to keep up-to-date with developments in nursing.

Occupational health nursing is a field that is becoming increasingly important. Many nurses find it a very satisfying occupation, particularly those who can be self-directing and can assume the role of a responsible, professional member of the health team.

NURSES IN PHYSICIANS' AND DENTISTS' OFFICES

The office nurse is defined as one "whose practice concerns patients receiving care in an office or clinic from one or more physicians or dentists and who holds responsibility for the nursing care of these patients and promotion of their health and welfare."[19]

[19] American Nurses' Association, Office Nurses' Section, *Functions, Standards, and Qualifications for the Practice of Office Nursing*, New York, The Association, 1962, p. 5.

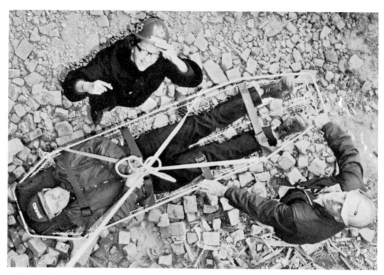

Fig. 9-8. A construction-gang nurse goes 3 stories down to give first aid and to supervise the transportation of an injured worker. (Chicago *Sun-Times* Photo)

That many nurses find office nursing a very satisfying type of work is seen by the fact that in 1966, some 47,000 registered nurses were practicing in this field, or about 8 per cent of the total registered nurses in the country.[20] The ANA Research and Statistics Unit made a survey of office nurses in July, 1964. They found that the typical office nurse was employed by a single practitioner and that 1/5 of the nurses were employed by medical or dental groups. A majority of the nurses surveyed had been in their positions for at least 5 years. About 13 per cent of the full-time nurses were in supervisory positions.[21]

Responsibilities of the Office Nurse

The office nurse may be the only professionally trained person working with the physician in his office or one of several nurses. In either case, her major responsibility is nursing, or the development and maintenance of a nursing program. This program should be based upon sound principles of nursing practice. It will be important for the office nurse to keep informed about the standards of practice as these are developed by the ANA Divisions on Practice.

The office nurse who uses her professional knowledge and skills well, will contribute to the quality of patient care, because her work serves to enhance that of the physician. For example, a nurse who, in addition to giving and

[20] American Nurses' Association, *Facts About Nursing: A Statistical Summary,* New York, The Association, 1968, p. 21.
[21] _____. *Facts About Nursing: A Statistical Summary,* New York, The Association, 1965, pp. 167-168.

helping with treatments and tests, sees her role as one of helping patients to make the best use of their office visit with the physician by preparing them for their visit and reinforcing instruction or interpreting directions following the visit, can do much to influence the quality of patient care. This nurse is indeed making use of her professional nursing knowledge and skills to extend and enhance the physician's care.

Health education of the patient and the family is an important function of the office nurse. She has as many opportunities to teach as there are patients. Patients, and their families, often will turn to her with their questions because she is a nurse and because they do not "want to bother the busy doctor." As indicated before, she has an important function to reinforce the physician's instructions.

Office nurses frequently have another teaching responsibility — that of on-the-job teaching, supervision and direction of the other personnel employed by the physician. Of course, the nature and the size of her employer's practice will affect the amount of responsibility she carries for other personnel.

While most of the work of the office nurse is, as her title implies, in the physician's or dentist's office, she may occasionally make home visits for the physician to give treatments or perhaps to observe a patient's conditions. However, she should have a knowledge of the community health agencies available to the patient and his family, so that she can refer them to the appropriate agency when necessary. In collaborating with other health and welfare agencies, she assists the patient to secure the services that the doctor has indicated to be helpful to patients and families. Generally, the office nurse is responsible for nursing and should not be expected to take over billing and other secretarial activities.

Factors Influencing the Work of the Office Nurse

The relation between the nurse and the physician is perhaps one of the most important factors determining her ability to function effectively. She will need to interpret correctly her nursing functions to her employer and to assist in developing policies and procedures guiding her work.

The nurse working in a physician's office should be one who can show initiative and judgment and be self-directing. She must be willing to spend some time on her own professional development. She should subscribe to at least one professional nursing journal, such as the *American Journal of Nursing,* in order to keep abreast of nursing advances.

Because she is so often the only professional nurse in the office, she needs to look elsewhere for the professional stimulation and guidance she needs. The ANA Divisions on Practice and the office Nurses' Section of the state nurses associations serve to provide the kind of assistance, stimulation and direction that the office nurse requires. Membership in the ANA and participation in professional association meetings, institutes and workshops becomes a major qualification for the job of office nursing.

The Office Nurse and Interpersonal Relations

An important role of the office nurse is that of serving as the liaison between the physician's office, the family, the hospital and community health agencies. In this role she can help the patient and his family make the best use of all of the available services, as well as facilitate the work of the physician and any other services involved.

The office nurse also has a unique opportunity to interpret nursing to the public and to the medical profession. In her daily contacts with patients, their families, and others who come to the physician's office, she influences many in their attitudes toward nurses and nursing. By her actions and the interpretation she gives, she can do much to promote better understanding of nursing and of the functions and role of nurses in our society today.

PROBLEMS

General

1. When a group like the nursing profession prepares statements on standards, qualifications and preparation for its various types of workers, it takes some time before these are accepted in practice. What would you do if you found yourself in a situation in which the approved standards had not been met? Would you leave? Would you try to effect a change so that the standards would be met? Would you accept the situation as inevitable and do nothing? What steps would you take to change the standards if those in the administration do not accept the profession's standards?

2. It is said that nurses have given away their most important nurturing and helping functions to auxiliary nursing personnel, especially in hospitals. If this is true, what suggestions do you have for changing this situation? Describe your concept of the role of the nurse in the hospital. Which nursing functions or responsibilities *should not* be turned over to auxiliary personnel?

3. (a) Make a list of the present foremost leaders in each of the nursing fields described in this chapter and in Chapter 10. (b) You may wish to prepare biographies on some of these leaders for information of the entire class and for filing for use of future classes.

Nurses in Private Practice

1. Some nurses in private practice are becoming specialists. What do you think of this trend?

2. The number of nurses in private practice, while still sizeable, has been gradually decreasing. Discuss the future role of the nurse in private practice. How might this differ from her present role?

3. There seems to be a variation in the attitude of nurses in private prac-

tice toward the families of patients. For example, there is the nurse who insists that the wife of a seriously ill patient leave as soon as she, the nurse, comes to take care of the patient. I have heard a nurse say: "He only needs one of us to take care of him, and that's why I am here." Yet in instances like this the relatives have been cooperative about limiting their visits and stepping outside the room if treatment is necessary. This is really an acute problem at times and a deterrent to good relationships. Sometimes the whole nursing profession is blamed for such a situation. What do you think can be done to correct these situations?

Nurses in Hospitals and Similar Health Facilities

1. Hospital economics is an important consideration, not only for the hospital administrator, but for all hospital personnel. (a) Why do you think hospitals are so expensive to administer? (b) Why is the cost of hospitalization so high? (c) How can hospital personnel practice economies?

2. Hospitals are rapidly becoming community health centers rather than institutions caring for the sick in isolation from the community. How do you see this new role of hospitals affecting the responsibilities of the nurses working within them?

3. A number of patients who have been in hospitals say that they received little or no professional nursing care because auxiliary personnel were assigned to care for them. Can this situation be remedied? How? Who is responsible? What are the legal implications?

Nurses in Public Health Agencies

1. Discuss the value of experience in nursing in public health agencies during preservice education in colleges or universities.

2. There seems to be a trend toward expansion of the role of the public health nurse in the clinic. Discuss the concept of the "nursing clinic" as described by Resnik (see references by Resnik and by Lewis and Resnik in the Suggested References" at the end of this chapter). What are the implications for nursing practice?

3. Discuss any one of the trends affecting public health nursing listed in the chapter in relation to what you see as its influence on the current practice of nurses in public health.

Nurses in School Health Programs

1. (a) Are the functions of the school nurse working in a program under the administration of the board of education different from those working in a generalized public health nursing agency that provides for school nursing? (b) Discuss the advantages and the disadvantages of each type of program to the community and to the schools.

2. Describe the characteristics of the person whom you believe would make a good school nurse in an elementary school setting; include both personal and professional characteristics.

3. What are the implications of the increased use of drugs, including marijuana, LSD and others, by teen-agers to the school nurse in the high school setting?

4. A new Department of School Nurses has been set up within the National Education Association. Of what advantage to school nurses is membership in this department?

Nurses in Occupational Health Services

1. (a) List the principal functions of a staff nurse in an industrial medical service. (b) List the major functions of the director of an industrial nursing service. (c) What are the desirable qualifications for nurses in these positions? (d) Why is occupational health nursing so important?

2. Plan a symposium on Occupational Health Nursing. Discuss the following topics in relation to this: (a) Effect of Occupational Health Nursing on Production in Industry; (b) Rehabilitation in Industry; (c) Mental Health in Industry; (d) Human Relations in Industry; (e) Student of Nursing in Industry.

3. How does the salary of occupational health nurses compare with that of nurses in other fields, such as those in public health, hospital, school and office nursing?

Nurses in Physicians' and Dentists' Offices

1. How do you account for the large percentage of nurses choosing to work in physicians' offices?

2. Discuss some of the disadvantages and the advantages of working in a physician's or dentist's office.

3. Visit an office nurse in your community and interview her about her work, covering such areas as the problems she encounters, her interpretation of the nurse-patient-doctor relationships, and what she considers her major responsibilities.

SUGGESTED REFERENCES*

NURSES IN PRIVATE PRACTICE

Caddell, E. B. "Growth and Development of the Private Duty Nurse." *Tar Heel Nurse,* **30**:30-32, Mar. 1968.

---

* In each chapter all citations are footnoted and are not included here. All starred references are recommended for additional reading.

Finer, H. "Evaluating the Private Duty Nurse's Performance." *American Journal of Nursing,* **56:**1564-1566, Dec. 1956.

Hadley, B. J. and Wenhold, B. K. "The Private Duty Nurse Teaches Cardiac Care." *American Journal of Nursing,* **62:**50-53, Jan. 1962.

Hansen, E. E. "Guiding the Practical Nurse in Private Duty Care." *American Journal of Nursing,* **63:**72-74, June 1963.

"Private Duty Nursing." (editorial) *American Journal of Nursing,* **62:**49, Jan. 1962.

Smith, E. J. "The Future Role of the Private Duty Nurse." *Tar Heel Nurse,* **30:** 32-33, Mar. 1968.

* Stone, V. "The Role of the Private Duty Nurse." *Tar Heel Nurse,* **30:**26-27, Mar. 1968.

NURSING IN HOSPITALS AND EXTENDED CARE FACILITIES

Barrett, J. *The Head Nurse: Her Changing Role.* New York, Appleton-Century-Crofts, 1968.

Benne, W. G., et al. *The Role of the Nurse in the Outpatient Department.* New York, American Nurses' Foundation, 1961.

Brockmeier, M. J. "Nursing in Two Community Health Settings." *Nursing Outlook,* **16:**55-58, Apr. 1968.

Brodt, D. E. "Where is the General Duty Nurse." *American Journal of Nursing,* **68:**1732, Aug. 1968.

Cartmill, G. E. "Presidential Address." *Hospitals,* **41:**62-65, Oct. 1967.

Davis, K. "The Delivery of Nursing Services: Twelve Areas for Experimentation." In *Research and Experimentation in the Delivery of Nursing Services.* New York, American Nurses' Association, 1968, pp. 6-13.

Dunn, H. "Facing Realities in Nursing Administration Today." *American Journal of Nursing,* **68:**1013-1018, May 1968.

Ehrlich, I. F. "Supervision: Process Not Position." *American Journal of Nursing,* **68:**115-119, Jan. 1968.

Gabrielson, R. C. "Utilization of the Technical and Professional Nurse Practitioner in Hospital Nursing Services." *National League for Nursing Conference Papers,* 39-46, Nov. 1968.

Gascoyne, R. A. "Supervisors of Nursing are Superfluous." *Canadian Nurse,* **64:**25, Jan. 1968.

Gordon, M. "The Clinical Specialist as a Change Agent." *Nursing Outlook,* **17:** 37-39, Mar. 1969.

Grapski, L. F. "The Hospital Health Care Service: Goals for Nursing Research." In *Research and Experimentation in the Delivery of Nursing Services.* New York, American Nurses' Association, 1968, pp. 14-20.

Hagen, E. and Wolff, L. *Nursing Leadership Behavior in General Hospitals.* New York, Institute of Research and Service in Nursing Education, Teachers College, Columbia University, 1961.

Haglund, E. J. "Community Nursing Services: The Shape of the Future." In *Research and Experimentation in the Delivery of Nursing Services.* New York, American Nurses' Association, 1968, pp. 21-36.

Johnson, D. E., et al. "The Clinical Specialist as a Practitioner." *American Journal of Nursing,* **67:**2298-2303, Nov. 1967.

Kriegal, J. *The Head Nurse: Thoughts and Decisions.* New York, Macmillan, 1968.

Olson, M. E. "Comparison of Head Nurse and Staff Nurse Attitudes Toward Various Aspects of Nursing Care." *Nursing Research,* **17:**349-353, Jul./Aug. 1968.

Ramphal, M. "Clinical Nursing Supervision." *American Journal of Nursing,* **68:** 1900-1902, Sept. 1968.

Sloan, J. "Ask the Staff Nurse." *American Journal of Nursing,* **67:**2362, Nov. 1967.

Smith, E. F. "Nursing Service Administration is Nursing Too." *Nursing Outlook,* **16:**19, Sept. 1968.

Tappan, F. M. *Toward Understanding Administrators.* New York, Macmillan, 1968.

Towner, A. M. "No More Supervisors?" *Nursing Outlook,* **16:**56-58, Feb. 1968.

Wolf, E. S. "Nurse Clinician in a Specialty Hospital." *Nursing Outlook,* **16:**41-43, June 1968.

See also references in Chapter 2 under ". . . Hospital Trends," "Trends in Extended Care Facilities" and "Nursing Trends."

NURSING IN PUBLIC HEALTH AGENCIES

Clack, F. B. and Wishik, C. S. "New Staff for Public Health." *Public Health Reports,* **83:**150-154, Feb. 1968.

Cohen, H. "Accreditation of Community Nursing Services." *American Journal of Public Health,* **57:**2138-2142, Dec. 1967.

Cotter, Sister Mary Dolora. "The Public Health Nurse and Community Mental Health." *Nursing Outlook,* **16:**59-61, Apr. 1968.

English, M. O. and Lee, R. M. "Planning for Community-Wide Patient Care." *Nursing Outlook,* **16:**38-42, Apr. 1968.

Helvie, C. O., *et al.* "The Setting and Nursing Practice." *Nursing Outlook,* Part I, **16:**27-29, Aug. 1968; Part II, **16:**35-38, Sept. 1968.

"Home Health Aide Services." *Nursing Outlook,* **16:**60, Nov. 1968.

Johnson, W. C. and Hardin, C. *Content and Dynamics of Home Visits of Public Health Nurses.* New York, American Nurses' Foundation, Part I, 1962. Part II, 1969.

* Lewis, C. E. and Resnik, B. K. "Nurse Clinics and Progressive Ambulatory Care." *New England Journal of Medicine,* **277:**1236-1241, Dec. 7, 1967.

* Lindberg, H. G. and Carlson, B. V. "A Public Health Nurse in the Physician's Office." *Nursing Outlook,* **16:**43-45, Apr. 1968.

McNeil, E. E. "Transition in Public Health Nursing." *University of Michigan Medical Center Journal,* **33:**386-391, Dec. 1967.

Mitch, A. D. and Kaczala, S. "The Public Health Nurse Coordinator in a General Hospital." *Nursing Outlook,* **16:**34-36, Feb. 1968.

Ostendorf, M. J. "The Public Health Nurse's Role in Helping a Family with Mental Health Problems." *Perspectives in Psychiatric Care,* **5:**208-213, Sept./Oct. 1967.

Parramore, B. and Yeager, W. "Team Nursing in Public Health." *Nursing Outlook,* **16:**54-56, June 1968.

Peese, E. M. "Public Health Nursing and Comprehensive Health Care." *Nursing Outlook,* **16:**48-52, Jan. 1968.

Rasmussen, S. "The Expanding Circle." *Nursing Outlook,* **16:**29-31, Feb. 1968.

* Resnik, B. A. "The Nursing Clinic: An Experiment in Ambulatory Patient Care." In *ANA Regional Clinical Conferences, 1967.* New York, Appleton-Century-Crofts, 1968, pp. 95-100.

Sheldon, A. and Hope, P. K. "The Developing Role of the Nurse in a Community Mental Health Program." *Perspectives in Psychiatric Care,* **5:**272-279, Nov./Dec. 1967.

Volante, R. S. "This I Believe . . . About the Clinical Teaching of Public Health Nursing." *Nursing Outlook,* **15:**49-50, Nov. 1967.

Wolff, I. S. "The Community Health View of Mentally Ill and Mentally Restored Patients." *Perspectives in Psychiatric Care,* **3(1):**9-23, 1965.

NURSING IN SCHOOL HEALTH PROGRAMS

Basco, D. "Evaluation of School Nursing Activities." *Nursing Research,* **12:**212-221, 1963.

Cromwell, G. E. *The Nurse in the School Health Program.* Philadelphia, Saunders, 1963.

Dunphy, B. A. "In Defence of School Nurses' Aides." *American Journal of Nursing,* **66:**1338-1341, June 1966.

Fitzgerald, H. "Full Use of Nurse Potential in a College Health Service." *Journal of the American College Health Association,* **16:**178-181, Dec. 1967.

Ford, L. C., *et al.* "New Perspectives in College Health Nursing." *Journal of the American College Health Association,* **16:**372-377, Apr. 1968.

_____. "The College Health Nurse—A Professional in Today's Society: A Panel Discussion." *Journal of the American College Health Association,* **16:**339-344, Apr. 1968.

Fricke, I. B. "The Illinois Study of School Nurse Practice." *Journal of School Health,* **37:**24-28, Jan. 1967.

Holden, L. W. "What Does the Administrator Need of His Nurse and Vice Versa." *Journal of the American College Health Association,* **16:**316, 319, Apr. 1968.

King, J. S. "A School Nurse in Bolivia." *Nursing Outlook,* **16:**37-39, Nov. 1968.

Olson, A. "Health Education and the Middle-age Child." *Journal of School Health,* **37:**467-469, Nov. 1967.

Robinson, C. M. *Handbook for Nurses—Secondary Schools.* San Jose, Calif., 1968.

Rosenthal, E. M. "We Have a Health Club." *American Journal of Nursing,* **68:**1946-1947, Sept. 1968.

Rosner, A. C. "Role Progression in School Nursing." *Colorado Nurse,* **67:**7-12, Dec. 1967.

* Shear, B. E. "Team Action in Pupil Personnel." *The Bulletin of the National Association of Secondary School Principals,* **52:**37-48, Jan. 1968.

Tipple, D. C. "Misuse of Assistants in School Health." *American Journal of Nursing,* **64:**99-101, Sept. 1964.

* _____. "The School Nurse as a Counselor." *American Journal of Nursing,* **63:**110-113, Sept. 1963.

Troop, E. "Sixty Years of School Nurse Preparation." *Nursing Outlook,* **11:**364-366, May 1963.

Troy, V. M. "The Role of the College Health Nurse During an Epidemic." *Journal of the American College Health Association,* **16:**121-124, Dec. 1967.

NURSING IN OCCUPATIONAL HEALTH SERVICES

* American Association of Industrial Nurses. *Standards and Criteria for Evaluating an Occupational Nursing Service.* New York, The Association, 1965.

* American Nurses' Association. *Guide for the Development of a Manual for an Employee Health Program.* New York, The Association, 1962.

American Nurses' Association. Occupational Health Nurses Section. *Selected Areas of Knowledge or Skill Basic to Effective Practice of Occupational Health Nursing.* New York, The Association, 1966.

* Bauer, M. L. and Brown, M. L. *Occupational Health Nurses: An Initial Survey.* Washington, D.C., Division of Occupational Health, Public Health Service, U. S. Department of Health, Education, and Welfare, May 1966.

Brown, M. L. "Nurse's Role in an Occupational Health Program for Hospital Employees." *American Association of Industrial Nurses Journal,* **15:**7-8, May 1967.

* _____. "Data on Occupational Health Nurses." *American Journal of Nursing,* **65:**120-123, May 1965.

* Colucci, B. L. "The Role of the Industrial Nurse in the Safety Program." *American Association of Industrial Nurses Journal,* **16:**17-19, Mar. 1968.

* "Committee on Education 1943-1968." *American Association of Industrial Nurses Journal,* **16:**10-11, Jan. 1968.

Courtenay, I. "Occupational Health Nursing." *Canadian Nurse,* **64:**36-40, Apr. 1968.

Donovan, H. M. "Nursing Service Administration." *American Association of Industrial Nurses Journal,* **15:**15-16, Nov. 1967.

Felton, J. S. "Medical Direction in Occupational Health Nursing." *American Journal of Nursing,* **66:**2019-2022, Sept. 1966.

* Henriksen, H. L. "Health Care of Workers in the United States." *Nursing Outlook,* **16:**32-33, May 1968.

"Her World's a Stage." *American Journal of Nursing,* **64:**78-80, Aug. 1964.

* Hershey, N. "The Nurse Who Works Alone." *American Journal of Nursing,* **62:**105-106, Nov. 1962; **62:**91-92, Dec. 1962.

Hughes, J. P. "Role of the Occupational Health Nurse Today and Tomorrow." *Nursing Mirror,* **72:**76, Oct. 20, 1967.

Hutchins, J. "Orientation of the Aerospace Nurse to Occupational Health." *American Association of Industrial Nurses Journal,* **16:**7-12, July 1968.

* Johnson, D. R. "Today and Tomorrow: The Occupational Health Nurse's Broadening Responsibility." *American Association of Industrial Nurses Journal,* **16:**17-19, June 1968.

Keller, M. J. "The Occupational Health Nurse and Short-term Illness Absences." *Nursing Outlook,* **16:**32-34, Sept. 1968.

La Roche, L. P. "The Missile Nurses at Cape Canaveral." *American Journal of Nursing,* **63:**54-58, Jan. 1963.

Levine, R. C. "The Nurse's Role in Management." *American Association of Industrial Nurses Journal,* **15:**16-18, Dec. 1967.

McMechen, A. "Daily Visits to the Launching Pads." *American Journal of Nursing,* **63:**58-60, Jan. 1963.

Nilsen, D. "The Man on the Job: A Challenge to the Sophisticated Health Team." *American Association of Industrial Nurses Journal,* **16:**14-16, Mar. 1968.

O'Brien, M. E. "Widening Horizons and Occupational Health Nursing." *International Nursing Review,* **15:**280-284, July 1968.

Peplau, H. E. "Interpersonal Relations and the Work of the Industrial Nurse." *American Association of Industrial Nurses Journal,* **15:**7-12, Nov. 1967.

* *Public Health Nursing in Industry.* Washington, D.C., Public Health Service, U. S. Department of Health, Education, and Welfare, 1968.

Rush, H. C. "Role of the Industrial Nurse Re-examined." *American Association of Industrial Nurses Journal,* **15:**10-11, Mar. 1967.

Sadusk, J. F., Jr. "Legal Implications of Changing Patterns of Practice." *Journal of the American Medical Association,* **190:**1135-1136, Dec. 20, 1964.

Saller, D. M. "The Varied Role of the Industrial Nurse." *American Association of Industrial Nurses Journal,* **15:**13-15, Dec. 1967.

Stanwick, A. M. "Nurse at Work." *American Association of Industrial Nurses Journal,* **16:**34-38, Feb. 1968.

Stewart, G. A. "The Nurse in a Small Company Views Her Responsibility." *American Association of Industrial Nurses Journal,* **15:**14-17, Jan. 1967.

Sturgis, K. R. "Implications of Current Social Changes for the Nurse in Occupational Health." *American Association of Industrial Nurses Journal,* **15:**12-15, Oct. 1967.

Wagner, S. P. "Role of Occupational Nurse in Efficient Worker Utilization." *Archives of Environmental Health,* 4:451-453, Apr. 1962.

_____. "Nurse-Management-Physician Relationships." *American Association of Industrial Nurses Journal,* 10:18-20, Feb. 1962.

Walker, M. "Today's Occupational Health Nurse." *Nursing Outlook,* 13:62-64, Nov. 1965.

Walton, A. "Working Inside Prison." *Occupational Health Nurse* (Aukland), 1:1-3, Oct. 1967.

Welch, J. R. "Construction Gang Nurse." *American Journal of Nursing,* 64:118-120, Jan. 1964.

Wetsel, F. C. "Management's Appraisal of the Nurse in Industry." *Nursing Outlook,* 13:65-67, Nov. 1965.

* Williams, E. V. "Graduate Programs for Occupational Health Nurses." *American Association of Industrial Nurses Journal,* 15:9-10, Dec. 1967.

See also publications on nurses' responsibilities, policy guides, standards and other relevant topics published by the AAIN, the ANA and the AMA.

NURSING IN PHYSICIANS' AND DENTISTS' OFFICES

Amacher, G. M. "Family-oriented Problems." *Tar Heel Nurse,* 30:41-44, Mar. 1968.

Austin, G. *et al.* "Pediatric Screening Examinations in Private Practice." *Pediatrics,* 41:115-119, Jan. 1968.

* Dodd, L. P. *Problems Arising From the Handling of Drugs in the Physician's Office.* New York, American Nurses' Association, 1965.

"Employment Conditions of Office Nurses." *American Journal of Nursing,* 65:111, Sept. 1965.

"Guidelines for the Office Nurse in Determining Her Relation to the Medical Assistant." *American Journal of Nursing,* 65:117, Mar. 1965.

Hershey, N. "Office Nurse." *American Journal of Nursing,* 65:108-110, May 1965.

Lindberg, H. G. and Carlson, B. V. "A Public Health Nurse in the Private Physician's Office." *Nursing Outlook,* 16:43-45, Apr. 1968.

Smith, J. W., *et al.* "Extended Use of Nursing Services and General Practice." *British Medical Journal,* 4:672-674, Dec. 16, 1967.

Spurling, B. "I'll Take Small-Town Nursing, Thank You." *RN,* 31:48-51, Feb. 1968.

CHAPTER

10

Nurses in Education, Consultation, Research and Professional Organizations

The major categories of employment for nurses are listed in Chapter 8. The positions chiefly described here are those held by educational administrators, teachers, consultants, research workers and nurses working in professional organizations. These positions require preparation at the graduate level or its equivalent.

EDUCATIONAL PROGRAMS FOR NURSING

Before describing the qualifications and the preparation of nurses who hold positions in educational programs for nursing, it may be helpful to give a brief description of the present and emerging types of educational programs for nursing in which nurses are employed.

The present system of education for nursing includes a variety of pre-service programs, that is, programs for students who have had no previous education in nursing. These include: (1) the program in practical nursing (vocational), (2) the program in the diploma school of nursing (semi-professional), (3) the program in the institution of higher education leading to an associate degree (technical) and (4) the undergraduate program in a college or university leading to a baccalaureate degree (professional). There are 2 types of educational programs for graduate nurses: (1) the under-graduate program listed under (4) above for graduate nurses from diploma schools of nursing and for those who have completed an associate degree in nursing and (2) graduate programs leading to higher degrees. In addition to these programs, there are a number of short-term courses (continuing education programs) provided by the nursing faculty in educational institutions. These short-term courses are aimed at enlarging the knowledge of the registered nurse in various special areas of interest, for example, in the care of the patient in coronary care units, or the care of the premature infant, to mention only 2. Programs of inservice education are provided by agencies offering nursing service.

Undergraduate education in nursing and graduate education for nurses were described briefly in Chapter 3, "Nursing as a Profession." The other types will now be described briefly. Also discussed in Chapter 3 is the influence of the ANA stand on education.

Among the 4 types of preservice programs preparing nurses for licensure as registered nurses, all but the hospital diploma program have been in-creasing in number of schools and in number of admissions—especially during the last 5 years. The ANA position paper on education, issued in 1965, has had an effect on this trend. Nursing education is in a period of reshaping. Many states now have blueprints calling for regional and state-wide planning for all types of preservice programs, including those pre-paring practical nurses. The latter programs have been increasing rapidly, despite the efforts of the ANA to encourage their replacement by the as-sociate degree programs. In 1967, the practical nursing programs produced more than 41 per cent of all graduates from preservice programs.[1]

As a result of the recommendations of the Surgeon General's Consultant Group in Nursing in their 1963 report, *Toward Quality in Nursing; Needs and Goals,* the ANA and NLN acted to establish an independent com-mission to study nursing education. The National Commission for the Study of Nursing Education, Inc., headed by W. Allen Wallis, president of the University of Rochester (New York), began its work in 1967.[2] The work of the Commission will no doubt have further influence on the direction of nursing education. You will want to study the report a summary of which appears in the February 1970 *American Journal of Nursing.*

Preservice Program in the Hospital School of Nursing

The preservice diploma program in nursing that is offered in a hospital school of nursing, which prepares students for licensure as registered nurses, places emphasis primarily on preparation for nursing practice,

[1] M. B. Harty, "Trends in Nursing Education," *American Journal of Nursing,* **68**:771, Apr. 1968.
[2] "Commission to Study Nursing Education," (news) *American Journal of Nursing,* **67**: 1181-1182, June 1967.

although many have included some liberal arts education. The hospital diploma program has been declining over the past few years. In 1957 there were 944 such schools, but in 1967 only 767 were operating.[3] However, diploma programs continue to prepare the largest percentage of registered nurses of any of the preservice programs. In 1966 to 1967 they produced 71.8 per cent of the total number of graduates.[4]

Changes are continuing to take place in the curriculums in hospital schools of nursing. Generally, however, learning experiences are included in the following areas of instruction: fundamentals in nursing, medical and surgical nursing, maternal and child health, mental health and psychiatric nursing, communicable disease nursing, including tuberculosis nursing, and rehabilitation nursing. Although learning experiences in nursing usually constitute the core of the curriculum, the following areas of instruction are included in many programs: religion, communications, interpersonal relations, and social science. The psychologic, physical and biologic sciences are included for attaining scientific understanding.

As in other preservice educational programs in nursing, there is a trend toward large groupings of content into fewer courses. Also, a number of schools have shortened their programs to less than 3 calendar years.

Preservice Program Leading to an Associate Degree

The preservice educational program in nursing leading to an associate degree has been evolving since 1952, primarily in junior and community colleges. This is the most rapidly growing of the programs preparing persons for licensure as registered nurses. In 1963 there were 105 programs; by 1967 there were 281.[5] Preparation in this program is based on the assumption that nursing functions can be differentiated and that they range from very simple to very complex.

The student in these programs is being prepared for technical nursing. The program is designed for those who want to study in a multipurpose collegiate institution and to prepare for nursing in a short period of time. The main characteristics of the curriculums are:

1. They consist of approximately 2 calendar years of study beyond high school.

2. They follow, in general, the educational pattern in the institution.

3. There are broad groupings of subject matter. The basic sciences are concentrated in the first year of the curriculum; general education courses extend throughout both years. The trend seems to be to incorporate principles and concepts of pharmacology, mental health and nutrition throughout the nursing courses where they are appropriate to nursing

[3] Harty, *op. cit.*, p. 767.
[4] American Nurses' Association, *Facts About Nursing: A Statistical Summary*, New York, The Association, 1968, p. 88.
[5] Harty, *op. cit.*, p. 770.

action. Emphasis is on 4 basic areas of nursing: (1) fundamentals in nursing or what is common to all illness regardless of where the patient is, (2) maternal and child health, (3) clinical nursing science based on the variety of health problems and illnesses of various age groups and (4) psychiatric nursing. There is approximately 50 per cent general education and 50 per cent special education, with some emphasis on communications, interpersonal relations, social science and nursing brought together in a unified curriculum in the 2 academic or calendar years. Learning experience in each clinical situation is planned as an integral part of the nursing courses. There are, of course, variations of patterns depending on general philosophies of the different institutions offering these programs.

4. They are based on a teaching process that emphasizes going from the simple to the complex in common nursing situations, and problem solving for the development of judgment.

5. They are based on the idea that the centering of an educational program around educational purposes will keep the student a student and not a worker while studying.

6. They are planned usually as occupational education and are complete in themselves, not requiring additional study for employment as general staff nurses.

7. They lead to an associate degree.

8. The graduates are eligible for licensing examinations in the state where the program is located.

For information on the experiment in programs of this type, read the following references:

Montag, M. L. *Community College Education for Nursing.* New York, McGraw-Hill, 1959.

Anderson, B. *Nursing Education in Community Junior Colleges.* Philadelphia, Lippincott, 1966.

Preservice Program in Practical Nursing

The curriculum for the preparation of practical nurses, like all other curricula in nursing, is undergoing change based on experimentations. It is conducted in independent schools, in public vocational education insitutions, in hospitals, in junior colleges and in universities. In 1967, there were a total of 1,149 programs with an enrollment of 41,077.[6] Programs are usually 1 year in length and lead to a diploma or certificate. The purpose is to prepare a worker for 2 roles: (1) to give direct nursing care under supervision of a registered nurse or physician to patients in uncomplicated situations and (2) to assist the registered nurse in a close working relationship in giving nursing care in more complex situations.

[6] American Nurses' Association. *Facts About Nursing: A Statistical Summary,* New York, The Association, 1968, pp. 164-166.

Emphasis in the curriculum is on learning to nurse patients in carefully selected situations, and clinical education experiences centering on direct bedside care are provided. Concepts from nursing and from biologic and behavioral sciences are related to patient care of all age groups with common nursing problems.

Inservice Educational Programs in Nursing

Inservice educational programs for induction and continuation of education based on the needs of professional and allied nursing personnel in all types of nursing service agencies have been developed or are being started. General on-the-job programs for the training of auxiliary personnel, such as aides, attendants and maids, and some specialized nursing services also are being developed in increasing numbers.[7] There is evidence that on-the-job training programs for auxiliary personnel need considerable study for general improvement.

MAJOR POSITIONS FOR NURSES IN EDUCATION

The main positions for nurses responsible for nursing educational programs leading to baccalaureate or higher degrees are as teachers in the following areas: fundamentals of nursing, general nursing or nursing arts; nursing in special clinical fields, such as medical and surgical, maternal and child health, mental health and psychiatric, cancer, coronary care, orthopedic, tuberculosis and rehabilitation. In graduate programs, teachers also are employed in major functional areas in nursing service and nursing education, such as administration, supervision, curriculum development and improvement, teaching, consultation and research as well as special clinical fields. Other positions in the institutions of higher education are: coordinator or supervisor of field work, director or coordinator of curriculum, dean,[8] associate dean, assistant dean, assistant to the dean or the director, associate director, assistant director or assistant to the director.

The main positions for nurses responsible for educational programs in diploma schools in hospitals are those of teachers in most of the areas listed for those in the undergraduate program in nursing in an institution of higher education. As pointed out elsewhere, because of the tendency for instructional areas in nursing to broaden, there may be, in the future, some changes

---

[7] According to the Report of the Surgeon General's Consultant Group on Nursing, *Toward Quality in Nursing: Needs and Goals,* a desirable ratio of nursing personnel giving direct patient care in hospitals is 50 per cent professional nurses, 30 per cent practical nurses and 20 per cent on-the-job-trained aides (p. 16). It would appear, however, that many nursing services have not reached this ratio.

[8] "Dean" is used if the unit in which the program is placed is a college or a school in a university. "Director" frequently is used if the educational program is in a department of a larger division of the university or a college. Sometimes, "chairman of department" or "chairman of faculty" is used. There are also other administrative titles used depending on the policy of the institution.

in areas of specialization, particularly for teachers of nursing. Other positions for nurses in these schools of nursing are: director, associate director, assistant director or assistant to the director. There is a trend toward employing a director or coordinator of curriculum, who sometimes is referred to by use of the title "educational director."

The main positions for nurses in programs leading to an associate degree in junior and community colleges are educational administrator (specific title depending on the one used in the educational institution for such position), field coordinator, and teacher of fundamental nursing, of maternal and child health, of clinical nursing science and of psychiatric nursing.

The major positions for nurses in educational programs for the preparation of practical nurses are nursing instructor, field coordinator, director and assistant director.

In addition to the preceding list of positions for nurses in education, there are several other positions in which nurses sometimes are employed, such as director of research program, research assistant, counselor or director of guidance service, director of or consultant in educational service divisions in national, state or local nursing organizations, such as counseling and placement services, executive secretary, state supervisor, or visitor for state boards of nursing. Positions also are available for nursing educators in such places as health departments, the health and hygiene divisions of city and state departments of education, industry, home nursing divisions of the Nursing Service of the American National Red Cross, and the various Federal nursing services, such as the Army, Navy, or Air Force Nurse Corps, or other Federal agency where educational advisers and special educational consultants are used.

You can see that there are many opportunities for nurses in which graduate education in nursing is a fundamental requirement. Actually, there is currently a critical shortage of qualified faculty in all types of nursing programs and it is hoped that some of you will consider the possibility of preparing for this important teaching area. Some of the positions available are discussed elsewhere in this chapter and in other chapters, such as in Chapter 11, "Nurses in the Federal Government."

Nurses in Teaching Positions

When you are on the instructional staff for the implementation of an educational program in nursing, you have individual as well as group responsibilities. The following are some of the important individual responsibilities:

1. Planning, teaching, supervising and evaluating the learning experiences of students
2. Advising students and building rapport so that students' problems can be solved and their goals can be attained
3. Developing a special area of instruction
4. Studying, keeping up to date, and doing studies as needed

5. Writing reports of meetings, book reviews, articles for publication in professional magazines, critiques of reports of studies in nursing and related fields

6. Participating in and contributing to nursing and allied professional organizations

7. Participating in community services activities

8. Participating in the educational unit of nursing and contributing to the goals and objectives

In addition to the individual responsibilities you may have as a teacher, there are certain responsibilities you will share with the instructional staff as a whole. Some of these are:

1. To bring to bear on the thinking and the development of the entire instructional staff the results of inquiry in your special area of instruction and to make recommendations for the development of policy and program toward the fullest achievement of the purposes of the educational unit in nursing and the institution of which this unit is a part.

2. To participate in the formulation of educational and personnel policies and to make recommendations through the appropriate channels regarding the development of the curriculum, the improvement of instruction and guidance of students and the promotion of the interests, the happiness and the welfare of the staff and the students. This involves working with other groups.

3. To seek, to devise and to adopt methods of working together that capitalize on and contribute to the further development of ability, initiative and creative leadership of staff members and that foster continuous adjustment to changing needs and to the progressive development of common goals.

4. To determine the instructional staff's procedure of group functioning, set up standing and special committees and make suggestions, when appropriate, about the delegation of responsibility for individual functions relative to curriculum and program development and improvement.

5. To share in curriculum planning for the school in all of its aspects, including continuous cooperative evaluation of the progress and results of the curriculum as a result of the particular curriculum improvement plan for which the staff has the responsibility. Such sharing involves all people concerned, including those in participating and cooperating agencies.

6. To participate, as an elected or assigned representative, on college or university committees.

With these responsibilities of the individual teacher and the instructional staff as a whole in mind, it appears that some of the major qualifications one would hope to find in the members of an instructional staff are:

1. Ability to think and stimulate others to think

2. Ability to use effective methods of working as an individual and within a group inside and outside the school situation

3. Intellectual curiosity and imagination

4. Critical judgment and social sensitivity

5. A sense of fairness

6. A spirit of acceptance

7. A sense of humor

8. A capacity for sympathetic understanding and insight into problems of students

9. Ability to respect the individuality of students

10. Sound personal and professional values

11. Ability to teach, which includes competence in a particular field of instruction and understanding the functions of planning, organizing, directing, coordinating, stimulating, and evaluating as related to curriculum improvement and teaching

12. Ability to plan and give expert nursing care if you are a teacher of clinical nursing

13. Knowledge of the functional and the administrative organization of the unit of nursing and of the institution as a whole and the channels of communication

14. Understanding of and skill in the use of the problem-solving approach in the nursing situation, if you are teaching in the clinical area

It is suggested that you read Eugenia K. Spalding's article, "What Is a Teacher," in the October 1963 issue of *Hospital Progress*.

No one person can possess the total of the qualifications suggested in this or in other parts of this section or book. It is an appropriate mixture of these qualifications that is desired. The important thing in any situation is to understand expectations. When areas of expected accomplishment are well understood, accepted and fully shared by instructional or other staffs, it appears logical to expect feelings of security to be high and feelings of frustration and anxiety to be low, with a high degree of job satisfaction and personal growth.

Programs for the preparation of teachers vary somewhat in accord with the place where the teacher is expecting to work. The two major aspects of education for the teacher concern preparation in her area of instruction, for example, in the nursing specialty she expects to teach, and preparation in principles and methods of teaching, learning and evaluation.

The practice is for programs for teachers to be planned on the doctoral level for those expecting to teach in graduate programs for nurses and at least on the master's level for those who expect to teach in preservice nursing education programs.

Nurses in Administrative Positions in Educational Programs

A principal job of the educational administrator is to provide the kind of climate or atmosphere in which people can work on their jobs. Generally, if an administrator says that something in relation to the curriculum has to be done and has to be done now and in a certain way, with the instructional staff's having no part in the decision reached, the job may get done but without satisfaction to the staff and the students. There even may be complete balking and absolutely no accomplishment. On the other hand, if the members of a staff have security and a real feeling that an administrator will back them up and give them support, morale can be very high. There must exist the feeling that a staff member can go to the administrator for help on new developments or plans being tried out.

An administrator should be able to see all the work to be done in its relationship to the purpose of the program, and be able to bring about and maintain an organization capable of accomplishing that purpose.

The administrator is concerned with such general responsibilities as listed below:

1. Studying the objectives, the policies, the facilities and the resources of the institution of which the educational unit in nursing is a part; the needs of society for nursing; the functions of the nursing profession; the needs of individual students and the group as a whole; and the provision of the educational services which might be developed in the institution as a means for reaching the accepted objectives

2. Selecting and arranging for the appointment of staff members who collectively can carry out plans for reaching the objectives

3. Arranging for and permitting free discussion of ideas, philosophy and methods

4. Interpreting the educational program and its needs to the instituition's administration in terms of budgetary and other requirements, such as personnel, facilities and negotiations with outside agencies

5. Finding and devising ways of carrying on the program, by providing the necessary organization, facilities, equipment, working space and secretarial and other assistance

6. Seeing that the system of communication is effective

7. Encouraging and facilitating the development of the best plan of organization for getting work done

8. Providing services so that members of the instructional group can do their jobs effectively

9. Evaluating cooperatively with the other members of the staff the progress being made

10. Reporting to the officers of administration of the institution the progress and needs of the educational unit

11. Providing educational leadership in all phases of the program.

The ability for administration might be based on a consideration of an appropriate combination of the qualities listed below. You can see that they are almost identical with those suggested for teachers, with the emphasis on good qualities of administration for this group and on teaching for the teaching group.

1. Ability to think clearly

2. Intellectual curiosity and imagination

3. Critical judgment and social sensitivity

4. Ability to use effective methods of working with or getting others to work

5. Sound personal and professional values

6. Competence in administration and in conducting studies for improvement of administrative practices

7. Ability to evaluate the progress of others

8. Ability to see the whole as well as its parts

9. A sense of timing

10. A sense of humor

11. A sense of fairness

12. Respect for others

13. Integrity

14. Tenacity

Programs for the preparation of administrators in education vary slightly in accord with the type of educational program to be administered.

The practice is for programs for educational administrators to be planned on the doctoral level for those expecting to administer graduate or baccalaureate programs for nurses, and on the master's level as a minimum for those who expect to teach in diploma or associate degree programs.

Nurses in Inservice Education Programs

Inservice education programs have been in existence for a long time in one form or another. Public health nursing services have had organized programs for a number of years, but these organized programs are a relatively new development in hospital nursing services. They are one way in which the agency can improve the nursing care of patients.

There is a need for career planning in nursing for the individual nurse and for inservice education to be based upon the triad of her preservice education, experience and career plans within the institution or agency.

Those concerned with inservice and on-the-job training programs need a special type of preparation. Several universities are working on experimental educational programs for such personnel. It generally is thought that nurses who are concerned with inservice programs could benefit by areas of instruction that would help them in the development or improvement of: (1) skill in nursing practice or whatever is to be taught; (2) understanding of and skill in teaching, supervision and consultation; (3) understanding of the relationship of these processes to the processes of administration and research; (4) understanding of the broad problems and desirable practices in patient-care planning; (5) understanding of and skill in the use of the problem-solving approach to everyday problems in the practice of nursing and inservice education in areas of concern; (6) understanding of the role and the functions of the director of or instructor in inservice education; (7) understanding of self and others involved in inservice education within the various service agencies in nursing and (8) ability to plan and implement programs for different kinds of nursing personnel.

Positions are available in universities for those who desire to prepare administrative and instructional personnel for inservice and on-the-job programs in nursing services, hospitals and public health. Positions for these people, so prepared, are open in hospitals and related institutions, and in public health nursing services, for conducting programs in inservice education.

How Are Trends in Nursing Education Affecting Occupational Opportunities for Nurses in Education?

There are many influences affecting occupational opportunities for nurses in education. Some are listed here. You may think of others.

1. Because there is a need to improve and broaden instruction in nursing, and because schools of nursing are expanding, there is a continuing and critical need for more and better prepared teachers in nursing for all types of educational programs for nursing, especially in graduate education.

2. There has been a definite trend to separate instructional and service positions in hospitals offering educational programs in nursing. However, there is still demand for personnel in clinical nursing who will administer patient units in hospitals and also serve as teachers in nursing in their special fields. Some administrators in university medical centers are beginning to feel that a combination of nursing service and nursing education is more likely to accomplish desirable goals. This means that these people holding dual positions must know the content of the special field and be able to teach as well as to administer, a big job for one person.

3. Curriculum patterns are changing in all types of educational programs for nursing. The trend toward larger groupings of content, based on over-all objectives of the curriculum, is a major one. This trend is changing the type and the scope of areas in nursing for which teachers of nursing will be prepared for both preservice and graduate programs. Preparation for teaching both maternal and child care in a single course is one example. However, in graduate education in clinical areas there also appears to be a trend toward increasing specialization.

4. Perhaps among the greater influences on opportunities for nurses in education is the expansion of rehabilitation and public health programs and the increase in psychiatric patients, as well as the changing concepts of what constitutes good care for these patients. Teachers and educational consultants are needed in increasing numbers in these as well as in all the clinical nursing areas, both in educational institutions and in service agencies.

5. Educational requirements for the appointment of nursing teachers are the same as for other teachers in institutions of higher education.

Without doubt, nursing education is developing along changed lines, and we need well-qualified nurses in it. Nursing education is an interesting, important and challenging task, and the openings for well-prepared candidates are numerous and challenging.

NURSES IN CONSULTATION[9]

An important position in many health and educational agencies is that of the specialized nurse consultant. With the expansion of knowledge required of all health workers, and especially of professional nurses themselves, no one person can know all there is to know in the various special clinical fields or other functional areas. It is the function of the nurse consultant to provide, through her consultation services, assistance to nurses and allied groups in her area of specialized competence. Her primary functions are advisory and educational. Some of her general responsibilities would seem to include surveying a specific situation in terms of the problem or the problems for which consultation was sought, in light of the purpose of the agency or the individual person seeking help and of the functions and the relationship between the people involved. The usual functions are:

1. Inquiring and fact finding
2. Planning consultation procedure concerning the actual help to be given on the basis of such inquiry and fact finding
3. Stimulating thinking of the people concerned with the problem or the problems that have grown out of a need in the specific situation
4. Coordinating consultation activities in terms of relationships expected in the situation
5. Using resources effectively
6. Contributing expertness of knowledge when indicated
7. Maintaining good interpersonal and group relations
8. Evaluating procedures used

Where Do Nurse Consultants Work?

The nurse consultant is usually employed in local, state and national health and educational agencies or institutions. Examples of titles in this category of position are: generalized public health nursing consultant, maternal and child health consultant, geriatric nursing consultant, occupational health nursing consultant, tuberculosis nursing consultant, consultant in chronic disease nursing, consultant in communicable disease nursing, nursing education consultant, consultant in nursing service and many others. As the titles indicate, the consultant is concerned with a particular

[9] This section is concerned with nurses who make consultation their specialty — not consultation by, for example, the registered nurse, the licensed practical nurse, the clinical nursing specialist with the registered nurse, and so on.

clinical specialty, or other functional area in nursing. Sometimes, however, she is a generalist.

What Qualifications Must Consultants Have?

In addition to undergraduate nursing education, consultant nurses are expected to have had education and experience in their special area of competence qualifying them as experts. Graduate education which includes both the clinical specialty and the functional area of consultation is necessary in order to carry consultation responsibilities adequately as a clinical expert. An educational consultant should have preparation and experience in clinical nursing and in education, as well as consultation. And a nursing service consultant should have preparation and experience in clinical nursing, in nursing service administration and in consultation.

The ability for consultation might be based on an appropriate combination of the qualities listed below. You can see that some of these qualities are identical with those suggested for teachers, administrators, supervisors and research workers.

1. Ability to think and communicate clearly
2. Ability to observe accurately and to make expert judgments
3. Ability to plan; the consultant should be a specialist in planning
4. Ability to stimulate others to think
5. Ability to work through others
6. Ability to size up people quickly
7. Understanding and ability to define and redefine the role of consultation
8. Ability to discover the expectations of consultees
9. Ability to make people "feel at home"
10. Understanding of and skill in interpersonal and intergroup relations
11. Vision in relation to nursing as a whole
12. Ability to live with the frustrations of people
13. Ability to write reports

If your long-range goal is to become a consultant in a specialized area, you should begin plans early to obtain the kind of broad experience that you will require and for the type of graduate program that will best serve your needs.

NURSES IN RESEARCH

Of increasing importance today is the place of the nurse in research. A profession depends on the research that its members carry out for the growth and the development of the scientific knowledge on which the profession rests. Nursing is no exception, and in recent years more and more concern has been expressed about the need for nursing research and for nurse scientists or researchers. Much research in nursing in the past has been directed toward the study of the nurse and of nursing education. This type of research is important and must continue. But in addition there is a critical need for more patient-centered research directed toward the study of nursing practice. The Division of Nursing, U.S. National Institutes of Health, recognized the critical need when it supported the need for nursing research fellowships and nurse-scientist programs.

One leader in nursing has expressed the opinion that more emphasis should be placed upon the use of research as well as the doing of it. She also cautioned against "half-baked" research by unqualified nurses. She thinks there is a need for a small number of qualified researchers and a vast number of intelligent consumers to put research findings into practical use.

How Does the Nurse Function in Research?

Generally speaking, nurses have always been expected to participate in research, but few until recent times have been engaged in scientific investigations in nursing. Mildred Newton, in her article, "As Nursing Research Comes of Age," defines 6 roles in nursing research: data collector, student of research, teacher of research, project team member, project director and research expediter.[10] Another role is that of the creative thinker—the innovator or inventor of the theory underlying various nursing practices or the definer of problems to be researched. Nurses working in research today are employed as research assistants, research associates, as research project directors and as directors of research programs or institutes. They may be working in institutions of higher learning or in local, state or national private or governmental agencies.

What Qualifications Must You Have for a Research Position?

All nurses should be qualified to serve as data collectors and to evaluate research findings and apply these in the practice situation—the findings of research must be put into action. The great need is for nurses qualified to teach research and to design and carry out independent studies for the improvement of nursing practice.

Nursing students who are interested in becoming nurse researchers should begin planning for graduate study as soon as possible after graduation from their preservice program in nursing. The number of graduate schools that offer programs at the doctoral level for nurse scientists is increasing, and opportunities for nurses in research will continue to expand.

[10] *American Journal of Nursing,* **62**:46, Aug. 1962.

NURSES IN PROFESSIONAL ORGANIZATIONS

Opportunities for nurses in professional organization work are increasing at all levels — local, state and national. Special programs are being developed to prepare nurses for their responsibilities in organization work. The first program for this purpose was started in the Division of Nursing Education, Teachers College, Columbia University, in 1950. In fact, the preparation of nurses for organization work has grown so important that the Shirley C. Titus Fellowship has been established to assist nurses in preparing for this field. This fellowship is administered by Nurses' Educational Funds, Inc.

Some nurses have been employed by nursing organizations for part-time work; borrowing nurses for a time from their regular jobs is becoming common. Both the borrowed and the part-time nurses have been utilized by nursing organizations for making surveys, for consultation service and for other special projects such as research. The emphasis on mass education, regional planning and field work by national nursing organizations also has increased the number of nurses in this occupational area of nursing. An extensive list of opportunities in this area can be found in Chapter 8, "General Survey of Occupational Opportunities for Nurses," in the section entitled "Positions Available in Professional Organizations."

Main Activities of Nurses in Professional Organizations

The main activities of nurses in professional organization work revolve around the objectives of the particular organization. In general, they have custody of the archives for the group. They direct the activities and the programs in accordance with the objectives approved by the members who compose the group or by their representatives, the elected officers. This means that they must keep in touch with problems in the field and make studies to assist in arriving at worth-while solutions of such problems. They also must prepare agenda, organize programs and see that conventions are conducted smoothly. They work with control boards, commissions, divisions, departments, councils, occupational forums, committees, regional, state, district and local associations and with individual members of the organization and allied groups. They are the principal public relations representatives of the organization, both within the organization and in their relations with the membership of other organizations. They prepare reports, bulletins, news releases and articles for publication. Some may need to be specialists in legislation; others may be specialists in education or in the various areas of nursing service. Some may need to know the intricacies of compiling statistics, and others must have the ability to review and edit. Almost all need to hold offices and to be active in civic groups as well as in other related organized groups. In fact, these workers must be versatile, since they never know when they will be called on to attend a meeting, speak in public, or work quietly behind the scenes, doing the many detailed jobs that are required to keep the wheels of the organization running smoothly over the rough roads that most of them must travel.

In regional or state nurses association offices, because the staff may be limited, the executive secretary or director of headquarters office may need to know how to do many of the things listed in the preceding paragraph. She needs to have knowledge about and an awareness of implications of legislation affecting nursing. In one year, an executive secretary in one of the larger states spent 50 per cent of her time on legislation when the legislature was in session. This did not count the time of the other members of the staff who worked on keeping members informed about current legislation affecting nursing. An executive director or secretary in a state nurses association must have a thorough knowledge of the nursing practice act in the state and be able to interpret it in an intelligent and unbiased way. She serves as a liaison between the board of directors of the organization and its membership and also between the board and the related national nursing organization. She also needs to know how to work with allied professional groups. She has to be constantly alert to the nursing problems on the national as well as the local level. She also has to be able to establish a working climate in which these problems can be approached and studied, so that recommendations for improving current untoward conditions in nursing can be made and implemented. She needs to be able to stimulate and promote thoughtful discussions of major issues in nursing. She needs an understanding of business procedures and personnel administration.

She must know how to acquire information on employment conditions and methods for getting good employment conditions for nurses, including information on industrial relations. In state nurses association offices that have a professional staff assigned to direct the various programs of the association, the responsibilities of the executive director includes coordination of all programs. She and her assistants need to participate actively in committees and hold offices in other organizations, in order to contribute to the work done and in turn learn much of value for use in their state. Participation in the activities of the boards of such associations as Altrusa, Soroptimist, or American Association of University Women or committees of allied professional or civic groups is an essential part of the work of these people, as is official representation for their associations at all types of meetings of these and similar groups.

The executive director of a regional or state league for nursing has responsibilities equally broad. She also works with similar groups, both within the organization and with allied groups.

It is suggested that you read the following references by Dr. Merton, in connection with this chapter:

Merton, R. K. "The Functions of the Professional Association." *American Journal of Nursing*, **58**:50-54, Jan. 1958.

_____. "Dilemmas of Democracy in the Voluntary Associations." *American Journal of Nursing*, **66**:1055-1061, May 1966.

How Does a Nurse Enter This Field?

As a rule, the first step is to become an active member of a district or a state nurses association or a local, regional or state league for nursing and then to participate actively in local committee work and organization projects. After that, the interested and capable organization workers soon are detected, as they stand out in any organization. It is from among this group of active workers that selections are made when positions are available.

Experience in various fields of nursing in different parts of the country and abroad is valuable to obtain the wide background required. Ability to adjust and work cooperatively with many kinds of people and in difficult situations with much tact and skill is an essential qualification for entrance into positions in this field.

The persons selected for specialized tasks are required to have the necessary qualifications for the particular work. For example, a person doing work in the field of curriculum would be required to have preparation in the area of curriculum development and improvement. The nurse working with the economic security program would benefit from preparation in industrial relations or personnel administration or both.

Almost all who are employed usually have at least a bachelor's degree, although increasingly a master's or doctor's degree is required, and experience and qualifications that make them suitable for selection for the particular work to be done.

One executive director of a state nurses association made this comment about her work: "It is a very stimulating experience, and there are many satisfactions as one looks back over the months and years and reviews the real progress made." There are also the ever-present challenges of the things yet to be accomplished for nurses and nursing.

PROBLEMS

Nurses in Education

1. (a) Consult the current *Facts About Nursing,* and report on the number and the distribution of the various types of educational programs in nursing and the estimated needs for administrative and instructional personnel for these programs. (b) If surveys of nursing needs and resources have been made in your state, discuss the estimated need for faculty in all types of programs.

2. If you wished to pursue graduate education in nursing, where could you locate pertinent information on (a) educational programs and (b) scholarships and traineeships?

Nurses in Consultation Work

1. What steps would you need to take if your goal was to become a consultant?

2. (a) Discuss what you believe would be the satisfactions of doing consultant work. (b) What do you think would be the problems that consultants face in working with nurses in service agencies or educational institutions?

Nurses in Research Work

1. Who do you think should do research in nursing? Why?

2. If there is a research division on nursing where you are studying, ask one of your group to confer with its director on the kinds of research underway or completed, and to report her finding to the class.

3. Where would you look for information on available research occupational opportunities for nurses?

Nurses in Professional Organizations

1. (a) Ask one of your group to interview the executive officer of your district or state nurses association to learn first-hand about her functions and what qualifications she believes a person in this position should possess. (b) Ask the student to report her interview to your class group.

2. (a) Study current issues of the *American Journal of Nursing, Nursing Outlook,* and newsletters issued occasionally by the national, regional or state nursing organizations. (b) From this study make a list of the emerging occupational opportunities for nurses in organization work.

SUGGESTED REFERENCES*

NURSES IN EDUCATION

* American Nurses' Association. Committee on Education. "ANA Position on Education for Nursing." *American Journal of Nursing,* **65:**107-111, Dec. 1965.
* "Characteristics of Baccalaureate and Graduate Education in Nursing." *Nursing Outlook,* **16:**36-37, July 1968.
Dustan, L. C. "Characteristics of Students in Three Types of Nursing Education Programs." *Nursing Research,* **13:**159-166, Spring 1964.
Hoyt, R. S. "Nursing Education and the Hospital School." *Journal of the Medical Society of New Jersey,* **64:**523-527, Sept. 1967.
Johnson, D. E. "Post-Masters Education." *Nursing Outlook,* **12:**33-35, Jan. 1964.
Kemble, E. L. "The Dean — Born or Made?" *Nursing Outlook,* **11:**737-749, Oct. 1963.
* Kibrick, A. "Summary: Associate Degree Programs." *National League for Nursing Conference Papers,* 1968, pp. 63-68.

* In each chapter all citations are footnoted and are not included here. All starred references are recommended for additional reading.

Millard, R., Jr. "Liberal and Professional Nursing Education." *Nursing Outlook,* **16:**22-25, July 1968.
* Montag, M. L. "Nurse Faculty in Associate Degree Programs." *Nursing Outlook,* **12:**40-42, July 1964.
* National League for Nursing. *Statements on ... Practical Nurse Education.* New York, The League, 1968.
* _____. Department of Baccalaureate and Higher Degree Programs. *Policies and Procedures of Accreditation for Baccalaureate and Higher Degree Programs in Nursing.* New York, The League, 1968.
New England Board of Higher Education. Regional Nursing Program. *Proceedings of the First Inter-University Faculty Work Conference.* Wellesley, Mass., New England Board of Higher Education, 1960.
* Notter, L. E. and Smith, K. M. *Community Planning for Nursing Education: Papers from the 1968 Convention of the American Nurses' Association.* New York, American Nurses' Association, 1968.
* Ozimek, D. "The Preparation of a Generalist." *Nursing Outlook,* **16:**28-29, Dec. 1968.
Smyth, Sister Mary Paul and Elder, Sister Nathalie. "Nursing Education Curriculums, 1968: Direction or Drift." *Nursing Outlook,* **16:**41-43, Dec. 1968.
* Spalding, E. K. "What is a Teacher?" *Hospital Progress,* **44:**178-202, Oct. 1963.
See references in Chapter 3 on professional nursing education and, also, in Chapter 16 on continued education.

NURSES IN CONSULTATION

Frank, Sister Charles Marie. "Consultation in Retrospect." *Nursing Outlook,* **10:**750-752, Nov. 1962.
* Gilbert, R. "Functions of the Consultant." *Teachers College Record,* **61:**177-187, Jan. 1960.
Johnson, B. S. "Psychiatric Nurse Consultants in a General Hospital." *Nursing Outlook,* **11:**728-729, Oct. 1963.
Lima, A. "A WHO Nurse Reports." *American Journal of Nursing,* **62:**100-103, Mar. 1962.
Poorman, A. "The Hospital Consultant Nurse." *Nursing Outlook,* **3:**382-385, July 1955.

NURSES IN RESEARCH

* Conant, L. B. "On Becoming a Nurse Researcher." *Nursing Research,* **17:**68-71, Jan./Feb. 1968.
* Davis, M. Z. "Some Problems in Identity in Becoming a Nurse Researcher." *Nursing Research,* **17:**166-168, Mar./Apr. 1968.
National League for Nursing. Council of Baccalaureate and Higher Degree Programs. *Extending the Boundaries of Nursing Education — The Preparation and Role of the Nurse Scientist.* New York, The League, 1968.
* "The Nurse in Research: ANA Guidelines in Ethical Values." *Nursing Research,* **17:**104-107, Mar./Apr. 1968.
* "The Nurse Researcher and the Nursing Profession." *International Nursing Review,* **14:**33-35, Dec. 1967.

OTHER NURSING OPPORTUNITIES

Alena, V. M. "Flight Nursing: Improving the Present ... Probing the Future: Meeting the Challenge Through Applied Research." *Aerospace Medicine,* **39:**292-295, Mar. 1968.

"ANA Statement of Nurse-Midwifery." *Bulletin of the American College of Nurse-Midwifery,* **13**:26-27, Feb. 1968.

Baum, A. Z. "Nurse to the Astronauts." *RN,* **31**:46-47, May 1968.

Campbell, M. B. "Pioneer and Perseverance." *Journal of the Association of Nurse Anesthetists,* **36**:111-119, Apr. 1968.

Cherescavich, G. D. "Role of the Clinical Specialist in Nursing." *Hospital Management,* **104**:78-79, Nov. 1967.

Gilzean, E. "My Nursing Has Paid Me Twice." *Nursing Times,* **63**:1723, Dec. 22, 1967.

Hellman, L. M. "Nurse-Midwifery in the United States." *Obstetrics and Midwifery,* **30**:883-888, Dec. 1967.

Hepner, J. O. "The Role of the Nurse Anesthetist in the Front Line Expertise Nursing Corps." *Journal of the American Association of Nurse Anesthetists,* **35**:446-454, Dec. 1967.

Newcomb, R. F. "Summer Camp Nursing." *RN,* **31**:30-34, Mar. 1968.

Runnerstrom, L. "Nurse Midwifery at the Crossroads." *Bulletin of the American College of Nurse Midwifery,* **12**:131-134, Nov. 1967.

CHAPTER

11

Nurses in the
Federal Government

Many nurses are employed by various governmental units, Federal, state and local. This chapter pertains especially to work under the Federal Government, which began employing contract nurses to serve with the Army during the Spanish-American War. These contract nurses demonstrated the value of women's services in the care of the sick and were the forerunners of the thousands of nurses now employed by governmental agencies, both military and civilian, in the USA and throughout the world.

Nursing in the Federal nursing services carries many advantages and a few disadvantages, some of which will be brought out here. Others you will learn as you make your own occupational investigation.

The next 4 sections deal with the nurses in the armed services. It is interesting to note that, in 1967, nurses were granted equal opportunity with men in these services. Figure 11-1 shows President Lyndon B. Johnson signing the equal opportunity bill.

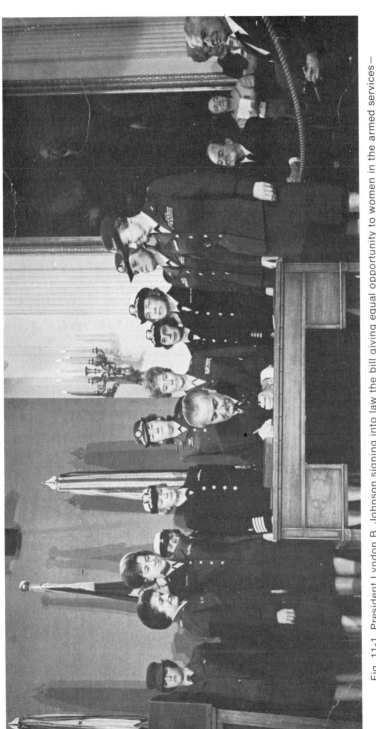

Fig. 11-1. President Lyndon B. Johnson signing into law the bill giving equal opportunity to women in the armed services—November 8, 1967. (Reprinted with permission from the *Quarterly Review* of the D.C. Nurses Association, Winter 1967-1968, p. 6.)

ARMY NURSE CORPS

Organized as a part of the Army Medical Department in 1901, the Army Nurse Corps (ANC) is the oldest of all the Federal nursing services. As early as July 27, 1775, the Continental Congress authorized the employment of women to care for the sick and the wounded. Although there were no professionally trained nurses at that time, some women were employed as nurses and others served without pay.

Again, during the Civil War (1861 to 1865), more than 3,000 women were authorized to serve in the Army hospitals. Dorothea Linde Dix was appointed superintendent of women nurses for the Union Army on June 10, 1861 and served throughout the war with limited authority over the women employed by the government. Many other women served in Army hospitals under the sponsorship of the U.S. Sanitary Commission and various voluntary societies. A limited number of the women employed by the Army received 1 month of training in a New York hospital, under the guidance of Elizabeth Blackwell, M.D., the first woman to graduate from a school of medicine in the USA.

It was not until the Spanish-American War (1898) that the first permanent organization of Army nurses was formed. Anita Newcomb McGee, M.D., was appointed Acting Assistant Surgeon (contract surgeon) on August 29, 1898 and served in the Office of the Surgeon General, in charge of women contract nurses, through 1900. She had no authority over men hired as nurses under the contract. As chairman of the DAR Hospital Corps Committee through August 1898, she examined credentials of some 8,000 women volunteers, sending the names of qualified trained nurses to the Surgeon General for a contract and duty assignment. The first women graduate nurses signed contracts on May 10, 1898, and nurses have served continuously in Army hospitals since then. Some 1,500 women – the majority trained nurses, a few women physicians and a number of women immune to yellow fever who had practical experience in nursing – served as contract nurses for varying periods of time up to July 1899, the peak duty strength being 1,158. The number decreased rapidly with some 200 on duty at a time through 1900.

Dr. McGee drafted the section of a War Department bill which, as Section 19 of the Act of Congress of February 2, 1901, created the Nurse Corps (female) as a part of the permanent military establishment (it was renamed the Army Nurse Corps in July 1918). Composed of a superintendent, chief nurses, nurses and reserve nurses – all graduate nurses – 202 contract nurses became charter members of the Corps on February 2, 1901. A former contract nurse, Mrs. Dita H. Kinney, had replaced Dr. McGee in The Surgeon General's Office on January 1, 1901. Appointed superintendent by the Secretary of War on March 15, 1901, she served through July 1909. The second superintendent, Jane A. Delano (August 1909 to March 1912), resigned to head the American National Red Cross

Nursing Service. Nurses were enrolled with the Red Cross for service when needed in meeting its national and international commitments and, in April 1912, were designated the primary source of reserve nurses for the military establishment. When the reserve nurse, with her own consent, was called to active duty in the Army, she served under the same provisions as the nurses of the permanent Corps, with the length of service dictated by the emergency.

There were 233 regular and 170 reserve nurses on duty in Army hospitals in April 1917 when the USA entered World War I. Then the nation-wide call for nurses by the American National Red Cross and other nursing organizations brought a peak strength of 21,480 nurses on duty on November 11, 1918. Over 80 per cent were nurses whose applications were screened and submitted to the Surgeon General by the Red Cross.[1] Over 10,000 nurses served overseas with the American Expeditionary Forces. Many received the citations of the French, the British and the USA governments.

In 1920, through the *Army Reorganization Act of June 4*, members of the ANC were granted relative rank from second lieutenant to major. They were authorized to wear the insignia of the relative rank and had some of the privileges of commissioned officers, but were granted neither the pay nor the authority of a commission. The relative rank span was increased to colonel in December 1942, when the pay of grade was authorized.

There were less than 7,000 nurses in the Corps on December 7, 1941, but over 57,000 in August 1945, before the demobilization started. Mrs. Julia O. Flikke, the superintendent from June 1937 to June 1943, and her assistant, Florence A. Blanchfield (superintendent from July 1943 to September 1947), were given temporary commissions as colonel and lieutenant colonel, respectively, in the Army of the USA on March 13, 1942 — the first women to hold commissioned status. In the latter part of 1943, *Bill H.R. 3761*, recommending actual permanent rank for Army nurses, was introduced to the Congress by Mrs. Frances Payne Bolton, but it was received unfavorably by the War Department and was withdrawn. In March 1944, a new bill providing temporary commissions for nurses during World War II and 6 months thereafter was introduced by Mrs. Bolton. This became law on June 22, 1944.

The contributions of the ANC in World War II are well known. Nurses served world-wide. Sixty-six were held prisoner by the Japanese; 16 lost their lives by enemy action. One out of every 40 was decorated.

On April 16, 1947, through *Public Law 36: The Army-Navy Nurses Act of 1947*, for the first time nurses were given permanent commissioned status in the USA regular Army, and an ANC Section was established in the Officers Reserve Corps. Florence A. Blanchfield was the first woman to be given permanent commissioned status in the regular Army (lieutenant colonel) and the grade of colonel as Chief, ANC.

---

[1] This source of military nursing supply was discontinued in 1947.

The *Army-Navy Nurses Act of 1947* was amended in 1955 by *Public Law 294*, 84th Congress. This authorized the appointment of male nurses as reserve commissioned officers. Since then male nurses have been assigned to active duty in the ANC. *Public Law 89-609* of September 30, 1966 authorized regular Army commissions in the ANC for men.

Passage of *Public Law 85-155*, in August 1957, brought added advantages and provided career opportunities for officers of the ANC. The law standardized the size of the Corps and the number of its officers, established new rules for retirement and initial officer appointment, and provided for an increasing number of nurses in upper grades, including limited permanent promotions to colonel. *Public Law 90-130* of November 8, 1967 removed artificial restrictions on grades of women officers in all of the armed services. It authorized the Service Secretary to prescribe the numbers in permanent grades through colonel (or captain, U.S. Navy). It removed statutory barriers to general or flag officer (U.S. Navy) rank for women, but did not prescribe such appointments.

How Does the ANC Function as Part of the Army Service?

The Chief of the ANC is appointed from Corps officers by the Secretary of the Army, upon the recommendation of the Surgeon General, for a period not to exceed 4 years. Currently serving in the grade of colonel, the Chief ranks over all other ANC Colonels during the Tour. Nurses are appointed in the rank of second and first lieutenant, and captain. Promotions to first lieutenant, captain, major, lieutenant colonel and colonel are determined by the professional qualifications of the individual nurse plus the amount of executive ability, judgment and tact exhibited, as well as the capacity to assume increasing responsibility. The higher the rank, the greater are the responsibilities. An ANC officer serves as Chief of nursing service in each Army hospital. The professional duties are comparable to those of a director of nursing service in a civilian hospital.

An 8-week basic program is conducted at the Medical Field Service School, Brooke Army Medical Center, Fort Sam Houston, Texas, providing military instruction for ANC officers entering active duty.

The Army nurse is responsible for the instruction and the supervision of the enlisted men and women who assist in the nursing care in military hospitals. ANC officers serve as instructors in formal courses conducted for enlisted personnel of the Army Medical Service. The Army nurse, like all nurses, is responsible to the physician for carrying out his medical care plan for the patient.

Services Rendered by the ANC

Nursing in the Army includes the care not only of members of the Army proper but also of their families and others entitled to care in military hos-

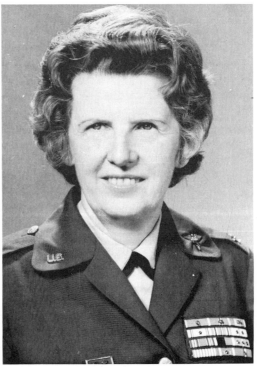

Fig. 11-2. Colonel Ruby G. Bradley, the Army's most decorated nurse, retired March 1963 as Director of Nursing Activities at Brooke Army Medical Center. (Official U.S. Army Photo)

pitals. The functions are comparable to those performed by nurses in civilian hospitals. The Army health nurse is the public health nurse of the military community. As a member of the Preventive Medicine team, she provides family-centered services.

Duties of the Army Nurse in Peace, War, or Disaster

In peacetime, Army nurses are assigned to military hospitals in the USA and in foreign countries wherever Army troops are stationed. Opportunity for experience is available in all nursing specialties. A few nurses are assigned overseas to selected Military Assistance Advisory Groups and USA missions. Army nurses may be assigned to a station type hospital located on a military post, to one of several larger general hospitals usually located near or in a large city, or to a general dispensary. Army nurses also work with medical teams or units sent to give medical assistance in time of major disaster, such as the Yugoslavian earthquake in 1963.

During wartime, nurses serve in mobile Army surgical hospitals, evacuation hospitals, or in field, station and general hospitals. They may serve on hospital trains or transport ships. Nursing of battle casualties provides unprecedented opportunity for experience in surgical nursing, preoperative and postoperative nursing care, a wide variety of medical conditions, and administration of rapidly expanding nursing units.

Figures 11-3 and 11-4 show Army nurses working in several types of situations.

Opportunities for Professional Growth and Development for the Army Nurse

The administrative officers of the Corps, believing that higher education in nursing and other fields is vitally important, have developed a greatly enlarged plan since World War II to assist the individual nurse in her professional advancement. Advanced courses are available to those who qualify and are conducted in anesthesiology, operating room, maternal and child health, psychiatric nursing, Army health nursing, medical-surgical nursing, nursing research and health care administration. At the Walter Reed Army Institute for Research, a department of nursing has been organized to carry out research studies in all fields of nursing practice. Army nurses who are interested and qualified in research may be assigned to this department or may be utilized in research projects in various geographical areas. Nurses prepared at a beginning level of public health nursing may participate in a developmental training program at one of several military installations.

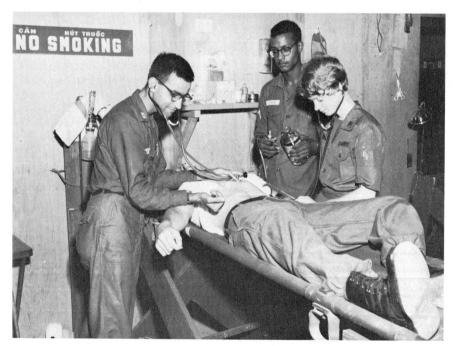

Fig. 11-3. Physician, nurse and medical corpsman in triage area, Third Surgical Hospital, Republic of Vietnam. (U.S. Army)

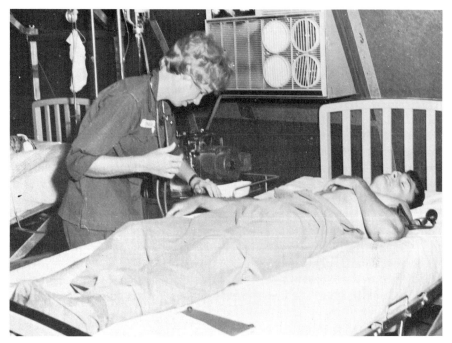

Fig. 11-4. Nurse caring for Vietnam war casualty, Twenty-fourth Evacuation Hospital in Vietnam. (U.S. Army)

By special arrangement, a limited number of career officers are sent to leading universities for graduate preparation in special branches of clinical nursing, education and administration, and receive tuition, full pay, and other allowances. Many other educational opportunities are provided, such as extension courses through USAFI and through the Medical Field Service School, workshops, institutes, and short courses in collaboration with university schools of nursing. Selected nurses attend the ANC Career Course or the Army Medical Service Officer Advanced Course at the Medical Field Service School. These courses prepare the Army nurse in administrative, staff and command procedures required for specific assignments.

Emphasis is placed on proper classification of personnel in terms of educational and experiential background so that ANC officers may be identified readily according to qualifications. This is considered most essential if personnel are to be utilized properly. Records of career officers are studied carefully, so that professional growth may result from planned professional progression in the form of educational opportunities or developmental assignments. The benefits from such career planning redound to the individual in terms of greater job satisfaction and to the service in the form of improved patient care.

How Do the Living and the Working Conditions of the ANC Compare With Conditions in Civilian Nursing?

Working conditions for Army nurses compare favorably with those of civilian nurses. Assignments and hours of duty are similar. Social life in the Army is especially attractive to nurses. Through status as an officer, the Army nurse may take part in all post activities—official, social and recreational.

Living conditions for Army nurses vary from post to post. Most nurses serving in the USA may live off post in a house or an apartment. Quarters are provided, should the nurse desire to live on the military post. In all overseas areas, quarters are provided for Army personnel.

Wherever an Army nurse lives, she gets a special allowance for food in addition to her base pay. If she dines with the Army, she is served appetizing, well-prepared food of highest quality, or she may choose to eat at the Officers' Club. If she likes to cook at home, she may buy food at a great savings at the post commissary.

Her income, comparable with or above civilian salaries, depending on rank and length of service, brings her far greater return. In addition to complete medical, surgical, hospital and dental care, she may shop at the post exchange and enjoy other fringe benefits.

Eligibility Requirements for the ANC

All candidates are appointed in the Army Reserve, ANC branch, before becoming eligible for service in a military hospital either as a reserve or as a regular Army nurse. The basic requirements for appointment are listed below. The nurse must:

1. Be of high moral integrity and possess excellent personal and professional attributes.

2. Be a citizen of the USA or Puerto Rico, or have been lawfully admitted to the USA for permanent residence.

3. Be a graduate of a hospital school of nursing or a baccalaureate nursing program, which is accredited and/or acceptable to the Department of the Army, and be currently licensed in the USA to practice professional nursing.

4. Have, if female, no dependents under the age of 18.

5. Meet certain age requirements. These are:

a. Appointment with concurrent active duty: Applicants must not have reached their 33rd birthday, except that this maximum age may be increased by up to 7 years prior active duty performed as a commissioned or warrant officer in the Armed Forces.

b. Appointment only: Applicants normally must not have reached their 35th birthday except that this maximun age may be increased by the amount of any creditable prior service, either active or reserve.

Nurses may apply for appointment in the U. S. Army Reserve or in the Regular Army. Eligible registered professional nurses are appointed in the grade for which they qualify, based on experience and education. Information concerning application may be obtained by writing to the Surgeon General, Department of the Army, ATTN: MEDPT-MP, Washington, D.C.. 20315.

Factors That Determine Eligibility for Promotion

Promotion to higher grade is based on nursing ability and potential leadership qualities.

Scale of Salaries in the ANC

Salaries in the Army Nurse Corps range from $5,449, the beginning salary for the general staff nurse (second lieutenant), to $16,465, the top salary for the chief of the ANC (colonel) or chief nurse, medical center or overseas command. These salaries include quarters allowance. Retirement provision is made for the reserve as well as the regular Army nurse. Now, women officers receive the same pay and allowance as men officers of equivalent rank. Leave accumulates on the basis of 2½ days per month for each month worked, and the individual nurse may accrue up to 60 days.[2]

After 20 years of active service in the ANC, a nurse may retire at the discretion of the Secretary of the Army. No salary deductions are made for retirement, but benefits are determined by multiplying the basic monthly pay at time of retirement by years of service by 2.5 per cent.

Army Nursing Student Program. The Army Nursing Student program provides for financial assistance to selected male or female nursing students, in acceptable schools of nursing, who have completed 2 years of a hospital or collegiate program in nursing. Participants receive the pay and allowances of their grade. Baccalaureate students receive tuition and fees and are commissioned in the ANC 6 months prior to graduation. Following licensure, participants are obligated to serve 2 or 3 years on active duty in the ANC, depending on the length of their participation in the program.

Walter Reed Army Institute of Nursing

The first group of outstanding high-school graduates was selected and entered 83 colleges in 37 states in the fall of 1964. Participants complete their first 2 years in the college where enrolled and must meet requirements for admission and transfer to the University of Maryland School of Nursing for their last 2 years. The University of Maryland is responsible for all academic and professional aspects of their program until the students

[2] Salaries for personnel discussed throughout this chapter are subject to constant change, sometimes large and sometimes minor. You will wish to note any changes made since 1970.

complete requirements for a bachelor of science degree in nursing. After graduation and successful completion of state licensure, the candidates will be commissioned as second lieutenants in the ANC, with an obligation, of 3 years as Reservists on active duty. Student participants receive tuition and fees, along with full pay and allowances of their grade, while in school. For this long range program, it is planned to select a limited number of male or female participants annually.

The purpose of this subsidy program is to assist in the Army's need for professional nurse officers for patient care activities, teaching and supervision.

Registered Nurse Student Program. Each year, also, a limited number of registered nurses are selected to complete the requirements for a baccalaureate or master's degree in nursing. Applicants must be eligible for appointment in the ANC and be able to complete the degree requirements in less than 24 months. Participants receive pay and allowances of officers of their grade and are obligated to serve on active duty in the ANC for 2 or 3 years following graduation, depending on their length of participation in the program.

Size of the ANC

In peacetime, the quota of nurses is in proportion to the number of military personnel; the size of the ANC fluctuates accordingly. Usually it is based on a ratio of 6 nurses per 1,000 men.

The strength of the ANC rose from 625 in 1939 to 57,000 in 1945 — a real tribute to the sense of responsibility of nurses for their country's need. As of June 1968, there were approximately 4,700 ANC officers on active duty.

Table 2. ARMY NURSE CORPS: NURSES SERVING, 1945-1968, AS OF JUNE 30 EACH YEAR

Year	Number	Year	Number	Year	Number
1945	54,291*	1953	4,692	1961	3,283
1946	13,617	1954	4,189	1962	3,402
1947	5,979	1955	3,757	1963	2,981
1948	4,317	1956	3,556	1964	2,969
1949	4,662	1957	3,384	1965	3,121
1950	3,401	1958	3,359	1966	3,735
1951	5,361	1959	3,364	1967	4,545
1952	5,323	1960	3,310	1968	4,700

* The peak of 57,000 was reached on August 14, 1945, V-J Day.

Source: American Nurses' Association, *Facts About Nursing: A Statistical Summary,* New York, The Association, 1964, p. 59, for all figures through 1963. Figures for 1964 through 1968 are from the ANC, Office of the Surgeon General.

It is suggested that you keep in touch with releases made by the ANC through the *American Journal of Nursing* and other sources regarding supply and demand in this Service.

AIR FORCE NURSE CORPS

The Air Force Nurse Corps (AFNC) was established as an integral part of the Air Force Medical Service on July 1, 1949, in accordance with the *Joint Army and Air Force Adjustment Regulation 1-11-62, May 16, 1949.*

At that time Army nurses were permitted to apply for transfer to the Air Force, and 1,199 transfers were made, of which 307 were from components of the regular Army. The others were members of the ANC Reserve on extended active duty. During World War II, nurses on duty at Air Force installations and those who participated in air evacuation activities were members of the ANC.

The AFNC has been increasing in size since its beginning.

Table 3. AIR FORCE NURSE CORPS: NURSES SERVING, 1954-1968, AS OF JUNE 30 EACH YEAR

Year	Number	Year	Number	Year	Number
1954	2,609	1959	2,880	1964	3,412
1955	2,289	1960	2,977	1965	3,488
1956	2,609	1961	3,113	1966	3,757
1957	2,949	1962	3,438	1967	4,102
1958	2,833	1963	3,409	1968	4,220

Source: American Nurses' Association. *Facts About Nursing: A Statistical Summary.* New York, The Association, 1964, p. 58, for all figures through 1963. Figures for 1964 through 1968 are from the AFNC, Office of the Surgeon General.

General Advantages of Being a Nurse in the Air Force Nurse Corps

An Air Force nurse has a career that is interesting and that utilizes and recognizes education and experience. The opportunities for a successful life as an Air Force nurse are many. The nurse's professional ability and experience will be enhanced through the variety of assignments and the wide scope of practice available. She will have the opportunity to take advantage of continued education that will bring progressive advancement. A number of occasions to travel both in this country and abroad are provided. Most of all, the nurse contributes her professional knowledge of excellent nursing care toward the constant well-being of the airman and his family.

How Is the Security of the Nurse Provided for in the Air Force Nurse Corps?

The Air Force nurse can enjoy economic advantages, at no personal expense. For example, medical and dental care during her career is provided at no personal cost.

Congress has provided retirement benefits for reserve officers as well as regular officers. The amount of money that the Air Force nurse receives is based on the length of service and the highest grade held. Should a nurse be retired for a physical disability incurred while in the Service, satisfactory monthly allowances are provided. The amount is based on a schedule for rating disabilities provided by Congress.

Salary Paid to an Air Force Nurse

Congress has established a pay scale for officers in the armed forces. A newly appointed officer is provided with a uniform allowance of $300 on original appointment. This allowance is the same as that allowed all officers when they first enter military service. While on active duty as a second lieutenant, the nurse's starting monthly pay and allowances are:

Base pay*	$343.20
Subsistence allowance†	47.88
Rental allowance‡	85.20 (single)
Total monthly pay	$476.28

* Pay increases are based on promotion and length of service.
† Subsistence and rental allowances are free from Federal tax.
‡ If quarters on military installations are not available.
(See also footnote 2, p. 259.)

There is extra pay for flight nurses assigned to aeromedical evacuation duties. The amount of this extra stipend depends on the individual's grade and years of service.

Opportunities for Personal and Professional Advancement

The Air Force nurse can look forward to progressive advancement. Criteria for temporary promotions for regular and reserve officers are announced periodically by the Department of the Air Force, depending on existing vacancies in the various grades. Important considerations in selecting officers for promotion are manner of performance of professional responsibilities, education, professional experience and aptitude. Members of the regular component are eligible for permanent promotions after completing established periods of time in each grade.

Living Conditions on an Air Force Base

A satisfying life can be found on almost every Air Force base. In off-duty hours the nurse finds opportunities for recreation, social activity and relaxation. Swimming pools, theaters, tennis courts, golf courses, bowling alleys and gymnasium facilities may be available at little or no personal cost. Then too, there are social activities to be found at the officers' clubs. Very often, groups organize beach parties, picnics and tours to historic centers and famous resorts found near many Air Force bases.

The Air Force undertakes to provide the nurse with as attractive and pleasant surroundings as possible. If living quarters are not available, the nurse may be permitted to reside in the civilian community. An Air Force installation resembles a well-planned community. There are commissaries and base exchanges—which duplicate department stores and super-markets—near at hand, where all articles needed can be purchased at approximate cost. Added to the places mentioned above are gasoline stations, banks, post offices, beauty salons, laundry and tailoring services and other conveniences.

Types of Positions Available to Members of the Corps

An officer in the AFNC, who can qualify through experience and educational preparation, may be assigned as a general staff nurse, a nurse administrator, an operating room nurse, a psychiatric nurse, a flight nurse, an anesthetist or an instructor.

In an assignment as a general staff nurse, full responsibility for bedside nursing care is assumed. The Air Force nurse administers various medications and treatments as ordered, assists the physician, maintains records on the progress of patients, conducts courses in convalescent care for airmen patients and their families. In addition, the nurse assists in educational programs and instructs auxiliary nursing personnel. Staff nurses may be assigned to medical, surgical, pediatric, obstetric, or communicable disease hospital units, as well as to dispensaries, clinics, aeromedical evacuation squadrons, teaching staffs. They also serve in units for intensive care, research, coronary care, school health, aerospace medicine, or as nurse advisors.

An administrative nurse in an Air Force hospital is responsible to the hospital commanding officer for nursing service in the hospital or may be responsible to the chief of service for nursing service in 1 or more units in a clinical section. She supervises all nurses and certain other related personnel in order to maintain constantly the highest standards of patient care. In addition, she conducts on-the-job training for nursing service personnel. Administrative nurses are responsible for directing nursing activities and for counseling nurses assigned to the hospital.

The operating room nurse makes preparations for and assists the surgeon in performing surgical operations. It is her responsibility to supervise the personnel assigned to the operating room.

The phychiatric nurse gives or supervises the professional nursing care of psychiatric patients, assists the physician in various procedures and keeps records of the patients' progress. Air Force psychiatric nurses participate in training and supervising allied and related nursing personnel.

Patient aeromedical evacuation is an outstanding contribution to the goal of saving lives. Over a million patients have been transported safely from such worldwide outposts as the Far East, Europe, the South Pacific and the Middle East. A tremendous contribution to this enviable record is the work of the flight nurse, who is a vital link in the chain of continued medical treatment of the patient evacuee. While aboard the aeromedical evacuation plane, the flight nurse exercises the same authority and has the same responsibilities as a hospital staff nurse. Before a flight nurse assumes her duties, she must learn special procedures to cope with the problems of aeromedical evacuation. The program is open to physically qualified Air Force nurses (age limitation, 36) who have expressed a willingness to participate in frequent aerial flights both during and after training. It is conducted at the U. S. Air Force School of Aerospace Medicine, Brooks Air Force Base, Texas. There the nurses are taught the theory and the practical phases of flight nursing. They complete basic courses on the care of sick and wounded

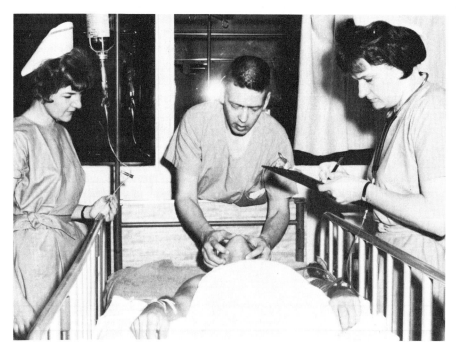

Fig. 11-5. Captain Herbert V. Staudenmaier (center) nurse in charge of the recovery room at the Wilford Hall USAF Hospital, instructs Captains Nancy J. Barron and Dorothy R. Novotny on the principles of maintaining an open airway. The Aerospace Nurse Residents spend 4 weeks of their 52 week Aerospace Nursing Course at the Wilford Hall USAF Hospital, Texas, to be especially prepared in emergency, surgical and postoperative nursing procedures. (USAF Photo)

in flight, become familiar with the equipment, and learn the aeromedical application of psychiatry, ophthalmology and otorhinolaryngology. They are given instruction in the use of respirators in flight, and learn the effects of high altitudes on the body and how to handle oxygen equipment. The nurses learn the importance of nutritional flight feeding and take further studies in preventive, aviation, global and space medicine. They study the principles of survival and the use of survival equipment. While gaining this flying experience, they receive remuneration in addition to regular pay. Figures 11-5 and 11-6 show the flight nurse in action.

As a nurse anesthetist, the Air Force nurse administers or supervises the administering of anesthetics to patients under the direction of the surgeon. She keeps the surgeon advised of the patient's general condition and reactions to the anesthetic during the operation. The nurse administers the necessary measures directed by the surgeon to eliminate shock, and keeps records of the patient's reactions during and immediately following anesthesia.

Opportunities for Travel

Nurses in the AFNC are assigned to interesting places. One of the exciting aspects of service with the Air Force is the world-wide extent of its activities. The Air Force nurse has an opportunity to request foreign service in such places as Hawaii, Alaska, Japan, the Philippines, England, Europe, Puerto Rico, and other parts of the world. The Air Force nurse's career gives many opportunities for sightseeing and visiting America's most important cities.

The Educational Programs

Two AFNC goals that reflect its high standards are:
1. To promote and ensure better patient care.
2. To develop and stimulate professional growth.

Every effort is made to keep the nurse current on new developments in aviation, global and space medicine and in nursing procedures and practices. Qualified Air Force nurses on active duty may apply for specialized courses in flight nursing, aerospace nursing, anesthesia, operating room management, advanced obstetrical nursing, and—for those who display leadership ability—nursing service administration conducted at Air Force schools and hospitals and cooperating civilian institutions. Also available at these hospitals is an abundance of clinical material, plus fine medical facilities and practice.

Each year a number of qualified nurses are sent to leading civilian universities to complete requirements for degrees in nursing. This is at government expense, and they draw full pay and allowances. In addition, those qualified Air Force nurses who desire to complete the final calendar year of

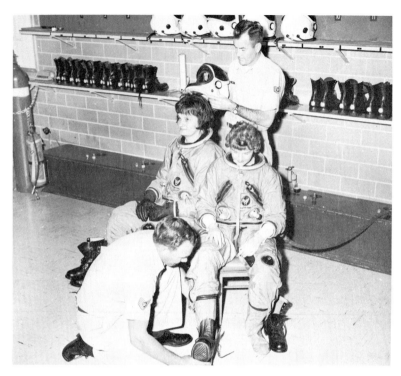

Fig. 11-6. Captains Dorothy R. Novotny and Nancy J. Barron (top), donning outer space gear and (bottom) making a pressure suit integrity check during their 52-week course in Aerospace Nursing. Donning pressure suits provides knowledge of physiological protection at altitude and in space. Maintenance, repair, and preflight validation of the pressure suit are also part of the course. (USAF Photos)

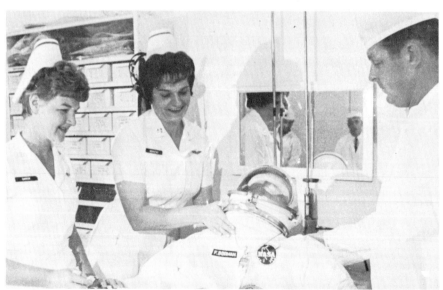

residence courses required for an undergraduate or graduate degree can complete this final year at any accredited university they prefer. While in attendance, they draw the full pay and allowance of their grade.

Each year a number of qualified nurses are sent to universities at government expense for workshops on subjects related to nursing. During off-duty hours they can earn credits toward a degree through correspondence and self-study courses offered by the U. S. Armed Forces Institute at a nominal fee. Additional courses may be taken at no extra charge. Colleges and universities also schedule extension courses for Air Force nurses conducted by their own instructors during off-duty hours at most Air Force installations. The cost to participate in these courses is shared by the Air Force and varies with the school and with the course.

The Air Force Nurse as a Social Force

War has been one of the forces that have helped to make professional nursing an essential social service. This has become increasingly apparent in the increased number of international health programs. Air Force nurses assigned to hospitals in foreign countries have been instrumental in promoting peace and relationships that have aided advancement in the nursing profession of those countries.

Rapid transition in the nursing profession has been noted especially in Japan since World War II. Professional nurses in Japan are gradually acquiring more status, better pay and better training. Undoubtedly, American nursing standards have also affected the profession in varying degrees in other countries through our military nurses.

The Air Force nurse is also instrumental in helping young women in their own countries to choose nursing as a career, by visiting the various schools and discussing with students their plans for the future.

Admission Requirements for Entrance into the AFNC

To obtain an appointment in the AFNC Reserve, a nurse must:

1. Be a graduate of a school of nursing acceptable to the Surgeon General, USAF.

2. Be currently registered in any state or territory of the USA.

3. Meet physical and professional qualifications.

4. Be at least 20 years of age but not over 35. Female applicants must be without dependents under 18 years of age.

5. Be a citizen of the USA.

6. Possess high moral qualifications.

The candidate who can qualify will receive an appointment in a grade ranging from second lieutenant to captain, depending on age, professional experience and educational attainment.

The correct application forms and necessary instructions may be obtained by contacting your local Air Force nurse advisor.

NAVY NURSE CORPS

The Navy Nurse Corps (NNC) is a staff corps of the Navy established by an Act of Congress, May 13, 1908, and organized within the Medical Department of the Navy.

The need for nurses in the Navy was realized and set down in writing long before 1908. In 1814, six years before the birth of Florence Nightingale, Dr. William Paul Barton, a young Navy surgeon, included in his recommendations to the Secretary of the Navy for conducting hospitals and institutions for the sick the following:

The nurses, whose number should be proportionate to the extent of the hospital and the number of patients, should be women of humane dispositions and tender manners; active and healthy.... They are to attend with fidelity and care upon all the sick committed to their charge; should promptly obey their calls and, if possible, anticipate their reasonable wants. They should administer all medicines and diets prescribed for the sick, in the manner and at the times specified in their directions. ... They should obey punctually all orders from superiors; and should exact a ready acquiescence in their commands, from the attendants under them.[3]

The Navy unfortunately was not yet ready for women in its ranks. It was not until 50 years later during the Civil War that nurses first appeared on the Navy horizon. In 1862 a confederate side-wheel river steamer, *The Red Rover,* was captured by the Union and converted into the first hospital ship to care for the sick and injured. Four Sisters of the Order of the Holy Cross were the first nurse volunteers to offer their services in caring for the injured Navy men. These and other Sisters of the Order continued to serve aboard this ship until November 17, 1865, the last day of service for *The Red Rover.*

Three decades later, the need again for nurses to care for war casualties of the Spanish American War brought women into the Navy institutions. At this time the nurses were hired on a contract basis and remained for 50 days.

Although nurses served in the Navy during times of great crisis, it was not until the turn of the century that efforts were successful in securing legislation to permit nurses to function as an integral part of the Navy. This was realized in 1908 when Esther Voorhees Hasson was appointed the first superintendent of nurses and 19 additional nurses accepted appointments in the Navy.

In 1908 the nurses entering Naval service did not hold any officer status. It was not until July 1942 when *Public Law 654* was enacted by the 77th Congress that they received relative rank in the grades of ensign to lieutenant commander. In February 1944, *Public Law 238* of the 78th Congress

---

[3] Information secured from the Navy Nurse Corps. It was taken from Dr. W. C. Barton's *A Treatise Containing a Plan for the Internal Government of Marine Hospitals in the United States Together with a Scheme for Amending and Systematizing the Medical Department of the Navy, 1814.*

authorized military commissioned rank for nurses for the duration of the war and 6 months; and the *Army-Navy Nurses Act of 1947, Public Law 36,* enacted by the 80th Congress, established the Nurse Corps as a permanent staff corps of the Navy.

In November 1967, *Public Law 90-130* of the 90th Congress materially augmented promotional opportunities for Navy nurses, to the grades of Captain and Commander, by equating promotional percentages with those of male line officers.

Functions and Activities of the Nurse Corps Officer

The primary function of nurses in the Navy is to maintain health and provide nursing care to men and women of the Navy and Marine Corps and, when facilities are available, to their dependents. In times of peace, nurses are generally assigned to hospitals and dispensaries both within and outside of the USA. A limited number are assigned to transport ships used to transfer men and their dependents to and from foreign duty stations. In time of war or emergency, nurses are sent wherever their services are considered necessary.

With the USA's entry into World War I in 1917, nurses were for the first time deployed to England, Scotland, Ireland and France to assist in

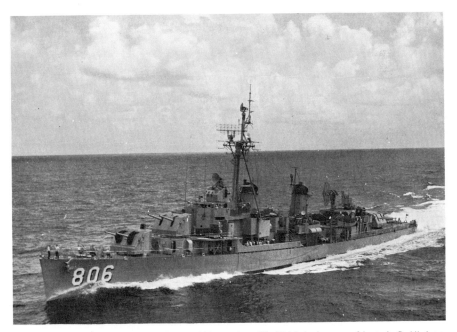

Fig. 11-7. U.S.S. *Higbee*, christened November 19, 1944, in honor of Lenah S. Higbee, NC, USN. (Official U.S. Navy Photo)

caring for the battle casualties. The number of nurses serving at this time totaled 1,835. Four of these nurses were decorated with the Navy Cross for valorous performance of duty; 3 were awarded posthumously. The 4th recipient, Lenah S. Higbee, NC, USN, received further recognition when the Destroyer, U.S.S. *Higbee,* christened November 19, 1944, was named in her honor (Figure 11-7).

On the fateful day of December 7, 1941, when Pearl Harbor was bombed by the Japanese, nurses were on duty at the Naval Hospital, Pearl Harbor and aboard the U.S.S. *Solace,* a hospital ship anchored in the harbor. Nurses were also located on the Philippine Islands and on Guam. Those at Pearl Harbor were able to give care to the casualties and were commended for gallant service during the attack. The nurses on Guam were taken prisoners when the Japanese captured the island and were held until August 1942. They all received the Bronze Star Medal (Army) and Silver Star Medal (Navy) for gallant service during attack and during the period when they were in the hands of the enemy. In 1942, 11 nurses were captured by the Japanese at Manila and interned at Santo Tomas; they were later moved to Los Banos, P.I. They survived 37 months as prisoners of war and were liberated in 1945.

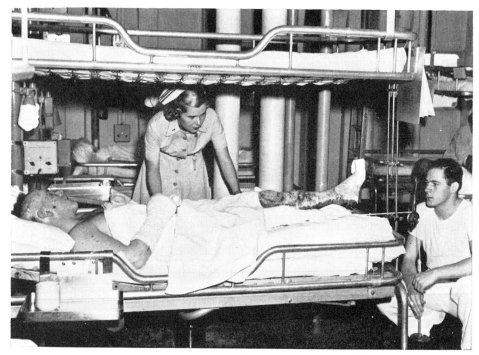

Fig. 11-8. A Navy nurse changes a patient's position while a corpsman adjusts weights on the right stump. The photograph was taken aboard the U.S.S. *Constitution.* (U.S. Navy photo)

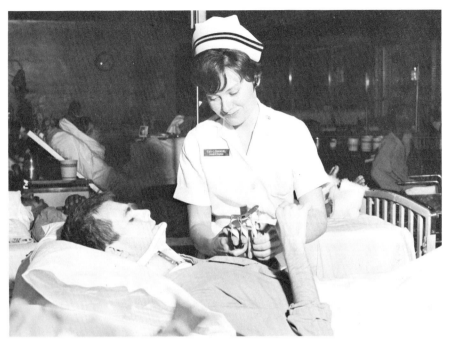

Fig. 11-9. Navy nurse giving care to a patient in the U.S. Naval Hospital at Portsmouth, Virginia. (U.S. Navy Photo)

From early 1942 until the end of World War II, Navy nurses were on duty at 21 foreign stations, on 12 hospital ships, at 40 naval hospitals and in 175 dispensaries in the USA. Nurses also were assigned to flight nursing, and in 1945 they landed on Guam, Iwo Jima and Okinawa to evacuate casualties by air. The number of nurses on active duty during the war reached approximately 11,000.

The number of decorations and awards presented to Navy nurses during World War II is representative of the outstanding performance of members of the Nurse Corps. Sue Dauser, the Superintendent of the Nurse Corps during World War II was awarded the Distinguished Service Medal, and Ann Bernatitis, who served with a surgical unit on Bataan, was awarded the Legion of Merit. Over 250 other nurses received commendations for their service.

After the cessation of hostilities in 1945 and subsequent to demobilization, the strength of the Corps was reduced to approximately 2,100. This strength has been maintained with the exception of the period between 1950 and 1953, when the numbers were increased to approximately 3,200 to care for casualties of the Korean conflict. Nurses were once again deployed to foreign shores and aboard hospital ships to treat and transfer the sick and wounded.

Navy nurses have also served in Vietnam. In 1965, 4 nurses attached to the Station Hospital, U. S. Navy Headquarters Support Activity, Saigon, Vietnam, were awarded the Purple Heart for injuries received during the Vietcong terrorist bombing of the Brink Bachelor officers' quarters. These nurses were the first women members of the U. S. Armed Forces to receive the Purple Heart Award for injuries in the Vietnam conflict.

The duties of the nurses in the Navy are not always confined to caring for military patients. Because of the geographic location of many Navy facilities, nurses are called on to assist neighboring communities with public health and emergency problems. In 1917 a nurse was assigned as welfare nurse in St. Croix, and another was assigned as supervisor at the Insane and Leper Asylum in the Virgin Islands. On Guam, nurses served as visiting nurses to various districts to follow up tuberculosis patients who had been discharged from the hospital. In 1956, nurses were assigned to the sea life to aid in bringing Hungarian refugees to the USA; and in 1961, they boarded the aircraft carriers U.S.S. *Shangra La* and U.S.S. *Antietam* to render assistance to hurricane disaster victims in Texas.

The NNC numbers have always been small in relation to the number of patients to be nursed. For this reason, and because nurses are not generally assigned aboard fighting ships, one of the important duties of nurses is to teach the hospital corpsmen to give nursing care. This is accomplished on the ward situation as well as in the Hospital Corps Schools.

When nurses first became a part of the Navy, the formal teaching of nursing to hospital corpsmen was meager. In 1915 a nurse was requested to lecture on nursing subjects for 1 hour a week at the U. S. Naval Hospital Corps School at Narragansett, Rhode Island. In 1917 this program was expanded, and nurses were assigned to full time teaching duties at the Hospital Corps schools. From that time, nurses have constantly been associated with the Hospital Corps Schools.

The NNC has been influential in advancing the practice of nursing in many of the isolated areas of the world through the teaching of nursing to the nationals. In 1911, Navy nurses developed a school of nursing for young women in Guam, the Mariana Islands. This school was operated until the attack on the island by the Japanese in 1941; it was reestablished in 1945 and operated by the Navy until 1950, when the Department of the Interior assumed responsibility for the government of the island.

Schools of nursing also were established by Navy nurses for women on Samoa in 1914, on St. Thomas and St. Croix, Virgin Islands in 1917, and on Guam in 1946. In 1945 nurses stationed on Saipan assisted in training native nurse attendants.

Admission to the Corps

Three avenues are available whereby one may gain admission into the NNC:

1. A graduate of an approved school of nursing may make application through the local office of the U. S. Navy Recruiting Station. If qualified, the request is forwarded to the Secretary of the Navy for approval. The applicant then is given a commission in the U. S. Naval Reserve.

2. Full-time students who are matriculated in a baccalaureate nursing program – approved by the NLN – may participate in the NNC Candidate Program when they are within 2 years of completion of degree requirements. Participation in the program may be for 1 or 2 years.

Applicants who are accepted into the program receive full tuition as well as pay and allowances of a hospitalman until they are within 6 months of completion of their degree requirements. During the last 6 months they receive a commission in the grade of ensign with full pay and allowances of their rank in addition to tuition. On graduation, candidates are obliged to serve on active duty for a period of time proportionate to the length of time spent in the candidate program. Application for this program also is made through the local office of the U. S. Navy Recruiting Station. (Registered nurses, if eligible, may apply for this program.)

3. Enlisted personnel on active duty in the Hospital Corps of the Department of the Navy may make application for the Navy Enlisted Nursing Education Program. If they meet the established criteria for the program, orders to a civilian university for full-time duty under instruction leading to a Bachelor of Science Degree in Nursing are authorized. At the completion of the program, the individual receives a commission in the Nurse Corps and orders to active duty. The Nurse Corps Officer then serves on active duty for a minimum of 4 years following completion of the academic program.

Requirements for Appointment in the Nurse Corps

An applicant must:

1. Be a graduate from a school of nursing approved by the appropriate State Board of Nursing or the NLN, and be currently registered in 1 state or the District of Columbia.

2. Be between the ages of 20 and 34.

3. Be either single, or married, but have no dependents under the age of 18, regardless of legal custody. There are no dependency restrictions for male applicants.

4. Submit professional credentials and employment records in order to establish mental, moral and professional qualifications and aptitude for military service.

5. Be physically qualified by standards set for appointment in the Nurse Corps, U.S. Naval Reserve.

A Career in the Navy

Initial appointment in the Navy is made in the grade of ensign, lieutenant (junior grade) or lieutenant, depending on the age and the professional qualifications of the applicant. All members of the Nurse Corps are commissioned officers.

On accepting a commission in the Navy, the Officer receives temporary duty orders to the U.S. Naval School, Officer (Women), Naval Schools Command, Newport, R. I., to receive officer indoctrination.

The objective of the 4-week indoctrination course is to aid the newly appointed officer to adjust to military life and to practice nursing within the naval establishment. Systematic instruction in naval subjects is provided to familiarize the officer with her position and responsibilities in the Navy and with the operation of the Navy Medical Department.

After completion of the indoctrination program, nurses are assigned to medical activities in accordance with their qualifications and with the needs of both the nurse and the service. Preference as to duty station is given consideration whenever possible.

The nurse who chooses to make the Navy a career can anticipate assignments in hospitals and dispensaries in a variety of geographic areas both within and outside the USA and aboard transport or hospital ships. A Navy nurse may also be assigned to a civilian academic program for full-time duty under instruction on both the undergraduate and graduate level. Unusual but interesting assignments available to the career Nurse Corps officer include recruiting duty, nursing research assignments, and assignment to radioisotope departments.

Advancement Opportunities and Economic Security

After a Nurse Corps Reserve officer has completed 18 months of active duty she is eligible to submit a request for transfer to the regular component of the Navy. If found qualified by the Board set up to review applicants, she then resigns her Reserve commission and accepts a commission in the regular Navy.

The present promotion system permits Nurse Corps officers to progress from the rank of ensign through captain after spending the required time in each rank and being selected for promotion on the basis of professional and personal qualifications.

Continuous education and training is provided for all Nurse Corps officers on active duty. This education is available through inservice and outservice programs.

Nurses in the regular Navy are given the opportunity to pursue further education both at the undergraduate and graduate level. Selection of nurses for participation in these programs is based on the officer's academic and professional record. Nurses who avail themselves of this educational opportunity are expected to remain in the Naval service for a period which varies in proportion to the duration of the schooling afforded them.

Nurses of the reserve and regular Navy are eligible to pursue a 2-year course in anesthesia, which is set up on a cooperating basis with a civilian university and selected large Naval hospitals. On completion of this course, students are eligible to take the national examination for certification as a registered anesthetist.

All nurses on active duty are encouraged to attend short courses, workshops, seminars and institutes conducted at civilian and military facilities and by professional nursing and allied associations.

The base salary for Naval officers is established by law. In addition, regular pay increases are granted, based on length of service. As of July 1968, salaries ranged from a minimum monthly rate of $343.20 for ensigns to a maximum monthly rate of $1,373.10 for captains. Subsistence and rental allowances are also given (see footnote 2 on page 259). Leave with pay is earned at the rate of 30 days for each year of active duty and may be accumulated up to 60 days.

A Nurse Corps officer may be eligible for retirement benefits under the following circumstances:

1. Voluntary retirement — after completing 20 years of active duty
2. Physical disability retirement — on acquiring a disability that is incurred in accordance with the conditions established for physical disability retirement
3. Statutory retirement — after completing 30 to 31 years of active duty for captain, 26 years for commander and 20 years for lieutenant commander, or on reaching age 62, whichever is earlier.

Social Security benefits are available to all officers of the Navy in addition to Navy retirement benefits.

U.S. Naval Reserve

After a Nurse Corps reserve officer has spent a specified amount of time on active duty, she may request extension of active duty and remain as a Nurse Corps reserve officer; she may request transfer to the regular Navy, or she may request release from active duty and return to civilian life. When released from active duty the officer remains a member of the Naval Reserve on inactive duty unless and until she resigns her reserve commission. Officers of the Inactive Reserve are available for recall to active duty in case of a national emergency and are eligible to request active duty at any time.

While in the Inactive Reserve component, members may participate actively in Reserve units in their areas, for which retirement points may be earned.

Nurses also may apply for a commission in the Inactive Naval Reserve without prior active duty. These officers may at a later time request active duty or they may remain permanently in an Inactive Reserve component.

NURSING IN THE PUBLIC HEALTH SERVICE, U. S. DEPARTMENT OF HEALTH, EDUCATION, AND WELFARE

An act of Congress signed by President John Adams on July 16, 1798, established a marine hospital service "for the relief of sick and disabled seamen," and created the first activity of what is now the Public Health Service (PHS). Establishment of the Marine Hospital Service was the first civilian health program of the young Federal Government. Today, the PHS, under the direction of the Surgeon General, is the Federal agency specifically charged with responsibility for protecting and improving the nation's health.

Some Highlights of PHS History[4]

The first marine hospital was established in 1802 in a repaired barrack on Castle Island in Boston Harbor and was authorized to "provide a steward, nurse, beds, bedding, and utensils." These early hospital facilities were moved to Charlestown, Massachusetts, in January 1804. There, with Dr. Benjamin Waterhouse of Harvard as the physician in charge, the Marine Hospital not only served sick seamen, but also became the center at which Harvard medical students learned to practice—the first teaching hospital in the USA.

During the next 50 years, marine hospitals were opened in key coastal and inland ports throughout the USA. Administration of these hospitals was centralized in 1870 under the Treasury Department.

In the last half of the 19th century, the Marine Hospital Service assumed 2 additional functions for which the PHS is still responsible. In 1887, a hygienic laboratory was established at the Staten Island hospital in New York as the principal research station of the Service. Later transferred to headquarters in Washington, D.C., the laboratory was the forerunner of the National Institutes of Health, today the principal biomedical research arm of the Federal Government.

For many years, physicians in the marine hospitals had helped communities to curb epidemics of diseases such as yellow fever, acting under the authority of a number of short-term laws. In 1893, the Congress gave the Service full responsibility for interstate and foreign quarantine, and provision was made for cooperation with state health agencies in this effort.

Reflecting the broadening responsibility, the name of the Marine Hospital Service was changed, in 1902, to the Public Health and Marine Hospital Service and, in 1912, to its current name of U.S. Public Health Service. Today (1970) the PHS is a component of the U.S. Department of Health, Education and Welfare.

---

[4] See also the previous (seventh) edition of E. K. Spalding and L. E. Notter, *Professional Nursing: Foundations, Perspectives and Relationships,* Philadelphia, Lippincott, 1965, pp. 192-198, for additional material on the history of the PHS.

Federal legislation, designed to assure all citizens access to quality health care, has shaped the modern history of the PHS, making it the principal Federal health agency.

The *Social Security Act of 1935* formally established a Federal-state partnership in health. Title VI of the act authorized Federal grants to the states to aid the development of public health services. The partnership created a network of basic public health programs throughout the nation. In the years that followed, other cooperative programs were launched against specific public health problems, including venereal disease and tuberculosis. The *Comprehensive Health Planning and Public Health Services Act of 1966* gave new direction to the partnership. Among the major provisions of this act is support for comprehensive health planning on a state and areawide basis.

The *National Cancer Act of 1937* created the National Cancer Institute, the first in the 8 categories of institutes which make up the National Institutes of Health. The act also set the pattern for Federal assistance to biomedical research. It authorized the National Cancer Institute to conduct research in its own laboratories and to award grants for research to nongovernmental institutions and to individuals. Financial support for the training of research scientists was also provided. Later legislation authorized Federal assistance for the construction of research facilities.

After World War II, significant legislation was also directed toward national shortages of health facilities, services and personnel. The *National Hospital Survey and Construction Program Act of 1946* authorized the awarding of Federal funds to the states to aid the construction of hospitals and health centers. Other kinds of health facilities, including nursing homes, were later covered under the program.

The *Health Professions Educational Assistance Act of 1963*, the *Nurse Training Act of 1964*, and the *Health Manpower Act of 1968* stand as landmarks in the development of health manpower resources. Under these acts, as amended, Federal funds are available to health professions schools for educational support and to aid them in building teaching facilities. Loans and scholarships for students are provided through Federal funds administered by the schools.

The health hazards of the modern environment — radiation, air pollution — have also been the object of a major health effort. The *Clean Air Act of 1963* is notable among the Federal laws which have stimulated action to reduce the impact of known environmental health hazards and to identify potential hazards.

Organization of the PHS

The PHS is made up of 3 operating agencies: the Health Services and Mental Health Administration; the National Institutes of Health; and the Consumer Protection and Environmental Health Service.

Programs of the Health Services and Mental Health Administration (HSMHA) promote the development of personal and mental health services throughout the nation. These programs include assistance to the states for the planning and development of comprehensive health services, and for the construction of hospitals, community mental health centers and other types of health facilities. Technical assistance is given to public and private health agencies in the control of chronic and communicable diseases. Research within the organization is conducted and administration of health services is supported. HSMHA is also responsible for the direct health care programs of the PHS. Merchant seamen still constitute one of the largest beneficiary groups. Since 1955, the PHS has also provided health care to nearly 400,000 American Indians and Alaskan natives.

The National Institutes of Health (NIH) conducts biomedical research and administers Federal support for research in nongovernmental institutions and for research training. The work of 6 of the 8 institutes is targeted against the major causes of death and disability in the USA—cancer, heart disease, allergy and infectious diseases, arthritis and metabolic diseases, dental diseases, and neurological diseases and blindness. Two other institutes are concerned with the broad areas of child health and human development and general medical sciences. The Bureau of Health Manpower, which administers Federal programs assisting health manpower development, is a part of the National Institutes of Health. So is the National Library of Medicine.

The Environmental Health and Consumer Protection Service conducts a wide range of programs, from the testing of drugs to the control of air pollution. Its mission is to protect the people in the USA from health hazards in the environment and in products and services used in daily life.

Each of these agencies uses a variety of mechanisms to accomplish its mission—training activities, statistical studies, research, demonstration of new methods and technology, and many others. Nurses employed by these agencies may act as consultants to hospitals, state and local health agencies, universities and other appropriate organizations; conduct or assist in research studies; prepare information materials; or administer research and training grants. Many assignments are in PHS headquarters in and around Washington, D.C. Nurses are also members of the PHS staff in the 9 regional offices of the U. S. Department of Health, Education, and Welfare and in a host of hospitals, clinics and field stations. Whatever the assignment, wherever the stations, PHS nurses, serving on interdisciplinary health teams, are building upon a proud tradition.

Highlights of PHS Nursing History

Hospital Nursing. Professional nurses—men as well as women—were first employed in the marine hospitals in the 1890's. They were assigned to the hospital for the care of immigrants arriving at Ellis Island in New York harbor. Professionally trained women nurses began to be employed generally in marine hospitals in about 1912.

The first superintendent of nurses was Lucy Minnigerode, who was appointed to the position in 1919. She also organized a nursing service for all the marine hospitals at that time.

Public Health Nursing. Even before World War I, a few nurses had been employed for special projects which today would be considered public health work. Notable among them were the pellagra and trachoma control programs, begun in the Kentucky mountains in 1914. During the next 14 years, public health nurses assigned to these programs covered 18,000 square miles of mountainous terrain in 27 counties, traveling on horseback, muleback or on foot to visit homes, examine families and teach personal hygiene and the fundamentals of good health.

Consultant Services. In 1934, a public health nursing section was added to the consultant service which the PHS provided to state health departments. Following the enactment of the *Social Security Act of 1935* and the authorization of grants to the states for public health programs, the nursing consultation service was greatly expanded. Among its more important accomplishments are the improvement of general qualifications for nurses in public health; the promotion, through state nursing directors in public health, of programs of inservice training; and the improvement of educational programs for the preparation of public health nurses.

In World War II, nursing consultants helped to develop civilian defense plans. By early 1945, nurses in public health, recruited by PHS, were serving state and local health departments in war impact areas in 39 states and Puerto Rico. PHS nurses served with the armed forces and, in the years after the war, with international relief agencies.

The administration of the U. S. Cadet Nurse Corps program during World War II, created by the acute need for nurses in civilian and military service, was a major wartime activity. Authorized by the *Bolton Act of 1943*, the Cadet Nurse Corps recruited 180,000 students for preservice programs and provided instruction to 17,000 graduate nurses.

Indian Health. Although nurses had worked with Indians as early as 1890, their services were performed largely in hospitals operated under the auspices of various mission groups. It was not until 1924 that Elinor D. Gregg was appointed to the position of supervisor of field nurses and field matrons in the Bureau of Indian Affairs (BIA), under the U. S. Department of Interior. In 1926, all BIA nurses—hospital and public health—were placed under the direction of Miss Gregg.

The nursing service for the Indians was transferred to the PHS in 1955. By June 1968, the Indian health program staff included approximately 1,050 professional nurses and 1,050 auxiliary nursing personnel, employed in all types of nursing positions—public health, clinic, school and hospital.

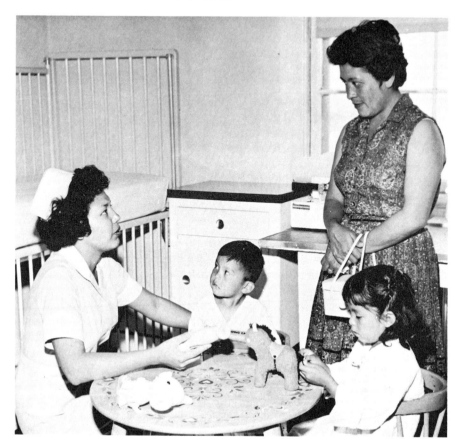

Fig. 11-10. The teaching of Indian families is one function of the public health nurse. (Public Health Service, U.S. Department of Health, Education, and Welfare)

Figures 11-10 and 11-11 show some teaching activities in the Indian health service.

Chief Nurse Officer. The Commissioned Corps of the PHS, established in 1889, is 1 of the 2 personnel systems through which members of the health professions enter the PHS. In 1949, the membership of the Commissioned Corps was expanded to include nurses and the position of Chief Nurse Officer, with the rank of Assistant Surgeon General, was established. Lucile Petry Leone was the first to hold this position. She was succeeded in 1966 by Margaret McLaughlin.

CURRENT NURSING PROGRAMS AND OPPORTUNITIES FOR SERVICE IN THE PHS

Most of the 2,500-member nursing staff of the PHS is assigned to the HSMHA and the NIH. Their work falls into 4 broad categories: hospital

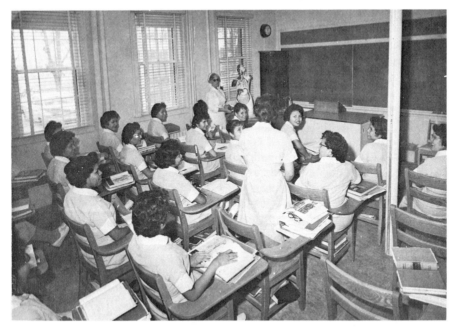

Fig. 11-11. The teaching of practical nurses is a major function in the Indian health program. (Public Health Service, U.S. Department of Health, Education, and Welfare)

nursing, public health nursing, consultation and research. Frequently, the categories are not strict. A nurse in a chronic-disease-control program, for example, may participate in a study of some new preventive technique and then go on to work with state and community health agencies in applying the knowledge gained in the study. Nor does the administration with which the nurse is employed limit the choice of function. One nurse at the Clinical Center, the research hospital of the NIH, may be engaged in patient care, while another is part of a laboratory research team investigating some aspect of cancer.

For some positions in the PHS, the completion of preservice education is the basic qualification. Other positions may require graduate education in public health nursing, education, hospital nursing service, or a clinical specialty. Whatever preparation the nurse brings to the PHS, there is always opportunity, through the career development program, for further professional development in line with her interests and capabilities.

Hospital Nursing in the PHS

General and specialized nursing skills are required in the installations maintained by the PHS in locations ranging from isolated Indian reservations to the nation's largest cities. A system of general hospitals and out-patient clinics, located in ports from Boston to San Francisco, serves merchant seamen and other legally designated medical beneficiaries of the

PHS. These include members of the U.S. Coast Guard and the Environmental Science Services Administration, and members of the armed forces and their dependents to whom military hospitals are not available. In addition to the general hospitals and cinics, a hospital at Carville, Louisiana, is devoted to the care of persons with leprosy, and to training and research in this disease.

All PHS hospitals are well equipped; some are new. The hospital nurse works a 40-hour, 5-day week. Whenever possible, qualified nurses are permitted to enroll for graduate education in specialized fields, in accordance with the needs of the nurse and of the Service. Orientation and inservice education programs also are provided. Participation in professional and community activities is encouraged. Great emphasis is placed on career development.

The PHS hospitals are affiliated with colleges and universities which have medical, dental and nursing schools. They offer internships and residencies in various medical specialities and in other health disciplines. Several are cooperating with the Office of Economic Opportunity in providing training programs for the poor. Research in clinical medicine is a third major activity of these hospitals.

The hospitals and clinics offer a wide variety of experience in clinical nursing, nursing service administration and education. Assignments for practice and education are planned in the interest of developing nurses for careers in the PHS.

Another group of hospitals, clinics and health centers serves American Indians and Alaskan natives — Indians, Eskimos and Aleuts. The 51 hospitals (in 1970) range in size from 12 to 400 beds and stretch from the reservations of the Navajos and Hopis in the West to Kotzebue, above the Arctic Circle, where a new 54-bed hospital was opened in 1964 with modern apartments for personnel. Many of these hospitals are in areas rich in scenic beauty and close to national parks and other points of interest.

In addition, there are 8 area offices. Two nurse consultants, one in hospital nursing and one in public health, are usually assigned to each area office.

In the Indian health program, nurses have a real opportunity to mesh preventive and curative nursing into total patient and family service. Often they participate in special study and action programs, such as mass immunization for measles, accident prevention, and trachoma control. Of unusual appeal to many people is the opportunity the programs offer to learn about and work with people of different cultures.

Specialized Facilities

The Clinical Center, located in Bethesda, Maryland (a suburb of Washington, D.C.), is the research hospital of the NIH. The hospital has over 500 beds on 23 nursing units, surrounded by 1,100 research laboratories.

Every patient is part of a research project. The fields of research may range from allergies to vascular diseases, and the work scope of a project from diagnostic procedures to chemotherapy or corrective surgery. Nurses are important members of the NIH research teams but at no time do they forsake their primary duty of caring for patients. There are opportunities to utilize all types of nursing skills and nursing knowledge, and to assist in the designing of new equipment and the development of advanced procedures in nursing care.

Three other specialized facilities are a part of the National Institutes of Mental Health (NIMH): St. Elizabeth's Hospital, located in Washington, D.C., an institution for treatment of and research in mental illness; and the NIMH Clinical Research Centers at Lexington, Kentucky, and Ft. Worth, Texas, where drug addicts are treated.

Nurses at St. Elizabeth's Hospital participate in a wide variety of programs for the care of patients. Opportunities to develop psychiatric nursing skills are provided through inservice and continuing education programs. Clinical specialists in psychiatric nursing conduct and direct research investigations and analyze problems, utilizing the findings as a basis for improvement of psychiatric nursing care.

Public Health Nursing and Consultation

In other assignments, nurses in the PHS assist in the development of general and specialized public health programs, in field training, in demonstrations and in special studies. They may provide direct service, but more frequently they assist organizations in the development of nursing service. This assistance is usually directed toward a specific goal. For example, nurses at the National Communicable Disease Center, which spearheads the PHS attack on infectious diseases, participate in program planning, training and consultation. As training specialists they help educational institutions and state and community health agencies to improve their inservice training programs and provide continuing education in epidemiology and communicable disease control. Nurses assigned to the areas of tuberculosis and venereal disease help service agencies to strengthen nursing care — emphasizing prevention, casefinding and control of these diseases.

Nurse consultants in another unit of the PHS contribute to the development of standards for the hospitals, home health agencies, and other facilities which participate in the Health Insurance Program for the Aged (Medicare). They continue to work with those responsible for these facilities and with the states to assure the availability and quality of nursing service under this program.

In the Consumer Protection and Environmental Health Service, nurses provide consultation for the development of such services as industrial health programs.

Headquarters offices in Washington are often the duty station for public health assignments. But these assignments may also take the nurses to foreign countries. (For international activities, see p. 536.)

Research

Biomedical research is concentrated in the NIH. In addition, many programs of the PHS offer opportunities to nurses for applied research. Nurses conduct or participate in community and epidemiological studies. They are often a part of the multidisciplinary teams conducting special studies in such areas as nutrition, glaucoma and cytological testing for cervical cancer. The PHS affords many opportunities for its nurses to learn research methodology.

The Division of Nursing

The Division of Nursing is the unit of the PHS which studies nurses, nursing education and nursing services, per se. It is responsible for maintaining a continuous review of national needs for nursing services, in and out of hospitals, including areas of special practice; for examining needs of nursing education as related to these services; and for the development and administration of programs to assure that these needs are met. The Division is the central source of information, including publications, and offers direct assistance with manpower needs and resources; with the recruitment, education, training and utilization of nursing personnel; with the organization and delivery of nursing services; and with nursing research and the application of research findings.

The Division's staff provides consultation and technical assistance to institutions and agencies on all matters related to the administration of nursing services and the ways in which these services are made available to patients. Sometimes this kind of help can be given by staff members with rich backgrounds of experience in hospital, other institutional or public health nursing; sometimes it is necessary to develop study methods in order to help organizations examine and measure the effectiveness of the service they provide. One example is the study of nursing personnel activities in order to identify inappropriate use of personnel and to show ways of extending the skills of the professional nurse.

The Division of Nursing also administers the *Nurse Training Act of 1964* (also discussed in Chapter 27), the aim of which is to increase the number of well-prepared nurses in the nation.[5] The act authorizes Federal funds not only to help defray the education expenses of undergraduate students in need of financial assistance, but also for construction of nursing school facilities, for limited basic support of the facilities and for the improvement of curricula within schools of nursing. In administering the *Nurse Training*

[5] The *Nurse Training Act of 1964* was extended under the *Health Manpower Act of 1968*.

Act..., nurses within the Division provide consultation on education problems as well as advice on matters relating to the school's application for funds. The *Nurse Training Act...* also extended the Professional Nurse Traineeship Program and added both long-term and short-term traineeships for graduate nurses to prepare as clinical specialists. Formerly, the traineeships were limited to study in teaching and nursing administration.

Continuing education for nurses, both degree and nondegree, is a developing area in which the Division of Nursing is actively involved. Of major interest to the Division is the promotion of scientific research in nursing. Division nurses with advanced educational preparation are engaged in a variety of studies encompassing all aspects of nursing. A part of the research is carried on by the Nursing Research Field Center in San Francisco, with cooperating institutions. In addition, the staff administers grants for research by qualified faculty groups and individuals throughout the country. Along with research, the staff assumes responsibility for bringing together, evaluating and communicating new nursing knowledge to the country's practicing nurses who can then apply it to improve patient care.

In recent years emphasis in research has shifted from studies of nurses and nursing to studies concerned with the effects of nursing care on patients. Specific subject areas of study include the effect of nursing care on postoperative vomiting, nursing care and pain patterns following heart surgery, autonomic responses to nursing comfort measures, nutrition as an aspect of nursing care and intensive nursing care in acute myocardial infarction. This last study was considered so significant that the Division of Nursing, with the cooperation of the investigators, incorporated the findings into multimedia teaching tools to make the information available for all those needing it.

Nursing manpower throughout the USA is another vital concern of the Division of Nursing. The staff not only is involved with the recruitment of new, inactive and part-time nurses, but also provides consultation to help hospitals and other health agencies affect the best possible utilization of the nurse supply they already have. The Division of Nursing consultants work with states and regions, assisting them with their studies of their various nursing needs and resources. These studies not only show numbers, locations and characteristics of nurses, but also contain useful analyses of the collected information which serve as a basis for sound state and regional planning.

Providing consultation to agencies or to educational institutions requires skill in working with groups and individuals, as well as expertness in the area—clinical or other functional area such as teaching, or educational or nursing service administration—in which the consultation is being given. Some of the Division's staff come prepared with these competencies; for others, with potential for professional development, the Division provides opportunities for career development to prepare for positions of greater responsibility.

How Appointments are Made

The qualified nurse may enter the PHS by appointment to the Commissioned Corps as a regular or reserve officer, or through the Federal Civil Service. Graduates of approved schools of nursing—diploma, baccalaureate and associate—are eligible for Civil Service appointments. Civil Service nurses hold positions classified at GS4 through GS7 for staff nurse, and from GS9 through GS14 for other positions. The nurse who wishes a Civil Service appointment may apply for a position at any facility she prefers and, if appointed, will be assigned to that station. There are often opportunities for transfer from one station to another.

Service in the Commissioned Corps is in some ways similar to Army and Navy service; in time of war or national emergency, the Commissioned Corps constitutes a part of the military forces of the USA. Salaries and ranks are identical to those of officers in the armed forces. The baccalaureate degree is required for appointment to the Commissioned Corps. Because of this requirement, appointments are not made to the lowest grades. Also, nurses with qualifying experience are appointed to the Corps at the highest grade for which they are eligible, which can include the higher grades. Salaries, including base pay and rental and subsistence allowances, are paid in cash with extra allowances for dependents. Increases in salaries are automatic with specified years of PHS experience. Salaries range from the beginning salary in the assistant grade (comparable Navy rank—lieutenant, junior grade) to the top salary of the assistant surgeon general.

A career development program emphasizes development of individual talents and interests of nurses with either Commissioned or Civil Service appointments. A planned program of progressive experience and education, including opportunity to undertake graduate study, is arranged for nurses whose capacity and interest indicate a development potential for the large number of key positions (administrative, consultative, research, international and other) required for achievement of the diversified missions of the PHS.

NURSING SERVICE OF THE VETERANS ADMINISTRATION

Origin of the Veterans Administration Nursing Service

The U. S. Veterans' Bureau was established on August 9, 1921, by an Act of Congress. On April 29, 1922, the President of the USA transferred from the PHS to the Veterans' Bureau 57 hospitals that had been operated for the care of disabled veterans. On May 1, 1922, when this transfer was effected, the 1,442 nurses who were transferred from the PHS constituted the original Veterans Administration Nursing Service. One of these nurses, Mary A. Hickey, became the first superintendent of nurses—a position she held until her retirement in December, 1942.

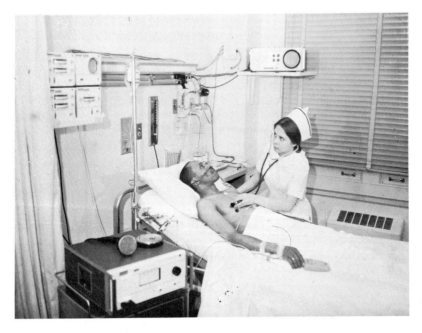

Fig. 11-12. (Top) A Veterans Administration Coronary Care nurse specialist gives expert nursing care. (Bottom) A Veterans Administration rehabilitation nurse encourages the nursing home resident to complete his personal care. (Veterans Administration)

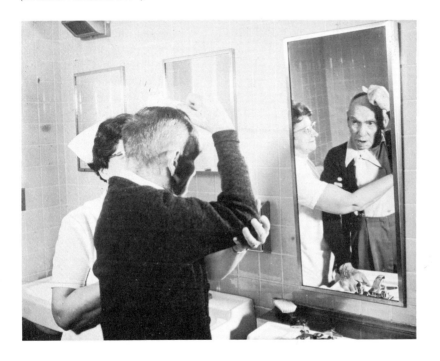

On July 3, 1930, *Public Law No. 536* was enacted (71st Congress), which authorized the President, by executive order, to consolidate and coordinate governmental activities affecting war veterans into an establishment to be known as the Veterans Administration (VA). The governmental agencies directly affected by this legislation were the U. S. Veterans' Bureau and the National Home for Disabled Volunteer Soldiers, both independent establishments, and the Bureau of Pensions in the Interior Department. On July 21, 1930, the President issued an executive order authorizing the consolidation of these agencies, and within a few days thereafter the Director of the Veterans' Bureau was appointed and confirmed as the Administrator of Veterans' Affairs.

On January 3, 1946, a basic change was made by *Public Law 293* (now *Public Law 85-857*), which took physicians, dentists and nurses out of Civil Service and placed them in a newly constituted Department of Medicine and Surgery headed by a chief medical director. The law provides for a director of nursing service who shall be a qualified registered nurse appointed by the administrator. The director of nursing service is responsible to the chief medical director through the assistant chief medical director for professional services. Dorothy V. Wheeler, the first director of nursing service, served from 1946-1954. She was succeeded by Cecilia H. Hauge who retired in 1966. Upon Miss Hauge's retirement, Mary J. McCarthy became director of nursing service.

How Extensive is the VA Nursing Service?

To meet the medical-care needs of eligible veterans, the Department of Medicine and Surgery operates a system of hospitals throughout the USA and Puerto Rico. Hospitals are of 3 types—general, neuropsychiatric and rehabilitation. There is a wide variety of clinical facilities, medical-care programs and research activities in VA hospitals. Nursing participates in multidisciplinary planning for patient care. Established clinics in hospitals and regional offices provide outpatient medical service to eligible veterans. In Hawaii and Alaska this service is given through regional office clinics. Public health nurses assigned to clinics participate in coordinating care between the clinic, the home and the hospital. They make a major contribution to the continued rehabilitation of the patient at home by participating in arrangements with community agencies for home nursing care and by teaching patients and families. Figures 11-12 and 11-13 show the nurse giving expert nursing care, helping patients with self-care, and conducting a group therapy session.

Requirements for Appointment to the Nursing Service

The basic requirements for appointment to the VA Nursing Service are:
  1. USA citizenship

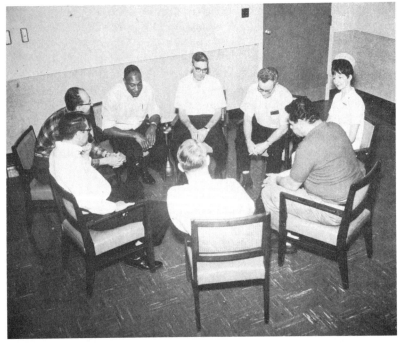

Fig. 11-13. A Veterans Administration Psychiatric–Mental Health nurse conducts a group therapy session. (Veterans Administration)

2. Graduation from an approved school of professional nursing

3. Current active registration as a graduate professional nurse

4. Meeting of the physical standards of the Department of Medicine and Surgery

5. A successful professional record

Some of these standards may be waived. Further information about appointment and waiver can be obtained at the time of application. A Civil Service examination is not required. New graduates may receive an appointment to a temporary position pending receipt of state registration on evidence that state board examination has been applied for or completed.

How Appointments to the Service Are Made

Nurses are appointed to the Department of Medicine and Surgery by a Professional Standards Board composed of nurses. This board determines the applicant's eligibility for appointment in terms of the basic appointment requirements. Selection for employment is made from eligible applicants by the director and chief of nursing service of the local field station. On employment, a nurse is assigned to responsibilities in keeping with patient-care needs and her interests, skills and preparation. Position titles used in the VA are similar to those used in any hospital or clinic nursing service. In the central office in Washington, D.C., are a director, an assistant director and 3 divisions with nurse specialists.

Assignments of nurses as chiefs of service and associate chiefs, one for education and one for research, are made by the Director, Nursing Service, Washington, D.C., in cooperation with the director of the local field station. Also, nurses prepared for and interested in research careers are assigned as Chiefs, Research in Clinical Nursing.

Newly graduated nurses may be given temporary appointments pending state registration if the state board examination has been applied for or completed.

Salary Range in the VA Nursing Service

Appointment grade and salary are based on the Nurse Qualification Standards established by the VA.

Major benefits include: 30 days vacation (120 days maximum accrual), 15 days sick leave (accumulates indefinitely), 8 holidays each year, cash allowance for uniforms, free uniform laundry, and retirement plans at low cost. Part-time employment up to 25 hours per week is available at many VA Hospitals. Cost of transfers, when made in the interest of the service, is defrayed by the Government and includes expense of transportation of the immediate family and, within some limitations, shipment of household goods and personal effects. As of July 1968, the salaries ranged from a minimum of $6,321 for the junior grade to a maximum of $22,031 for the assistant director. In some localities, salaries for all grades are higher than the established minimum (see footnote 2 of this chapter, p. 259).

Staff Development Program and Opportunities for Advancement

As a career VA nurse, you will find ample opportunity for advancement. You can advance through training by participation in continuous inservice educational programs, attendance at workshops and institutes or meetings and conventions of the professional organizations, and the opportunity to pursue university education.

You may also advance within the field of your choice. The VA progressive nursing care is firmly anchored in an educational program that permits you to achieve your goals in either clinical or administrative areas. Well-planned inservice education programs provide opportunity for increasing your professional knowledge and earning ability through:

    1. Individualized orientation.

    2. Continuing education and training in clinical specialties and assignments.

3. Head nurse and supervisory courses.

4. Contribution to the education of health workers.

5. Attendance at regional, national, international workshops and conferences.

6. Leave to complete advanced degrees.

7. Preceptorship training for chief nurse and associate chief of nursing service for education position.

Staff development programs are designed to help you to prepare for more responsible positions before actual assignment. Inservice education programs are considered a pivot for hospital work in VA nursing service. Such programs may be arbitrarily divided into 2 types, the 2nd being an evolvement from and a continuation of the first: (1) those that introduce the nurse to the position and the organization where the work is to be done, and (2) those that are intended to provide increasing competence in nursing skills and to broaden professional understandings, thus creating job satisfaction.

Development of the professional nurse through participation with nursing groups in the community is encouraged. Approach to planning for patient care, rehabilitation, discharge and follow-up is multidisciplinary in nature, with the professional and allied nursing personnel looked on as valuable, contributing team members. Preparation for contribution to the health team's effort has taken place through planned multidisciplinary conferences on a regional basis, and through the aforementioned inservice programming, individualized to meet each hospital's needs.

The cause, the prevention and the treatment of diseases are constantly being investigated in VA hospitals through organized research projects which, in many instances, directly involve the nurse. Nursing research designed to search out and test the bases of nursing practice is assuming its proper position, along with patient care, as a continuing function of VA nurses. Chiefs, Research in Clinical Nursing are assigned to selected hospitals. The nurse-clinician is encouraged to identify nursing care problems and to initiate investigational studies seeking solutions to these problems. Also, VA nurses are engaged in studying administrative practices, role definition, nursing service organization and the delivery of patient care services, as well as other areas associated with program development.

The facilities of VA hospitals in 1967 were being used by 163 preservice nursing education programs for their student learning experiences in psychiatric nursing, general medical and surgical nursing, operating room nursing, nursing of chest diseases, and care of patients with chronic illness. This offers to the nurses in these hospitals, used as educational field centers, stimulating opportunities to participate in teaching and supervising students and trainees. In addition to the preservice nursing student programs, VA hospitals provide clinical experience for students from graduate programs, from practical nurse and vocational schools and from other programs concerned with preparation of health workers.

How and Where Applications Are Made for Appointment to the VA Nursing Service

The nearest VA hospital, center, or regional office, or the Nursing Service, Veterans Administration, Washington, D.C., 20025, will furnish information and copies of VA Form 10-2850a, "Application for Nurses in the Department of Medicine and Surgery." Two copies of the completed form should be submitted directly to the field station in which the applicant is interested.

CHILDREN'S BUREAU, SOCIAL AND REHABILITATION SERVICE, U.S. DEPARTMENT OF HEALTH, EDUCATION AND WELFARE

Parts 1 and 2 of Title V of the *Social Security Act,* approved by the President, August 14, 1935, provide for maternal and child health services and for services to crippled children to be administered by the Children's Bureau. Amendments included in *Public Law 88-156* of October 1963 provide for assistance to

states and communities in preventing and combating mental retardation through expansion and improvement of the maternal and child health and crippled children's programs, through provision of prenatal, maternity, and infant care for individuals with conditions associated with childbearing which may lead to mental retardation, and through planning for comprehensive action to combat mental retardation, and for other purposes.[6]

In addition to providing for funds for additional services, funds are provided for research aimed at improvement of maternal and child health and crippled children's services.

The Children's Bureau, formerly a part of the Welfare Administration, is now a part of the Social and Rehabilitation Service in the U.S. Department of Health, Education, and Welfare. At the time the Maternal and Child Health Division and the Crippled Children's Division were established in the Children's Bureau, a Section of Public Health Nursing was created to serve all divisions. Naomi Deutsch was the first chief of the Nursing Division. Her successor was Ruth G. Taylor, who was succeeded, upon her retirement, by Agnes Fuller. When Agnes Fuller retired, the present (1970) chief of the Nursing Section of the Children's Bureau, Katherine W. Kendall, was appointed.

Nursing consultants serve in each of the regional offices which are geographically the same as those to which the nursing consultants of the PHS are assigned. The Nursing Section is responsible for the development of the nursing aspects of maternal and child health and crippled children's services administered by the Children's Bureau. This includes both com-

[6] *Public Law 88-156,* 88th Congress, H.R. 7544, October 24, 1963, p. 1.

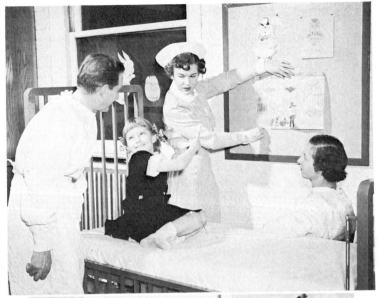

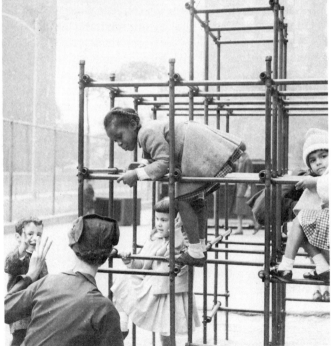

Fig. 11-14. Comprehensive nursing care in the hospital and the community is the concern of the Children's Bureau. (Top photo by Arch Hardy; bottom by Esther Bubley; Children's Bureau, Social and Rehabilitation Service, U.S. Department of Health, Education, and Welfare)

munity and institutional nursing services, as well as education for nurses in maternal and child care and services for crippled children.

The chief function of the regional nursing staff of the Children's Bureau is to consult on the nursing aspects of maternal and child health and crippled children's services with the state agencies that are administering these services under the Social Security Act. Consultation is given as a member of the regional team which includes a physician, a nutritionist, a medical social worker, an administrative methods consultant and the nurse. They are concerned with all aspects of comprehensive service to meet the health and related social needs of mothers and children. Other activities include assistance to nursing schools in developing programs related to maternal and child care, preparing articles and other material for publication, participating in studies and research related to nursing care of mothers and children, serving on committees of national, regional, and state nursing and allied organizations, and participating in conference programs of nursing and other organizations.

The Nursing Section has been given special attention to parent education, child growth and development, curriculum development in maternal and child health and research in all of these areas. While special attention to these areas has continued, the following also have had special emphasis in recent years: mental retardation, school health, children in day care and problems of unmarried mothers. These services relate particularly to the health and the medical care of high-risk mothers and children in socially deprived areas. Despite the affluence, and the medical and technical advances in our country, far too many mothers still have no prenatal care, far too many infants still do not live to see their first birthday, and far too many other infants still suffer neurological damage.

New programs receiving much emphasis today (1970) are those in mental retardation and special projects: (1) Maternal and Infant Care and (2) Children and Youth, designed to reach high-risk mothers and children from socially deprived areas. The newest program, with limited funds, is that of Family Planning. Grants are made to universities for the training of personnel to work in the above fields, and grants to assist in the development or expansion of nursing education programs in maternal and child health.

Requirements and Salaries for Nursing Consultants in the Children's Bureau

Most Bureau nursing positions are in the general salary range of $13,500-$16,000. (See footnote 2 of this chapter, p. 259.) Qualifications for the positions are established by the U.S. Civil Service Commission and include specialized training in public health and in nursing in maternal and child care with specialized experience in consultative activities related to comprehensive programs for mothers and children. Details of the requirements appear in the announcements published by the U.S. Civil Service

Commission of nursing consultant examinations to be held for Bureau positions; examinations are given from time to time as the needs of the service require.

Provisions of the Social Security Act for Improving the Services of Nurses in the Children's Bureau

The Social Security Act provides for grants in aid from the Children's Bureau to the states for maternal and child health and crippled children's services and to institutions of higher learning, especially for the preparation of the clinical specialist in nursing.

Stipends for study in nursing are granted by state agencies having responsibility for administering services under the Social Security Act; such stipends are granted to nurse educators and to public-health, hospital and other institutional nurses for additional preparation in the various fields of nursing in maternal and child care and in services to handicapped children.

HEALTH OCCUPATIONS EDUCATION, OFFICE OF EDUCATION, U.S. DEPARTMENT OF HEALTH, EDUCATION, AND WELFARE

The program of Health Occupations Education (HOE) is operated as one area of occupational education within the Federal-state program of vocational and technical education. Under the administration of the Division of Vocational and Technical Education, Federal legislation authorizes a permanent program of Federal aid for purposes of extending, improving and maintaining quality programs that prepare youth and adults for the world of work. All persons who need and can be benefited by such training (including auxiliary nursing), are to be served—the disadvantaged, the handicapped, the unemployed, the school dropout, the underemployed—as well as those who can succeed in regular vocational programs at high school and posthigh school levels. Programs offered under these funds must be vocational in orientation, must prepare people for gainful employment in occupations that are not classified as professional and must relate to manpower needs in all fields of employment.

A brief outline of Federal legislation for vocational and technical education, relevant to the training of health workers, follows:

George-Barden Title I (P.L. 79-586)

Purpose: To authorize matching grants to states for vocational education in agriculture, home economics, trades and industries

Provisions: Based on state plans, funds may be used for training in useful occupations, for administration and supervision programs, for teacher education and for guidance

George-Barden Title II (Title III of P.L. 84-911; amended by Sec. 11, P.L. 88-210)

Purpose: To authorize matching grants to states for training practical nurses and other similar health workers in hospitals and other health agencies

Provisions: Funds may be used for administration, promotion, instructional programs and inservice teacher education

George-Barden Title III (Title VIII of the National Defense Education Act, amended by Sec. 11, P.L. 88-210)

Purpose: To authorize matching grants to states for training highly skilled technicians essential to the national defense

Provisions: Funds may be used for training highly skilled technicians in all occupational fields

Vocational Education Act of 1963

Purpose: To authorize Federal grants to states to expand, improve and maintain existing programs, as well as develop new programs, of vocational and technical education

Provisions: Based on approved state Plans, funds are used on a matching basis for training in any bona fide gainful occupation as defined in the regulations; for teacher education, construction, guidance, work-study programs, research and special projects; and for state and local administration of the programs

Appalachian Regional Development Act of 1965 Title II (P.L. 89-4)

Purpose: To authorize Federal grants for educational facilities in Appalachia

Provisions: Individual grant awards, providing 50 to 80 per cent as the Federal share for construction, are made to local boards of education through state boards for vocational education

Vocational Education Amendments of 1968 (P.L. 90-576) (This Act replaces the George-Barden Act and the Vocational Education Act of 1963.)

Major provisions of the amendments:

State Grants, for use in training youth and adults for the employment; special emphasis given to training the handicapped and the disadvantaged

Research, funded by both Federal and state grant programs

Innovative Programs, directed toward experimenting with new approaches to training

Curriculum Development, particularly in new occupations; strengthening existing curriculums

Vocational Education Personnel Development, providing grants to support the preparation of teachers, supervisors, administrators and other education personnel

Other provisions cover: Residential Schools, Consumer Education, Cooperative Vocational Education and Work-Study Programs.

The amount of aid authorized from 1969 through 1972 totals $3,180,050,000.00

Aid by occupational area was eliminated from the Vocational Education Acts by the 1968 amendments. State plans that set forth priorities for use of funds under the Acts will determine the programs to be offered in each state. Identification of health manpower needs, including the need for more nurses at all levels, will play a significant role in a state's decisions on distribution of these Federal monies and their matching state monies.

From 1956 to the present time, the Office of Education (OE) has employed specialists (persons with competency both in education and in the health field) to provide leadership in implementing the provisions of the vocational education legislation. Initially, professional nurses were selected and assigned to staff a section within the Division of Vocational and Technical Education. Following enactment of the *Vocational Education Act of 1963*, renewed emphasis was given to expanding the program to include curriculums serving the broad range of health occupations, from short-term courses through associate degree or technical level offerings.

During the years 1964 through 1969, regionalization of the OE's programs initiated the use of program officers serving in Health Occupations Education (HOE) in regional offices of the OE. These program officers were recruited from various health professions, including nursing. In the 1969 fiscal year, education specialists, with professional nursing backgrounds, who were serving the OE totaled 6 — 3 at headquarters and 3 in regional offices (Boston, New York and Chicago). Two regional offices — Dallas and Kansas City — employed specialists whose preparation for the health field was in an allied health profession. To supplement the headquarters staff for HOE, consultant services by 8 persons for up to 30 days per year were authorized. The list of consultants for the health area included, among others, individuals selected from the fields of medicine, education, guidance, school administration and professional nursing.

Organization

A program officer is assigned responsibility for the Division's activities relating to HOE, and functions in a national leadership role for the program authorized under the vocational education acts. In addition, the specialist or program officer serves as a focus for the OE in matters pertaining to education for health manpower. This entails coordination with other Federal agencies, representing the OE in advisory councils established by other agencies, serving as a resource person for this area, and maintaining liaison with national associations, schools, and others as indicated.

Program of Work

In accord with provisions of the vocational education acts, program officers for HOE function within the Federal-state program of vocational and technical education and serve in an educational leadership role. The functions of these program officers include:

1. Promotion and development of training programs that prepare for health service occupations under public vocational education.

2. Consultation services to state vocational education staffs in state-wide planning; and to regional, state and local vocational education personnel in planning, establishing and operating programs.

3. Leadership in the national program of health occupations training under public vocational education funds.

4. Coordination with national health organizations and agencies.

5. Evaluation of the total program.

6. Stimulation of research; promotion of studies, experimentation and pilot projects; and dissemination and implementation of the results of research.

7. Preparation of publications that will assist state and local vocational educators in the promotion, organization and operation of training programs.

8. Gathering and disseminating information on the status of vocational education's training programs as these relate to health personnel.

9. Preparing reports, as required, under the Vocational Education Act.

10. Serving as OE's liaison to other Federal agencies and programs concerned with health manpower.

Appointment of Program Officers

Qualifications for program specialists in vocational and technical education include broad experience and preparation in education and in one or more occupational fields related to the program area in which the specialist will function. Successful experience as a teacher, a supervisor and, possibly, an educational administrator at the local or state level would be desirable. Advanced preparation in education, preferably with emphasis on vocational and technical education, would be necessary. Professional nurses whose education and career have included both nursing service and nursing education are often particularly interested and effective in the position of specialist. A background of experience in nursing education, in supervision or teaching in public health nursing, or in nursing service supervision and administration can be valuable to the specialist in fulfilling the responsibilities of the office. Preparation in other health professions may also serve as effective preparation for the specialist position in view of the expanding scope of the program.

Applications may be filed with the program officer or with the division director, vocational and technical education. Appointments are made in accord with civil service standards and procedures. Inquiries or applications may be mailed to the Director, Division of Vocational and Technical Education, Office of Education, U. S. Department of Health, Education, and Welfare, Washington, D.C. 20202.

VOCATIONAL REHABILITATION NURSING IN THE SOCIAL AND REHABILITATION SERVICE, U. S. DEPARTMENT OF HEALTH, EDUCATION, AND WELFARE

Historical Background

The work of the present Social and Rehabilitation Administration[7] began in 1920 when the President, on June 2, signed the *Vocational Rehabilitation Act (Public Law 236*, 66th Congress) commonly known as the *Smith-Fess Act*. The law authorized an experimental program for a temporary period to provide, through a joint Federal and state financial program, the services of special assistance in job training, counseling and guidance for disabled persons, artificial limbs and other prosthetic appliances where needed and placement in a suitable job. The program was continued by legislative acts that extended the authority until it became permanent with the passage of the *Social Security Act* in 1935 (*Public Law 113*, 78th Congress), which expanded the scope of services and authorized for the first time the provision of medical services, services to individuals who had suffered psychiatric illness and vocational rehabilitation of the blind.

The *Vocational Rehabilitation Act,* signed by the President on August 3, 1964 (*Public Law 565*, 83rd Congress), continued the basic provisions for services to handicapped people and broadened the scope of the program by authorizing changes in its professional, fiscal and technical aspects. It authorized: (1) a new system of grants for extension of grants and improvement of services, (2) grants for research to improve rehabilitation methods and to conduct demonstration projects to spread new knowledge to communities and (3) grants to educational institutions to selected trainees to stimulate the training of additional professional personnel for rehabilitation services.

The *Vocational Rehabilitation Act Amendment of 1965 (Public Law 89-33)* broadened the scope of existing vocational rehabilitation legislation by making possible more flexible financing and administration of state vocational rehabilitation programs, establishing a new 5-year program of grants for the construction of rehabilitation facilities and workshops, authorizing a 5-year program of grants for the staffing of rehabilitation facilities and creating a National Commission on Architectural Barriers to Rehabilitation of the Handicapped. Specific authority for intramural research was given to the Vocational Rehabilitation Administration.

The *Vocational Rehabilitation Act Amendments of 1967 (Public Law 90-99)* extended and expanded the authorization of grants to states for rehabilitation services, also authorizing assistance in the establishment and

---

[7] From 1943 until January 1963 the agency was known as the Office of Vocational Rehabilitation. From February 1963 to August 1967, the Agency was known as the Vocational Rehabilitation Administration.

operation of a National Center for Deaf-Blind Youths and Adults. The 1967 amendments further provided funds for projects which would extend rehabilitation services to handicapped migrant agricultural workers.

The *Vocational Rehabilitation Act Amendments of 1968 (Public Law 90-391)* again gave authority for extension and expansion of existing programs with emphasis on new funds to recruit and train handicapped individuals.

The Nursing Program in the Social and Rehabilitation Service

Nursing was one of the professional groups designated to receive training grants. The program of training grants for nursing was developed by the Division of Training with consultation of an advisory group of nurse specialists from the PHS and the Children's Bureau. Mrs. Vera Hansel was lent to the Office of Vocational Rehabilitation by the Public Health Service for approximately a year and a half to assist in the development and the implementation of the nurse training grant program. Miss Margaret Taylor, a member of the Nursing Advisory Panel, served as needed as special consultant and field visitor from 1958 to 1961. In January 1961, the first full-time rehabilitation nursing consultant, Miss Helen C. Anderson, was employed by the Vocational Rehabilitation Administration in the Office of Health and Medical Affairs—a division established with the administration in 1960. This position was later discontinued.

At present (1970), no nurses are employed in this agency. Nurses from other Federal agencies are used as consultants serving on a 3-member Nursing Advisory Panel that makes recommendations on nurse training policies and reviews and recommends action on rehabilitation nursing training grant requests.

The responsibilities of nursing are to encourage the development of policies and practices of rehabilitative nursing throughout the country; to promote the establishment, the expansion, and the improvement of rehabilitation nursing training programs; to encourage, recommend and evaluate research projects in the field of nursing related to rehabilitation; to consult with regional and state vocational rehabilitation agency personnel in matters pertaining to nursing resources, practices and training; to maintain relationships with public and voluntary agencies, professional organizations and educational institutions and work with them to promote and improve the rehabilitative practices of nursing and the rehabilitation of the disabled. The traineeship program is small, with only 9 universities participating. All programs offer a master's degree in rehabilitation nursing; one offers a doctoral degree.

OPPORTUNITIES THROUGH THE U. S.
CIVIL SERVICE COMMISSION

The *Civil Service Act of 1883* created the U. S. Civil Service Commission. It directs recruitment and examination programs for certain of the Federal Government agencies. However, the agencies themselves determine the positions to be filled and the number and kind of employees they need. The agencies also determine the duties and the pay grade of each position. Ruth A. Heintzelman was appointed nursing consultant, Medical Division of the U. S. Civil Service Commission, on March 1, 1944. She was the first nurse to fill this position. When she retired, the position was abolished. The Commission has professional nursing personnel available to it from a number of government agencies, as well as from the ANA, for advice and assistance.

Nurses Employed Through the U. S. Civil Service Commission

Nurses in the Division of Indian Health of the PHS, the Children's Bureau, hospitals in the Panama Canal Zone government, St. Elizabeth's and Freedmen's Hospitals, Washington, D.C., and in the District of Columbia government are employed through the Commission. Nurses in the PHS not in the Commissioned Corps also are employed through Civil Service. Employment of these nurses in the different Federal services under Civil Service has been discussed throughout this chapter.

Army, Navy, and Air Force hospitals employ civilian nurses under Civil Service procedures. A few positions exist in other Federal agencies in the employee health programs.

We suggest that you review some of the examination announcements, which give details about requirements, duties, pay, working conditions and the like.

What Are Excepted Appointments Under Civil Service?

Excepted appointments are those excepted from the competitive requirements of the *Civil Service Act*; that is, these appointments are not made from Civil Service registers. Nurses in foreign service with the U. S. Department of State and nurses in the VA are in the excepted group.

Some Characteristics of Employment Under Civil Service

Under the personnel policies of the Federal Government, each position is classified according to grade and each grade has a specific salary. Currently (1970) approximately 7,000 civil service nursing positions are covered by the general schedule. The title of *Nurse* is used for all nurse positions at

Grades GS-4 and GS-5, where the requirements are completion of a professional nursing education program and registration to practice. The titles Clinical nurse, Operating Room Nurse, Psychiatric Nurse, Occupational Health Nurse, Research Nurse and Consulting Nurse cover positions above GS-5.

The *Federal Pay Reform Act* passed in October 1962 established salary scales for civilian nurses in the Federal Government. It provided for a 2-stage, general level increase, one in October 1962 and another in January 1964. New schedules, effective in July 1969, were passed by Congress in 1968. It is important to remember that salaries are reviewed frequently and recommendations for changes are made to Congress as needed. In addition, the Civil Service Commission has the authority to establish special salary rates, higher than the regular rates provided by statute, when the government is significantly handicapped in recruiting and retaining well-qualified personnel because of substantially higher rates paid by private employers. Special rates were in effect in some 15 metropolitan areas across the nation in 1968. A nurse making a decision on employment in the Federal Government on the basis of salary considerations should, therefore, be sure to determine the salary rates in the geographic area in which she is interested, as well as the current grade levels of the Civil Service.

Appointments to jobs are made on the basis of ability as demonstrated in competitive examinations. Appointments are made without regard to race, religion, color, national origin, sex, politics, or any other nonmerit factor.

It is suggested that you read references about the U. S. Civil Service Commission listed at the end of this chapter to secure further information. You may also desire to review announcements on positions from the merit system in your state.

Announcements about employment opportunities in the Federal Government can be secured from the U. S. Civil Service Commission in Washington, D.C., or from regional offices.

THE COUNCIL OF FEDERAL NURSING SERVICES

The Council of Federal Nursing Services was organized in 1943 to meet the need for cooperation among Federal nursing personnel during World War II. Its objectives, as stated at that time, were:

1. To provide a means of easy exchange of information about the Federal Government nursing services.

2. To provide mutual assistance in the consideration of the nursing problems presented by the Federal Government nursing services.

3. To formulate recommendations concerning Federal Government nursing problems for which consideration by the National Council for War Service is desired.

In 1946, the third objective was revised to read: To formulate recommendations concerning Federal nursing problems for which consideration by professional nursing organizations and other groups is desired, and to receive recommendations from professional groups and others. Also in 1946, a fourth objective was added which reads: To serve as a source of information on Federal nursing services and on promotional activities in relation to Federal nursing services.

The organization is informal, with no official government status. The membership is from Federal agencies responsible for nationwide nursing services, and includes the chief nurses of the Army, Navy and Air Force Nurse Corps, the Chief Nurse of the PHS and the Director of Nursing Services of the VA, with liaison representation from the Director of Nursing Services, American Red Cross, and from the ANA and NLN. Nurses in other Federal units are invited to participate when appropriate, as programs in these agencies develop.

IMPORTANCE OF KEEPING INFORMED ABOUT NURSING IN THE FEDERAL GOVERNMENT

The Federal Government nursing services which increase during time of war are the military services. During wartime many new sections or divisions are developed to meet emergency needs. Some are dissolved at the end of the emergency, and others may continue and become permanent services born through emergency needs. During peacetime the Nursing Service of the VA usually increases.

As suggested throughout, it is important to keep in touch with the latest occupational developments in the Government nursing services by reading the *American Journal of Nursing, Nursing Outlook, Military Medicine,* and other pertinent periodicals. Announcements of examinations of the U. S. Civil Service Commission will keep you up to date on current developments in connection with nurses under Civil Service in the Federal Government. To learn about requirements for nurses in the Commissioned Corps write the Army Nurse Corps, the Air Force Nurse Corps, the Navy Nurse Corps, and the Public Health Service.

It is important to remember that as nurses we have the responsibility of providing adequate and efficient nursing service to the civilian as well as to the military population.

PROBLEMS

1. If you wished to write to a Federal Government nursing service, where would you find the address in the *American Journal of Nursing? Nursing Outlook?*

2. Search 5 journals in nursing, in public health, and in hospital administration for the last year for articles written by nurses in the services of the Federal Government. In what areas were these articles written?

3. What are the opportunities in the Federal nursing services in: (a) nursing education? (b) hospital nursing service? (c) nursing in public health? (d) clinical nursing? (e) research?

4. What are the emerging occupational opportunities for nurses in the Federal nursing services that are due primarily to political influences during the last 2 to 3 years such as, for example, the passage of Federal legislation?

5. How does the selection of nurses employed by the Department of Medicine and Surgery of the VA differ from other Federal services?

6. Compare activities of nurses in the PHS with those of nurses in the Ministry of Health in the United Kingdom of Great Britain and Northern Ireland.

7. Review the current "Official Directory" of the *American Journal of Nursing* and make a list of the nurses who head the various divisions in the Federal nursing services.

8. If you are interested in working as a consultant of the Children's Bureau, how could you plan your professional career?

9. (a) What is the name and the address of the nursing consultant of the Children's Bureau in your state? (b) How could she help you learn more about programs for high-risk mothers and infants in the USA?

10. What Federal legislation affecting the Federal nursing service has been passed since 1969?

11. Which Federal agencies provide traineeships for graduate education in nursing? Undergraduate education?

SUGGESTED REFERENCES*

GENERAL

* American Nurses' Association. *Facts About Nursing: A Statistical Summary,* New York, The Association, 1964, pp. 58-60, 180-185. Read also each succeeding edition.
Leone, L. P. "Nurses in the Federal Government." *Nursing Outlook,* 9:227-229, April 1961.
Ritter, J. "An Historic Signing at the White House." *Weather Vane,* 36:13,28, Dec. 1967.

ARMY NURSE CORPS

"Army and University Establish Nursing School." *American Journal of Nursing,* 64:8, May 1964.
* Austin, A. L. *History of Nursing Source Book.* New York, Putnam, 1957, pp. 364-427.

* In each chapter all citations are footnoted and are not included here. All starred references are recommended for additional reading.

Belote, M. A. "Nurses and the Army Build-up." *American Journal of Nursing,* **62:**84-85, Feb. 1962.
* Dannett, S. G. L. and Jones, K. M. *Our Women of the Sixties.* Washington, D.C., U. S. Civil War Centennial Commission (Press of Byron S. Adams), 1963.
Dock, L. L., *et al. History of American Red Cross Nursing.* New York, Macmillan, 1922.
Flikke, J. O. *Nurses in Action.* Philadelphia, Lippincott, 1943.
Harper, M. "Army Nurse—Ambassador-at-Large." *Nursing Outlook,* **9:**88-90, Feb. 1961.
Haynes, I. "Commissions and Men Nurses." *American Journal of Nursing,* **56:**775, June 1956.
Jenicek, J. A. "Vietnam—New Challenge for the Army Nurse Anesthetist." *Journal of the American Association of Nurse Anesthestists,* **35:**347-352, Oct. 1967.
Nichols, G. A., *et al.* "Supportive Nurse Roles in Army Nursing." *Military Medicine,* **133:**57-62, Jan. 1968.
* "Satisfaction in Serving: Army Nurses in Vietnam." *AORN Journal,* **7:**86-89, Jan. 1968.
Stimson, J. C. "The Army Nurse Corps." In *The Medical Department of the United States Army in the World War.* vol. XIII, part 2. Washington, D.C., Government Printing Office, 1927.
_____. "Earliest Known Connection of Women Nurses with Army Hospitals in the United States." *American Journal of Nursing,* **25:**18, Jan. 1925.
_____, and Thompson, E. C. S. "Women Nurses with the Union Forces During the Civil War." *The Military Surgeon,* **62:**1-17, Jan. 1928; **62:**208-230, Feb. 1928.
_____, *et al.* "The Forerunners of the American Army Nurse." *The Military Surgeon,* **58:**133-141, Feb. 1926.
* Werley, H. H. "Different Research Roles in Army Nursing." *Nursing Outlook,* **11:**134-136, Feb. 1963.
* _____. "Army Nurse Participation in and Contribution to Research." *Nursing Outlook,* **11:**52-55, Jan. 1963.
_____, and Verhonick, P. J. "Experimentation in Nursing Practice in the Army." *Nursing Outlook,* **11:**204-206, Mar. 1963.
"You're in the Army Now." *RN,* **31:**32-37, Aug. 1968.

AIR FORCE NURSE CORPS

"Air Force Nursing." *Nursing Outlook,* **7:**408-409, July 1959.
* Albert, J. "What's Different About Flight Nursing?" *American Journal of Nursing,* **56:**873-874, July 1956.
* Chandler, C. H. "The New Air Force Nurse." *Nursing Outlook,* **12:**36-37, Aug. 1964.
Gersema, V. M. "When You Choose Air Force Nursing." *Nursing Outlook,* **3:**380-381, July 1955.
Goddard, M. A., and Arrington, A. M. "Is Missile Nursing Different?" *American Association of Industrial Nurses Journal,* **9:**8-11, Aug. 1961.
Lay, F. "Next Step—Outer Space." *American Journal of Nursing,* **59:**971-973, July 1959.
Martin, A. M. "We Earn Our Wings." *American Journal of Nursing,* **57:**894-896, July 1957.
* Popiel, E. S. "The Air Force Nurse Corps: Try to Remember Our Heritage." *Colorado Nurse,* **67:**7-9, Nov. 1967.
* *The Professional Nurse in the United States Air Force.* Washington, D.C., Government Printing Office, 1967.

NAVY NURSE CORPS

Bowman, J. B. "History of Nursing in the Navy." *American Journal of Nursing,* **28:**883-889, Sept. 1928.

Casaregola, M. "The Nurse in Navy Blues." *American Journal of Nursing,* **54:** 594-595, May 1954.

Elliott, J. "Nursing Touring Cape Kennedy." *Nursing Outlook,* **16:**59, Feb. 1968.

———. "Nursing with the Navy in Malta." *Nursing Times,* **63:**1683-1685, Dec. 1967.

Handbook of the Hospital Corps of the United States Navy. Washington, D.C., Government Printing Office, 1969.

Harrington, E. "Aboard a Hospital Ship." *American Journal of Nursing,* **53:**584-586, May 1953.

Jackson, W. L. "We've Reached the Golden Year." *American Journal of Nursing,* **58:**671-673, May 1958.

Lindelof, J. G. "Action Aboard USS Repose." *Weather Vane,* **36:**39-41, Oct. 1967.

McKeon, W. "Back from Vietnam." *American Journal of Nursing,* **67:**2120-2123, Oct. 1967.

McKown, F. C. and Lee, A. "International Ward." *American Journal of Nursing,* **69:**772-773, Apr. 1969.

Mitchell, R. J. "Training Hospital Corpsmen in the Navy." *Nursing Outlook,* **3:**281-283, May 1955.

* Morin, A. E. "Navy Hospital in Saigon." *American Journal of Nursing,* **66:**1977-1979, Sept. 1966.

* "The Navy Nurse Corps Launches a Nuclear Nursing Program." *Nursing Outlook,* **7:**216-217, Apr. 1959.

Recicar, C. "I Nursed Aboard a Refugee Ship." *American Journal of Nursing,* **57:**300-302, Mar. 1957.

"Training Program for Military Nurses From Friendly Allied Armed Forces." *Nursing Outlook,* **8:**84-85, Feb. 1960.

U.S. Department of the Navy. Bureau of Medicine and Surgery. *Handbook of the Hospital Corps, United States Navy, 1959.* Washington, D.C., Government Printing Office, 1959, pp. 4-1 to 4-166.

———. "The Navy Nurse Corps." *Manual of the Medical Department, U.S. Navy.* Washington, D.C., Government Printing Office, 1958, pp. 1-5.

———, Nursing Division. *Navy Nurse Corps Candidate Program.* Washington, D.C., The Department, Oct. 1957. Mimeographed.

NURSING IN THE PUBLIC HEALTH SERVICE OF THE U.S. DEPARTMENT OF HEALTH, EDUCATION, AND WELFARE

"Congress Votes $35,913,000 for Aid to Nurse Education." (News) *American Journal of Nursing,* **68:**2503, Dec. 1968.

"Contracts for Refresher Courses Continued to November 30." (At Press Time) *American Journal of Nursing,* **68:**2289, Nov. 1968.

Gardner, M. S. *Public Health Nursing.* New York, Macmillan, 1936, pp. 42-44.

"HEW Reorganization Affects Division of Nursing." (At Press Time) *American Journal of Nursing,* **68:**940, May 1968.

Lorent, M. "Nurses are Highly Trained Professionals at World's Most Cosmopolitan Hospital." *South African Nursing Journal,* **34:**24, Sept. 1967.

Loughlin, B. W. "Aide Training Reaches the Navaho Reservation." *American Journal of Nursing,* **63:**106-109, July 1963.

Petry, L. "One Hundred Fifty Years of Service." *American Journal of Nursing,* **48:**434-435, July 1948.

"President Signs Bill Aiding Nurse Education." (News) *American Journal of Nursing*, **68**:2063-2064, 2092, 2096, 2098, Oct. 1968.

The Public Health Service. *Background Material Concerning the Mission and Organization of the Public Health Service, Prepared for the Interstate and Foreign Commerce Committee, United States House of Representatives, April 1963*. Washington, D.C., Government Printing Office, 1963.

Shriver, B. M., *et al.* "Follow-up on Mental Health Trainees." *American Journal of Nursing*, **67**:2569-2572, Dec. 1967.

U. S. Department of Health, Education, and Welfare. Public Health Service. *Nurse Training Act of 1964. Program Review Report*. Washington, D.C., Government Printing Office, 1967.

* *The United States Cadet Nurse Corps and Other Federal Nurse Training Programs*. Washington, D.C., Government Printing Office, 1950.

Vreeland, E. M. "Nursing Research Programs of the Public Health Service." *Nursing Research*, **13**:148-158, Spring 1964.

See current issues of *Public Health Reports*.
See also references in Chapter 25, in the section entitled "Office of International Health, Public Health Service."

NURSING SERVICE OF THE VA

Veterans Administration. *A Guide for Inservice Education Activities in VA Nursing Service*. Washington, D.C., The Administration, Aug. 1963.

_____. *There Is a Star in Your Future*. Washington, D.C., The Administration, July 1963.

_____. *Nursing Care of the Long Term Patient*. Washington, D.C., The Administration, Apr. 10, 1963.

NURSING SECTION OF THE CHILDREN'S BUREAU OF THE U.S.
DEPARTMENT OF HEALTH, EDUCATION, AND WELFARE

* Anderson, E. H. "Commitment to Child Health." *American Journal of Nursing*, **67**:2076-2080, Oct. 1967.

Deitrick, S. H. and Bradbury, D. E. *The International Activities of the Children's Bureau*. Washington, D.C., Government Printing Office, 1961.

Holtgrewe, M. M. *The Role of the Public Health Nurse in Mental Retardation*. Washington, D.C., Government Printing Office, 1964.

Leckner, E. J. "The Public Health Nurse in a Program for the Mentally Retarded." *Children*, **2**:70-74, Mar.-Apr. 1964.

* U.S. Department of Health, Education, and Welfare. Social Security Administration. Children's Bureau. *It's Your Children's Bureau*. Washington, D.C., Government Printing Office, 1964.

* Wolff, I. *Nursing Role in Counseling Parents of Mentally Retarded Children*. Washington, D.C., Government Printing Office, 1964.

See also the many folders and pamphlets of the Children's Bureau published by the Government Printing Office on the various phases of maternal and child health and welfare, especially the magazine *Children*.

HEALTH OCCUPATIONS EDUCATION, U.S. OFFICE OF EDUCATION,
DEPARTMENT OF HEALTH, EDUCATION, AND WELFARE

U.S. Department of Health, Education, and Welfare. Office of Education. *Digest of Annual Reports of State Boards of Vocational Education, Fiscal Year Ended*

June 30, 1962. Washington, D.C., Government Printing Office, 1963.

———. *Practical Nurse Education: Report of a National Conference on Practical Nurse Education, February 3-7, 1958, in Chicago, Illinois.* Washington, D.C., Office of Education, 1958.

* "Vocational Education Act Seen as Nurse Opportunity." (News) *American Journal of Nursing,* **69:**13, 30, 34, Jan. 1969.

West, M. D. and Crowther, B. *Education for Practical Nursing, 1960.* New York, National League for Nursing, 1962.

OPPORTUNITIES THROUGH THE U.S. CIVIL SERVICE COMMISSION

U.S. Civil Service Commission. *Futures in the Federal Government.* Washington, D.C., Government Printing Office, Dec. 1967.

———. *Federal Careers for Women.* Washington, D.C., Government Printing Office, Oct. 1967.

———. *Working for the U.S.A.* Washington, D.C., Government Printing Office, May 1967.

———. Your Retirement System. Washington, D.C., Government Printing Office, Jan. 1967.

Announcements of examinations for positions in the different Federal nursing services can be secured by writing to the U.S. Civil Service Commission, Washington, D.C., 20025.

CHAPTER

12

Nurses in a National Disaster or Emergency

Planning for civil defense is a way of life and will be for some time to come. Every citizen has a responsibility for planning adequate civil defense measures, and the professional health disciplines have specific additional responsibilities. Civil defense is a professional way of life for the health disciplines, including nursing. Nurses must be prepared for their dual role in civil defense—as private citizens and as professional persons.

BACKGROUND OF CIVIL DEFENSE LEGISLATION

Even when the words "Hiroshima" and "Nagasaki" were still accepted definitions of the ultimate in man-made disaster, American men of vision predicted that the secret of atomic fission would not long remain unshared. Nuclear weapons would one day be a part of enemy arsenals, to menace both the armed forces and the civilian population of our country. Realizing that the threat of war would be with us for some time, these farsighted men proposed a system of civilian defense to complement military preparedness. Largely as a result of their recommendations, initial efforts were made to secure civil defense legislation. With the *National Security Act of 1947,*

Congress created the National Security Council, a nonmilitary agency intended to advise the President concerning the integration of domestic, foreign and military policies relating to national security.

Further attempts to make civil defense a vital force included the *Federal Civil Defense Act of 1950*. This act (Public Law 920), as amended, vested the responsibility for civil defense in the states and their political subdivisions, with the Federal Government providing coordination and guidance. Since the passage of Public Law 920 in 1950, many changes in defense planning have occurred.

FEDERAL AGENCY RESPONSIBILITIES

As of 1970, 2 main government agencies are concerned with defense planning—the Office of Emergency Preparedness and the Office of Civil Defense.

The Office of Emergency Preparedness (OEP) is a staff agency in the executive office of the President. Briefly, its responsibilities are:

1. To advise and assist the President relative to civil defense policy and coordination of defenses.

2. To plan for and expedite postattack rehabilitation.

3. To carry on other functions, such as strategic stockpile and manpower adjudication.

In other words, the OEP is responsible for functions that will enable us to recover more easily from an attack and begin rebuilding.

The Office of Civil Defense (OCD) in the Department of the Army, U. S. Department of Defense, is the agency responsible for all Federal civil defense functions except for those reserved to the President or delegated by him to other agencies. In addition to preparing and directing national civil defense plans and programs, the general functions of the agency also include assisting state and local governments in the development of their civil defense capabilities. OCD has an active role in developing the national fallout shelter system, the civil defense warning system and the radiological monitoring and reporting system.

National responsibility for the medical health aspects of the civil defense programs was assigned to the U. S. Department of Health, Education, and Welfare through 2 Executive Orders issued by the President. *Executive Order 10958* granted full authority to develop requirements, plans and operations for the management of the national stockpile of emergency medical supplies and equipment. *Executive Order 11001* directed the programs covering health services, civilian health manpower, health resources and educational programs to the U. S. Department of Health, Education, and Welfare. The Secretary of the Department, in turn, redelegated responsibility for these health activities to the PHS.

The PHS, in its normal role as improver, protector and restorer of the nation's health, has grown accustomed to operating within a framework of actual or impending disaster. Its role now includes the functions of emergency planning and preparedness. The overall emergency-health-preparedness goal established by the PHS is to prepare and help carry out a program that will assure the availability of adequate health services for our civilian population in a national emergency. Activities to achieve this goal are grouped into 3 major areas:

1. Preparation of the civilian to meet his own health needs when deprived of the services of a physician

2. Assistance to states and local communities in developing the capability to implement their emergency health operational and survival plans

3. Development of a coordinated emergency program for Federal agencies with health or health-related responsibilities

EMERGENCY HEALTH SERVICES

Planning the Program

Present planning (1970) calls for the development of plans and programs which cover all aspects of emergency health and medical services and resources, and which are applicable to all unexpected events ranging from highway accidents to thermonuclear attack. The continued growth and mobility of the population increase the possibility of the involvement of larger number of casualties in the event of natural disasters or accidents, as well as in enemy attack. The increased nuclear capabilities of other nations and the existing political situations in the world continue the threat of nuclear war.

Community survival plans must be flexible, including those for emergency health services, and alternate plans must be provided to meet the existing situation. These plans will vary according to the community's size, the amounts and kinds of resources normally available and the disaster situations most apt to occur. The community's health resources can be organized in a number of ways, but whatever the organization, it will be responsible for utilizing all available resources in providing medical care and public health services, and for performing the necessary administrative functions to meet the additional resource needs of health operating units.

Medical Stockpile Program

Originally the Medical Stockpile Program was predominantly a casualty care program that could become operational almost immediately and remain in operation for a relatively short period of time. The supplies and the equipment for the original Packaged Disaster Hospitals (PDH) were based upon this planning. With the later program it became necessary to add items to the PDH to increase its capabilities from primarily a traumatic surgical unit to one that could provide medical care to all types of serious sickness and injury. This 200-bed unit consists of hospital supplies, equipment and pharmaceuticals which are packed for long-term storage. At least 1 medication is included for each important therapeutic category. The supplies and equipment are sufficient to provide a 30-day operational capability, after which it is planned that back-up supplies will be available from medical supply depots located throughout the country.

The PDH's are assembled by the PHS and are stored in affiliation with local hospitals in carefully selected communities. In the event of a disaster the PDH can be used to: (1) expand the assigned hospital or (2) establish a separate 200-bed hospital in a preselected building and operate as an adjunt to its assigned hospital. If an actual postdisaster situation does not require the use of the PDH for one of the above purposes, selected supplies and equipment may be readily utilized in accordance with actual needs. Thus, it may serve to supply first-aid teams, first-aid stations, or emergency-treatment stations, or it may be used as a source of back-up supplies for all community medical care activities.

As the use of supplies and equipment from the PDH's continued following natural disasters, it was recognized that a smaller and more mobile unit was needed. Such a unit could be dispatched rapidly into a disaster area to provide initial emergency medical care for disaster victims. Components were then selected from the PDH to form the Natural Disaster Hospital (NDH). The NDH consists of pharmaceuticals, hospital supplies and equipment, surgical supplies and equipment, intravenous solutions, electrical equipment and other vital supporting supplies. This short-term medical facility can be set up as a complete 50-bed unit and can operate for up to 24 hours. It can be used to expand a hospital's facilities, or set up in a church, school, community center or other available building. It has been estimated that the emergency needs of approximately 300 casualties can be met by the unit. The NDH's have been stored in areas with a high natural disaster potential.

Hospital Reserve Disaster Inventory units (HRDI units) are being placed with selected community hospitals to increase their capability to provide care to disaster victims for a period of time without relying on outside sources. These 50-bed units contain a 30-day supply of essential emergency medical supplies commonly used in casualty care. The units are kept ready for use at all times through the rotation of the HRDI supplies with the daily operational supplies of the affiliated hospital.

Medical Care in Community Fallout Shelters

Many variables will determine the areas affected by the hazardous effects of radioactive fallout. If such a disaster should occur, survivors in many areas of the nation will not suffer from the direct effects of the detonation, because they will not be near an area of destruction. Depending on the existing wind patterns, others will escape the secondary effects of the detonation—the hazards of radioactive fallout. Still others will be in areas affected by fallout and all survivors will be exposed to health hazards and health problems.

The effectiveness of the management of a fallout shelter and the emergency medical care is directly related to public preparedness by planning, organizing, training and testing. These form an operational preparedness assuring the availability of medical supplies and health manpower in proportion to the desired level of medical care. Individuals should be designated for specific assignments which involve the movement of material from outside resource points to shelter sites, and also provide essential health manpower.

Medical care in fallout shelters may be austere, aimed to provide survival care for the sick and injured and measures to prevent the spread of disease. In order that the best possible preventive and health conservation measures be carried out, it is essential that the shelter manager and his staff work closely with the health officer and his group in:

1. Designating the location and area of the Health Unit (sick bay or infirmary).

2. Providing that area with the best available equipment and supplies necessary for its operation.

3. Maintaining maximum security measures for such equipment, supplies and the privacy required for its successful operation.

4. Making clear at the onset with the health services personnel that conservation of all supplies, dressings, drugs, food and water is essential and must be carried out in every respect.

5. Establishing a duty roster around the clock for the Health Unit.

6. Setting definite hours for daily sick call and sanitary inspections.

7. Establishing complete understanding that certain prescription drugs and medical items contained in the kits, and designed only for physicians' and allied health workers' use, will not be available for lay workers.

The Federal Government is stocking an austere medical kit in shelters. It is the responsibility of the community to add any item designed to improve the level and extent of medical care. The drug supply could be increased if pharmacists planned ahead of time to have an emergency kit available for persons to take with them to the shelter. Persons with particular dietary needs should bring the special foods they require; parents should bring infant formulas and other appropriate baby foods; and persons needing special medicine, such as those with diabetic and cardiac conditions, should bring their medicine with them.

Postdisaster Incidence of Illness

In any postdisaster period it is assumed that the normal incidence of illness will increase greatly. This estimate is based on:

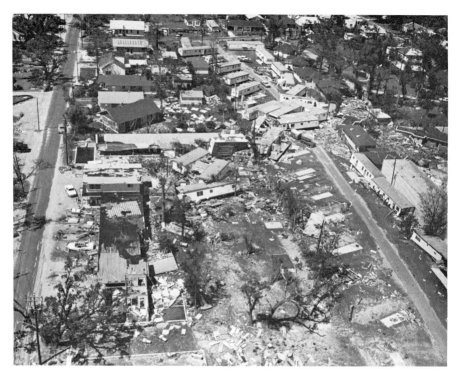

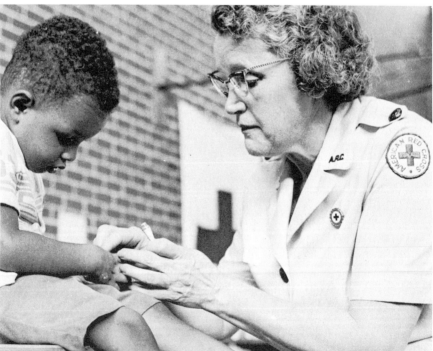

Fig. 12-1, a *(top)* and b *(bottom). (Caption on facing page)*

Fig. 12-1 (a) An aerial view of some of the extensive damage created when Hurricane Camille stormed ashore with monstrous tides and winds in excess of 200 miles per hour along the Gulf Coast between Mobile, Alabama, and lower Louisiana. (b) A nurse concentrates on a child with an injured hand. (American Red Cross photos taken by Ted Carland). (c) A nurse checks the condition of an elderly patient who was airlifted back to the Gulfport area after being evacuated earlier to a hospital in Meridian, Mississippi.

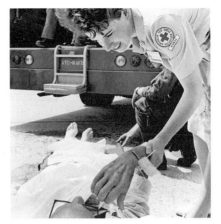

Fig. 12-1, c.

1. A breakdown or deterioration of the environmental factors which control the peacetime health status. This includes disruption of normal water supplies; excreta disposal systems and disposal of other wastes; increase in water pollution and in the rodent and vector population.

2. Crowded living conditions, which invite the spread of disease.

3. Extremes of temperature—due to climatic conditions and aggravated by lack of heating and cooling facilities.

4. Nutritional problems. The supply of food may be limited. Milk and other perishable food products may be contaminated. Lack of refrigeration may be a contributing factor.

5. Emotional pressures that may precipitate heart attacks, strokes and premature births, and may aggravate peptic ulcers, existing cardiac diseases and asthmatic conditions.

6. Lack of drugs for the treatment of chronic conditions—which could aggravate existing chronic diseases and possibly precipitate acute complicating conditions.

7. Increase in accident rate—caused by loss of emotional control or panic, and an increase of accident proneness.

8. Continuation of the usual emergency surgery requirements; people will continue to have acute appendicitis, ruptured ulcers, strangulated hernias and other types of acute surgical conditions.

Because of the time required to allow radiation to decay to permissible levels, there could be a delay, varying from hours to weeks, before an emergency health services program would become operational. Thus the patient load and the types of conditions may vary. The patient load characteristics will be of a type falling somewhere between the true casualty patient and the more traditional peacetime hospital patient, but will also include patients suffering from complications resulting from the delay in treatment.

DISASTER NURSING

What is disaster nursing? It is nursing practiced in a situation where professional personnel, supplies, equipment, physical facilities and utilities are limited or not available. Disaster situations vary in magnitude—from a small to a major natural disaster, to one in which the continental USA is attacked with nuclear weapons. In addition to disasters occurring as a result of nuclear accidents, there are many other kinds of national disasters. Pictures showing nursing activities following Hurricane Camille in 1969 may be seen in Figure 12-1.[1]

If a nuclear disaster should occur, medical care will probably be austere, and medical treatment procedures will be based on the following principles:

1. Lifesaving measures in the treatment of traumatic injuries, acute infectious diseases and chronic diseases with acute complicating factors

2. Preventing the spread of disease to others to keep the incidence of illness at as low a rate as possible

3. Controlling and shortening the period of illness, so that a patient may join the work force as soon as possible

4. Preventing crippling or hazardous complications of illness

5. Alleviating suffering to give patient comfort and to help to prevent emotional situations from arising

Medical care in a fallout shelter will be aimed to provide survival care for the sick and injured and measures to prevent the spread of disease. Nurses may be the only persons available to cope with the health problems, and they will be responsible for providing care with only the available supplies and equipment. Nursing functions and responsibilities will increase and broaden with the establishment of emergency medical and health services. Nurses will be required to recognize signs and symptoms of illness or injury, and make appraisals based on their professional judgment. Nursing judgment will also need to be used to determine when a treatment or medication should be discontinued or modified.

Nursing functions will have to be expanded to meet the austere situation, where automation will not exist and improvisation will be required. There will be early discharge of patients, those occupying a hospital bed will be critically ill, requiring intensive care, insofar as possible in an austere situation. The health needs of the surviving population will increase enormously due to disruption of water supplies, sewage disposal treatment facilities, increase in insect and rodent population, and a general deterioration of environmental sanitation. There will be less direct medical supervision, and nursing management may include 3 or 4 wards, instead of the usual 1. Many trained and untrained volunteers will be giving nursing care and will require greater supervision. These are a few of the broad responsibilities that nurses will have in a disaster situation.

[1] See also Chapter 26 for further discussion of national disasters that are the responsibility of the American National Red Cross.

NATIONAL NURSING ORGANIZATION ACTIVITIES IN DISASTER OR EMERGENCY

The ANA

The ANA has assumed responsibility for national defense activities in 2 major areas: (1) advice to the Office of Civil Defense in the U. S. Department of Defense and the Division of Emergency Health Services of the PHS in the U. S. Department of Health, Education, and Welfare; and (2) provision of basic information for the profession to aid nurses in understanding and carrying out their role in national preparedness. An ANA Committee on Emergency Health Preparedness and National Defense[2] has been at work since 1950, implementing these responsibilities.

Some of the important results of this committee's work include:

1. Development of a *Statement of Committee's History, Philosophy, Purpose, and Functions* to serve as a framework for action of the national committee. The statement was developed in 1954 and revised in 1959, 1964 and 1968. (The predecessors of this statement were called *1954 Document, 1959 Document*, and *Statement of Assumptions, Purpose, and Functions*, in 1964.)

2. Preparation of *The Role of the Nurse in Disaster*, first published in 1960 and revised in 1964.

3. Preparation of *Guidelines for SNA-DNA Committees on Emergency Health Preparedness*, published in 1967.

4. Preparation of *List of Films and Film Catalogs for Use in Preparing for Nursing in Disaster and National Defense*, released for publication in 1963 and revised in 1968.

In 1968, the committee prepared a new position statement on selective service for nurses. This *Resolution Regarding Planning for Civilian and Military Needs and Selective Service* provides for long-range military and civilian manpower requirements and effective means for meeting these needs.

In 1968, the ANA prepared a memo for all state and district nurses association committees entitled, *Emergency Health Preparedness and Your Nursing Service: An Action Program for Hospitals, Community Agencies, and Nursing Homes*. The memo called attention to Standard No. 7 and the Assessment Factors of the ANA *Standards for Organized Nursing Services* which states:

The nursing department has clearly delineated responsibility in the health care facility's disaster plan.

Assessment Factors

a. The nursing department assumes responsibility for effective execution of those phases of the plan which affect nursing services.

b. Each member of the nursing staff has information about the health care facility's overall disaster plan.

[2] Formerly called the Committee on Nursing in Disaster and National Defense.

c. Each member of the nursing staff knows, understands, and has practiced his own role in the event of a disaster.[3]

A disaster plan which is simple and flexible was recommended. Also included were recommendations for activities of state and district nurses association committees.

The NLN

When the NLN was organized in 1952, it took over the disaster programs of the organizations that became a part of it. In assuming its share of responsibility in the matter of preparation for national defense, the NLN expressed its primary objective as leadership in interpreting the philosophy and content of disaster nursing to institutions employing nursing personnel. Three major tasks were accepted: (1) to help schools of nursing recognize the need to teach disaster nursing skills, (2) to assist nursing services in making the teaching of disaster nursing a part of their inservice education and (3) to help nursing services and communities in developing plans to follow in the event of natural or enemy-caused disasters.[4]

In 1958, the NLN undertook a project in disaster nursing designed to improve the preparation of nurses for the functions they are expected to assume during disasters. It was financed through a contract with the Federal Civil Defense Administration (now the Department of Defense, Office of Civil Defense) and was in effect from January 27, 1958 to September 6, 1961.[5] Figures 12-2 and 12-3 show work groups of individuals interested in the project.

The project was designed to investigate and to demonstrate ways of preparing students of nursing and personnel in hospital nursing services to cope with the unusual nursing problems presented by disaster situations, and to assume certain additional functions of medical practice, as expected of nurses in the absence of physicians in such situations. In broad outline, the problem encountered by nurses in disaster situations consists of the interruption of planned nursing service in existing institutions, agencies and homes by a sudden intrusion of great numbers of sick and injured, and the use of shelters and other structures for disaster victims.

The major approach of the investigation was through demonstration studies conducted in a hospital nursing service and in educational programs of various types. The institutions and the programs in which the studies were carried out were:

1. Massachusetts General Hospital—hospital nursing service and diploma program.

[3] American Nurses' Association, *Standards for Organized Nursing Services*, New York, The Association, 1965, p. 11.

[4] "The National League for Nursing and National Defense," *Nursing Outlook*, 7:233, Apr. 1959.

[5] M. V. Neal, *Disaster Nursing Preparation, Report of a Pilot Project Conducted in Four Schools of Nursing and One Hospital Nursing Service*, New York, National League for Nursing, 1963.

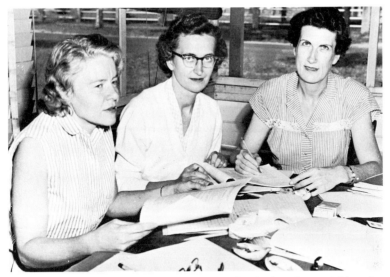

Fig. 12-2. First work session of participants developing plans to initiate the disaster nursing study of the National League for Nursing and the Office of Civil and Defense Mobilization, August 1958, at the home of R. Louise McManus, Bass River, Massachusetts. *Left to right*, they are Miss Mary V. Neal, NLN; Lt. Col. Harriet Werley, ANC; and Catherine M. Sullivan, Office of Civil and Defense Mobilization.

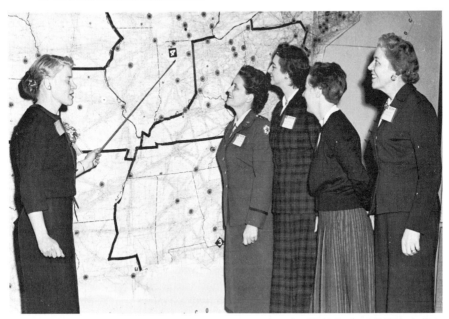

Fig. 12-3. Disaster Nursing Project Directors discuss the NLN Project (1959). *Left to right:* Mary V. Neal, NLN staff, and Project Director; Capt. Drusilla Poole, University of Minnesota, Minneapolis, Minn.; Grace Davidson, Skidmore College, New York, N.Y.; Capt. Virginia Farrell, Massachusetts General Hospital, Boston, Mass.; and Lt. Col. Ida Graham Price, Teachers College, Columbia University, New York, N.Y. (Office of Civil Defense)

2. University of Minnesota—practical nursing program and basic baccalaureate program.

3. Skidmore College—basic baccalaureate degree program.

4. Teachers College, Columbia University—baccalaureate degree program for registered nurses and graduate programs.

The accounts of the demonstration projects include a wealth of specific data—outlines of course content and teaching methods, charts showing the placement of learning experiences within the curriculum and tests for measuring students' knowledge before and after the learning experience. Some of the conclusions of the project were:

1. Disaster nursing is not a clinical specialty.

2. Students in nursing are inadequately informed about national and world affairs that have direct implications for national security and indirectly for disaster nursing.

3. Disaster nursing instruction may be included within the usual nursing courses.

An essential part of the project was the development of a standardized achievement test in disaster nursing by the NLN Test Construction Unit. Unlike other NLN achievement tests, this test is available for use by graduate professional nurses, as well as by professional nursing students who are nearing graduation. In addition to a total score, the test is constructed to provide 2 subscores: (1) general nursing knowledge applicable to disaster situations and (2) facts and principles peculiar to disasters and disaster nursing.

The general belief continues to be that content applicable to disaster nursing should be integrated within the appropriate clinical courses in the basic nursing curriculum. It is recommended that emphasis be on the basic principles which are applicable to any stressful situation in nursing, in a wide variety of settings.

COORDINATION OF PLANNING

Your institution or agency cannot operate in an actual disaster without the help of supporting services such as welfare, police, transportation and communications. Therefore, its activities must be coordinated with the community's survival plan. All levels of government must be included in plans for disasters or emergencies national in scope. Therefore, planning must be coordinated through the community, the state, and the Federal Government, and this formulates the "national plan."

Health services planning is coordinated through the country or local health departments and the state health departments. At the Federal level of government, this planning is coordinated with the PHS, U. S. Department of Health, Education, and Welfare. Within the PHS, the Division of Emergency Health Services is responsible for the preattack planning and programming of emergency health services and for coordinating them with the Office of Civil Defense.

ROLE OF THE PROFESSIONAL NURSE

Professional nurses need to be oriented to and psychologically prepared for disaster work. In disaster operations, nurses will find themselves working in heterogeneous groups of persons with wide ranges of preparation, skill and stability. Nurses must also develop the attitude that, in a disaster, they will be able to "do the best for the most with the least."

As a professional nurse you will want to prepare for your disaster nursing responsibilities by knowing the disaster plan of your institution or agency and particularly your nursing service section. Knowing the plan is not enough, however. You should know also your specific disaster assignment and the additional functions or areas of responsibility that it includes. Your disaster assignment may include more than clinical activities. It may include management skills and teaching responsibilities. In an actual disaster, professional nurses will be responsible for the management of personnel, supplies and equipment, and they will be teaching both trained and untrained volunteers by various on-the-job methods.

You, the students of nursing, are living in a period of varying national and international tensions. Various crises have brought the possibility of nuclear war close to us as a nation. It can happen, and we must be prepared. Also, natural disasters are always a threat, as are those disasters caused by civil tensions. Disaster nursing preparedness is important for emergencies of all magnitudes. Students of today are the professional nursing leaders of tomorrow — and leadership in your community is essential for disaster nursing preparedness.

PROBLEMS

1. What are the survival plans of your community for emergency health services?

2. What are the plans for coordination and mutual aid in your local community and who will be the chief nurse for emergency services in the event of an enemy attack?

3. (a) Does your institution have a fallout shelter? (b) Where is it located and what is its capacity? (c) List the medical items stored in the shelter by the Federal Government. Check with your local civil defense office to secure this information.

4. What is the role of the following in disaster planning: (a) American Red Cross? (b) American Hospital Association? (c) American Psychiatric Association?

5. What is the role of the following in determining general standards and educational plans for nursing in civil defense programs: (a) ANA? (b) NLN? (c) AMA?

6. What are the committees concerned with national disaster and their membership in the following organizations: (a) ANA? (b) AMA?

7. List 5 situations, other than war, in which disaster nursing principles are applicable.

8. How would you, a student of nursing, "go into operation" in a mass emergency in your community? What measures would you take: (a) For self-protection? (b) To help your classmates? (c) To help your neighbors?

9. (a) What have been the major national disasters in the USA during the past 3 years? (b) How would you, if you were a registered nurse, assist in such disasters?

SUGGESTED REFERENCES*

* American Hospital Association. *Principles of Disaster Planning for Hospitals.* Chicago, The Association, 1967.
_____. *Check List for Hospital Disaster Planning.* Chicago, The Association, 1964.
* American Nurses' Association. Special Committee on Emergency Health Preparedness and National Defense. *Statement of Committee's History Philosophy, Purpose, and Functions.* New York, The Association, 1968.
_____. *List of Films and Film Catalogs for Use in Preparing for Nursing in Disaster and National Defense.* New York, The Association, 1968.
* _____. *Guidelines for SNA-DNA Committees on Emergency Health Preparedness.* New York, The Association, 1968.
* _____. *Action Program for SNA and DNA Committees on Emergency Health Preparedness.* New York, The Association, 1967.
_____. *The Role of the Nurse in National Disaster.* Washington, D.C., U. S. Department of Health, Education, and Welfare, Public Health Service, 1965.
American Psychiatric Association. Committee on Disaster and Civil Defense. *First Aid for Psychological Reactions in Disasters.* Washington, D.C., The Association, 1964.
Brooks, E. A. "Preparation for Emergencies." *Nursing Outlook,* **12:**47-49, Sept. 1964.
Executive Office of the President. Office of Emergency Preparedness. *The National Plan for Emergency Preparedness.* Washington, D.C., Government Printing Office, 1964.
Frazier, D. S. "The Function of the Professional Nurse in Event of a Nuclear Attack." *American Association of Industrial Nurses Journal,* **10:**12-14, Feb. 1962.
Hundley, J. M. "National Disasters: Types and Effects." *American Association of Industrial Nurses Journal,* **11:**26-28, June 1963.
Magnussen, A. "Who Does What—In Defense, In Natural Disaster." *American Journal of Nursing,* **65:**118-121, Mar. 1965.
Mahoney, R. F. *Emergency and Disaster Nursing.* New York, Macmillan, 1969.
Nabbe, F. C. *Disaster Nursing.* New York, Little-Field, 1960.

* In each chapter all citations are footnoted and are not included here. All starred references are recommended for additional reading.

* U. S. Department of Defense. Office of Civil Defense. *In Time of Emergency.* Washington, D.C., Government Printing Office, 1968.

————, *et al. Family Guide Emergency Health Care.* Washington, D.C., Government Printing Office, 1966.

* ————. *Medical Self-Help Training . . . For You and Your Community.* Washington, D.C., Government Printing Office, 1965.

* U. S. Department of Health, Education, and Welfare. Public Health Service. Division of Emergency Health Services, *et al. The Role of Medicine for Emergency Preparedness.* Washington, D.C., Government Printing Office, 1968.

————. *Establishing the Packaged Disaster Hospital.* Washington, D.C., Government Printing Office, 1966.

————. *Check List for Developing a Packaged Disaster Hospital Readiness Plan.* Washington, D.C., Government Printing Office, 1966.

————. *Nurses' Ward Management Guide for the Packaged Disaster Hospital.* Washington, D.C., Government Printing Office, 1965.

————. *Austere Medical Care for Disaster.* Washington, D.C., Government Printing Office, 1964.

————. *Community Emergency Health Preparedness.* Washington, D.C., Government Printing Office, 1964.

* U. S. Navy. Bureau of Naval Personnel. *Disaster Control: Ashore and Afloat.* Washington, D.C., Government Printing Office, 1968.

CHAPTER

13

Choosing
a Field
of Nursing

Early in your preservice nursing education, or at least during your last year before graduation, you will wish to ask yourself: What particular type of nursing shall I choose? As you know, it is important to choose wisely both for your sake and for that of the patient. Satisfaction in your work is one of the fruits of a wise choice. Also, if you are doing work you like and for which you are fitted, the chances are that you will be more effective in carrying out your responsibilities. This chapter includes suggestions to help you make a choice of a field of nursing.

REEVALUATING MOTIVES FOR CHOOSING A FIELD OF NURSING

Persons have different reasons for entering the occupation of nursing. Because your motives may change as you gain knowledge and experience, it is wise to stop once in a while and take stock of yourself to see exactly why you are in nursing and why you have selected the special field of nursing in which you work.

Socioeconomic factors are also considered in choosing a special field in nursing. Salaries, fringe benefits, hours of work, opportunities for advancement and retirement plans are often critical factors in vocational choice. They are important factors but they are not the only factors to be considered.

One student of nursing said: "Being an administrator pays well, and good administrators are scarce." Another said: "Going into the armed services is a job with a pension; that is the field I am going to enter." The fact that these choices are not choices in the true sense of the word, when they are the only reason for selecting a position, is not always recognized.

Another reason for a certain choice is to gain ability and training. This is an important reason for the nurse who is concerned about her long-range vocational planning. One type of work may be used as a steppingstone to another or as a basis for further education. A graduate of an associate degree or diploma program may look for a position where she can combine work with attendance at a college or university where a baccalaureate degree can be obtained. Some institutions allow time off to attend school and others may include tuition as a fringe benefit. This type of benefit is growing more common, particularly in large medical centers where promotion is limited to nurses with baccalaureate degrees.

Today, when so many nurses are married either before or soon after graduation from a school of nursing, the choice of a position will no doubt be influenced by the plans both she and her husband have. The job may need to be selected because of its proximity to their home. Even so, it will be important to think in terms of long-range goals. With the current trend toward clinical specialization, should the young nurse look for a job in a field where she feels she might later specialize? One young nurse, a recent graduate of a baccalaureate program, decided that she was interested in psychiatric nursing. She selected a position in a psychiatric service in a general hospital in a city where there was also a university offering graduate work in psychiatric nursing. She began attending the university on a part-time basis. Later, with a fellowship, she completed her work at the university. Meanwhile, she married the young man of her choice and is starting her family. She may need time off from nursing for awhile to care for her family. But, when she is ready to return to nursing, her careful planning toward her long-range goals will serve to give direction to her future role in nursing.

Still another reason for choosing a certain field of work in nursing springs from altruistic or humanitarian motives or from a religious feeling. The altruistic or humanitarian motive is based on a desire to give a social service to mankind. The religious reason is based on the love of God and the desire to serve Him directly and, through Him, to serve fellow-men.

A combination of several of these reasons may be found by one person.

With the shortage of qualified professional nursing personnel, the newly graduated nurse frequently is offered and, perhaps because of pressure exerted by the employer, accepts a position for which she is not prepared by education and experience. As a result, she feels inadequate and is frustrated in trying to meet the demands of the position. Therefore, she fails to gain job satisfaction, which is essential to her happiness and well-being. Once the nurse accepts such a position, influencing factors, such as desire for prestige and economic considerations, interfere with her reevaluating her choice and doing further vocational planning.

Different people vary in their reactions, depending on their psychologic traits. As people mature, they seem to become more realistic in their choices. Interest seems to have a firmer basis in experience and a growing philosophy of life, as well as in economic factors. These factors are seen and evaluated truly. Ability and training required are judged more accurately. Sometimes, only after a nurse has experienced several types of work can she make an intelligent career choice based on an accurate estimate of her talents and interests. Today's graduate has broad vistas before her in clinical nursing, in nursing education, in nursing service and in nursing research.

CHOOSING A SPECIFIC TYPE OF NURSING

The first consideration, in choosing a specific type of nursing, should be the tentative crystallization of work and life objectives, immediate and long-view. A long-time consideration of what you may want to do or be or where you desire to go 5 or 10 years hence, is important. This involves self-analysis and occupational analysis.

Choosing your specific field of nursing constitutes not only 1 decision. It involves making a large number of decisions over a fairly long period.

IMPORTANCE OF SELF-EVALUATION

Self-analysis is helpful in order to see how you are fitted potentially for the field of your choice. A satisfactory choice can usually be made if you consider your capacities, interests and goals.

It is important to seek counsel from one who is able to help you find relevant personal and social facts, understand them and make appropriate decisions. Such counsel could be sought from your adviser or instructor, or special vocational counselor, if one is available. However, the counselor does not do your thinking and give you a prescription.

Some items that you might consider in making a systematic study of yourself prerequisite to an occupational analysis are:

1. Consider your age. In general, age is indicative of degree of maturity and the amount of experience to build on. The very young may be limited in experience as well as in preparation for certain types of work, such as administration. On the other hand, the older person, without adequate preparation and experience, may likewise be limited. Nevertheless, age is a factor that cannot be overlooked in any self-analysis.

2. Consider your experience and the amount, the type and the quality of education needed. Completion of your work in a hospital nursing school, a college, or elsewhere may be an influencing factor on future

decisions. Grades may be indicative of potential special abilities and interests. Preferences for particular courses and reasons for likes and dislikes for certain areas of instruction may reveal abilities and interests. Cocurricular activities, such as offices held and committee work, are sometimes proof of abilities and interests in certain types of nursing work.

The authors have discussed educational plans with many nurses who have realized suddenly, with regret, that their nursing school records were a genuine handicap for graduate work. These students have wondered why no one ever had told them earlier about the items that are looked at in admission applications on entering an educational program. Some graduate nurse students have been shown disfavor because their records evidenced lack of ability to get along with other students or no interest in cocurricular activities that might have helped in the development of social and other skills. The student is often not aware that her willingness to carry her share of student activities is an indicator of her willingness to carry her share of extras in the world of work. All students would find it valuable, for future reference, to keep a record of cocurricular activities in which they engaged, such as offices held, committees served on, and honors received.

3. Consider your understanding of present reactions to previous experiences and of plans and future ambitions. Ambitions often differ from interests and expectations. If you realize this, you may be better able to analyze and solve some of your problems.

4. Consider your aptitudes, physical condition, disabilities. Psychologic and other test data, such as from NLN Tests, throw light on intelligence, special aptitudes and achievement.[1] This kind of information helps you and your counselor to round out the picture of yourself and needs to be obtained in order for you to choose a field in nursing intelligently. Universities with colleges or departments of nursing also provide counseling and will assist in your self-evaluation, particularly with advice about additional preparation that may be required for specific positions. You may wish also to refer to the *Directory of Approved Vocational Counseling Services,* published by the American Personnel and Guidance Association, to learn where, in your locality, special vocational counseling services are available.

It might be helpful for you to consider some of the following questions in making a self-analysis:

1. What are my intellectual capacities? How do I think? Do I learn new things rapidly? Do I learn best from reading the printed page? Do I make good decisions rapidly? Do I need time to make good decisions? How can I change my pace of thinking? Am I satisfied on a job where the

---

[1] The performance of applicants on the League tests is reported only to the director of the school. The student who wishes to use this service would need to work, therefore, through the director of the school. It should be pointed out, however, that only a few schools are now using these tests.

day-to-day problems are relatively the same? Do I need constant, significant, new learnings to be happy?

2. What is my physical self like? How much physical energy and vitality do I have? Can I work long hours without too much tension? Do I wear out easily and need to rest each day?

3. What is my emotional and spiritual self like? Have I tried to determine my philosophy of life? What do I believe about myself in relation to self and others? What do I practice in my daily life toward self and others? Do I know where to go for help if emotionally upset?

You will think of other questions that could be used in making a self-analysis.

OCCUPATIONAL ANALYSIS

It is not enough to know your aptitudes, abilities and interests when making a choice of a field of work in nursing. These need to be related to conditions in nursing, occupational trends, and requirements that are likely to affect your ability to make use of aptitudes and to express interests.

What Should Guide You in Making a Choice?

Develop an appreciation of occupational trends and survey the scope of opportunities in nursing as a whole. Occupational trends and shifts in numbers and percentages of nurses in different fields reveal expanding and contracting fields and when the demand is exceeding the supply. It is not easy for everyone to make interpretations about occupational trends. It takes rare talent to exercise judgment about these items. Consequently, you will need to get this kind of information from reliable sources such as your school counselor or the state nurses association.

Learn the requirements of each type of nursing which interests you as a possible choice. If any field reveals definite shortages, you may desire to fit yourself for it if you are potentially suitable and like it sufficiently. Finally, compare the opportunities from which you will make your final selection in relation to what you have learned about yourself in the self-analysis.

Useful Sources for Getting Acquainted With Fields of Nursing

There are several ways to get acquainted with available fields of nursing; the following are some of the more important:

Study the U.S. Census Bureau reports, *Facts About Nursing* published annually by the ANA, and reports of nurse inventories made by such agencies as the Division of Nursing of the Bureau of Health Professions Education and Manpower, U.S. Department of Health, Education, and Welfare, the U.S. Office of Civil Defense, and the American Hospital

Association. Several references at the end of this chapter and articles in current professional nursing journals, also could give you valuable information about occupational needs in nursing.

Read career pamphlets and what others have to say about different fields of nursing.

Talk with those in particular fields to learn what they like about the work; the disadvantages of the work; considerations regarding health and physical demands; scholarship requirements; salaries; religious, ethical and disciplinary aspects; interpersonal relationships required; relationships to the community; living conditions; or any other phases suggested in the outline in the next section for making an occupational analysis (p. 330).

Relate all experiences in your preservice program to occupational planning and use every opportunity to observe and learn about kinds of nursing positions in various settings. Make personal investigation of the work, if possible.

Secure available information from headquarters of nursing organizations — national, state, or local.

Review the publications of the ANA on clinical practice and the development of standards. Examine qualifications stated in job descriptions for nurse personnel.

Review the employment standards recommended by state nurses associations.

Who Should Decide Which Field You Will Enter?

You, yourself, will need to make the final decision as to which field you will enter. Study the whole situation. Get all the counsel and help you can, but reserve the final decision for yourself and attempt to make it as intelligently and unemotionally as possible. Prayer for spiritual guidance helps many people.

After a Choice Has Been Made, Does It Necessarily Follow That You Will Stay in That Kind of Work?

No, the idea that there is just one place for each person is false. Frequently, one type of work becomes a steppingstone to another. It is quite possible that it may even lead into an entirely different occupational area in nursing or into a field other than nursing.

GUIDE FOR MAKING AN OCCUPATIONAL ANALYSIS

The following suggestions may be useful as a guide for making an analysis of 1 or 2 types of work of interest to you.

In presenting the report in writing or orally, state how your data were gathered, by library work, interviews, or other methods, and the date of gathering them.

Each school could save these reports. They could be filed, added to by students each year, and thus become very useful as references.

THE SUGGESTED GUIDE

A. Brief history of particular type of work.
B. Demand for the particular type of work.
  1. What is the total number of nurses employed in this country?
  2. How many nurses are employed locally in this work?
  3. Is it in a growing or a diminishing field?
  4. Is it overcrowded, or is there a shortage of workers?
C. Regularity of employment.
  1. Is it stable or fluctuating?
  2. Is it found only locally, or is it representative of the state, section of the country, the nation, or the world?
D. Work done.
  1. How is the particular field defined?
  2. What functions are involved? With what people will the association and functional relationships be closest? What is the relationship among people in the same field or place where work will be done?
  3. Does it require nursing skill, social skill, administrative skill, teaching skill, all of these, or other skills?
  4. Is it subject to any hazards, health or accident?
  5. Does it require much or little physical activity? Which do I prefer?
  6. Does it require extensive travel?
  7. Do I have to own and drive a car?
E. Qualifications.
  1. Are there opportunities for both men and women?
  2. Does age influence success in the work?
  3. Is any particular church affiliation required? Is church affiliation a barrier?
  4. What are the physical, the mental and the social requirements?
  5. What are the specialized skills required?
  6. Are there special tests to be taken? What are these?
  7. Does it require unusual tact and leadership?
  8. Are there any legal limitations? What are they?
  9. Do I qualify?
F. Preparation required.
  1. What initial preparation is necessary for this work?
  2. What special or graduate preparation is necessary? Desirable?
  3. What experience is essential? Desirable?

4. Where can education and experience be procured? What educational institutions offer special preparation? Are there on-the-job training opportunities? How long will it take? How much will it cost? What entrance requirements, if any, must be met? Are scholarships, traineeships, fellowships, or loan funds available for the preparation required?
5. Is time allowed for attendance at school? With tuition allowance?
6. Does the work require experience in some related field before one can enter the chosen work? What types of work serve as steppingstones for promotion? Is such experience basic to further preparation?
7. What is the opportunity for promotion? Are there opportunities to advance in clinical specialties, in administrative or teaching or other positions?

G. Methods of entering.
1. Do you enter through the Civil Service Commission?
2. Is it best to obtain information from the state nurses association? A professional nurses' registry?
3. Can you get help from the placement services at the educational centers?
4. Do you apply to an office of a military nurse Corps, such as the Army Nurse Corps? Navy Nurse Corps? Air Force Nurse Corps?

H. Earnings.
1. What is the beginning salary? The most common salary? The maximum salary?
2. What are the life earnings, as a rule?
3. Is salary paid weekly, monthly, by the day or hour, or how?
4. Is there an increase for further experience? For more education? What provision is made for increments? What is the basis for such salary increments? Is it additional preparation, experience or what?
5. How much vacation and other leave are granted?
6. Is there a retirement plan?
7. Is hospitalization or other health insurance provided?
8. Are earnings controlled by laws, labor boards, unions, or collective bargaining?
9. Is there additional compensation for evening and night work? For overtime? For special assignments?

I. Advantages and disadvantages.
1. Are the hours of work reasonable? Is there much overtime work? Night work?
2. Does the work offer advancement?
3. Do many of the workers attempt to get into other nursing fields after the first year of experience?

4. Are inservice education programs available?
5. What is the vacation period?
6. What social and professional relations does the worker have with the community? With physicians? Supervisors? Patients? The general public?
7. Is there time, place and adequate income for recreation? For enjoyment of home life and participation in social and civic affairs? Where do nurses in the special type of work usually live? What kinds of friends do they tend to have? What are the living conditions?
8. Is there an opportunity for continuing education? Is there provision for educational or sabbatical leaves in educational institutions? For attendance at professional and related organization and educational meetings?
9. Is the type of work likely to change because of change in social or economic conditions or public need?
10. Are there many students preparing for this work?
11. What are the real opportunities for service to society?

J. Other considerations.
1. Who are some of the leaders in the field?
2. What are the typical places of employment?
3. What is the significant literature in the field — books, magazines, other?
4. What are the nursing and other organizations that you might join with profit?

IMPORTANCE OF WISE CHOICE OF A FIELD OF NURSING

One of the outstanding characteristics of our culture is the right of the individual person to choose his work. Another is the high degree of specialization. The number of fields in nursing from which to choose is growing. Therefore, the correct choice is important.

Occupational choice is affected by the kind of person you are, and by coworkers, society and others, such as parents, teachers, friends and advisers.

The key to making an occupational choice appears to be in the way you appraise yourself and the work you want to do. Much depends on your future goals — goals for practice, goals for continuing education and goals for your future life in general.

Decisions on choice of work generally are not made overnight, although it sometimes seems as though they are. They are more likely to be decisions reached after the problem has been lived with a long time. They are often one-step-at-a-time decisions. At one point the question is, What field in nursing do you want to go into? At another point you will consider the educational institution you want to attend for continued education and the kind of courses to take. At another point it may be the specific job to look for. Decisions are made gradually as increasing self-knowledge permits and as circumstances dictate.

It is suggested that you refer to references in Chapter 8, "General Survey of Occupational Opportunities for Nurses" as well as Chapters 9, 10, and 11. The suggested references in these 4 chapters are not comprehensive or all-inclusive. They are merely given as a starting point. You may wish to start your own collection on any field or type of work in which you become interested.

Chapter 16, "Continued Education for Nurses," will give further clues that may be helpful to you in choosing a field of work in nursing. So will Chapter 14, "Obtaining, Filling, and Resigning From a Position."

PROBLEMS

1. In which of the following fields of nursing are the opportunities expanding or contracting: (a) private practice? (b) public health? (c) office nursing? (d) school health work? (e) hospitals? (f) occupational health? (g) organization work? (h) education? (i) consultation? (j) research?

2. Choose a field of nursing you think you might like to enter upon graduation. State the reasons for your choice, including your qualifications and the relationship of the position or field to your future goals. You might have an out-of-class session with members of your group and make comparisons. You could ask the school counselor to be a consultant to the group.

SUGGESTED REFERENCES

Hoppock, R. *Occupational Information*. New York, McGraw-Hill, 1967.

Secure current materials from the ANA-NLN Committee on Nursing Careers, American Nurses' Association, 10 Columbus Circle, New York, N.Y. 10019.

CHAPTER

14

Obtaining, Filling and Resigning from a Position

How are you, as a young nurse, to find a place among the thousands of women and men making up the nation's reservoir of nurses? How can you obtain work that will offer full scope to your education, interests and abilities and be productive of real values? You have been examining various fields of nursing and types of positions as well as the general employment picture; the next step is to select the type of work you want to do. Although a great deal of the material in this chapter relates to the nurse who is seeking a permanent position or is employed in one, many of the principles are also applicable to the nurse in private practice.

OBTAINING A POSITION

Fundamentally, success in obtaining employment depends on the supply and the demand for personnel in the field of your choice and your ability to fill the type of position available. Employers are interested in your professional competence, in your skill in interpersonal relationships, in your preparation and experience and in your intelligence, personality and health. Some or all of these militate for or against every nurse when she applies for a position. Study the market to make sure that the services you expect to offer will be in demand.[1]

MEANS OF LOCATING A POSITION

Channels Through Which Positions Are Located

The way you go about finding a position depends to some extent on your field of interest in nursing. In general, the channels are professional nurse placement offices, placement offices in educational institutions, announcements of Civil Service examinations, advertisements in professional periodicals, relatives, friends, acquaintances and direct contacts with employers, physicians, patients and others. If you desire a commission in the Army, Air Force, or Navy Nurse Corps, or in the PHS of the U.S. Department of Health, Education, and Welfare, write directly to the service of choice for information. The VA hospitals also employ a large number of nurses.

Not all the channels listed here are recommended for indiscriminate use, although the channel really matters much less than the care and wisdom with which the person chooses a job. Theoretically, the professional placement service should be of greatest assistance. It is important for the nurse to investigate a position thoroughly. Personal acquaintance with the prospective employer, his strengths and weaknesses, and his situation, is a vitally important factor, as is similar acquaintance on the part of the employer with the strengths and weaknesses of the applicant. You will be particularly interested in the philosophy of the agency, the philosophy of nursing care and the philosophy underlying the organizational structure. Sometimes your educational adviser can guide you into exactly the right situation.

Auspices Under Which Nurse Placement Services Are Conducted

Nurse placement may be conducted by hospitals, other health institutions and educational institutions; national, state and district nurses associations; other professional groups; employment centers operated by the state or local offices of the U.S. Employment Service; and by commercial agencies. Not all of these are professionally sponsored services.

The placement services that have seemed to be the most satisfactory for nurses are those sponsored and conducted by the professional nurses associations.

[1] See Chapter 13, "Choosing a Field of Nursing," for factors to consider in making an occupational choice.

Assistance from the Professional Association

Nurse placement services may be national, state, or local. Professional registries for nurses in private practice are organized by, affiliated with and approved by district nurses associations and approved by state nurses associations.[2] The American Nurses' Association Professional Credentials and Personnel Service, Inc. (ANA PC&PS) is located at 10 Columbus Circle, New York, N.Y., 10019.

The ANA PC&PS

On September 1, 1945, the Nurse Placement Service's Midwest Bureau was acquired and reorganized as the office of the ANA PC&PS. This office was moved to New York City in 1959 and now serves as the center of the professional record service for nurses in all states. The ANA PC&PS and state PC&PS offices formerly provided both record service and counseling and placement service. State offices served nurses and employers in their states, and the national office served nurses and employers in the 32 states that could not afford to establish their own PC&PS office.

In 1964, in an effort to reduce the cost of the ANA PC&PS while continuing to provide the same service to nurses in all states, the ANA House of Delegates voted to limit the functions of the ANA PC&PS to professional record services. Counseling and placement assistance became the responsibility of the state nurses associations. The ANA PC&PS office discontinued listing and referral of positions in 1965, and began compilation of PC&PS records for nurses in all states in 1966. Transfer of state PC&PS records to the national office began in 1966 and continued into 1969.[3]

Service from the ANA PC&PS

The professional record service consists of compiling a cumulative record of professional education and experience, including references from previous employers; sending biographies; updating records and biographies as needed; and safe-keeping and storage of the records. Completion of the PC&PS application form provides the basis for compilation of a record. Confirmation of diplomas and degrees awarded, dates and titles of positions held, and evaluation of performance (references) are obtained by PC&PS directly from the schools and employing organizations. From 2 to 6 weeks are required to compile a new record, depending upon the speed with which references are returned. The PC&PS record remains on file throughout the nurse's professional career.

References are obtained by PC&PS from former employers and educa-

[2] State approved registries are listed in the back of the May and November issues of the *American Journal of Nursing.*
[3] "The New PC & PS," *American Journal of Nursing,* **68:**328-331, Feb. 1968.

tional institutions, with the nurse's permission. Reference requests are automatically sent to the head of the department of nursing in the school or employing organization; it is important that the evaluation be supplied by someone to whom the nurse has been administratively responsible. Usually only one reference is obtained for each period of employment. PC&PS policy permits sharing a reference with the nurse on request, if the reference was obtained after this policy became effective in October 1967. It is expected that references will be based on periodic evaluations of performance discussed by the supervisor and nurse during employment. It is suggested that the nurse, planning to leave a position, should ask her employer for a final evaluation before she leaves.

The PC&PS biography is a summary of the PC&PS record and contains the following information: a list of educational programs completed, including confirmation and evaluation of progress in these programs, date of diploma or degree awarded and major program of study; R.N. licenses and state certificates held; foreign language skills; professional activities, publications, workshops and institutes attended; titles of positions held, including confirmation of dates, clinical area where indicated, name and address of employing organizations and evaluation of performance. Unless otherwise indicated, only references covering the last 10 years of employment and at least 3 employment periods are included in a biography. If desired, the nurse may supply a statement to be sent with the biography describing professional interests, expectations and goals.

Biographies are released only on authorization sent to PC&PS by the nurse; they are not released on request from the employer without prior permission from the nurse. The request to send a biography must include the name and title of the recipient, with his responsibility in the employing organization clearly indicated. Also needed is the title of the position for which the nurse is applying, or the reason for sending the biography.

Service from State Nurses Associations

State nurses associations develop their own professional counseling and placement services with assistance from the ANA PC&PS. By 1968, 43 states provided service, including:

1. Information about positions open in the state.

2. General information about employment opportunities and standards in the state, including salaries; license to practice; and names and addresses of principal hospitals, public health agencies, schools of nursing, professional registries, public schools and business and industrial organizations that employ nurses.

3. Information about cost of living, residence accommodations, climate and recreation facilities.

4. Assistance to nurses with plans for professional growth and development, including information about educational programs and finan-

cial aid for study, and help with questions related to professional practice and employment conditions.

Employers of nurses are assisted by listing position openings, and referral of openings to nurses interested in employment in the state. The state office also provides employers with current information about salaries and employment conditions, which will help to attract and hold qualified nurse personnel. Periodically, state associations send a list of position openings to the ANA PC&PS office for duplication and distribution to all states. This provides a method for distributing information about employment opportunities in all states to nurses throughout the country.

Employers also appreciate receiving the professional biographies prepared for nurses by the ANA PC&PS. The value of reviewing professional credentials of candidates for positions prior to employment, and of retaining credentials of employees in confidential personnel files, is increasingly recognized.

Responsibility of the Nurse in Using PC&PS

Any ANA member or associate member can have her record compiled by the ANA PC&PS and receive counseling and assistance with placement. When requesting service from PC&PS you should:

1. Enclose your current ANA membership card (member or associate) in your letter requesting service from the ANA PC&PS or from a state nurses association (SNA) office.

2. Include your PC&PS file number (Social Security Number), and former name, if name has changed since last contact with PC&PS.

3. When requesting assistance from an SNA office, be specific about interests in regard to type of position desired, preferred location within the state, minimum salary acceptable and date of availability.

4. Investigate positions carfully. Although the SNA office provides preliminary information about positions, detailed information should be obtained from the employing organization. If interested in a position, write a letter of application or further inquiry.

5. Send *written* request to the ANA PC&PS office to release your biography, and enclose a check for the required fee.

6. When your need for service is ended, inform the SNA offices that provided assistance.

7. Keep the ANA PC&PS informed of additional education programs completed and changes in employment.

The ANA assumes financial responsibility for operation of the national office, and the state nurses associations assume responsibility for support of state services. However, in order to obtain additional resources to assist the ANA in providing record service to nurses in all states, the ANA House of Delegates approved the charging of fees for service by the ANA PC&PS, beginning July 1, 1968. A charge of $10.00 is made to begin a new record and send 1 biography. A fee of $2.00 is required to send a biography at other times.

There is no charge to update a record already on file, and the compilation fee includes safe-keeping and storage of the record. Since assistance with counseling and placement is provided by SNA offices, there is no charge to send a biography to an SNA office for use in assisting the nurse.

PC&PS is a tangible benefit of membership in the ANA. Membership dues make it possible for the ANA to offer professional record service; fees help to meet the cost of the service provided. The quality, professional aspects and personal nature of the service support the policy that the individual member who uses PC&PS should participate in paying for the service received, over and above membership dues.

Principles Underlying Service from the National Professional Association

A statement of principles of the former ANA Professional Counseling & Placement Service can be found in the January 1952 issue of the *American Journal of Nursing,* pages 48-49. These principles are still useful in describing service by PC&PS and understanding the development of good employer-employee relationships as well as nurse-patient relationships, and include the following:

A primary purpose of professional service is to improve the quality of nursing practice through service to the individual nurse. Professional credentials on file and ready to use help the nurse with application for a position, admission to a college or university, and application for license to practice in another state. Employers find the PC&PS biography of considerable assistance in selection of qualified nurse personnel.

Basic to provision of professional record service and assistance with counseling and placement is respect for the nurses as individuals. Skill in the technique of counseling is helpful. Nurses with special employment problems are referred to appropriate sources of assistance.

Nurses are encouraged to accept responsibility for making their own decisions, investigating positions thoroughly, business-like conduct of negotiations with employers, accepting employment for which they are qualified and utilizing opportunities for keeping abreast of current knowledge and trends.

Employers of nurses are encouraged to establish sound personnel policies and employment conditions that will attract and hold qualified nurse personnel.

Employers are encouraged to write references which present complete and objective evaluations of the person being rated, based on periodic evaluation during employment. In order to assist the nurse with professional growth and development, references obtained after October 1967 are available for review by the nurse on request, unless otherwise stipulated by the writer.

PC&PS cooperates with other programs of the professional association in supporting the need for college preparation and continuing education in nursing, upgrading professional practice and promoting the economic and general welfare of nurses.

Professional record service and assistance with counseling and placement are unrestricted by considerations of nationality, race, creed, color, or sex.

Effective counseling and assistance with placement may pay long-term dividends in the adjustment of the nurse. The effectiveness of this service can be measured ultimately by the adjustment of nurses, by their fitness for the positions they accept, and by their understanding of and appreciation for their responsibility for continuing to develop their professional skills and knowledge and for making their work successful.

Help You Can Expect From the Nursing School Which Graduated You

It is general practice that the nursing school, unless it is in an institution of higher education, does not operate a placement service, but it may well assist its graduates, whenever possible, to secure positions, and provide information and advice on selection of a field, employment in it, and the possibility of advancement through supplemental or advanced study and experience. Sometimes arrangements are made for conferences with prospective employers. However, the most important function of the school in this connection is to help students to discover their special aptitudes while they are still students, to teach them how to make occupational studies, and to refer them to the appropriate professional counseling and placement services in the state and the community where the school is located. If the school is a part of an institution of higher education and it has a placement division, the student can be guided to seek counseling and placement from the appropriate personnel of that division. When the student is guided to seek expert counsel as to her abilities, aptitudes, or interests, or how to use the counseling facilities available, she can gain a rather comprehensive and systematic concept of her abilities and how best to use them.

Civil Service Applications and Examinations

Civil Service announcements provide information about nursing positions and vacancies with certain government agencies. These announcements are made some time before the date of the examination and include information on the required qualifications, the nature of the examination, the salary, where to obtain application blanks, and the period for filing applications. The application itself contains directions for completion and filing. The announcements of Federal agencies are published in post offices and other government buildings in the USA and its territories. They may be secured from the Civil Service commissions of the Federal and the state governments, occasionally from counties, and in a few instances from large cities, such as New York. They also may be secured from government nursing services, but it is better to write directly to the Civil Service commissions, requesting that announcements of examinations of interest to you be sent. Information about the U.S. Civil Service Commission is included in Chapter 11.

Advertisements Regarding Positions

Each month the *American Journal of Nursing, Nursing Outlook,* and other health periodicals publish classified advertisements of positions available. Position openings also are listed in the bulletins of the state nurses associations.

Usefulness of Relatives and Friends in Establishing Employment Contacts

Relatives and friends can be most helpful when they know your qualifications and preferences. As employers of nurses we have secured very well-qualified personnel through friends who knew of potential applicants for special types of positions.

Disadvantage of Relying on Outside Influence

If you secure a position through political or other influence, the people with whom you work are likely to resent this fact, especially if you are not qualified for the job. There is danger, too, of losing the position when your influential friends lose their power. On the whole, it seems wiser to make your own way and not depend too much on politicians to obtain a position. You have the satisfaction then of being independent and of knowing that your success is due to your own preparation and ability.

Obtaining Employment Through Direct Contact With Employers

The nurse in private practice may register with a few physicians and be kept busy by them; however, should they retire she may be out of employment for a time. She may also work independently, receiving her calls directly from patients. From the economic standpoint, however, this is sometimes risky and unsatisfactory. The really good nurse will usually be called from many sources, whether definitely registered with all of them or not. Registration with a nurses' professional registry approved by the professional association is considered advisable.

A nurse seeking a hospital position may make personal application to the director of nursing service, and the nurse in public health may communicate with the head of the nursing service of a public health organization. In fact, a position in any of the nursing and allied fields may be secured through personal application to the employer.

Cooperating With Placement Service While Seeking a Position

Let us suppose that you have registered for a position with the PC&PS of the nurses association. Reply promptly to any calls or letters pertaining to positions, and remember that it is up to you to make application to the employing agency if you are interested in a position. Follow up as many desirable contacts as possible without being too aggressive. The more contacts a nurse can establish, the better known she will be. It is important, too, to notify those who have assisted you when you have accepted a position.

Methods Used in Applying For a Position

The 2 most common methods of applying for a position are the written application, which may be either a letter or a formal application form, and the personal interview. The second often results from the first.

A letter of application should be written to a prospective employer, even though you plan to ask a placement office to send your professional credentials to the employer. If you wish to have ANA PC&PS send your biography to a prospective employer, you, not the employer, must make this request to the ANA PC&PS office and send the required fee. Telephone requests are accepted in an emergency, but must be confirmed in writing. PC&PS sends credentials only on request from the nurse applying for the position.

It is helpful to an employer to know that your credentials are on file with PC&PS. Many employers include on their application forms this question: Do you have an ANA PC&PS file? It is an advantage to you to mention, in your letter of application, that your credentials are on file with ANA PC&PS and that you will ask that they be sent to the employer.

THE WRITTEN APPLICATION

Why Is the Letter of Application Important?

A letter of application is important because it helps the prospective employer to judge your scholarship and ability, much of your personality, and possibly how you would keep his records. If it is well written, it may open the way for further consideration which often is prevented if it is poorly written. Employers assume that the letter represents the best work of which you are capable. Therefore, writing it carefully, observing correct form and content, is important.

Good Form for Letters of Application

Make sure that you have followed the principles of correct letter writing and have used a good grade of plain, dignified stationery. See that your letter is clear, complete, concise, and courteous and that it conveys your exact meaning, with correct spelling, punctuation and paragraphing. There are numerous publications that include guidelines on how to prepare application letters to secure a position. Your counselor or librarian can assist you to locate a suitable reference on this topic.

What Data Should the Letter of Application Contain?

The letter should include no nonessential details but should give all necessary information, such as:

A clear, definite statement of application for the particular position, including your interest in applying for the position, pending receipt of additional information about the position and/or the organization.
The reasons for applying and the source of your information concerning the vacancy in question.
A concise account of your credentials, both general and professional, including education, experience and other qualifications; or referral to your professional credential file.
A few important, authoritative references, but not too many, and not those already on file in your PC&PS credentials.
A request for a personal interview, if possible.

When an employer's application form is used, or if a placement service is putting you in contact with an employer, only the specified forms need to be completed.

Consider the following points when making your own list of credentials. In giving educational qualifications, include the complete and correct location of all schools you attended, dates of attendance, the diplomas or degrees received; mention also any special preparation, formal or informal, which you have had that might be helpful. In presenting information on education and experience, it is advisable to follow a chronologic order. The general practice is to begin with the most recent and date back to the beginning.

Only such qualifications need be included as are significant to the position or usually are given in any letter of application: age, health, matrimonial status, licensure by state boards of nursing, and affiliation with professional and other relevant organizations and honorary societies.

As a rule, there should not be more than 3 to 5 names for references, unless additional ones are requested. Include the names of those people who are qualified to evaluate your scholarship, professional ability, character and personality. Usually, the most acceptable references are past instructors and former and present employers or their representatives. Give the complete address of each reference.

It is advisable to get permission from a person to use his name as reference. The tone of the letter asking for use of a reference name varies according to your relationship with the person. On the whole the letter should indicate what you are doing now, what application you intend to make, why the position is desired, and how the reference will be helpful. A stamped addressed envelope should be enclosed for a reply. If permission is granted to use someone's name for reference, it should be acknowledged. It is a courteous gesture to let all who have sent recommendations know whether or not you have been successful in securing the desired position.

When requesting an interview, ask to have it arranged at the convenience of the employer or indicate when you will be free to call. Include your complete address and telephone number.

Completing the Application Form

You cannot be too careful in completing application forms, because frequently inexactness and carelessness in this respect have been the chief causes of failure to secure desirable positions. To show how important this is, the following case is related:

Annabelle Sisson was applying for a position in which she was greatly interested and for which she was exceptionally well qualified. But when she completed her application blank, she used many abbreviations, including "pt." for "patient" and "ı/c" for "with." The answers were pencil-written with apparent erasures, and as a climax, she completely forgot to sign her name. Needless to say, she lost an opportunity.

Some guides for completing an application follow. Answer the question that is asked and keep to the point. Avoid ambiguity. Keep the form neat and clean. Do not change the question asked; but if you have additional remarks, reserve them for the space allotted for that purpose or make a special-remarks section. Be consistent in your answers. Be sure to answer all the questions. Observe the rules of good composition. Give accurate dates regarding employment. Write legibly or print if you cannot type the form. Make sure that you have followed carefully all directions. Insert all enclosures requested.

Many candidates for positions leave significant gaps in their history and experience. Some are hesitant to include age. Gaps in employment history always should be explained, at least by some brief reference. There is no point in concealing any relevant fact from a prospective employer. Age, for example, is never without significance, and the omission of a birth date may lead the employer to draw the wrong conclusions.

THE PERSONAL INTERVIEW

A personal interview, when seeking employment, is very important, not only for the employer but because it gives you an opportunity to visit the employing organization or person, to meet some of the people with whom you would be working in the situation and to learn about the philosophy, policies, and practices of the employer or association. Likewise, it gives the employer an opportunity to become acquainted with you and your philosophy. Distance, of course, may sometimes prevent you from going for an interview.

There are 3 steps to be taken in making a personal application through an interview: preparing for the interview, having the interview and following up the interview.

Preparing For the Interview

In preparation for the interview, find out all you can about the position in view, the organization, if there is one, and the prospective employer. Make a definite appointment and assemble beforehand general information about yourself on which the employer may ask questions.

Find out the requirements of the prospective position and decide how well you fulfill them and can fit yourself into the situation. You may need expert counsel on this.

You might learn something about the history of the employing agency, its philosophy and purposes, its founders, salient facts in its development, its physical facilities, and environment, its written personnel policies, and who are its contemporary personnel, particularly those with whom you will work most closely. It is advisable also to read any literature that it issues, such as annual reports and special publications.

Try to get some impression of the prospective employer through the correspondence you have received. Make sure of his correct name, title, and position. If possible, find out his approximate age, the qualities he prefers in employees, and all you can about his methods, characteristics, reputation, likes, hobbies, and prejudices. Try to find out whether he is fair and progressive. If he is, there will be advantage in working for him, and you will profit by association with him. Such inquiry is worth while, because you should consider your own time, service, and reputation, and your professional, personal, social and economic future.

Have your questions ready in advance.

Make a Definite Appointment

A definite appointment may be obtained by a letter, by telephone, or by telegram. The communication should be sent sufficiently far ahead to allow for an answer. If a letter is written, it should follow the general principles of correct business procedure suggested for the letter of application.

If a definite appointment is made, the interviewer, whether he is a counselor at the placement agency or an employer, will be sure to be in his office when you call, and he will have reserved time for you. The appointment brings you directly to the attention of the employer as a definite personality, a person who has a particular aim and a concise reason for coming to see him. It raises the status of the visit from one of casual encounter to one of business appointment. It gives you the opportunity to meet personnel with whom you would work and also to review facilities and other work equipment.

If considerable travel is involved to keep the interview, find out whether the employer is willing to pay all or part of the cost of the travel.

How May You Prepare Yourself to Present Your Qualifications?

This may be done by thinking through all the questions that are likely to be brought up, so that you are prepared to reply most advantageously. Do not try to answer the questions in a static way, but thinking them over beforehand should help to clarify your thoughts and prepare you to answer readily when questioned. If your professional biography has not been submitted by a placement agency, it is helpful to prepare a written statement of your credentials in such form that it can be left with the interviewer. In this outline the same information should be included as was suggested for the written letter of application. It is important, also, to have with you other credentials such as state registration card, membership cards of the ANA and NLN, and evidence of naturalization or birth certificate.

Getting Ready for the Interview

You will want to appear for the interview in good physical conditon. A poor physical appearance sometimes results from self-pity, worry, insufficient sleep, or loss of appetite. Good grooming, which is very important, includes cleanliness, carefully arranged hair, well-manicured nails, and appropriate dress.

It is suggested that you allow yourself ample time to arrive at the appointed hour, so that you will be neither late, too early, nor hurried. If you are obliged to wait, do not show impatience but be courteous to all with whom you come in contact. This will display poise, will lessen any nervousness, and will react favorably on others.

If it has been arranged for you to see the instituion and any of your potential coworkers when you have an employment interview, plan sufficient time to do so. It is not possible to do such sightseeing and visiting if only an hour or two is planned for your visit. Sometimes it is wise to plan for an overnight stay.

During the Interview

When you are being greeted by the interviewer, it is important to use his correct name and title and to observe the rules of courtesy. As a rule, it is better to let the interviewer ask the first questions. This will give you time to study the interviewer, to decide on what you wish to say, and to follow his line of thought. While answering the questions that are asked, also bring in whatever information you wish to convey. Occasionally an interviewer may wait for you to begin.

In any case keep his viewpoint before you and adjust your conversation to his, being careful not to run ahead. By studying him you can determine what points of your conversation interest him most, and it may be wise then to dwell on those to some extent.

Stick to the essentials and cover them. The interviewer is not interested in long stories about your past experiences, for his time is valuable. Avoid the personal element as far as possible. Answer all questions clearly, honestly, and without boasting, remembering to keep in mind the essentials. Admit any failure, if necessary. Show that you recognize the problem and tell what constructive efforts you have made to improve yourself because of past failure. Past failures are not necessarily handicaps for future employment. Make no rash promises. Tell no hard-luck story. Make no complaint about a former employer. Do not beg for the position. Inquiries as to the program of the organization and where you would fit in if you were employed will help both you and the employer to come to an intelligent decision.

The Question of Salary

It is best to let the interviewer introduce the subject of salary. If he first decides he wants you for the position, it is easier for you to get what you think you deserve. Moreover, after talking over the conditions and the prospects of the position, you are able to judge better what should be an adequate compensation.

Amount of salary will depend on the nature of the position, what standard of living is required of it, the responsibilities of the position, your capacity and skill in doing the work and the personnel policies of the employing agency.

If the employer states the salary he expects to pay, probably the best thing to do is to think it over. If he should ask how much you want, instead of naming a definite salary, you might say that you expect one proportionate to the requirements of the position and your ability to fulfill them, and that you will be glad to consider any reasonable offer. If he asks what is the least you will take, you may inquire whether there is a salary policy and on what basis increases are made, or what was the starting and the last salary of the person who held the position previously. Of course, you should be familiar with the employment standards, including salary, established by the state nurses association in the state in which the employing agency is located, for the type of position you are seeking. If it is an institution of higher education, you might ask about the salary range for the different faculty ranks. The salary recommendations of the state nurses association may be used as a guide in other situations.

Remember that salary is not the most important thing in the beginning. What you will be receiving in a few years is of far greater significance. A satisfactory salary usually accompanies success in a position and depends on your fitness for it, your growth in it, and the salary conditions of the time. Also find out what some of the other benefits, such as insurance, retirement plans, vacation, sick leave, inservice education, sabbaticals, and so forth. Most agencies have booklets describing their personnel policies and will give you a copy. Additional questions you may want to ask during the interview will relate to opportunities for advancement and for continuing education, types of assignments, and opportunities to participate in professional organization activities, to mention a few.

The Interview Follow-up

After your return home, write the interviewer a short letter expressing again your appreciation of his courtesy, and if further interviews seem advisable, arrange for them, using as much tactful persistence as possible.

If you are appointed to the desired position, your letter of acceptance is important because it gives you the opportunity of defining your interpretation of what already has been decided concerning salary, functions and the exact date of beginning your service. This letter should be kept as a matter of record, and it may become your contract. The letter offering you the position, if one has been received, should be saved also. It is equally important to write a follow-up letter even though you are not accepted for the position. Such a letter should be written because good losers are admired and also because the employer may have a position for you some other time.

Defeat in securing a position may lead to success. Defeat may be a good beginning if you study the procedure you followed to discover why you failed or why someone else was appointed. Then you can use this experience to improve your skill in applying for another position.

FILLING A POSITION AND THE MEANING OF SUCCESS

Obtaining a position is merely one of the preliminary steps in occupational success. More important is success in the job and attainment of the recognition which leads to professional advancement and personal gratification.

What is Success? How Is It Measured?

There are many definitions of success, varying from those which are purely materialistic to those of an entirely spiritual nature. Genuine success depends on the harmonious development of the whole personality. It is not measured by apparent external success or achievement. The real criterion is not money, culture, or fame. Inward satisfaction and peace are inherent in true happiness and are brought about by courageously facing and solving daily problems and living as well as you know how, doing the best you can under the circumstance, and continually seeking to improve.

On What Is Occupational Success Founded?

The prime requisite is a well-developed personality. Without it, exceptional abilities cannot be utilized to their fullest extent; and with it, ordinary talents can effect extraordinary results. Some traits found in the person with a well-developed personality are enthusiasm, sincerity, tact, self-control, ability to adhere to business and social amenities, sureness of self, cheerfulness, dependability, courage of convictions, dedication, consideration of others, sense of social and moral responsibility, dynamic force, magnetism, power of expression (written and spoken), social compatibility and pleasing appearance.

Opportunities will not be lacking for the well-prepared nurse who has the ability to adjust personality to the job situation, regardless of what it may be. Such adjustment means not only becoming used to work and liking it, but also becoming accustomed to social conditions at work, to working conditions other than social, and to the life pattern characteristic of the particular occupation and community.

After taking a position, do not think that you are prepared without further study to handle every problem that arises. That additional preparation is necessary you will learn through experience. All life is a learning process. Participate in inservice education programs in your employing organization. Keep up with advances in medical, nursing and related sciences or other relevant areas by reading professional periodicals and by participating in the activities of your professional organization. The responsibility for your continuing education is yours.

Causes of Failure

The causes of failure in a position hinge around you or the situation. Aside from the matter of technical ability and fitness for the particular job, success or failure depends largely on the emotions. Faulty mental habits resulting in social maladjustment and inability to adopt the right attitude toward life are the principal causes of failure. A common cause is lack of cooperation. This may arise because you are not aware of your role in the organization or because you fail to see the viewpoint of others. Cooperation may be defined as working with others in such a way that they are able to work with you.

Other important causes of failure are hot temper, sensitiveness and touchiness, intolerance of the shortcomings of others, tendency to hold resentment, insincerity, unreliability, dishonesty, nervousness, conceit, envy, discourtesy, sarcasm, intolerance, boastfulness, being too glum, sullenness, being argumentative, obstinacy, diffidence, lack of tact, failure to plan your work and do your share and unwise choice of friends.

Unwholesome recreation is also a causal factor in occupational failure. Many well-qualified persons have lost good positions because they were too much in love with pleasure or were "burning the candle at both ends," and thereby not only brought disaster to themselves but also caused great unhappiness to their families and friends. On the other hand, not taking sufficient time for relaxation and recreation is equally unwise and may lead to failure.

Although poor health or physical defects may be used as an excuse for failure, success may be possible in spite of such handicaps. The accomplishments of Helen Keller and others prove this point.

Other factors in the situation which may cause failure are petty jealousies, unfairness, animosity on the part of those with whom you work, or poor organization and administration of work.

We all need to recognize that we build our own professional record. References in our placement biographies are usually fairly objective. The past employer, on the whole, attempts not to handicap future employment of an employee by writing damaging references. Poor references, however, can be overcome by improving performance in the next position and with proper counseling. Some nurses vocally blame others — employers, colleagues, and people in the placement service — instead of understanding that they build their own professional records.

Turning Failure Into Success

How can you capitalize on a failure and become successful? The only real failure is acceptance of defeat. Sometimes a good, sound defeat at the beginning of a career can be a real challenge. It may show you your failings and limitations in time for you to do something about them, and it may keep you from thinking that you can succeed without working. An occasional defeat, even though a serious one, will tend to prevent you from overestimating your ability and asking more for yourself than anyone will give you.

It seems safe to say that probably there was never a big success in living, or a small one either, that was not founded in good part on some defeat.

If the failure should result in dismissal, the first thing to do is to ascertain the cause and to correct it. Then muster as much courage and confidence as you can, and go out at once to secure another job. No matter how unimportant the new one may be, it is better to accept it, meanwhile continuing to look for a better one. It is almost always to the person already employed that the opportunities for the best positions come. However, do not accept a job that holds no interest or future for you and yet keeps you tied down so that you will have no time to look for a desirable positon.

HOLDING OR FILLING A JOB

What is the difference between holding and really filling a job? *Holding* a job consists merely in doing the minimum amount of work in the maximum amount of time, showing little or no interest. If you are concerned with actually *filling* your position, you will know and like your work, take personal pride in it and do your best at all times. You will not be afraid of doing something that may seem to be a little out of your line. If you are a nurse in private practice caring for a patient at home, it may be necessary sometimes to perform certain acts that ordinarily are not considered nursing functions but become so because of the nature of the circumstances. Such activities as driving a patient to church, reading aloud, playing tennis, or even washing dishes may become nursing functions if they help in effecting a cure or relieving the situation. We believe that any activity that helps a patient spiritually, emotionally, mentally, or physically is a nursing function.

The willingness to see things from your employer's point of view and to be loyal to him is important in *filling* a position. Disloyalty is shown in criticizing employers or supervisors or their opinions, discussing confidential matters, or disregarding their instructions while appearing to follow them.

In the last analysis, then, to achieve real success it is necessary to *fill* the position and not merely to *hold* it. Many times the person of average ability who works hard to do this will succeed, while the brilliant person who lacks concentration, loyalty, or stability may fail.

RESIGNING FROM A POSITION

When inclined to resign from a position it is well to remember that probably no position is perfect and that it takes time to become completely adjusted to a new one. Unless there is unmistakable evidence that you are in the wrong position, or there are other serious reasons for changing, it is often advisable to remain for at least 3 years if the position is a responsible one. The first year probably will be spent in adjusting yourself to the job; the second year probably will help you to find your real place; in the third year you will be better able to decide whether or not you are in the right job. Even then, you should take ample time to think things over. Analyze the whole problem to determine the cause of the difficulty — to decide whether it lies in the situation itself or whether you are blameworthy. Before taking any decisive step, talk things over with your employer. This is only fair to him, and it is possible that he may have in view something better for you. If you neglect to do this, you may make the mistake of resigning just before you are about to receive an important promotion.

On the other hand, if you are certain that you are in a position for which you are not suited physically, mentally, emotionally, or technically, or in which there is no possible opportunity for advancement, you might be wise to make a change. However, do not resign until you have secured expert counsel.

Of course, if you are offered a more desirable positon, you might accept it even though you are satisfied with your present one, but first be sure that you are making a wise change. The new job should offer more in one or more of the following aspects: salary, opportunities for advancement, congenial and satisfying work, self-expression, and creative work.

In resigning from a position the "open-door" policy is the best to observe. Leave with a friendly feeling toward your directors, supervisors and colleagues. Some day you may wish to return, and their good-will undoubtedly would be an asset.

Interest in your work should be sustained to the very day of leaving. Work should be left in good condition even if it may necessitate your return for a few days after your resignation goes into effect.

When you decide to resign give notice within a reasonable time, the length depending on the type of position you hold, so that someone may be secured to replace you. In a position of some responsibility, a month usually is considered sufficient time, but the importance and the nature of the work should be considered as well as the rules of the organization. As a rule, a faculty member should give notice of a term. In an emergency the officers of administration are generally considerate and arrange for a short notice. It is also advisable to request a terminal interview for the purpose of discussing the employer's overall evaluation of your work during your employment with the organization.

If you are nursing in the field of private practice, never leave a patient until you have notified the physician and another nurse or some satisfactory type of relief has been secured.

The letter of resignation should include the intended date of leaving and the reasons for leaving. It should express regret, no matter what the causes for resigning may be. It is important that the letter be courteous, for it usually is kept on file. In the securing of a new position the reference of your former employer is most important. It will be influenced by his last impression of you, created partly by your letter of resignation.

As soon as you have decided to make a change in your employment, it is advisable to notify ANA PC&PS or other placement service that you will terminate your current employment at a stated time and ask that a reference be secured to add to your professional record. This insures that your professional record is kept current and that the reference is secured from someone who will write your evaluation from personal knowledge and not from a written record.

PROBLEMS

1. Why is it important for every nurse to have her biography compiled by the ANA PC&PS?

2. A counselor in a state nurses association, wrote that one of the major problems that she observes is:

Inadequate educational preparation for past and present positions and for the level of position for which the nurse wishes to apply. Because of insufficient numbers of nurses qualified for supervisory, teaching, or administrative positions, employers have promoted or employed inadequately prepared persons. Therefore, the nurse often experiences severe frustrations and may make a poor adjustment. This is detrimental to the nurse, the employing organization, and the patient. Yet, having once held such a position, the nurse finds it difficult to accept one in which she thinks she has less prestige and is frequently resistant to the suggestion that additional educational preparation is desirable. The counselor often hears the statement: "I know of many nurses no better qualified than I who are holding top positions. Why can't I do the same?"

(a) What suggestions would you make for overcoming this problem? (b) Why should you avoid accepting a position for which you do not have the required preparation? Discuss the legal implications involved if the position requires the delivery of direct nursing care.

3. A prominent nurse educator wrote to us recently saying: I find that our graduates are quite annoyed with directors of nursing they interview for positions. They go to the interview expecting to be asked about their philosophy and ideas about nursing. All that is discussed relates to the personnel policies in the situation. They wonder if they are being interviewed as "nurses" or as "hands and feet." If you had this kind of experience, what could you do to change the nature of the interview? How could you secure the kind of information you want about the nature of the work or the philosophy of the agency, in order to know whether or not you are really interested in the position?

4. If you ever found yourself in a situation where the standards of nursing were lower than you had been taught were essential, what would you do?

SUGGESTED REFERENCES*

* Erickson, J. L. "How Nurses Feel About Their First Experience." *Nursing Outlook,* **12:**62-65, May 1964.
Frey, M. "A Look at Job Description." *American Journal of Nursing,* **60:**1782-1783, Dec. 1960.
"If You Ask Me." *American Journal of Nursing,* **63:**62-63, May 1963.
* "The New PC and PS." *American Journal of Nursing,* **68:**328-331, Feb. 1968.
Sheppard, H. L. and Belitzky, H. A. *The Best Way to Find a Job.* Baltimore, Johns Hopkins Press, 1966.
Sleeper, R. "When You Apply for Your First Position." *Nursing Outlook,* **9:**230-231, Apr. 1961.
Wilkins, M. C. "Fitting the Individual to the Job." *Nursing Outlook,* **11:**291-293, Apr. 1963.

See References in Chapter 11, entitled "Opportunities Through the U.S. Civil Service Commission"; also, see announcements of positions from your own state Civil Service Commission.

* In each chapter all citations are footnoted and are not included here. All starred references are recommended for additional reading.

CHAPTER

15

Planning Economic Security

Every day of your life you are engaged in the most important business in the world—the task of managing your life so that you will maintain a sense of security. To keep a sense of security, a field of work for which you are prepared and which offers personal, professional and economic advantages is essential. Opportunity to develop and maintain a well-balanced life is equally important. This is attained through the satisfaction of spiritual, physical, mental, emotional, social and financial needs and is provided if there are desirable relationships in church, home, school and with friends and professional colleagues. Contributing as a nurse and a citizen to your profession and to society is also a means of satisfying your desires and thereby gives a sense of security. Worry and a sense of insecurity create inefficiency.

In this chapter, emphasis is given to your economic problems and their solution, because your economic condition has a great effect on your feeling of security. All of this is influenced greatly by your salary level and by your personal money management.

Since the status of nursing finances are affected by other medical care costs, we shall first look at total health-care costs.

HEALTH-CARE COSTS AND NURSING

Probably no country, today, is more health conscious, or is more concerned about the rising costs of health care than our own USA. The scope of health care made possible by improved medical care has greatly expanded during the past quarter century, and individuals have learned to expect much more from the members of the health team. However, the increasing use of hospital care, the complex equipment required for diagnosis and treatment, the increasingly expensive lifesaving drugs, and the rising cost of labor and services generally—including nursing service—all have tended to raise the cost of medical care.

It has been estimated that, in 1966, the total expenditures for health services in this country was $45.4 billion. During this same period, the per capita health expenditures came to $230.69. Thirty-two per cent of the consumer's expenditures for personal health care were met by insurance, which met 68 per cent of his expenditures for hospital care. In 1967, Federal funds paid for 28 per cent of the cost of hospital care.[1] Since the introduction of medicare and medicaid these expenditures have increased even more dramatically. It is suggested that you follow this situation in the daily newspapers.

The growing interest in health and sickness insurance as well as other forms of prepaid medical-care plans is testimony of the public's concern about the cost of medical care. Today, most people accept the concept of health care as including prevention and rehabilitation as well as sickness care. In turn, they expect increasingly broader coverage from health-care plans, both private and governmental. They have accepted broader, more comprehensive tax supported public health programs. Unions have grown increasingly interested in providing comprehensive health care for their members, and the principle of government responsibility for provision of medical care to certain groups, such as the American Indians, migratory workers, merchant seamen and military personnel and their dependents, is generally accepted. The government also assumes responsibility for certain illnesses or conditions, such as tuberculosis and mental illness.

Both Medicare and Medicaid have had and continue to have a tremendous impact on health care resources, particularly on expansion of facilities, including extended-care facilities, and on health-manpower needs. For example:

At the end of the second year of Medicare's existance [in the summer of 1968], the record shows that 20 million Americans aged 65 and older—some 10 per cent of the nation's population—[were] covered by the program. More than a million elderly people have received post-hospital care in nursing homes, as well as in their own homes attended by visiting nurses, physiotherapists, and other health specialists. Almost a million and a half older citizens have benefited from hospital outpatient diagnostic services.[2]

[1] American Nurses' Association. *Facts About Nursing: A Statistical Summary*, New York, The Association, 1968, pp. 214-215.
[2] "Medicare at 2nd Anniversary," *Nursing Outlook*, 16:65, Oct. 1968.

The financial status of nurses, who form the largest group of health workers in this country, is related intimately to the finances of health care. The altruistic tradition and the fact that nursing, predominately a woman's profession, has suffered from the social status accorded women, have worked to the economic disadvantage of nurses through the years and also have proved disadvantageous, in many instances, to patient care. However, today's nurse is working more effectively, through her professional association, toward achieving an adequate monetary recognition of her contribution to health care, at the same time that she works for optimum patient care and for recognition of the role which modern nursing can play in implementing this care. She must do this responsibly without jeopardizing in any way the high ethical standards of the profession and with knowledge of the relation of the cost of nursing to the total health-care costs. In a later section of this chapter, the ANA Economic Security Program will be discussed. However, every nurse has the responsibility for helping to raise the social and economic standards as well as that of maintaining high standards of professional practice. To do this responsibly she must keep herself reasonably well informed regarding trends in costs and financing of health care and trends in the general conditions of employment.

Nursing is one of the services included in health-care insurance and in many prepaid medical-care plans. You might want to study your own health insurance plan, or other prepaid plans, to determine the amount of nursing care provided and whether or not you think that it is adequate. You also will want to watch Federal legislation regarding actions which may be taken in the future and which may affect nursing. The ANA watches Federal legislation and, through its publication, *Capital Commentary,* advises state nurses associations on pending bills.

NURSES' INCOMES

The earnings of nurses vary. The amount earned by a nurse in a year depends on the type of work she does, the responsibilities involved in it, the salary policy of the particular organization or individual employer, and the geographic sections of the country where nurses are employed. Nursing has had excellent advances in salaries during the last few years. A current aim is to increase the salary of the clinical specialist so that increases are not so closely tied with promotions to administrative positions.

You easily can find the salary ranges for nurses employed in government public health agencies, Federal, state, or local, through reviewing the announcements of merit system units. Salaries for nurses in the commissioned military Corps are included in Chapter 11, "Nurses in the Federal Government." State nurses' associations and state PC&PS are sources of information on recommended salary ranges as well as on salaries in effect in the various types of places where nurses work. Your state nurses association also has available minimum employment standards, established by sections, for each occupational group in nursing.

The ANA collects, compiles and analyzes salary and related data from a variety of sources, and at each biennial convention establishes a national salary goal for the beginning practitioner in nursing. In 1968, this national salary was set at $8,500 for nurses with a baccalaureate degree and $7,500 for those with a diploma or an associate degree in nursing. For complete information you may wish to read the latest edition of *Facts About Nursing* and other references listed at the end of this chapter. New publications are coming out continuously, so you will wish to keep up to date on these. Also, you should take into consideration the fact that nurses have been experiencing salary increases on a fairly regular basis.

Earnings of Nurses in Education

A survey of salaries of nurses in education was made by the Research and Statistics Unit of the ANA in September 1968. At that time the median annual salary of all teachers and educational administrators was $8,820. In collegiate programs this median salary was $9,200, the median for those in hospital schools of nursing was lower, $8,530. Registered nurse faculty in schools of practical nursing earned a median salary of $8,400.

Earnings of Nurses in Hospitals and Similar Institutions[3]

The Bureau of Labor Statistics of the U.S. Department of Labor made a survey of employment conditions of employees in nongovernment, non-Federal, short- and long-term hospitals in the USA (excluding Alaska and Hawaii) in July 1966. The weekly salaries of registered professional nurses ranged from $100.50 for general staff nurses to $154 for directors of nursing. Salaries in state and local government hospitals were generally higher than in nongovernment ones; they were also higher in the larger metropolitan areas. In 1967, the ANA estimated that staff nurses in hospitals of 200 beds were earning $117 per week.

Nurses' salaries vary by location and size of institution. In general, salaries are highest in the West and lowest in the South; and highest in metropolitan areas with populations of 1 million or more.

Earnings of Nurses in Private Practice

Nurses in private practice are self-employed persons. Their fees usually are paid directly by the patient or his family, or in some instances by major medical insurance or Workman's Compensation Boards. Their fees

[3] American Nurses' Association, *Facts About Nursing: A Statistical Summary*, New York, The Association, 1968, pp. 130-131.

comprise their total income and they must pay a percentage of their social security tax out of this income. They are not covered by the benefits, such as vacation, sick leave and holidays, ordinarily allowed in other nursing positions. According to the ANA Research and Statistics Unit, standard fees established by state nurses associations for private practice nurses, in 1968, ranged from $38 per day in one state to a low of $24 in another state. In California, a higher fee is charged if the nurse is a clinical specialist.[4]

The fee charged by nurses in private practice varies somewhat by geographical area. Higher fees may be paid for the care of patients within certain conditions, such as alcoholics, and for patients in intensive care units. Group nursing of 2 patients for 8 hours generally is done for a fee of the usual rate for one patient plus one half, which is shared by both patients.

Earnings of Nurses in Public Health

In the continuing upward trend of salaries of nurses in public health, salaries paid in local official health units remain generally higher than in nonofficial agencies. According to the NLN annual survey in 1968, the median salary of staff nurses in official units was $7,225; in nonofficial agencies it was $6,938. Nurses employed by boards of education fared somewhat better with a median salary of $7,611.[5]

Most agencies provide paid annual sick leave and cumulative sick leave. Most agencies also provide workman's compensation while some carry unemployment insurance, and health insurance plans.

Most of the agencies provide for social security coverage, while many provided both social security and some other retirement plan.

Because of the trend toward requiring a nurse to drive her own car at work in public health, most agencies reimburse the nurse on the basis of a rate per mile driven. Some agencies also pay the additional business insurance.

Earnings in Occupational Health Nursing

Beginning in 1960, salary data for occupational health nurses on a national basis have been available through the U.S. Bureau of Labor Statistics. The average weekly earnings of industrial nurses increased 16.1 per cent between 1963 and 1967. In February 1967, these nurses earned an average of $119 weekly. These earnings ranged from $92.50 in Greenville, South Carolina and Portland, Maine, to $138 in Beaumont-Port Arthur, Texas. Salaries generally were higher in the West and lowest in the South.[6]

[4] *Ibid.*, p. 129.

[5] "Salaries Paid by Public Health Nursing Services – 1968," *Nursing Outlook,* **16**:54-57, Dec. 1968.

[6] American Nurses' Association, *Facts About Nursing: A Statistical Summary,* New York, The Association, 1968, p. 151.

Summary

In all occupational fields in nursing, the better salaries are proportionate to preparation, professional or technical efficiency, work experience and personal qualifications. Also, the area of the country where you work will affect your salary. Higher salaries are more common in the Western and the Great Lakes areas, and in the larger cities; they are lowest in the South. Promotions to positions of greater responsibility and increased salary come as you grow in experience and obtain additional educational preparation. Recognition also is increasing for the expert practitioner, the clinical expert.

THE ANA ECONOMIC SECURITY PROGRAM

The ANA economic security program, adopted in 1946, is designed to help nurses to attain economic security and a standard of living in line with the educational preparation required and the professional services that they provide. The program is based on the belief that professional nurses share the responsibility for promoting high quality nursing service of the amount and the kind required. Inherent in this, if the supply of nurses is to be increased, is concern for economics, or the protecting and the improving of the economic status of nurses.

The program has as its broad goal the obtaining for nurses of the right to have a voice in determining the conditions under which they will practice their profession.

The employment standards for the economic security program are set by the various sections of the state nurses association and the implementation of the economic security program is carried out through the state association within the general framework established by the ANA. Under this program, nurses in a given institution or agency may designate the state association to act as their bargaining agent in employee-employer negotiations.

Collective bargaining involves mutual negotiation of a written contract embodying the agreement reached on salaries, hours, working conditions, pensions, holidays, vacations and other matters of common interest, including standards of practice. The ANA views collective bargaining as the means of communication and negotiation for better patient care. Also involved is recognition of employee representation and bargaining in good faith by representatives of employees and management. Basic to all of this is the freedom and the right of employees to form a group or an association, and to choose a representative to speak for them.

Because nurses are employees for the most part, they cannot decide unilaterally on their conditions of work, yet it is reasonable to expect that professional nurses should have a voice in determining the conditions under which they will practice their profession. Beginning in 1968, the ANA Commission on Economic and General Welare, with the support of the Board of

Directors of the ANA, launched an expanded economic security program. Under this program, the ANA provides direct assistance to state nurses associations in organizing and representing nurses. Assistance with state and local projects are determined by mutual agreement of the ANA and the state nurses associations involved.[7]

It is suggested that you read the references on economic security at the end of this chapter and follow the work of the economic security program by reading new articles as they appear in the professional journals. Remember, when considering economic security, to maintain your perspective by considering it alongside prevailing social and economic factors that of necessity affect nursing.

PERSONAL FINANCIAL PLANNING

Wise use of income is possible only by good planning. There is a plan that will suit your needs, tastes and available funds. Your problem is to determine just what that plan is. Any method of life that fails to take into consideration some scheme of financial planning may cause as many difficulties as trying to build a house without a set of specifications.

One's goals are essential to consider. Should I continue my education this year or wait until next year? Can I afford to get this extra dinner dress or am I already spending too much for such extras? Is it more fun to entertain frequently than to spend money for clothes? Should I buy a garbage disposal unit and a color television set or trade in the old car for a new one? Should I take a trip to Hawaii this year or wait until my savings reserve is larger? Am I spending wisely and putting aside as much as I should? What have I to show for what I have earned in the past? What will I probably have 10, 20, or 30 years from now? These are some of the questions confronting everyone who faces the future honestly. You may want luxuries and pleasures. You may desire to travel. You realize that money saved wisely now means greater independence in the future, that it means security when out of work, or that it may mean greater professional and social opportunities. You decide to save regularly and build up a surplus by developing a financial plan, or budget, that provides for spending less than you earn.

Whatever choices for spending you make, your guiding principle should be to use your money in such a way as to provide the greatest satisfaction and benefits to all concerned. If you spend your money according to a long-range plan, you will usually get more out of life and will be secure in the knowledge that you have a better chance for security. During a period of rising economy and high cost of living, such as we have been experiencing, thrift has a different meaning than it has during periods of economic stress. Furthermore, an age geared to a high level of spending will influence your habits.

[7] "ANA Commission Launches Expanded Economic Security Program," *ANA in Action*, 2:5, Mar./Apr. 1968.

Budgeting

There are sample budget forms obtainable from banks and other sources such as the Bureau of Home Economics in the U.S. Department of Agriculture and the Institute of Life Insurance. It is important, however, to realize there is no such thing as a standard budget that will fit all cases. As living expenses and taxes increase, budget plans necessarily change. Budgets also vary in accordance with living standards — low, moderate or high.

Successful money management requires 3 considerations: (1) determination of a definite plan, (2) consistent adherence to it and (3) wise laying-aside of funds for future security.

Some people manage their money well without keeping accounts. Others put their plans on paper — the budget — and they keep a record of all expenditures.

How an income is managed depends on personalities, the individual's interest or abilities in financing, the number in the family to be considered, mode of living, health needs, education costs, responsibilities and other factors, such as whether to own your home or rent.

The variation in cost of living in different cities and localities naturally affects the budget. By keeping a record of actual expenditures under different divisions, you get some idea of what you must allow when budgeting. Taxes, food, shelter and household, clothing, personal operating, advancement and entertaining, church and charity contributions, and savings are the principal ones for distributions of an income.

It is advisable to indicate food expenditures first. The amount provided will depend on whether you take your meals out or at home and whether you do your own cooking or live with others on a cooperative basis. After making the food estimate, add (1) the amount paid for rent and taxes and (2) your estimate of what you will spend for clothing. If you live in an apartment or a house, estimate what it costs to operate it, such as probable cost of heat, light, water, gas, cleaning, household supplies, replacements and improvements. Apportion whatever is left to such other uses as personal expenses, advancement, church and charity contributions, and savings.

Base your estimate of what you will spend for clothing on the clothing you have on hand and what you expect to buy. Cleaning, pressing, and alterations also should be considered. A careful investigation of your wardrobe to determine your needs for work and play, the purchase of garments that are durable, appropriate and attractive, and the taking advantage of worthwhile sales are points that should be kept in mind in making your clothes budget. Determine what you need and buy only that. Probably everyone needs to "splurge" now and then, and if in general you budget wisely, you can afford to go off the budget once in a while.

Personal expenses include such items as carfare, postage, toilet articles, hairdress and manicures. These extras count up rapidly, so they need to be watched carefully. Under advancement, estimated expenses of education,

Table 4. SUGGESTED DISTRIBUTION OF MONTHLY INCOME

Monthly Income[a]	No. in Family	Savings	Food	Housing[b]	Clothing	Trans- porta- tion[c]	Personal, Medical, and Other[d]
300	2	$ 15	$ 75	$ 85	$ 22	$ 36	$ 67
	4	7	93	86	35	33	46
350	2	20	87	97	29	45	72
	4	11	105	100	40	42	52
400	2	24	95	112	34	50	85
	4	14	116	116	45	44	65
450	2	32	99	125	38	59	97
	4	18	130	130	52	54	66
500	2	37	105	140	43	66	109
	4	23	135	145	59	60	78
550	2	47	112	155	49	71	116
	4	28	142	160	63	66	91
600	2	60	120	165	55	77	123
	4	35	150	175	68	72	100
700	2	84	135	175	63	90	153
	4	49	157	200	77	85	132
800	2	105	145	190	70	103	187
	4	60	165	220	90	103	162
900	2	130	153	205	81	126	205
	4	78	180	230	103	126	183
1000	2	155	160	215	90	140	240
	4	100	190	235	125	140	210

[a] After taxes and payroll deductions.
[b] Includes shelter, fuel, furnishings, appliances, and equipment.
[c] Includes automobile purchase and operation, and public transportation.
[d] Includes advancement, recreation, gifts, education, and other.
Source: American Bankers Association. Savings Division. *Personal Money Management*. New York, The Association, 1967, p. 22.

recreation, newspapers, health, professional association dues, and clubs are calculated. Savings is one of the most important items and is considered a social and a personal obligation. This item needs to be divided into at least 4 sections: (1) provision for illness, (2) provision for emergencies, (3) provision for retirement and (4) provision for dependents (if any). Having a reserve for entertainment, vacation and "Christmas money" may be considered a temporary saving.

Obviously, where the total income is small the greater share of it goes necessarily for taxes, food, rent, clothing and operation of a car, church and charity contributions, leaving a limited marginal allowance for personal expenses and advancement and entertaining, with savings probably covering no more than insurance premiums and a small emergency fund. As a rule, when income increases, living expenses advance, but then there is a larger opportunity for savings, advancement, entertainment and personal operating expenses.

After you work out a tentative financial plan for a year, you probably will find it helpful to adjust your plans to suit the expenses of the different months. A suggested distribution of income for families of 2 and of 4 members after income taxes are deducted can be found in Table 4. Savings goals in this example have been set high, as a challenge – a target for maximum effort. Marriage will affect your budget, of course, since the plans you make together must meet the goals and values of each of you.

In the March 17, 1969 issue of *The Washington Post* (pp. 1, 6), there is an article on model budgets issued by the Bureau of Labor Statistics. For the first time these are designed to help those living on lower, moderate and higher standards. These budgets are expected to be updated in the Spring of each year. Copies of the present survey, *Three Standards of Living: For an*

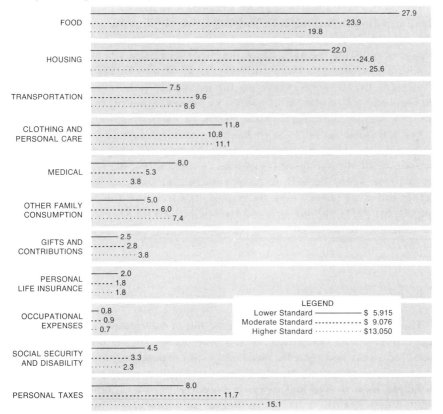

Fig. 15-1. Breakdown of the family dollar in model budgets issued by the Federal Government. (Courtesy of The Washington Post)

Urban Family of Four Persons, Spring 1967, can be purchased for $1.00 from the Government Printing Office, Washington, D.C., 20402, or from the regional offices of the U.S. Bureau of Labor Statistics. It is anticipated that these budgets will be of assistance to public assistance agencies, voluntary social and welfare agencies and other similar groups. Figure 15-1 shows the breakdown of the family dollar in current budgets issued by the government.

Budgeting for Church and Charity Contributions

What each individual contributes and to whom is a matter of personal choice. Most of us feel an obligation to contribute to our church, to the community fund and to a variety of charities. The important consideration, from the standpoint of the budget, is that the item be included.

The Checking Account—an Aid in Budgeting

One of the best aides in keeping a budget is to pay by check. Your checkbook can almost become your account book. A checking account has many advantages. It is useful primarily for the convenience it affords and as a means of reducing the hazards of theft or loss of cash. If a check is lost, you can stop payment and issue another check. Money lost is rarely returned. Canceled checks serve as receipts for payments, and a canceled check is a receipt that will stand up in court. As an indication of financial responsibility, a regular checking account also is an aid in obtaining credit.

For checking accounts with balances under a certain minimum, banks charge a fee, called a "service charge." Since additional charges are frequently made if large numbers of checks are written, the nurse having such an account would be wise to have enough cash on hand for small requirements and issue checks only for important purchases, for regular payments such as for the telephone, gas and electricity, and for payments on accounts, on insurance or in cases where receipts are desirable but are not likely to be given.

PROBLEMS AND METHODS OF SAVING

The reasons for saving are numerous, but in their general aspects, at least, they are probably similar for all. We save for the future, hoping to educate ourselves, rear and educate our families or dependents, supply necessities and comforts during illness and old age, and thus to enjoy peace of mind and sufficient time to live and develop properly. A special effort to save may mean a new television set, a trip abroad, or a new car. It may mean getting married or putting aside funds for Christmas spending, insurance, taxes, or vacation. For many it means money in reserve for emergencies.

One of the chief reasons for saving is to provide for security in old age. Although the Federal Government's social security plan provides for a small basic old-age retirement for many people, all people who receive benefits under the plan need to supplement it in order to have a sufficient income. Many organizations have pension or retirement plans, over and above social security, which usually require contributions from employee and employer. If by some chance you are in one of the very few positions where you do not benefit under the social security program or a plan of the organization which employs you, the need for giving consideration to some plan for future protection is even greater. To all, saving means funds for use when needed and a sense of security.

One can, of course, overemphasize economic security as a way of life. While economic problems can create worries, economic security may not solve all your problems. Furthermore, your philosophy of life can be a major factor in helping you to maintain a true security regardless of economic status.

When to Save

The sooner that saving is started the better. Begin saving now and save regularly. It is so very easy to put off saving until tomorrow, with the result that sickness or old age may come along and you will not be prepared to care for yourself or your dependents. After preparing a budget, it is a good idea to determine how much should be saved each pay day and to begin at once to save. If you are about to graduate, make up your mind to start your savings by using a part of your first salary. Saving should be a regular habit instead of an occasional whim or fancy. It is the steady plodder who puts a little aside each month as a part of a regular, well-organized plan who gets ahead and builds security, not the person who saves only at irregular intervals whenever she happens to sense the obligation and plans at the same time when and how she will spend it. Some points for consideration are: (1) determine what you need to save for taxes, (2) set a minimum amount to save for the future and (3) fix your standard of living on the balance of your income.

Saving should be planned in accordance with a well-rounded program of: (1) short-term investments to provide funds to be used in case of immediate need or emergency and (2) long-term investments that can be held as sound, regular income-producing security for old age and for possible unpredictable economic emergencies or calamities.

The most common forms of short-term investments are: (1) savings accounts (with Federal Deposit Insurance Corporation coverage up to $15,000), and (2) government bonds (preferably U.S. Government). For these there is usually a ready market, so that they may be converted into cash within a short period of time to meet any emergency needs.

The most common forms of long-term investments include: (1) stocks; (2) annuity and retirement insurance; (3) state, municipal and industrial bonds;

(4) mutual funds; (5) real estate and real estate mortgages and (6) sound business investments. It should be borne in mind that stock prices are usually less stable than bond prices, and emergency sales of stocks may create losses.

A well-rounded program of investments for the average working person might include: (1) savings through banks or building and loan funds and Government bonds, (2) social security insurance and (3) a program for supplementary annuity through insurance and pension plans. As a single nurse, just starting out in the profession, you might want to be sure you have at least the following plan to begin with: (1) social security coverage, (2) term insurance for a minimum of $1,000 or $2,000 and (3) a savings bank account that you build up until a reserve of at least 6 months' salary is achieved. Later, as it becomes possible, you might augment savings through either or both of the following: (1) a variable annuity insurance and (2) securities, preferably common stocks of investment quality. Mutual funds or the monthly investment plans offer ways of investing monthly.

The Savings Account

Usually, the first step in building a financial plan is to start a savings account. One of the greatest values of a savings account is the security that it ensures in such crises as illness, accidents, or other emergency financial demands. Everyone should maintain a savings account even though the amount of money involved is very small.

How much should you keep in a savings account? That depends on whether you are responsible for yourself only or for a family. Some banks have suggested that as an initial reserve fund, for a moderate income the savings account should be built to an amount equal to at least 3 to 6 months' income. Some experts suggest that you try 5 to 10 per cent of your take home pay as a starting basis for your savings plan. However, even small sums *regularly* set aside in a bank, multiplied by compound interest, will grow rapidly.

Where and How Savings Accounts Can Be Kept

There are 4 places where savings accounts are generally opened: commercial banks, mutual savings banks, savings and loan associations and credit unions.

Savings accounts in banks pay interest compounded quarterly or semi-annually. Some savings banks pay from the day of deposit if savings are left on deposit for the entire interest period. Up to $20,000, these savings are as safe as the U.S. Treasury if deposited in a bank or building and loan association insuring them in the Federal Deposit Insurance Corporation.

The "club" method of saving is a popular form of saving. It consists in making weekly deposits in a bank of from 25 cents to $5 for a certain period of time, usually about 50 weeks, at which time the club matures and the total deposited is then available. There are many objectives for club savings accounts, such as Christmas or vacation funds, the payment of insurance premiums or taxes, and savings for education.

A popular method of savings is through the purchase of bank certificates in units of $1,000 or more. These pay 5 per cent or more and are available at banks and savings and loan associations. In savings and loan associations (also known as building and loan associations), a number of shares are purchased, ranging in cost. Interest usually is paid quarterly or semi-annually. The interest rate ranges from 4 to 6 per cent.

Credit unions generally are organized among employees in an industry, or by occupational groups, such as teachers. They are in effect cooperative societies that take savings from and make loans to their members.

Savings Through Government Bonds

U.S. Government bonds are recognized as one of the safest investments. This method of saving is combined sometimes with a payroll savings plan. Bonds also can be bought directly from the U.S. Treasury Department, and in some communities such bonds are sold by banks and dealers. Similar to a savings account, savings bonds are a source of ready cash. Series "E" bonds, bought since February 1, 1957, earn $4\frac{1}{4}$ per cent when held to maturity — 7 years and 9 months. Interest is at a lower rate if the bonds are cashed before maturity.

Series "H" savings bonds pay $4\frac{1}{4}$ per cent when held to 10-year maturity. Interest is paid on these bonds by a U.S. Government Treasury check every 6 months.

Series "E" bonds may be held beyond maturity, and interest continues beyond maturity date. Series "H" bonds issued between June 1, 1959 and November 1, 1965 may be retained an addtional 10 years past maturity, and interest will continue.

In some instances the bonds may be left with the nearest Federal Reserve savings bank, free of charge. There is otherwise some danger of loss unless a safety deposit box is used.

For further information about Government savings bonds, you can obtain current materials on "E" and "H" bonds and treasury notes (paying high interest in 1970) from the U.S. Treasury Department or from any Federal Reserve bank.

Savings Through Home Ownership

There seems to be a difference of opinion on the value of home ownership as a means of saving. Some people believe it is a good way to invest money, particularly as a hedge against inflation. Before deciding on whether to buy or rent, it is important to study the various aspects of your situation: your personal inclinations, the permanence of your position, the size of your family, your health, how much time you will spend in your home, your income and what each will mean to you. Reading Chapter IV on "What You Should Know About Housing," in the 1967 edition of *Personal Money Management,* published by The American Bankers Association, may help you in making a decision on whether to rent or own a home.

Savings Through Stocks and Bonds

Other investments for consideration are stocks and bonds. Stocks are securities that represent an ownership interest in a corporation. If a company has issued both preferred and common stocks, the preferred has the prior claim on dividends and, in the event of liquidation, assets. Claims of both common and preferred stockholders are secondary to claims of bondholders or other creditors of the company. Common stockholders assume the greater risk, but they generally exercise the greater control and may gain greater reward in the form of capital appreciation or growth and protection against inflation. The terms *common stock* and *capital stock* often are used interchangeably when the company has no preferred stock. A bond is basically an IOU or promissory note of a corporation, usually issued in multiples of $1,000 although $500 denominations are not uncommon. A bond is evidence of a debt on which the issuing company usually promises to pay the bondholder a specified amount of interest for a specified length of time and to repay the loan on the expiration date. In every case, a bond represents debt; its holder is a creditor of the corporation and not a part owner as is the shareholder.

Popular forms of investing for many people are through the monthly investment plan of the New York Stock Exchange member firms or through the purchase of mutual funds on a regular basis. These 2 forms of investing provide for monthly payments. Dividends credited to your account may be reinvested automatically or paid to you directly. The plans are noncontractual; that is, you can discontinue them at any time. Mutual funds offer the features of diversification and professional management.

Before investing in any form of securities, it is vitally important to secure competent advice and full information. Every properly equipped broker's office has an efficient research department. Do not accept guidance from any individual without knowing his connections, his experience and the record of his firm. Check it with your bank. Many financial tragedies have occurred through misplaced confidence. Avoid speculation unless you can take the risk. No matter what securities you are considering, as an investor you should know the facts about the company you are investing in—the nature of the business, the suitability of the investment for you, the past performance of the company, the earnings over a period of years, and the future prospects of the company. Stock prices, in particular, fluctuate according to the business situation, political situation and many other factors. So, if you invest, you have to be prepared to take some risks and invest only if you can afford it; that is, if you have sufficient income, savings and other forms of protection such as life insurance.

Investing Through an Equity in Business

Going into or investing in business is another way to make money and to save if you have built up substantial savings. In this case, it is important to secure expert advice from commercial bankers and other successful business persons. When agreements need to be made, it is advisable to consult a lawyer. Nurses would do well if they could convert their hobbies into businesses at retirement, but they should be sure of their prospects of developing a clientele.

If you have not had much experience in investing, it may be advisable to consult your banker or insurance broker in order to work out a well-balanced investment plan. Or, if you have considerable money to invest, you may wish to open an agency account with a bank.

Protection Through Insurance

Insurance is a system of collective security through which the individual, in consideration of (or in exchange for) regular contributions, called premiums, is afforded a degree of protection against the financial crises arising as a result of injury, sickness, old age and death.[8]

All insurance companies are offering very attractive policies, and you can secure those which will fit your needs after you have investigated the different types and have learned what is expected of you in each type and what return you can expect, when and how. Those insurance plans that are probably of greatest interest to you are endowments; retirement annuity incomes; life, accident and sickness insurance; and the various hospitalization, surgical and medical care insurance plans. Some insurance may be secured through individual purchase of policies. Other types may be obtained through group plans with various insurance companies. Some are obtained through mutual insurance of a group itself, with the members creating their own insurance protection, while others are provided through legislative acts such as workmen's compensation acts (employer financed), the *Social Security Act* and other similar laws, such as the law that provides Medicare. Not all these insurance or protection plans are available to or satisfactory for all nurses, but it is advisable to know about them so that you may assist others to obtain the security they need.

Endowment Plan

An endowment policy is a method of insuring and saving and is payable to the insured at the end of a definite period. If the insured dies before the

---

[8] As defined by Alfred W. Oliphant when he was Senior Administrative Analyst, Bureau of State Services, U.S. PHS, Federal Security Agency.

policy matures, the face value of the policy is paid to her beneficiary or estate. When the endowment policy is paid up, the face value may be collected or left with the company, electing one of the options provided for future payment.

Many nurses, after carrying for from 10 to 20 years endowment policies maturing for sums of $1,000 and up, unfortunately then have collected and spent this money for unsound investments and thereby lost what they saved. Their experience emphasizes the wisdom of leaving the money with the company, exercising one of the options for future payments, or carefully reinvesting the proceeds, if they are not urgently needed, in another endowment, an annuity, government bonds, high-grade stocks and bonds, or a sensibly priced home, rather than dissipating them on luxuries or poorly selected investments.

Annuity Plan

The retirement or annuity income is a form of insurance contract that makes positive financial provision for old age. It guarantees the payment of a stipulated income beginning at an age selected by the insured and continuing as long as life lasts. Policies also may be written to provide regular incomes for surviving children or other dependents. It is probably one of the best systematic savings plans.

The combination of life insurance and annuity provides a most economical method of life insurance, savings, and old age retirement — truly a good investment. Cash value is always there for emergencies and can be borrowed on without affecting the plan and can be repaid in small sums and at any time, depending on the situation. Of course, should death occur, the amount borrowed will be deducted from the face amount prior to paying a beneficiary.

It is important to realize that all endowment and annuity plans have 4 or more settlement options: (1) payment in cash, (2) leaving with company at interest and withdrawal rights in part or total amount, (3) annuity life income guaranteed for 5, 10, 15 or more years and (4) a certain number of dollars for a certain period of time. It is also important to remember that the purchase of retirement insurance while you are young reduces the annual premium, since payment can be spread over a greater period than if purchased late in life.

Nurses teaching in colleges or universities are eligible for annuity plans such as the Teachers Insurance and Annuity Association (TIAA) and the College Retirement Equities Fund (CREF). Information regarding these can be obtained from TIAA-CREF at 730 Third Ave., New York, New York, 10017.

Social Security Insurance

The *Social Security Act* sets up a system of Federal old-age and survivor benefits financed by compulsory contributions from employers and employees. This is designed to pay retirement annuities to all qualified workers except those in certain exempted employments. Social Security insurance also provides disability payments and monthly payments, or a lump sum death payment to certain survivors. One of its great advantages is that, unlike employer sponsored pension plans, it is completely portable. The passage of the 1950 amendments increased benefits and extended coverage to nurses in private practice (under the self-employed classification) and to nurses employed in nonprofit institutions under certain conditions. Professional nurses who had been excluded from benefits now may secure coverage. The 1967 amendment to the Social Security Act improved and extended the 1965 amendments to the law. The references on the Social Security benefits at the end of this chapter describe these benefits.

Under 1967 amendments to the Social Security law, contribution rates for 1969-70 are 4.8 per cent for the employed worker and 4.8 per cent for the employer, making a total of 9.6 per cent. Self-employment tax is 6.9 per cent. In addition, the amount of earnings taxed were increased to $7,800 annually. The law provides for a gradual increase until 1987. By 1987, the employee and employer tax will each be 5.9 and the tax for self-employed persons will be 7.9 per cent. It is wise to keep informed about social security tax payments and benefits as they change from time to time.

Although social security benefits do not give nurses complete retirement security, state nurses associations through their economic security programs ask employers to provide both social security and supplementary retirement plans for nurses. These associations also sponsor individual retirement insurance plans for the self-employed nurses in private practice to supplement social security. The ANA consistently has supported legislation to increase social security benefits, so that nurses will be more adequately protected.

Some states also provide old-age annuities, the nature of which varies from state to state.

Straight or Regular Life Insurance

A straight (or whole) life policy is one of the least expensive forms of life insurance in terms of annual premiums per $1,000 of protection for dependents. For the young nurse with one or more other persons dependent on her continued earnings, it affords great protection for the money. Although a straight life policy requires the payment of premiums every year until death, most companies provide that it can be converted on the basis of cash surrendered, paid-up insurance, or an annuity at the option of the insured when the burden of paying the annual premiums becomes too great or when the need for insurance is reduced on the death of parents or the growth of children to maturity. While the limited payment plans provide higher cash values than straight life, their cash value can be used to provide an annuity for life under the income option of policy. For younger nurses a policy paid up at 65 is a good plan. Both plans will accumulate a cash reserve value that may be used as a basis for borrowing.

If there are no dependents, it is advised that one have a policy adequate to provide for the necessary expenses of the insured at the time of her death. A popular life insurance policy is the initial payment life type in which the premiums are paid only until the insured is 65, the usual age of retirement. A straight or limited payment life policy is just the opposite of an annuity; the former protects someone else if you die, while an annuity takes care of you at retirement for life.

Term Insurance

Term insurance is the least expensive of all insurance. Nurses with young dependents or disabled older nurses might find this the answer to their protection problem. It is usually obtainable for 5-, 10-, 15-, or 20-year periods, sometimes renewable, almost always convertible to regular insurance. It has no cash value as a rule, that is no savings value that can be taken in a lump sum. You cannot borrow on it, and it cannot become paid up. However, it offers the largest face value for the outlay. Term policies may be either convertible or nonconvertible. If convertible, they act to insure insurability in later years — on conversion into permanent plans. You should be sure that your term policy is renewable and convertible. This kind of insurance should be considered by the person who needs extensive protection for a limited time, such as during the years of carrying a mortgage or other type of loan. Although insurance agents sometimes ignore this policy, it is one with which all nurses should be familiar.

Health and Accident Insurance

Sickness or accident insurance pays on the investment only in the event that the insured gets sick or has an accident. Compensation for accidents or illness resulting from conditions of employment is provided for some by workmen's compensation laws. While there are still some gaps in coverage in nonfederal government employment, most nurses are now covered by workman's compensation.

It is wise to study the offerings on accident and health policies of reliable insurance companies and make comparisons. You might investigate to see whether there is any provision where you are working or through your nursing organization for group insurance, and if there is, you may wish to avail yourself of one or more of these plans. Most employers provide for some form of hospitalization and medical-surgical insurance, which provides coverage for medical and hospital bills and for some form of insurance that will replace, at least in part, lost income resulting from illness or accident.

Through some of the state nurses associations, nurses now have the opportunity for securing insurance for hospitalization, medical care and retirement plans at advantageous rates. Reduced group rates for automobile insurance, discount buying, and other items also provide economies for the nurse.

Group Insurance Plans

Group insurance plans, carried by some employers for the benefit of their employees usually, represent the cheapest form of insurance that it is possible to obtain. Group insurance usually is allocated to employees on a basis of monthly salary, and the contributions usually are paid either in full or in part by the employer. This type of insurance is generally discontinued at the termination of employment of the employee, but it usually may be converted at a slightly higher rate on a personal basis. As pointed out elsewhere in this chapter, group insurance is available for all types of nurses now, because even the nurses in private practice can benefit from group plans sponsored by state nurses associations.

In 1962, the Minnesota Nurses Association negotiated a contract with the Twin-City Hospital Council (Minneapolis-St. Paul), which provides for a pension plan that remains in effect as long as the nurse works in any of the 21 hospitals under contract. This was a break-through toward the idea of portable pension plans privately financed.

PROFESSIONAL LIABILITY PROTECTION

Professional liability insurance protects you as an insured nurse against possible claims or damage suits for alleged carelessness and negligence in the performance of your nursing functions. Remember: all persons are liable for their own negligence that causes injury to another person on his property.

Professional liability insurance was authorized by the House of Delegates of the ANA in May 1950 because of the increasing trend of the public to sue the nurse and of the courts to hold the nurse responsible for her professional acts. The policy includes personal liability in all states except Texas and Louisiana.

Protection is available to you, when you become a nurse, under the ANA group professional liability insurance plan which is underwritten by the Globe Indemnity Company. All registered nurses are eligible—there are no age restrictions. Liability coverage may be purchased starting from a minimum of $5,000. There is no limit on the amount of coverage that may be purchased. In 1964, rates began at $5.50 for minimum coverage for 1 year. Also available are 3-year rates. The application for this insurance can be secured from the ANA Economic Security unit, 10 Columbus Circle, New York, N.Y. 10019.

PLANNING FOR RETIREMENT

When we are young we seldom think about the idea of retiring. However, later on most of us look forward to the time when we can retire and enjoy the leisure to do some of the many things we cannot do during our working lives. While by far the majority of nurses marry and have families, most of them, as is true of women in other professions, return to their professional occupation of nursing when the children are old enough to permit this. Therefore, many nurses enjoy working up to, and sometimes beyond the generally accepted retirement age of 65 years.

Whether or not you plan to work until you are 65, it is wise to plan for the older years of your life. We have already talked about various ways of planning your financial security. However, it is not enough to be financially secure; we should also plan our lives so that we have a variety of interests, social, civic and cultural, which will make our older years pleasant and happy ones. The person with broad interests, who enjoys not only the active sports and activities, but also those that are more intellectually and socially focused, will have more varied interests to enjoy throughout life.

Many nurses who have been active in their professional nursing association find that after retirement they can continue to make a contribution to their profession. They now have the time to serve on committees and to enter into interesting activities in the association more extensively than was perhaps possible when they were busy working, or raising a family, and they enjoy the opportunity of serving.

PLANNING AN ESTATE

All of us will be concerned, at some time, with estate planning, or in counseling patients to plan their estates. Therefore, knowing about wills is helpful. A will is a declaration of what a person wishes to have done with his property after his death. Preparation, content and various items concerning wills differ from state to state.

Why You Should Know the Essentials of Wills

It is important to know about wills so that, if it is necessary for you to assist in making or probating a will, you can carry out the procedures correctly. If no lawyer is available, you may be called on to draft a will for a patient.[9] The fact that you are able to assist a patient in making his will may contribute greatly to his peace of mind.

Although you seldom, if ever, may be called on to draw up a will, it will not be unusual for you to be asked to witness one. Therefore, it is important to be familiar with the procedure and your responsibilities.

Since any undue influence brought to bear on the testator (the maker of the will) can invalidate the will, one of your duties in this connection is to

---

[9] The nurse should remember that the practice of law is hedged about with the same sort of legal restrictions as the practice of medicine.

try to prevent such influence. The beneficiaries should have nothing to do with drawing up and witnessing the will. In some instances it might be better for them not to know of the will until after it is executed. The question of undue influence is especially important where a physician, a nurse, or a lawyer is concerned, because of their usual confidential relationship with the patient.

Requirements of a Valid Will

The *English Wills Act,* which has been adopted by the states of the USA sometimes with slight changes, provides:

That no will shall be valid unless it shall be in writing and executed in manner hereinafter mentioned: (that is to say) it shall be signed at the foot or end thereof by the testator, or by some other person in his presence, and by his direction; and such signature shall be made or acknowledged by the testator in the presence of two or more witnesses present at the same time; and such witnesses shall attest and shall subscribe the will in the presence of the testator, but no form of attestation shall be necessary.[10]

The testator must be of age, of sufficient mental capacity and free from any undue influence. For the testator to have sufficient mental capacity he must be aware that he is making his will and realize what property he possesses, how he wishes to dispose of it and the relationship to him of those to whom he gives it. It is not essential that he should have sufficient mental capacity to carry on other usual business transactions. Peculiarities and mental weaknesses common to old age are not considered a lack of testamentary capacity.

No essential form is required for making a will, provided that the intention is expressed clearly. However, various formalities of signing and witnessing are defined by law. Although the underlying principles are the same, since they differ in details in various states it is well to find out exactly what is required by law in the state in which you are practicing, as failure to observe any of the statutory rules can invalidate an entire will. A will written on a scrap of paper, provided that it expresses the wishes of the testator and that it is properly signed and witnessed, may be as effective as one carefully drafted by a lawyer. However, it is always best to secure legal assistance. Otherwise, while the will may be valid, it may also be ambiguous, and long, costly court action may be necessary to determine what it means.

While the usual provision is that a will must be in writing, the printed or typewritten form is acceptable in general practice today. There is the instance in which a woman in a hospital in Indiana, realizing she was dying, called a nurse, wrote her will on a piece of the morning newspaper, and asked the nurse to witness it. This will was recognized as legal. In the instance of soldiers and sailors in action and in some states under certain very re-

[10] F. W. Marshall, *The Layman's Legal Guide to Essential Laws,* New York, Funk & Wagnalls, 1934, p. 297.

stricted conditions, oral wills are considered valid. This type of will is called a *nuncupative* will.

It is suggested that you do not undertake, under any conditions, to write a will unless the services of a lawyer cannot be secured. The penalties for illegal practice of law are similar to those for illegal practice of medicine. In addition, you are likely to commit errors in draftsmanship or in the execution of the will that could defeat the intention of the testator and result in an entirely different disposition of his property.

PROBLEMS

1. Plan a symposium on "Health Care and Nursing," using the following or similar topics: (a) Causes of the Rising Costs of Health Care; (b) What Nurses Should Know About Health and Sickness Insurance; (c) Current Medicare and Medicaid Plans.

2. (a) Study the most recent reports of studies on nurses' incomes, and make a comparison of the earnings of nurses employed in the different fields. (b) Compare the current earnings of nurses with those in other professional fields and of people in business.

3. (a) What is the meaning of recession? inflation? fixed dollar value? equities? (b) How can your financial plan balance fixed dollar value and equities? (c) On what does a balancing of your equities and fixed dollar assets depend?

4. What group insurance and retirement plans are available to you on graduation through your state nurses association?

5. (a) How should a woman ex-member of the military forces proceed in order to receive free hospitalization? (b) If you were a member of the military service and a veteran of the Vietnam War, where would you write to secure information on the National Service Life Insurance plan? (c) Why should every veteran carry National Service Life Insurance?

6. (a) Read the references concerning the Teachers Insurance and Annuity Association and the College Retirement Equities Fund at the end of this chapter under "Retirement," and learn how these programs serve nurses in universities and colleges. (b) How do the American Association of Retired Persons (AARP) and the National Retired Teachers Association (NRTA) serve nurses?

7. (a) What is collective bargaining? (b) How is this a part of the economic security program of the ANA? (c) Describe the economic security program of the ANA in detail. (d) Does your state have such a plan? (e) If so, what is it? (f) Describe paternalism in employer-employee relationships.

8. (a) Study the present income tax requirements and report those pertinent for nurses to your class. (b) How would you file an income tax return?

SUGGESTED REFERENCES*

HEALTH CARE PREPAYMENT AND OTHER INSURANCE PLANS

* American Nurses' Association. *Either Way . . . At Work or Play.* New York, The
    Association, n.d.
* _____. *So You Think You Can't Be Sued.* New York, The Association, n.d.
The Health Insurance Institute. *Of Health Insurance.* New York, The Institute, n.d.
Mattison, W. J. *Life Insurance and Annuities from the Buyer's Point of View.*
    Great Barrington, Mass., American Institute for Economic Research. Revised
    annually.
* Popick, B. "Social Security Disability Insurance Benefits." *American Journal of
    Nursing,* **69**:553, Mar. 1969.
_____. "The Social Security Disability Program: How It Can Benefit You and Your
    Patients." *American Association of Industrial Nurses Journal,* **15**:23-24,
    Nov. 1967.
Report of the National Advisory Commission on Health Manpower. vol. 1. Wash-
    ington, D.C., Government Printing Office, 1967.
Report of the National Conference on Medical Costs, June 27-28, 1967. Washing-
    ton, D.C., Government Printing Office, 1967.
*Report on the National Conference on Private Health Insurance, Washington,
    D.C., September 28-29, 1967.* Baltimore, Social Security Administration, 1968.
U.S. Department of Health, Education, and Welfare. Public Health Service. Health
    Manpower Bureau. *Health Manpower Perspectives: 1967.* Washington, D.C.,
    Government Printing Office, 1967.

See references in Chapter 2 on "Medicare and Medicaid." See also leaflets on
health insurance plans sponsored by your work organization, professional association or other organizations in your community.

ECONOMIC SECURITY PROGRAMS IN NURSING

* American Nurses' Association. *The New Approach to Economic Security,
    January, 1968.* New York, The Association, 1968.
_____. "A Glossary of Industrial Relations Terms." *American Journal of Nursing,*
    61:97-98, Mar. 1961.
Belote, M. "Nurses Are Making It Happen." *American Journal of Nursing,* **67**:284-
    289, Feb. 1967.
Conlon, A. "Bargaining Rights for Nurses—Convincing the Legislature." *American
    Journal of Nursing,* **66**:545-548, Mar. 1966.
"Conversation With: Jo Eleanor Elliott, Anne Zimmerman, Virginia M. Paulson,
    and Rozella Schlotfeldt." *American Journal of Nursing,* **68**:792-799, Apr. 1968.
Heneman, H. G., Jr. "Collective Bargaining: Major Instrument for Change."
    American Journal of Nursing, **68**:1039-1042, May 1968.
Kelly, D. N. "Equating the Nurse's Economic Rewards with the Service Given."
    American Journal of Nursing, **67**:1642-1645, Aug. 1967.
Killam, L. "In Good Faith." *American Journal of Nursing,* **67**:1883-1885, Sept.
    1967.
* Kruse, M. "The Right to Negotiate." *International Nursing Review,* **11**:10-12,
    Apr. 1964.
Lewis, E. P. "The New York City Hospital Story." *American Journal of Nursing,*
    66:1526-1535, July 1966.

*In each chapter all citations are footnoted and are not included here. All starred references
are recommended for additional reading.

Sister Maureen. "The Benefits of Bargaining." *American Journal of Nursing*, **63**:108-110, May 1963.

INCOME TAX

The USA Government publishes each year what you should know about the preparation of your income tax return. Write the Government Printing Office, Washington, D.C. You might also look at your state nurses association journals for information on reporting of income tax.

EMPLOYMENT CONDITIONS AND EARNINGS

Bunch, J. B., *et al.* "Nurse Anesthetists Conditions of Employment." *Journal of the American Association of Nurse Anesthetists*, **35**:253-261, Oct. 1967.
* *1968 Salary Pronouncement: Adopted by ANA House of Delegates, May 1968.* New York, American Nurses' Association, 1968.
"PNA Examines Some Employment Conditions in Pennsylvania." *Pennsylvania Nurse*, **22**:22-25, Dec. 1967.
"Salaries Paid by Public Health Services — 1968." *Nursing Outlook*, **16**:54-57, Dec. 1968. Similar reports are published annually.
Stafford, M. "Will Increased Economic Benefits Really Improve Patient Care?" *Chart*, **64**:242-245, Oct. 1967.
   Watch for reports of the latest salary studies by the ANA in *Facts About Nursing*, and by other agencies.

MONEY MANAGEMENT AND CONSUMER PROBLEMS

* The American Bankers Association. Savings and Mortgage Division. *Personal Money Management.* New York, The Association, 1967.
* Blair, L. L. *Your Financial Guide for Living.* New York, Prentice-Hall, 1963.
Doane, C. R. *How to Invest Wisely.* Great Barrington, Mass., American Institute for Economic Research, 1963.
Federal Savings and Loan Insurance Corporation. *Answers to Questions About Insurance of Savings.* Washington, D.C., The Corporation, n.d.
* *The Marketing Story.* Washington, D.C., Government Printing Office, 1968.
* New York Stock Exchange. Department of Public Information. *Fact Book.* New York, The Exchange. Published annually.

RETIREMENT

* American Association of Retired Persons. *Why AARP Is So Important to You.* Washington, D.C., The Association, 1963.
Annual Report of Teachers Insurance and Annuity Association of America (TIAA). New York, TIAA. Issued annually.
* Barbaccia, J. C. "Pre-retirement Planning." *American Association of Industrial Nurses Journal*, **16**:11-14, May 1968.
Brammall, R. "Pension Provisions and Safeguards." *Midwives Chronicle*, **80**:338-339, Oct. 1967; **81**:12-13, Jan. 1968.
Buchanan, K. "Combined Association's Superannuation Committee's Report." *Lamp*, **24**:8-9, Nov. 1967.
La Ganga, R. "To Nursing With Love." *American Journal of Nursing*, **67**:2556-2557, Dec. 1967.
* Mitchell, W. (ed.). *Preparation for Retirement: A New Guide to Program Development.* Washington, D.C., American Association of Retired Persons, 1968.

* "Planning for the Later Years." *Canadian Journal of Psychiatric Nursing,* **8**:11-12, Dec. 1967.
* *A Report to Participants: CREF Its First Fifteen Years.* New York, Teachers Insurance and Annuity Association—College Retirement Equities Fund, Nov. 1967.
* Schulz, J. H. *The Economic Status of the Retired Aged in 1980: Simulation Projections.* Washington, D.C., Government Printing Office, 1968.
Social Security Programs in the United States, Washington, D.C., Government Printing Office, 1968.
* U.S. Department of Health, Education, and Welfare. *Rights and Responsibilities of Those Who Receive Social Security Retirement or Survivor Benefits.* Washington, D.C., Government Printing Office, Sept. 1968. Revised when changes in legislation are made.
* _____. *Social Security Benefits: How You Earn Them. . . . How Much Credit You Need.* Washington, D.C., Government Printing Office. Published annually.
* _____. *Your Social Security.* Washington, D.C., Government Printing Office. Published annually.
* Ward, R. "Retirement for the Private Duty Nurse." *American Journal of Nursing,* **68**:806, Apr. 1968.
* Ware, G. W. *The New Guide to Happy Retirement.* New York, Crown, 1968.

CHAPTER

16

Continued Education for Nurses

Education continues throughout life for everyone. When you have been graduated, you may think that you have finished with the learning process. But you will quickly find in life situations and in nursing practice that your education has only begun. We must continue to learn throughout life if we are to be competent and successful in our chosen fields. Today, continued education is a must for all.

The question which cannot always be answered easily is, Do I need to continue formal education, or can I learn what I need in some other way? Although experience is often an excellent teacher, we all realize sooner or later that some things are learned better through organized courses and others through work and social experience.

Horizons widen after graduation from preservice education. For example, the nurse who has had a technical preservice education may find that her goals require that she seek a baccalaureate degree in nursing. The nurse who wants to enter a specialized field seeks graduate education because she finds she requires additional preparation, additional knowledge and specialized skills.

You will ask, What type of additional preparation do I need—in undergraduate work or in graduate education? Do I meet the requirements for graduate work? Where can I get graduate work? Where can I find an appropriate undergraduate program? Can I fit into such a program? Shall I do full-time or part-time work at the university? Where can I secure financial aid? Should I really continue formal education at all? By answering these and similar questions wisely and honestly you will be in a better position to plan.

The emphasis in this chapter is primarily on problems connected with education at a university after completion of a preservice program.

MEANING OF EDUCATION AND NURSING EDUCATION

Education is the cultivation of qualities and talents that help the human being to grow in the harmonious development of all his powers — physical, intellectual, social, esthetic and spiritual. Therefore, nursing education in its broadest sense includes all efforts and activities which prepare for complete living, as well as for a career in nursing.

TYPES OF EDUCATION FOR NURSES

As pointed out elsewhere, there are, in general, 3 types of education for graduate nurses:

1. Education leading to the baccalaureate degree in nursing. Nurses graduating from a hospital school of nursing or an associate degree program may obtain a baccalaureate degree (1) by applying for advanced standing in a preservice baccalaureate program in nursing and completing the requirements for the degree, or (2) by attending a university offering a generalized baccalaureate program for graduate nurses. Generalized baccalaureate programs have almost disappeared.

2. Graduate education for nurses leading to a master's or a doctor's degree. One type of graduate education for nurses is geared toward increasing the clinical knowledge and the skills of the nurse in nursing practice. Other types are geared toward developing knowledge and skills in other functional areas, such as: administration, curriculum development and improvement, teaching, supervision, consultation, or research in nursing. All types of graduate education are directed toward increased scholarship and include offerings concerned with investigative skills. All types are concerned with the improvement of nursing practice.

3. Inservice education, which may consist of on-the-job learning, learning through participation in problem solving and participation in policy-making conferences at work. It is important for all nurses to continue to study and to learn while they are employed, regardless of the type of educational program from which they have been graduated. Continued interest in learning is one of the marks of a truly professional person. Today, many places of em-

ployment provide an inservice education program in which the nurse may participate, the aims of which are to improve professional skills and ultimately to improve patient care.

Other common sources of education are personal experience; planned program in reading; lectures; observation; study at home; advanced study not leading to any degree or diploma; and participation in work conferences, workshops, institutes, study groups, meetings sponsored by nursing organizations and other groups, and the like. Many nurses take advantage of the short-term traineeships offered by colleges and universities and funded by the Division of Nursing of the PHS. Travel has cultural as well as professional value and is an excellent source of continued education. Opportunities through exchange programs for study abroad, through the Fulbright and other exchange plans, are also important sources of education.

The professional nurse, regardless of the number of graduate degrees she may have, will need to plan for continuing education. The explosion in knowledge characteristic of the 2nd half of the 20th century places increasing demands on all professional persons. It is encumbent upon nurses to accept responsibility for the quality of their practice and for the advancement of their nursing knowledge. Participation in institutes, workshops and short-term courses will be increasingly important as methods of keeping up-to-date. Nursing associations such as the ANA, the NLN and other national and state groups, offer unique opportunities for continuing education of this type through program meetings and by means of regional conferences, workshops and institutes. In some communities, nurses have access to university extension programs via video-tape lessons, or to such programs as the "Nursing Dial Access" of the University of Wisconsin, which provides an around-the-clock taped library available by phone to all nurses in the state. Other groups, such as the Western Interstate Collegiate and Higher Education in Nursing, the Southern Regional Education Board, and the New England Board of Higher Education, also plan and coordinate continuing education activities on a regional basis.

UNDERSTANDING THE SYSTEM OF EDUCATION FOR NURSING

The present system of education for nursing in the USA is in a state of transition. Therefore, some nurses seem to be confused about how to articulate their preservice education with graduate education for ensuring a sequential educational plan so that they will find the educational opportunities best suited to their talents, their needs and their professional objectives.

Because the objectives and the educational program in a hospital school of nursing or an associate degree program are different from that of baccalaureate education, orderly progression from one to the other is not possible. Therefore, much time may be lost in the process of articulation. A hospital school graduate who wishes to enter a baccalaureate program, often will find it necessary to plan for an additional 2 or more years of preparation for her degree. Each college or university sets up the requirements for a degree within the institution, and these requirements must be met before the degree can be conferred — in nursing or in any other field for which education is provided by the institution.

The student who desires to prepare eventually for a field such as teaching in nursing, which requires graduate preparation, would save time and effort if she enrolled in the preservice program leading to the baccalaureate degree at the start of her nursing career.

The young student who is interested in making a progressive vocational and educational plan could profit from studying the various types of educational programs for nursing. If she understands the current system of nursing education, she will be less likely to take the wrong educational road. A letter was received by one of the authors from a student who was very concerned about the lack of information some nurses seem to have about what type of preparation to pursue for teaching and other fields in nursing which require specialized preparation. She wrote:

Many graduate nurses do not seem to understand the various types and purposes of degree programs in nursing. I, myself, have encountered a number of nurses who have been bitterly disappointed to learn that the degrees they have received have not adequately prepared them for positions of teaching or administration in schools of nursing. For example, one nurse had a B.S. degree with a major in music; another had a major in history and political science; and a third, a major in religious education.

Some nurses have thought in the past that any degree would do — only to find when they arrive on a job they are not prepared for their special assignments.

POSITIONS FOR WHICH NURSES PREPARE IN GRADUATE PROGRAMS

The practice is for curricula for preparing clinical specialists and administrative and supervisory nursing personnel in hospitals and public health agencies, as well as for preparing personnel for inservice education in such agencies, to be on the master's or doctoral level.

The holding of a doctoral degree is common practice for appointments to administrative and instructional positions in nursing divisions of colleges and universities. This is also true for appointments to positions involving research and consultation in nursing.

A doctoral degree for all nurses in administrative and instructional positions in graduate educational programs in nursing is now a definite requirement. The following are positions nurses prepare for in graduate programs.

Positions in Nursing Service Programs

Hospital Nursing Service Positions
1. Director of nursing service, associate, assistant
2. Supervisor or divisional administrator
3. Clinical specialist
4. Head nurse
5. Director of inservice education (includes on-the-job training and on-going inservice education)
6. Consultant, generalized and in the various clinical areas

Public Health Nursing Service Positions
1. Director of nursing service, associate, assistant
2. Supervisor, assistant supervisor
3. Clinical specialist
4. Educational director, or director of inservice education
5. Consultant, generalized and in the various clinical areas

Occupational Health Nursing Service Positions
1. Director of nursing service
2. Supervisor
3. Consultant in occupational health nursing

School Health Nursing Service Positions
1. Administrator of school health nursing program
2. Supervisor
3. School nurse
4. Consultant in school health nursing

Positions in Nursing Education Programs

Vocational, Hospital, and College or University-Controlled Educational Program in Practical Nursing Leading to a Certificate or Diploma
1. Educational administrator (exact title depends on policy of the institution)
2. Teacher of nursing
3. Field teacher in clinical nursing practice

Hospital-Controlled School of Nursing Offering an Educational Program in Nursing Leading to a Diploma
1. Director, associate director, assistant director
2. Educational director or instructional leader
3. Teacher of fundamentals of nursing
4. Teacher of nursing in the various clinical fields
5. Teacher of science (physical, biological and social)
6. Field teacher in the various clinical practice fields

Junior or Community College Educational Program in Nursing Leading to an Associate Degree

1. Educational administrator, associate, assistant, instructional leader (title depends on policy of institution)
2. Teacher of fundamentals of nursing
3. Teacher of nursing in the various clinical fields
4. Field teacher in the various clinical practice fields

University or College Educational Program in Nursing Leading to a Baccalaureate Degree (Undergraduate)

1. Educational administrator, associate, assistant, instructional leader (exact title depends on policy of institution)
2. Teacher of fundamentals of nursing
3. Teacher of nursing in the various clinical fields

University Educational Program in Nursing Leading to a Graduate Degree

1. Educational administrator (exact title depends on policy of the institution)[1]
2. Teacher of nursing in the various clinical fields
3. Teacher of educational administration
4. Teacher of consultation
5. Teacher of curriculum development and instructional improvement, and of teaching
6. Teacher of inservice education (hospital and public health)
7. Teacher of physical and biologic sciences
8. Teacher of school health nursing
9. Teacher of nursing service administration
10. Teacher of supervision in nursing services
11. Teacher of problems of the profession
12. Teacher of research in nursing[2]

Positions in Governmental Organizations (State, National, International)

Some examples are:

1. Educational supervisor of practical nurse education
2. Program specialist in practical nurse education
3. Administrator, assistant, of state board of nursing
4. Consultant in various clinical and other areas of nursing
5. Administrator in various areas of nursing
6. Teacher in various areas of nursing
7. Director of nursing research activities

---

[1] Administrators of many graduate programs are also responsible for administration of the preservice undergraduate program; therefore, graduate preparation for administration of graduate programs may be combined with preparation for administration of preservice programs.

[2] Preparation for these teaching positions may combine the content of several areas in a single program.

Positions in Nursing and Allied Voluntary Organizations (State, National, International)

Some examples are:
1. Executive secretary, or director of local, state or national nursing organization
2. Administrator in various areas of nursing
3. Field worker in various areas of nursing service and nursing education
4. Counselor (vocational and educational)
5. Registrar of professional placement service
6. Consultant (nursing service, nursing education, special clinical field, community planning, legislation, other)
7. Magazine editor (nursing periodical, nursing section of health or hospital periodical)

Positions in Research

1. Director of research institute (nursing)
2. Researcher in nursing (various nursing fields)
3. Consultant in research in nursing
4. Research project director or principal investigator
5. Research assistant

Where Can You Secure a List of Institutions Offering Continuation Studies in Your Field?

The NLN publishes in *Nursing Outlook* each year, a list of educational programs for nurses which are currently accredited by that organization. This list shows in what institutions of higher education the different types of education programs in nursing are offered: preservice program leading to the baccalaureate degree for students with no previous preparation in nursing; a baccalaureate program with a major in nursing for graduates of hospital and associate degree programs; and those leading to master's or doctor's degrees, including clinical specialties and all other functional areas – teaching, curriculum development and improvement, supervision, administration, consultation and research.

ATTENDING A UNIVERSITY

Before you decide to apply for admission to pursue graduate study at a university, it is important to consider some points about yourself and also about the university.

How Can You Analyze Yourself to Ascertain That You Are Making a Wise Decision?

You might ask yourself:

Am I interested in current events in nursing and the world in general?

Have I selected the field of nursing for which I am best fitted and in which I prefer to work?

Have I the personality and other qualities necessary for success in my chosen field?

Do I feel the need to secure additional knowledge and practice?

Have I the proper foundation for graduate work? If not, how can I get it?

Was my achievement sufficiently high in the schools I attended? If not, was it because I lacked ability or was lazy or disinterested?

Do I really enjoy studying?

Am I capable of doing original or independent work without constant supervision?

Am I self-directing and able to practice self-discipline?

Do I desire general cultural as well as professional knowledge?

Is university attendance financially possible for me?

Will the return I get from this investment justify the use of my time and money?

The most important consideration, however, is whether you are willing to devote time and effort to work, both in and outside the classroom. It is safe to say that if you are the passive type or want merely to get by, a university is no place for you.

If, after analyzing yourself with the help of the best counselor you can consult in your school or community, you are still uncertain of your fitness to do work of graduate level, and if you meet requirements for admission, you might attend a summer session and find out. At the same time the university faculty would have an opportunity to evaluate your ability.

If You Desire to Take a Few Courses While Working, What Special Factors Should You Consider?

The principal factors that will influence your decision regarding part-time work are your general health and emotional stability, the requirements of your regular occupation, the amount of time you have for study, rest and recreation, the proximity of the university facilities, and the nature and the amount of work required in the courses you desire. After all, to get a degree at the expense of your health or your job or both is wasteful and unwise.

What Information Concerning the University is Necessary? How Can You Secure It?

Learn the size and the reputation of the instructional staff and the student body, the accomplishments of the graduates, the tuition, the type of library facilities, the accommodations for room and board and their cost, the admission requirements, the courses and the curricula offered, the method of evaluating credits and the university's standing. Accreditation and standing among other universities is highly important. A good procedure is to consider these items about several universities and compare them. You may find it helpful to discuss the university programs in which you are interested with someone who is in a position to help you judge them — perhaps the director of your school, or a graduate of the particular university.

Prospective universities should be looked at from other angles. Answers to the following questions usually can be found in the school's catalog:

1. Do the requirements for admission indicate that the graduate courses in nursing are built on a sound basis?

2. Do the programs provide for general and cultural preparation as well as sound professional preparation?

3. Are the organization and the design of the graduate programs and the faculty responsible for these programs flexible enough so that adjustments can be made for nurses who come from a variety of undergraduate preservice programs in nursing?

4. Are there field centers for guided experience in the area of instruction in which you are interested?

To make the most effective arrangements for entering the selected university you also may desire to get information on the following through personal conference at the university:

1. Amount of credit that will be allowed for your previous education in nursing. Many universities evaluate past nursing preparation and experience on an individual basis. They may allow credit or exemption by examination, or they may give transfer credit. Do not select a university that gives exactly the same amount of credit to all students. Remember that the educational institution which offers the lure of a large amount of credit for the program in a hospital school of nursing is not necessarily the best one to choose.

2. Approximate length of time it will take to complete the selected program.

3. Type of plan that can be made if you cannot complete the desirable program during one unbroken period.

4. How to make up prerequisites if entrance requirements cannot be met at once. Perhaps you can plan to work in your own community and at the same time remove deficiencies or take required courses in general education before actually enrolling at the selected university. If you plan to do either of these at another university before enrolling at the selected university, be sure to get a statement on the acceptability of such courses taken elsewhere. This can be obtained from the proper admissions official at the university you expect to enter eventually.

It is advisable to study several bulletins in order to compare their offerings. The quality and the methods of instruction, the morale of the students and the opportunities for cultural and spiritual advancement through association with worth-while people are important to the student. This information is obtained best by personal contact with the faculty, the students and the alumni. Personal interviews are also extremely important. If you live within the vicinity of the university of your choice, arrange for an interview with the adviser for students in the selected program either by telephone or through correspondence. *Do not take a chance and go for an interview without making a previous appointment.*

Even in this day when counseling is so readily available, some students actually go to the university without having chosen a special field in nursing or given serious thought to their personal assets, liabilities and interests. Naturally, it is difficult for a busy faculty adviser who does not know these students well to guide them at registration time into curricula most suitable to meet their needs.

What Are the Next Steps?

Fill in completely and correctly all application forms and assemble your credentials according to the instructions given in the university bulletin and on admission forms. Be sure to send your application to the university far enough in advance for complete evaluation before the date you expect to begin your studies. This is important, because it takes time to locate credentials, and it saves time and trouble for you on admission.

After your application has been accepted, make your educational plan. Become thoroughly familiar with the school's catalog, and make a tentative written outline of your anticipated educational plan before discussing it with the university adviser. You then will have a better concept of what you wish to do and of what he is trying to plan with you.

Should All Professional Nurses Work for Higher Degrees?

A college education for nurses is of real importance in our society. There is, however, too great a tendency for nurses to overrate the value of a degree, as such. A degree is merely a symbol, indicating that a certain type of preparation has been acquired by the student. It means nothing unless the person who holds it has the background and the ability to lead a well-balanced life in carrying on her occupation.

Working for a master's degree is important for those who wish to prepare themselves further in clinical areas or for certain positions in teaching, administration, consultation or research in nursing. Some of the questions you might ask yourself, if interested in preparation leading to the master's degree, are similar to those listed on pages 390-391 for consideration of doctoral study, especially 1, 2, 3, 4, 5 and 7. Many more nurses with master's degrees are needed to fill the demands.

The desire to work for a doctoral degree is commendable, but you should do so only if you have actually found yourself, have decided on a definite line of work that requires such a degree, have truly shown marked ability in your particular field, and, of course, if you enjoy the experience and can profit by it.

The number of nurses with doctoral degrees needs to be markedly increased if nursing is to reach professional stature. Professional stature is directly related to the extent of sound education which the practitioners have achieved and to the number prepared by advanced education to do the basic research needed to develop the scientific bases of nursing. For example, a great need is for a group of nurses, educated in the biologic, behavioral and physical sciences on the Ph.D. level. Much of the early research in nursing was directed by social scientists, and involved studies of nurses, their education, roles, functions and attitudes. As more nurse-scientists are prepared in the physical, biologic and behavioral sciences, more basic research in clinical areas dealing with patient care should result. Doctorates in all functional areas also will be important.

A decision to secure a doctor's degree has wide ramifications. Some questions you may ask yourself if you are considering a doctorate as part of your plan for continuing study are:

> What are my professional purposes and goals? In which field of nursing do I plan to work? Do I have the potential competence needed? Will the doctorate help me to develop that competence? Is the kind of doctoral program I desire available to me? What values may I expect from pursuing a program of doctoral study?

Some students want a doctorate because it is a requirement for the type of position they are seeking or holding. For example, if one wants to teach in or administer a graduate program, a doctorate is imperative. Some want it for the sake of prestige or because they believe it will bring greater monetary returns. These are all legitimate reasons. More fundamental questions are:

> What professional competencies may be secured through the doctorate? Do I need these special competencies in my work?

As you ask and get answers to the foregoing questions, you also will need to ask whether you have the potential qualifications for successful and satisfying work. Answers to some of the following questions may help you in arriving at a decision.

1. What has been the quality of your past professional experience? Can you make independent and significant decisions on the basis of principle and interpretation? Can you deal successfully with problems involving a variety of factors?

2. What is the quality of your scholarship? It is known that course marks are not highly reliable and should not be the sole factor to consider. However, marks are probably the best measure of your capacity for intellectual work of the type required in a doctoral program. Therefore,

try to attain satisfactory marks, even though marks are only one criterion.

3. Can you write? Writing of doctoral quality is more than pure mechanics. It involves the ability to do creative writing that will explain, interpret and stimulate thinking and action.

4. How do you react in difficult situations? Can you take criticism, resolve conflicting recommendations and still retain your self-control, personal integrity and objective point of view? Or do you get emotionally upset and blame others for your errors?

5. Are you a "self-initiator"? Can you analyze a problem, map out a plan of procedure for doing it, and get under way on your own "steam"? Or do you expect teachers or advisers to tell you what to do? Do you procrastinate and put off doing assignments until the deadline is reached and then ask for an extension of time?

6. Have you plenty of drive? Balance of work and recreation are important to maintain continued energy. Achieving a doctorate requires a great deal of drive which you yourself need to supply.

7. Do you know where and how to secure counsel of others in your self-evaluation? Who is best acquainted with you and your work where you completed your baccalaureate and master's degrees? Can he help you decide? Are you willing and able to make available to whomever you consult as full information as you can about your abilities, interests, experiences and competencies?

Even though you may not intend or desire to work for a higher degree, some attendance at a university is good for everyone who can profit from the courses taken and the association with faculty and students.

FINANCIAL AID FOR NURSES SEEKING EDUCATION

The main sources of financial aid to further your education are scholarships, fellowships, loan funds and part-time work.

A scholarship or fellowship is a gift, usually awarded to those who stand highest in competition. Ordinarily, it is expected that such a gift will be repaid later by one's professional contribution to the profession and to society. A loan is an advancement of money and must be repaid with or without interest, as agreed.

Alumni associations frequently establish scholarship and loan funds for the use of their own members. A number of preservice nursing schools, as well as certain public health nursing agencies, have provided scholarships for their faculty and staff members. Some of these scholarships and loan funds are specified for use at a particular university, while others may be used for attendance at any approved university of the applicant's choice. Frequently, scholarships and loan funds are secured by applying directly to universities. Other grants are available through nursing organizations, sororities, lodges, churches, philanthropic and educational foundations and the state and Federal governments.

Federal Government grants were made possible through certain provisions in the *Social Security Act* (1935). The *Training for Nurses Act* (1941) and the *Bolton Act* (1943) not only provided generous funds for educational programs for graduate nurses, but also influenced the planning of programs, so that they were established on a sounder basis and made more effective. Emphasis was placed on the need for practical field work. *Public Law 346: G. I. Bill of Rights* passed June 22, 1944, *Public Law 16* passed March 24, 1943, and *Public Law 550: Korean Bill of Rights* approved June 16, 1952, giving educational and other assistance to veterans, have provided large sums of money. Such measures as the *Mental Health Act* and other similar acts now incorporated in the *Public Health Service Act,* and the *Maternal and Child Health Acts,* have made it possible for many graduates to continue their education. Impetus has been given to the preparation of nurses for positions requiring specialized preparation by the passage of *Public Law 911, the Health Amendments Act of 1956.* It established a yearly program for each of 3 years to assist qualified nurses to prepare for teaching or administrative positions or for specialized training in public health. The *Nurse Training Act of 1964,* (Public Law 88-581) provided a balanced program of and for nursing education, and included loans and long-term traineeships for graduate students, as well as short-term traineeships.[3] In 1968, the *Nurse Training Act of 1964* was amended and continued by the passage of the *Health Manpower Act of 1968* (Public Law 90-490). The new legislation provided Federal aid to nurse education through the fiscal year 1970-1971[4] These programs are administered through the Public Health Service of the U.S. Department of Health, Education, and Welfare, and individual grants are obtained through application to approved institutions.

Other pertinent legislation is discussed in Chapter 27.

Beginning in 1955, a Nurse Research Fellowship Program has been administered by the Division of Nursing of the PHS. Special fellowships for research training are awarded by the Surgeon General for those recommended by the Nurse Scientist Graduate Training Committee. Later in 1962, a Nurse Scientist Graduate Training Grants Program was started. It not only helps to expand doctoral programs in universities but also provides training stipends to nurses working toward doctoral degrees in the biologic, physical, or behavioral sciences.[5]

Another source of government funds for aiding graduate nurses is the state governments. A number of states have made legislative provisions for granting financial aid to nurses for continuing their studies.

Nurses Educational Funds, Inc., is another important source of financial assistance. A successor to the Isabel Hampton Robb Memorial Fund

[3] U.S. Department of Health, Education, and Welfare. Public Health Service, *Nurse Training Act of 1964: Program Review Report,* Washington, D.C., Government Printing Office, 1967.
[4] "President Signs Bill Aiding Nurse Education," (News) *American Journal of Nursing,* **68:**2063-2064, Oct. 1968.
[5] E. M. Vreeland, "Nursing Research Programs of the Public Health Service," *Nursing Research,* **13:**148-158, Spring 1964.

founded in 1910, it was incorporated in 1941. For many years it was maintained almost entirely by gifts from nurses. Since 1954, contributions also have been sought outside the profession. Nurses Educational Funds' purpose is to provide scholarships, fellowships and loans to nurses for study in nursing leading to a baccalaureate or higher degree. In 1970, it administered the following awards:

American Journal of Nursing Fellowships

C. V. Mosby Scholarship

Mead Johnson Scholarships

Nurses' Scholarship and Fellowship Fund

National Student Nurses' Association Scholarship

Pet Milk Fellowship (for study in maternal and child health or pediatrics)

Isabel Hampton Robb Scholarship

W. B. Saunders Scholarship

Squibb Scholarship (for specialization in medical-surgical nursing)

Shirley C. Titus Fellowship Fund (for study in professional organization work)

American Journal of Nursing Company Scholarships

Paralyzed Veterans of America Inc. (for specialization in rehabilitation nursing)

Nurses Educational Funds is an independent corporation associated with the NLN. Further information can be obtained by writing to Nurses' Educational Fund, Inc., 10 Columbus Circle, New York, N.Y., 10019.

The requirements and the provisions of scholarships and fellowships vary according to their purposes. Some provide only for tuition, while others include funds for full maintenance and other expenses. They may vary from very small amounts of not more than $250 to larger ones of $5,000 to $6,000. Lists and general information on most of the available scholarships, fellowships and loan funds can be secured not only from the various colleges and universities offering nursing programs, but also from the counselors in state professional nurse placement services, the ANA PC&PS, and the ANA-NLN Nursing Careers Program.

You may secure financial assistance by doing part-time work in universities, local nursing schools and hospitals, and other places within the vicinity of the university. The work in which you are employed need not necessarily be in nursing but may be whatever opportunity offers. At universities the demand is usually for library, bibliographic, or stenographic work, for waiting on tables or dining room service, and sometimes for tutoring or teaching. However, the nurse usually can earn more working as a nurse than by doing the unskilled work available on most campuses. Opportunities may be found in local nursing schools. Opportunities for general staff or special nursing in a hospital frequently are available. Any of this work may be done in return for maintenance, tuition and other considerations or a definite salary or fee.

Because the sources of financial support for continued education are constantly changing and new ones are developing, it is wise to inform yourself frequently regarding them. An excellent source of information will be your adviser at the university of your choice.

SPECIAL EMPHASES IN PLANNING CONTINUED EDUCATION

The need for continued or adult education, whether formal or informal in nature, is imperative if you are to keep up with the changing world and to carry on effectively everyday nursing and living.

In the planning for additional professional education there are 2 important considerations: self-inventory and the securing of adequate information about institutions of higher education offering the educational programs you desire to enter.

When you have examined the factors that influence you in deciding whether you will continue your education in a university and where you will go, the next step is to see that all of your credentials are filed properly. Your educational plan should be determined also in the light of your choice of a field.

While at the university, do not work for a degree only, but try to focus your work and your thinking on problems, principles and solutions that will prepare you well for complete living and the work which you expect to undertake on graduation. Think of the degree as a mere symbol of what it represents in ability and not as an "open sesame" to anything you may desire to attain after you leave the university.

If you think you are not of the academic caliber to work for a degree beyond a baccalaureate, discuss your potential with your adviser. Those who go on for higher degrees should be those who will enjoy and profit by the experience. Those who, for varied reasons, do not take graduate courses can do much in the way of continued self-education by attending institutes, review, supplemental and adult courses, and professional organization meetings, or by reading and attending lectures. A good reading program will include current events, professional and recreational literature. Every nurse should read at least one professional journal regularly.

With the present emphasis on general adult education, there are many opportunities for the wise use of leisure, and nurses may find interesting and profitable ways of rounding out their lives in such fields as music, drama, or the other arts and crafts, and through wise selection of social experiences.

PROBLEMS

1. What is the difference between education for graduate nurses and graduate education for nurses?

2. Plan a symposium on the topic "Opportunities for Continued Preparation for Graduate Nurses." This might be divided into the following subtopics for discussion by the members of the symposium: (a) "Types of Graduate Educational Programs in Existence for Nurses," (b) "Steps in the Development of an Educational Plan Best Suited to Individual Needs of Nurses" and (c) "Value of Broad Experience for Professional Nurses."

3. What general type of content should be included in the curriculum designed to prepare nurses for each of the following positions: (a) head nurse in a unit of an obstetric division in a hospital? (b) clinical specialist in maternal and child health? (c) the nurse in a coronary care unit? (d) supervisor of a medical division in a hospital and instructor in medical nursing? (e) principal investigator or project director of research in a hospital or university? (f) teacher in general or fundamental nursing or one of the special nursing areas in a school of nursing? (g) supervisor of a nursing service in a public health agency? (h) supervisor of an intensive care unit in a hospital? (i) administrator of a university school of nursing? (j) administrator of a nursing service in a public health agency? (k) executive of a national nursing organization?

4. (a) Where in this country can nurses secure preparation in nurse midwifery? (b) For what purpose would you want this type of preparation?

5. How would you go about preparing yourself as a nurse-scientist?

6. (a) Make a list of Federal, other national, and local scholarships, fellowships and educational loan funds for which graduates of your school are eligible. (b) Indicate where information on these can be secured.

SUGGESTED REFERENCES*

CONTINUED EDUCATION

* American Nurses' Association. *Avenues for Continued Learning*. New York, The Association, 1967.
* _____. *Guide for the Establishment of Refresher Courses*. New York, The Association, 1968.
Armstrong, D. M. "Inservice Education and Postgraduate Courses." *AORN Journal*, **7**:57-59, Feb. 1968.
"Back to Nursing." *International Nursing Review*, **15**:141-143, Apr. 1968.
Boyle, R. and Peterson, F. "The Registered Nurse Seeks a College." *Nursing Outlook*, **10**:652-654, Oct. 1962.
Brodt, D. E. "College Bound – But Why?" *Nursing Outlook*, **17**:48-49, Jan. 1969.
Caddell, E. B. "Growth and Development of the Private Duty Nurse: How to Be a Continuous Learner." *Tar Heel Nurse*, **30**:30-32, Mar. 1968.
Calnan, M. E. "Inservice in Nursing Homes." *Nursing Outlook*, **16**:43-45, Feb. 1968.
Cohen, P. F. "Teacher-To-Be: Nursing Education?" *Educational Horizons*, **46**:123-126, Spring 1968.

---

* In each chapter all citations are footnoted and are not included here. All starred references are recommended for additional reading.

Ellison, D. "Staff Development—Developing Individual Potential." *AORN Journal*, **7**:77-81, Mar. 1968.

Graham, L. E. "Are We Motivating Students to go on for Graduate Education." *American Journal of Nursing*, **6**:48-50, Aug. 1968.

Hassenplug, L. W. "Going on for a Bachelor's Degree." *American Journal of Nursing*, **66**:83-85, Jan. 1966.

* Lambertsen, E. C. "Does Education Mean Exodus." *AORN Journal*, **6**:48-49, Dec. 1967.

Larson, V. S. "Education on Wheels." *American Journal of Nursing*, **67**:2554, Dec. 1967.

Lucek, D. "Refresher Course—the First Step." *Nursing Outlook*, **16**:23-25, Sept. 1968.

MacDonald, G. "Baccalaureate Education for Graduates of Diploma and Associate Degree Programs." *Nursing Outlook*, **12**:52-56, June 1964.

McClellan, M. "Staff Development in Action." *American Journal of Nursing*, **68**: 298-300, Feb. 1968.

Martin, L. P. "Orientation with Tapes and Slides." *American Journal of Nursing*, **68**:1032-1033, May 1968.

* Metcalf, M. L. "Clinical Rotation for New Graduates." *Nursing Outlook*, **16**:44-46, Sept. 1968.

* Myers, E., *et al.* "An Internship for New Graduates." *American Journal of Nursing*, **68**:96-98, Jan. 1968.

* National League for Nursing. Department of Baccalaureate and Higher Degrees. *Nursing Education—Creative, Continuing, Experimental.* New York, The League, 1966.

* Oram, P. G. and Routher, W. R. "Research as Inservice Education." *Nursing Outlook*, **18**:20-22, Sept. 1968.

Popiel, E. S. "The Many Facets of Continuing Education in Nursing." *Journal of Nursing Education*, **8**:3-13, Jan. 1969.

Schmitt, E. "Transition from Student to Graduate." *American Journal of Nursing*, **67**:2573-2575, Dec. 1967.

Shoben, E. J., Jr. "Means, Ends, and the Liberties of Education." *Journal of Higher Education*, **39**:61-68, Feb. 1968.

Smith, H. H. "An Experiment in Continuing Education for Nurses." *International Nursing Review*, **15**:134-139, Apr. 1968.

FINANCIAL AID

National League for Nursing. *Scholarships, Fellowships, Educational Grants, and Loans.* New York, The League, Sept. 1967.

Nurses' Educational Funds, Inc. *Information for Applicants.* New York, Nurses' Educational Funds, Inc., 1968. Revised periodically.

Check with your state nurses association to learn what scholarships are available within the state.

CHAPTER

17

Leadership Role of the Professional Nurse

The significance of the leadership role of the professional nurse as a major area of concern to the profession is being emphasized throughout the world. For example, the 1965 program at the ICN Congress in Frankfurt, Germany, was centered entirely on this topic. Courses on leadership have been introduced into nursing curricula. The words *leader* and *leadership* and the phrase *leadership role of the professional nurse* also have appeared with increasing frequency in nursing literature. These terms, particularly the last one, may be causing you some worry. Perhaps you, as a senior student of nursing, are apprehensive at the prospect of changing from a student who has been looking to others for leadership into a nurse who is expected to give leadership.

Possibly some of your anxiety stems from your idea of what a leader is. You may be picturing a person who walks alone—in front of a procession of followers who are entirely dependent on him for deciding their destination and finding a path to it—a person who is the group's only resource for selecting and achieving its goal. However, this is not the concept of leadership we have when we think of the leadership responsibilities of the registered nurse.

As a student of nursing, and even before you became a student, you have participated in activities wherein you, or your classmates, have assumed leadership roles. To mention only a very few, consider your student council activities, any committee work that you may have been involved in, and other student activities, such as planning for social affairs, not to mention such opportunities for leadership as participation in patient-care groups. And remember, leadership does not always reside in the chairman of the committee, the officers of the council, or the team leader.

Professional leadership as a process and as a responsibility of the nurse will be the focus of this chapter—primarily in terms of her role at work and in the community.

DEFINITION OF LEADERSHIP

Leadership, as currently used in professional literature, has been defined as the "process of helping a group achieve its aims and goals." Another frequently used definition is "the process or act of influencing the activities of an organized group in its efforts toward goal-setting and goal-achieving." Neither of these definitions, you will note, is in key with the concept of the solitary leader. Rather, they reflect a person who is part of his group, the other members of which have abilities and competencies that contribute toward the attainment of the group's goals.

As a matter of fact, in some groups the leadership is divided among several persons, in accordance with various aspects of the group's tasks and the specialized abilities of the individual members. Thus, a member of such a group may sometimes be a leader, at other times a follower. In still other groups, all of the members share the responsibility of leadership; in these instances, the leadership is said to be "group-centered."

If you will think about the leadership role in this light, you will agree with the conclusion that in certain instances you already have acted and are now acting in a leadership capacity, because you are influencing the activities of others. These instances will increase as you progress through your educational program. By the time that you make the transition from student of nursing to nurse, you will be used to assuming some leadership responsibilities and will be well prepared to take others in your stride.

This thinking about your leadership activities will in itself help you in your preparation for your future leadership obligations. Although different phases of leadership are discussed throughout this book, this chapter is intended to stimulate you to consider consciously the various aspects of your leadership role.

GROUPS—ROLES—QUALITIES

You assume many roles throughout your day. In some circumstances you take on your "student" role, which consists of listening, writing and thinking behaviors. You expect a person having a "teacher" role to behave in the way you have come to associate with that function. But during the day you also accept, for example, the role of "mother" with young children left in your charge; the role of "tutor" when helping a fellow classmate with a math problem; or perhaps a role with aggressive attributes while attending a football game and a role with pious attributes while at a service of worship. The groups in which you find yourself will change, depending on the roles you assume.

You will come to understand the various roles in the hospital or health setting. A patient (though a bank vice-president in the community) may have the role of sufferer, during his illness. The nurse (though a customer in his bank when outside the hospital) exerts a leadership nursing role to facilitate his comfort and recovery. Or as another example, perhaps the student herself is still "mothered" in her own home, and through thoughtful calls and packages, is assisted by her mother even though while away to study nursing. This same student, however, is the "mothering one" to a lonely child or older person who has feelings of separation not unlike her own.

The nursing student may also be in a role of "follower" under the direction and supervision of another nurse; yet, when needed, she is able to assume the role of team leader and can change her behavior accordingly. She learns which leadership actions bring about the desired goals of the health team. She combines knowledge and skills learned in her classes with the understanding and appreciation she probably began to learn in her own home. She tempers efficiency with the human qualities of understanding, patience and respect for the opinion and privacy of others.

One way to start thinking about your leadership activities is to list in a column all of the groups with which you, when you graduate, will be likely to be associated. These groups will probably fall into 3 categories: (1) the groups with which you will work as part of your job, (2) the organizations to which you will belong because you are a member of the nursing profession and (3) the groups of which you will be a member because of your citizenship responsibilities and your personal interests.

Next to this column, which might be labeled "Groups," make one headed, "The Nurse's Leadership Role." It will take considerable thought to fill in this column, but it could be most helpful if you do so. In fact, each entry represents the first essential of leadership — the leader's recognition that he has leadership responsibilities, his seeing himself as a leader.

Then, in a third column, jot down notes about the skills, attitudes, and other behaviors that are required for carrying out each of the leadership roles. It is doubtful that you can complete this column immediately. You might keep it and add to it also after you are graduated. The entries in it may well increase throughout your life.

The discussion that follows may help you to begin this compilation. It should be emphasized, however, that any list which you derive from it is only the start of a list and should not be regarded as final or complete.

NURSING LEADERSHIP ON THE JOB

The Health Team

One group of which practically every newly graduated nurse is a member is the health team — that is, the group of workers who are directly engaged in the care of a patient or a group of patients. In its basic form, this group consists of a patient, a nurse and a physician, but most health teams include other personnel, also. The patient is the first diagnostician. If he doesn't seek medical advice, no health care ensues. He becomes the primary implementer of the health-care plan when he seeks medical and nursing care. It is he who has to take the necessary steps in accepting medical, nursing and other help if his health condition is to improve.

The physician usually is regarded as the leader of the health team, because his judgment concerning the patient's health problems and his decisions about the patient's medical regimen have considerable influence on the activities of the other members of the group. However, there are other influencing functions for which other members of the health team have primary responsibility, so that, in reality, the health team is one of the groups in which more than one member has a leadership role. As a matter of fact, nursing leadership on this team is a prerogative of the nurse. By that we mean that she is expected to bring to any situation her own special nursing knowledge and skills and to assume leadership on the health team when nursing is the focus of concern. The physician takes "medical leadership." In fact, even the patient takes "patient leadership" at times, and the family takes "family leadership" when the situation requires this. One writer has expressed the idea that the physician is the goal setting or instrumental leader, while the nurse is the interpreter or expressive leader.

The nurse who has responsibility for the nursing care of patients 24 hours a day, 7 days a week, carries responsibility for almost all of the direct and indirect care of these patients. She also is responsible for much of the training and supervision of the auxiliary personnel working with her.

One of the most essential of the extramedical responsibilities is that of maintaining communications between the patient and the members of the health team. The patient, through his physiologic signs, his verbal remarks about how he feels and his nonverbal behavior, is constantly providing information about his health status, much of which has an important bearing on both the goals and the activities of the health-team members. Also, if the team is to achieve its goals, the conclusions of its members about what the patient should do must be communicated to the patient and sometimes to members of his family, and their reactions or feelings communicated back to the various team members. As you know, the nurse is the person who is chiefly responsible for receiving and transmitting messages from the patient to the members of the health team and for seeing to it that the patient and his family receive and understand the information and directions that emanate from the various team members — as well as for interpreting the messages, verbal and nonverbal, of the patient and the family. Thus in a very real sense, the nurse is the leader of the health team insofar as its communications with patients are concerned.

The importance of this role has been receiving increasing recognition in recent years. Social scientists as well as nurses have been studying the effectiveness of the communications system of the health team, and articles and even books on how the nurse can improve her competence in this area have been published. The student of nursing might well read some of these studies and articles as she prepares herself to assume her responsibilities as "chief communicator" on the health team.

Patient-to-Health Personnel Communications. One of the first steps toward readying yourself for this leadership role is to learn how to communicate the patient's messages in writing—through charts, records and nurses' notes. The value of these written communications—particularly the nurses' notes—has been illustrated in a study of patients who committed suicide while in Veterans Administration hospitals.

From the records of patients who had committed suicide, a selection was made of a number of cases ... [which] were then matched, man for man, with controls who were similar with respect to certain population factors.

The case records of these two sets of patients were then abstracted and presented "blind" to a conference of research personnel and psychiatric, medical, and nursing consultants, who were asked to commit themselves to a judgment as to whether each case was a suicide or a control and to give the reasons for their answer. The identity of the case was then revealed, and discussion was held as to the reasons for the right or wrong answer.

The case records utilized had been abstracted from psychiatric case histories, social work reports, psychological test data and reports, ancillary therapy reports (such as occupational, education, industrial therapy reports), laboratory reports, doctors' notes, and nurses' notes. Of these various sources of information, the observations in the nurses' notes, especially those pertaining to patients in general hospitals, were the most important in providing information which was useful for indicating which patients had committed suicide. ... Frequently, it was from these notes only that some picture of the personality of the patient was obtained.

In these studies, it also became clear that it is primarily through the nurse's activities and behavior that the patient obtains his impression of the emotional tone of the hospital, that is whether the hospital is felt to be supportive, helpful, and effective, or rejecting and unconcerned. A feeling of support from the hospital was frequently crucial in the nonsuicidal outcome of seriously ill patients.

The nurse's influence on the emotional climate of the hospital is magnified by her significant role in its communications system. It is because of her observations and recordings that the physician can treat the patient with added awareness of and sensitivity to his reactions. ... Through her communications, she can facilitate appreciation of the patient as a person rather than merely a collection of medical symptoms and thus contribute to the patient's feeling of being considered worthwhile.[1]

The report of this study emphasized that the really useful notes were those that described the patient's feelings, behavior and interactions with other patients and the staff. Unfortunately, not all nurses' notes contain this kind

[1] N. L. Farberow, and R. A. Palmer, "The Nurse's Role in the Prevention of Suicide," Nursing Forum, 3(1):94-96, 1964.

of useful information, as is brought out in another report, also on a suicidal patient.

This case report will quote two sets of nursing notes. The patient was a borderline schizophrenic man who was being treated on a rehabilitation ward for an orthopedic problem. The first set of notes was written shortly after it became apparent that he was decompensating and had become suicidal.

12/15   4:45 a.m. Darvon, 65 mg. Aspirin gr. X
            10:30 a.m. Darvon, 65 mg. Aspirin gr. X
            12:15 p.m. Seconal 100 mgm.
            6:45 p.m. Darvon, 65 mg. and ASA gr. X
            11:00 p.m. Darvon, 65 mg.

After the patient was transferred to the psychiatric service, the character of the nursing notes changed.

7/22   12:00-8:00 a.m. Slept well, was seen smoking in bed by the female aide, he was told by male aide that this would have to stop (said he was sorry).
            7:00 a.m. Said he doesn't care about clean clothes, whether he has any or not. "I haven't cared for a month."
            7:30 a.m.-4:00 p.m. Patient not talking very much. Stated he felt tired.[2]

Experiments in the use of automated nursing notes, such as the one reported by Rita Stein in the Jan./Feb. 1969 issue of *Nursing Research*, are being done in an effort to improve nurses' notes. The development of automated notes is an attempt to meet the need for accurate, consistent and comprehensive reporting. According to Dr. Stein, automated notes give more information than do traditional narrative reports. They also tend to be generally more useful in predicting impending crisis situations. Automated nursing notes are a part of the trend, especially in hospitals, toward computerizing all clinical data about the patient.[3]

Several types of skills are involved in producing useful notes: skill in finding out what is bothering the patient, physically and emotionally; skill in identifying the responses that will be significant to the members of the health team; and skill in presenting this information accurately and succinctly to those who can make use of it.

The ineptitude of many nurses with respect to the first of these skills — drawing from the patient information about his problems — has been receiving considerable attention in the last few years. Studies have brought out that the nurse often considers herself too busy — sometimes with relatively unimportant paper work — to take the time for more than a superficial "How are you?" inquiry about the patient's concerns; the patient perceives what he considers to be the nurse's indifference and does not even try to tell her of his complaints. Even nurses who make an effort to communicate with patients may not always know how to listen to what the patients, through words, actions, and demeanor, really are saying. However, many examples of good communications are also in evidence, where the nurse's ability to listen and to communicate make a difference in patient care. Studies have

[2] B. Bursten, "The Psychiatric Consultant and the Nurse." *Nursing Forum*, **2(4)**:16-17, 1963.
[3] R. F. Stein, "An Exploratory Study in the Development and Use of Automated Nursing Reports." *Nursing Research*, **18**:14-21, Jan./Feb. 1969.

been made that demonstrate the effect of communications on patient care.

Learning how to listen is therefore becoming one of the important objectives of educational programs in nursing. The student who is conscious of the need to prepare herself for her future leadership responsibilities might well concentrate on the achievement of this objective. Empathy and awareness of the patient's and his family's feelings and problems are basic to the provision of good nursing care. The nurse can achieve these only by listening and by encouraging the patient and his family to express their concerns and problems. Chapters 4 and 7 also discusses relationships in nursing practice.

Meetings of the various members of the health team to discuss patients constitute another opportunity for the nurse to communicate significant information to the professional personnel who need it. It is not likely that you will attend many of these meetings while you are a student, but you may well find that they have become a part of the routine activities of the institution or the agency in which you will be practicing when you have graduated. At these meetings, individual patients are discussed, and the patient-care plans of the various health specialists, including the nurse, are decided.

Since data about the patient are important material for these meetings, the nurse has a real leadership responsibility in them. Yet, some observers have reported that she is likely to be the least active participant. Here is an incident that has been reported by one such observer—a nurse:

The head nurse was concerned because the professional team ward conferences were of little value to her. She went into them with her Kardex in hand, wanting a nursing plan of care for the patients, and she never did get this plan. In fact, she never got around to saying anything. By the time the other members of the professional team had had their say, time was up.
Why did this happen? Who gives us permission to speak? What gives us the authority to speak? Did this nurse really act as a member of the professional team? Or by her lack of contribution did she communicate to the professional team that she was not in tune with them—that she had nothing to share—and so no authority to speak? Did she act like she was the ward clerk sitting there with pencil and paper taking notes?[4]

This comment points up one of the cardinal rules of effective leadership— a leader must have a belief in his ability to lead. As one authority has put it:

You have to be comfortable about saying to yourself, "Yes, I am good," "Yes, I can help other people" and "Yes, I am a good leader." Now this may sound conceited. The difference is that it's based on reality.[5]

So—face reality. As a nurse you, of all members of the health team, will be in the best position to relay information about the patient. You will be prepared to do this. Have faith in yourself and do it. Of course, as mentioned before, it is important to know when it is best to listen—all good leaders are also good listeners. But also, learn to gauge when it is your turn to make a

---

[4] G. Cherescavich, "Blocks to Communication in Professional Groups," *Perspectives in Psychiatric Care,* **2(2):**39, 1964.
[5] F. J. Rubenstein, "Discovering Your Talents," In *Leadership Development for Nurses.* Denver, University of Colorado School of Nursing, 1961, p. 56.

contribution. At first you may find this difficult, but remember that we all make mistakes as we learn. When you make mistakes, examine them to see why you failed, and then try again. Also, you might learn by watching others who you think carry this responsibility well. As a nurse, you are an expert about nursing and well equipped to assume leadership when nursing is the concern of the group, or should be their concern. Your ability to assume leadership at the right time is not so that you will shine as a leader but so that the patient will receive the best of care.

Health Personnel-to-Patient Communications. Nurses, particularly those in hospitals, are being accused also of remissness in their responsibility to channel information from the other members of the health team to the patient and his family. For example, one article opens with this statement:

> The prevailing practices in hospital nursing guarantee to a patient that he will be securely wrapped in a protective cocoon from which no information regarding his condition will emanate to relatives and friends.[6]

The article goes on to charge that many nurses refuse to divulge to the patient's family such simple information as his temperature and bowel-functioning.

The effect of this behavior on patients can be seen in the report of a study of hospitalized patients:

> Patients frequently refused to ask nurses questions related to their illness because when they did, they rarely received satisfactory answers. . . .
> [Do you ever ask the nurses for any information?] *Oh, come on now, this would be pretty silly. The nurse does not know anything. Nurses never give you answers.*[7]

Even those nurses who are eager to perform their role of explainer to the patient are not always successful at it. Here again, there may be a listening problem: the nurse may limit her information to the facts that she has decided in advance should be made known to the patient and may not try to find out, by listening to him, what other things he is asking her about. She also may talk to the patient and his family in language that they do not really understand.

How much explanation a patient should receive and when he should receive it are areas of needed nursing knowledge that have received little investigation.[8] Such decisions probably should be made on an individual basis according to the preconceptions and level of understanding of each patient, but it is possible that some basic principles could be discovered that would guide the nurse in making them. A search for these principles might well be an activity in which you, as a professional nurse, will want to participate.

Even as a student, you can begin to tackle the problems of health per-

---

[6] D. E. Little, "The Say Something Tell Nothing Concept of Nursing," *Nursing Forum,* 2(1):39, 1963.

[7] J. K. Skipper, Jr., *et al.,* "Some Barriers to Communication between Patients and Hospital Functionaires," *Nursing Forum,* 2(1):19, 1963.

[8] M. Aasterud, "Explanation to the Patient," *Nursing Forum,* 2(4):36-44, 1963.

sonnel-to-patient communications. At one school of nursing, two students compiled a list of all the questions that the patients on one service had been asking the various hospital personnel with whom they came in contact — ward clerks, ward maids and food-service employees as well as nursing personnel. They then put the most frequently asked questions and the answers to them in a booklet, which was given to each patient admitted to this service. Another pair of students, noting that some diabetic patients cared for by the public health nursing service, who did not speak English well had difficulty in understanding directions about how to administer insulin to themselves, prepared a booklet that described this technique in pictures.

These students have demonstrated another requirement of the leader — awareness of a problem and creativeness in finding a practical means of meeting it.

The Professional Nursing Service Team

Preparation as interpreter of the patient's needs also will help the beginning practitioner in nursing to assume her leadership obligations on the professional nursing team. Most newly graduated nurses will work on such a team in a hospital or in a public health nursing agency. As in the case of the health team, they may think that they have only a follower role on this team — that all of the leadership functions are carried by the director and assistant directors of the nursing service, the supervisors and, perhaps, the head nurses.

True, the administrative nursing personnel, by determining policies and practices, have a considerable influence on the goal-setting and goal-achieving activities of the professional nursing team. But, in carrying out these standard-setting functions, they must take into consideration the effect of the policies and practices on the comfort and well-being of the patients. And who on the team is in the best position to identify the patients' needs and to note when a policy, current or proposed, is at cross-purposes to these needs? The staff nurse, of course. Thus, the staff nurse is in a position to influence the policy- and practice-setting activities of the team — by definition, a leadership function.

The influence of the statement, "This would be best for the patients" on administrative routines should not be underestimated. For example, not so long ago it was common practice for all hospital patients to be roused at dawn. This arrangement was advantageous from the administrative point of view because it helped to equalize the nursing tasks of the personnel on the various tours of duty. But think of the discomfort to the patients, most of whom were not used to seeing the sun rise! No one can say for certain what is causing the disappearance of this custom, but it is not unlikely that staff nurse reports of patients' misery and complaints have been playing a large part in its elimination.

Sometimes there are occasions in which a policy that is appropriate for most patients should be modified for one patient. Again, it is the staff nurse who can identify such a situation and call it to the attention of administrative nursing personnel. Here is an instance in which a staff nurse recognized this leadership obligation:

A primipara was spotted by the nurse in a mothers' class as a conflicted and highly anxious person. She feared deformity of the baby and mental retardation; she did not seem to gain any reassurance from talking about it in the group. The same concern came up again and again. The reasons for this woman's hesitancy towards motherhood were clear from what glimpses she gave from her own childhood, from her talking about the highly promising career she had given up, from the quality of the marriage as it was observed.

The public health nurse gained her agency's consent to her meeting the demands of a dependency relationship this woman required. Daily bathing of the baby and making of the formula seemed necessary for weeks, in complete contrast to customary practices.[9]

If you become a staff nurse, you may identify ways in which you think that procedures might be improved, particularly if the procedures in the hospital or community health agency in which you are practicing vary from those in the institutions in which you are now receiving your clinical learning experiences. Before recommending changes, however, it is well to stop and ask yourself: "Do I think my way is best merely because it is the way I learned? Is the difference between my way and the way it is being done here an essential one?" If the difference is nonessential, you may decide that it is not worth the conflict that may arise if you proclaim, "My way is best. We must therefore do it my way."

A letter from a USA nurse who is working in an industrial clinic in Argentina illustrates this point:

I do not propose to speak with authority, but from observation and from personal experience during the several years in which I have been doing industrial nursing in foreign countries. It seems to me that those factors which decide the difference between a good nursing service program and a mediocre one might fall into three groups:
(1) The ability to work with the equipment and the supplies at hand
(2) The investigation and evaluation of the methods and practices already in use
(3) Attitudes and adaptation to personalities and customs
You will very likely agree that the nurse who is trained in the USA comes readily to the conclusion that equipment and supplies made in the states are superior in quality and durability and that their use in some cases results in the saving of much time. Not everyone, however, is of this opinion. Doctors and nurses like the equipment with which they are familiar. If it works effectively for them, why should they change? Many times it is the discerning nurse who can put to good use the "just as good" and yet persevere till she obtains the best in such things as sterilizing agents that make the difference between good technique and second-rate performance. . . .
In investigating different methods so as to evaluate them, it is wise to find out "why they do things that way" before condemning; there may be a good reason. I'll admit it takes patience, but you can get your point across by enlisting the goodwill of the people with whom you work and sort of studying together something that perhaps

[9] I. S. Wolff, "The Psychiatric Nurse in Community Mental Health—A Rebuttal," *Perspectives in Psychiatric Care*, **2**(2):15, 1964.

you already know in order to create a learning situation. (You can almost never get your point across by pointing out the merit of your system.) This method is far from easy, but if you succeed without losing your perspective, your company will have a good industrial nurse.[10]

The Nursing-Care Team[11]

The beginning practitioner in a hospital or community health agency setting may find herself frequently in charge of a team of nonprofessional nursing personnel to which the care of a group of patients has been assigned. In view of the importance of the small group in the achievement of the agency's goals — one authority views closely coordinated, small work groups as probably "the most important locus of decision in the hospital"[12] — the importance of the role of the leader of the nursing-care team cannot be overemphasized.

It is quite possible that you will have some learning experiences in this leadership position before you graduate and will be helped by your instructors to identify and develop the skills needed for it. A brief summary of some of the requirements for this leadership role may help you in these experiences.

First of all, it is important to recognize that unlike many of the other teams to which nurses belong, the nursing-care team often has only one professionally prepared member — the nurse herself. Therefore, the responsibility for leadership is likely to be centered in her and not divided among the members of the group. Although she can delegate tasks, and expect them to be carried out responsibly, she cannot delegate her responsibility for seeing to it that these tasks are accomplished.

This is not to say that the team leader stands apart from the group and issues orders. She works *with* the members and stimulates them to do their work well, not because they are driven to it, but because they want to achieve the group's goals.

Team nursing, if carried out well, combines the best thinking of all the team members about the patient's problems. The team is able to affect both climate and continuity of care. One team member, perhaps a nursing student, may suggest why a patient is uncomfortable. A nurse's aide may add her observations. The team leader is able to gather these opinions and adapt group thinking as she designs the nursing-care plan to meet the specific communicated needs of the patient. Team nursing could encourage each member of the team to contribute his best thinking to patient care.[13]

The team leader must realize, however, that the existence of appropriate

[10] E. M. McCloud, "A Letter From Tierra del Fuego," *American Association of Industrial Nurses Journal*, **12:**23-24, Jan. 1964.
[11] See reference to nursing-care team in Chapter 4.
[12] R. N. Wilson, *Newer Dimensions of Patient Care: Part 2*, by E. L. Brown, New York, Russell Sage Foundation, 1962, p. 48.
[13] R. C. Swansburg, *Team Nursing: A Programmed Learning Experience*, vol. 1, New York, Putnam, 1968, p. 13.

goals among the members of this group cannot be taken for granted, especially in the case of those members who have not chosen nursing as a career to the extent of investing effort in preparing for it. As Esther Lucile Brown has pointed out:

> Although many nursing aides are drawn to hospitals because they want to do something for the sick, probably much larger proportions are looking merely for a job, under the most pleasant conditions possible, where they can earn a living. . . . Such persons come without any work model, created and fostered by a training school or membership association, that emphasizes the importance of emotional commitment to their work as a social obligation, or as a prerequisite to personal growth and development and to possible advancement on the job. . . .
> Because they are primarily interested in the pay envelope, they have little identification with the goals of the institution.[14]

Helping the members of the nursing-care team to commit themselves to suitable goals is, therefore, one of the primary tasks of the team leader. One way that she accomplishes this is to demonstrate her own value system—to show, through her own actions, what tasks she considers most important. In a study of nurses in general hospitals, Elizabeth Hagen and Luverne Wolff found that some of the nurses "appeared to be thing-oriented, that is, they valued getting the work done quickly, keeping the unit neat and tidy, having records completed accurately and promptly, and having concern about equipment and supplies. Others tended to be person-oriented whether this person was a patient, a member of the patient's family, a visitor, a professional nurse, or an aide or other auxiliary person."[15] The nurses in this second group were, of course, the ones who considered giving direct care to patients more important than any other task. Perhaps you would like to think through whether one could, or should, ever be all "person oriented" or all "thing oriented." If not, what proportion of each would you care to suggest?

In evaluating your abilities as a team leader, you might take note of whether you tend to behave in a person-oriented or a thing-oriented way. Will the aides who have you as their work model see the giving of good care to patients as their most important goal? This self-evaluation need not await the day when you have your first team-leader assignment. You can undertake it in your clinical assignments this week.

And remember, person-oriented people respect the integrity of all persons —aides as well as patients—and try to help them to meet their needs. For clues about how to help your team members in this respect, you might well study Dr. Brown's book, *Newer Dimensions in Patient Care: Part 2.* She points out that most people like to work, but they want to feel that their job is important and to experience a sense of accomplishment in doing it.

No case has to be made for the importance of the aides' work. They perform one of the most essential services in the hospital, but they may not be

---

[14] *Newer Dimensions of Patient Care, Part 2,* New York, Russell Sage Foundation, 1962. p. 112.

[15] *Nursing Leadership Behavior in General Hospitals,* New York, Bureau of Publications, Teachers College, Columbia University, 1961, p. 143.

aware of this fact. One way to help them to recognize their importance is to make full use of the information that they acquire about patients and involve them in planning the group's work. Although most of the final decisions about nursing-care plans will be the responsibility of the team leader, her decisions will be better – and more likely to be implemented – if she listens to the information that her team members can provide and takes into account their suggestions.

She should also make it clear that she recognizes that it is the group – not herself alone – that accomplishes the tasks. *We*, rather than *I*, is a good word for a team leader to use. Praise for a task well done also gives a sense of accomplishment – and very often results in a repetition of the good performance. It may be that an aide will be more proficient than the nurse in some way – for example, in communicating with certain patients. Not only should the nurse make use of this ability in her assignments, but she might well comment on the aide's superiority to her in this respect.

Inservice education is one means of stimulating interest in, as well as providing the necessary training for, doing a job well. In addition to the programs provided by the hospital, frequent opportunities will occur for the team leader to help the members of her team to develop their capacities. Such teaching will include demonstrations of procedures, of course, but it should not stop there. Although aides cannot be expected to acquire the scientific background of the professional nurse, a rudimentary understanding of the *whys* as well as the *hows* of certain approaches is not beyond their grasp. Not only will this understanding help them to do a better job, but it also will give them the satisfaction that comes from learning.

In carrying out her teaching responsibilities, the team leader must prepare her team members for the new practices and procedures with which they may be confronted. Great changes are taking place in hospitals – changes that affect patterns of nursing care and medical and nursing procedures. Members of patients' families are being added to some nursing-care teams – a development that requires a repatterning of patient-care assignments, the establishment of new lines of communication, and, most important of all perhaps, the development of new attitudes. Electric monitoring devices and intercommunication systems are being introduced. New medical approaches – hypothermia, hyperthermia, hyperbaric therapy and kidney dialysis, to name a few – are making it necessary for nursing personnel to learn about complicated pieces of equipment.

Keeping abreast of new developments in one's field is, of course, one of the requirements of a professional person. The importance of this requirement is magnified when the work of other people, as well as one's own work, will be affected by these developments.

The professional literature is, of course, one of the important sources for the nurse to use in her continuing self-education. The nursing journals will help her to keep abreast of new developments. Also, she probably will find that for further understanding she will want to turn to books – both new ones and those that she has read previously. For example, a review of the principles of physics may be necessary for understanding the operation of a new piece of equipment, and a review of physiology for understanding its effect on the patient. It might be wise, therefore, for the nursing student not to dispose of her current textbooks but to utilize them as the foundation of her own professional library.

The nurse who is a team leader must be on the watch also for information appearing in newspapers and popular magazines that explains new health measures in terms that will be understandable to the members of her team. She cannot rely entirely on written materials, but they sometimes can be a useful addendum to her own explanations.

These, then, are some of the behaviors that characterize a good leader of a nursing-care team. They do not constitute an exhaustive list; the team leader may find herself confronted with problems that have not been dealt with here. For example, she may be in the position of working with aides who have been in the situation many more years than she has and who therefore tend to resent the leadership of a "youngster." Or, she may find that some of her team members never had any intention of working more than a few weeks in that particular situation and are immune to any enthusiasm-building efforts. In searching for ways of handling difficult situations like these, the nurse has one guideline: to treat the members of her team with the same consideration and respect that she shows toward her patients. By following this guideline she may not achieve completely successful results, but the results will be as successful as could be expected.

The Management and Educator Teams

Some nurses are members of teams that are not entirely, or even primarily, concerned with health. For example, the nurse in an industrial company may be a member of a management team that, although it is responsible for determining the scope and the policies of the company's health service, is not composed of people who are members of any health discipline. In some instances, the industrial physician is also a member of this team, but often the nurse is the only full-time health worker in the company and is therefore relied on to provide leadership in the company's health activities. Similarly, a nurse is often the only representative of the health disciplines on the faculty of a school.

Both of these nursing positions—that of occupational health nurse and that of school nurse—have developed far beyond the finger-bandaging and first-aid stage. Increasingly, businesses are recognizing that the worker who has been on the job for some time represents a capital asset and that it is to the company's benefit to keep him in maximum "running order." Their interest in his welfare, therefore, is being extended beyond the stage of treating and preventing occupationally caused disabilities to the prevention of other diseases and the maintenance of health. Similarly, schools are recognizing that the education of students in healthful living is among their important preparation-for-life responsibilities.

However, the majority of the members on management and faculty teams cannot be expected to know how to develop a health service that will implement these broad philosophies. The leadership role of the nurse on these teams is therefore obvious. She must develop her own job and interpret the importance of her activities in terms of the team's primary goals and values.

Since the nurse is prepared in programs that hold a health-for-health's-sake philosophy, the role of health leader on a team with other major goals requires some adaptation on her part. The occupational health nurse must take into consideration not only the health hazards of her company and the major health problems of its employees but also the means by which remedies can be instituted at minimal expense. She must, therefore, arm herself with knowledge about the employees' health problems and with information concerning the out-plant and in-plant resources that are available for attacking these problems. For example, data concerning the number of employees who have died of cancer, plus information that the local cancer society is willing to cooperate in a diagnostic program, might well influence the management team to agree to a program of cancer detection among the plant's employees. The same example applies to heart and other diseases.

A study of lunches in textile factories, which was made by a state nutrition committee, will serve as an example of a nurse's alertness to the health resources in her community. The report of this study brings out that 1 garment factory was included in it, along with 165 textile companies. Moreover, this garment factory was 1 of the 2 companies in the group in which a detailed study was made of the vitamin and mineral content of the lunches which the employees purchased from vending machines (the only food service available to them). One might wonder why a garment factory was included in the study and why the lunches of its employees were studied in detail. Then, this statement appears: "Absenteeism from minor illness and accidents on the job was so high that the company nurse requested help from a nutritionist. Skim milk was recommended as an addition [to the vending machine foods] because it is a good source of calcium and protein and is easily vended." [16] The nurse in this company saw the possible relationship between one of the company's problems — absenteeism — and a community health project and visualized a way these two situations could be coupled for the benefit of the employees' health.

School nurses are also in the process of identifying their appropriate role and activities for other members of the faculty. Because most of the members of this faculty team do their teaching in a classroom, they may not recognize that health principles often are taught "in the doing" when health problems arise and that parents as well as children should be included sometimes among the persons to be taught. Also, their concept of the content of

[16] E. J. Lease, *et al.*, "Industrial Lunches," *American Association of Industrial Nurses*, **12**:9, Feb. 1964.

health education may be limited to information about physical health, and they may not realize that the inculcation of mental health principles might well be part of the school's objectives.

Since these other teachers are in a position to identify children with health problems, including emotional disturbances, it is important that the school nurse help them not only to visualize her job in all its ramifications but also to become active participants in the school's health program. The methods that she uses to prepare them for this participation probably will depend on the customs of the particular faculty group. If it has an inservice education program, the nurse might well recommend a meeting or a series of meetings devoted to the detection of health problems and suggest appropriate resource persons. In other instances, she may decide that it is best to work on an individual basis with the teachers. In other words, the school nurse must take into consideration the prevailing attitudes and customs of the other members of the team—another requirement of the good leader.

NURSING LEADERSHIP OUTSIDE OF WORK

As a professional person, your responsibilities for providing leadership will not be confined to the groups with which you work as part of your job. Because the professional nurse has more than average knowledge in the field of health, she has an obligation over and beyond the regular duties of a citizen—that of bringing her influence to bear on the development of the health programs that serve the people in her local community, her state, the country and even the whole world. Moreover, this obligation does not cease if she withdraws, either temporarily or permanently, from nursing practice. There is really no such person as an inactive nurse; whatever the nurse's employment status, her leadership is always needed in public affairs.

Though a nurse begins the continuing responsibility for self-development during her preparation for nursing practice, she must always continue to expand herself with a broader, deeper preparation to meet and care for others.[17] Such development evidences itself in her ability to be sensitive to her coworkers and to anticipate the needs of her patients.

Your responsibility as a nurse-citizen will be broader in scope than that connected with your job. Your concern will be for the welfare of all your fellow-citizens, not merely those who are your patients. Thus, you will take cognizance of such widespread health problems as alcoholism, drug addiction and the hazards of smoking, even though you may not meet these particular problems in your work situation.

The fulfillment of this nurse-citizen obligation will enrich your life greatly, broadening your horizons and widening the circle of your personal contacts. For your own sake, it is important that you develop this aspect

[17] J. D. Copp and L. A. Copp, "Look to the Pattern of Relationship," *American Journal of Nursing,* **60**:1284. Sept. 1960.

of your leadership role. It is understandable, however, if at first you are over-whelmed by the idea that you can contribute to the solution of the health problems of society-at-large. Nonetheless, there are ways by which you can make your influence felt in these matters.

Political Leadership

A citizen of voting age automatically belongs to several political groups — the groups of people who are entitled to vote for elective officials in the citizen's local community, in his state, and in the USA. Although, except in the case of referendums, these voters usually do not vote for or against specific proposals, the persons for whom they vote make known their stand on important issues before the election. It is your responsibility as a citizen to study the records and the expressed views of the candidates for office and the platforms of the political parties with which they are affiliated and to vote for the candidates who are most likely to promote the programs that you think are in the best interest of the public.

You also may wish to work actively for the election of these candidates. One way of doing so is by participating in the activities of a young people's political club.

However, it would be unrealistic to assume that you, as an individual, will be able to influence the outcomes of elections to any great degree. Your chief means of influencing political decisions is through the elected officials who have a voice in these decisions. To do this, you will need to:

1. Inform yourself about the bills concerned with health matters which are currently under consideration, and develop your own position on the issues involved. Among your resources will be the daily newspapers, particularly the editorials; periodicals, especially the *American Journal of Nursing* and the magazine of your state nurses association; radio and television programs; and the literature of such organizations as the League of Women Voters and the AFL-CIO.

2. Learn about the legislative process — that is, the groups and the individuals through which a piece of proposed legislation passes before it is enacted into a Federal or state or local law. Find out which committee or committees of the legislative body will study the bill in which you are interested and the name of the people on these committees. Follow the bill as it proceeds along its route; know when it is under committee study, when it is coming up for vote by the entire legislative body, when it is sent to the Chief Executive for signature or veto.

3. Make known your stand to your elected representative or some other person, such as the chairman of a legislative committee, who has a voice in the passage or defeat of the bill. A personal visit is a good way of registering your opinion; so is a letter. In either event, make your presentation in a way befitting a professional person who is qualified to speak with authority and whose concern is for the public welfare. Do not merely state your position,

but explain the reasons for your stand and, wherever possible, document your points with facts from reliable sources.

Another way of making known your ideas about legislative proposals is through letters to the editors of newspapers and magazines and through participation in public forums and on radio and television programs.

Leadership Through Nursing Organizations

Although you will want to use every opportunity to promote your causes by political means, the political influence of one individual is admittedly limited. In particular, influencing action on proposed legislation is not equivalent to bringing into being new, needed programs for which no legislation has been proposed — a task that is beyond most individuals who are acting alone. However, groups do have considerable power in this direction. Associating yourself with organizations and clubs that include the promotion of social welfare among their objectives is one of the ways by which you can fulfill your leadership responsibility as a nurse-citizen.

The nursing organizations constitute major channels through which you, an individual, can effect improvement in the health care of all citizens. Through participating in the activities of these organizations you will achieve two ends. First, such participation will help you to see the range of nursing problems in perspective; in addition to the microscope through which you view the problems in your work situation, you will be furnished with a telescope that will enable you to examine other important problems in the world of nursing. For example, if you are employed in a general hospital, association with other members of a nursing organization will help you to understand the problems confronting psychiatric hospitals, nursing homes, community agencies — problems that are your problems too.

Then, membership in these organizations will enable you to participate in the shaping of programs that are directed toward the improvement of nursing care throughout the country. You need not be an office holder or the chairman of a committee to exercise your influence, because the nursing organizations are examples of groups in which leadership is group-centered. Any member who participates *actively* in the group's affairs is fulfilling a leadership obligation.

Part 3, which contains a description of the various national nursing organizations, can help you to decide on the ones that you should join. Membership in your professional association — the ANA — might be regarded as a "must" for a professional nurse. Many professional nurses also believe that a professional nurse should belong to the NLN — another national organization that is concerned with all fields of nursing.

Leadership Through Citizen Groups With Social Welfare Programs

In addition to the nursing organizations, there are many other organizations that are concerned with the improvement of the nation's health — the

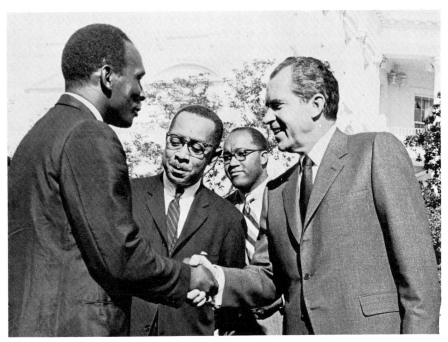

Fig. 17-1. Neil Butler, head nurse at University of Florida's J. Hillis Miller Hospital, being welcomed by President Nixon at the White House. Mr. Butler, a member of the Gainsville City Commission, was attending a Presidential meeting with a number of Negro leaders from across the country. Mr. Butler is also a member of the ANA BE-INvolved Membership Committee. (American Nurses' Association)

National Association for Mental Health, the American Cancer Society, the National Tuberculosis Association, the American Heart Association, to name only a few. In these organizations, health personnel and other citizens work together to promote the improvement and the development of health services.

You may wish to join some of these national organizations and thereby lend your support to their large-scale educational and research activities. However, you may find that you can participate more actively in their programs by associating yourself with the chapters or the branch organizations in your community. You may also wish to join other organizations in your community, such as business and professional women's clubs and church groups, that include social welfare projects among their activities. For an illustration of one nurse's participation in civic activities see Figure 17-1.

These groups will offer you an opportunity not only for studying community health problems and making recommendations about ways that the community should go about solving them but also for actually tackling some of them. Participation in such activities is particularly rewarding to those nurses who, because of family obligations, have left the work-a-day world of nursing and want some useful outlet for their professional abilities.

One such wife-and-mother nurse, whose field is psychiatric nursing, has told about her participation in a program that helps long-term psychiatric patients about to be discharged from state hospitals to become reacquainted with their community before they return to it.[18] In this "homecoming" program, groups of citizens take groups of patients on trips to the community over a period of several months, and help them to relearn to shop, find their way about on buses, and enjoy themselves in museums and zoos. Someone with a psychiatric background is needed as a liaison between the hospitals and the volunteer groups—thus the nurse leader. However, as this nurse leader points out, the other volunteers—all lay persons—can contribute to the program in ways that she cannot: when associating with them, the patients feel that they are mingling with normal human beings, not with hospital personnel who are watching their every move.

This recognition of the contributions that lay persons can make is an important attribute of the nurse who is participating in citizen organizations. Education in the health field places the nurse in one leadership role, but the other members of a project team are likely to have abilities that qualify them for leadership in other aspects of the project.

Leadership in Interpreting Professional Nursing to the Public

Throughout this chapter, some of the essentials of leadership have been identified in connection with various group situations in which you, as a professional nurse, may find yourself. In an effort to avoid boring repetition, a leadership characteristic usually has been mentioned in relation to only one of the several situations to which it applies. For example, although keeping abreast of current developments in nursing has been discussed in connection with only one team situation, it is a requirement of the nurse leader in any group.

Another omnipresent leadership function that deserves special emphasis is the interpretation of professional nursing—what it is and what it can and should be. Ideas about the potentials and the appropriate goals of nursing have been changing rapidly in recent years—so rapidly that many people, including in some cases members of other health disciplines, have not grasped all the implications of the newer concepts. It will be up to you, as a registered nurse, to define *modern* nursing and its role in health practice for all of the people with whom you come in contact.

The public-at-large also is entitled to this interpretation. As Mary C. Rockefeller, a member of the public who knows a great deal about nursing, has pointed out, all citizens have a great stake in the development of nursing, first as patients, and secondly as the sources of support for the health services. Mrs. Rockefeller also makes it clear that the public is bewildered by the changes that are taking place in health care, not all of which are "advances" in the eyes of many citizens.

[18] J. Rappeport, "Homecoming—A Volunteer Program," *Perspectives in Psychiatric Care,* 2(2):41-45, 1964.

One way that you can interpret what modern nursing is, is through your practice of nursing. No amount of talk about "the patient as a person" and "comprehensive nursing care" is as effective as actual demonstration of these concepts. However, some of the questions that the public is asking require verbal answers and explanations. For example, here are some of the questions raised by Mrs. Rockefeller:

Why all this education? Where is the bedside nurse? Where is the nurse who is supposed to take care of me? Why are there not greater rewards for the bedside nurse? How about all the nurses everywhere who are sitting at desks; what are they doing? Do they *all* have to be nurses?

. . . . .

As for nursing research, the public has no idea what is going on. What kinds of questions are being asked in nursing research and what are the investigators finding out? What is the difference between research and a study? What is meant by basic research? applied research? action research?[19]

It is doubtful if you, a student, are prepared as yet to answer all of these questions. You can, however, prepare the foundation on which any interpretation of nursing must be built. This foundation is your philosophy of nursing — what you believe it is, and is not, and what it can and should be. You could, of course, copy a statement of philosophy from a book or a nursing school bulletin. However, if you develop one yourself, as suggested elsewhere, it will have more meaning for you, and you will be able to explain it more effectively to others.

The formulation of a philosophy of nursing and the interpretation of this philosophy to others — through both actions and words — is one of the most important leadership responsibilities of the professional nurse. You, the student of professional nursing, can begin preparing for this responsibility now.

PROBLEMS

1. (a) Select from this chapter what you consider to be the underlying principles of leadership. (b) Explain or illustrate why you selected each statement.

2. Develop your own definition of leadership, making use of your readings and the ideas presented in this chapter.

3. (a) Review the past week and list the various roles you have assumed. (b) What do you think others expected of you when you assumed these roles?

4. (a) How many times in the past month have you been a part of group activity? (b) In what way was the group different because you joined it? (c) In which groups did you take active leadership? (d) In which groups did you shun leadership? (e) Do you know why you behaved as you did?

[19] M. C. Rockefeller, "The Why of Citizen Involvement in Patient Care," *Nursing Outlook,* **11**:581, Aug. 1963.

5. Prepare a paper in which you compare the health team and the nursing-service team in terms of the various leadership responsibilities of the professional nurse.

6. (a) During your clinical experiences, what hospital policies, practices, or procedures have you noticed that interfere with the comfort or the well-being of the patients. (Confine yourself to these three: policies, practices, and procedures; do not list conditions, such as personnel shortages.) (b) Take one of the items on your list and think through the ways in which it could be modified to the greater comfort of the patients, of their families. (c) What other problems, if any, would be created by this modification? (d) List the pros and the cons for making a change and decide whether, in your opinion, it should be made; how would you proceed to get your proposal adopted?

7. Assume that you are the team leader of a group of practical nurses and aides on a children's ward in which a mother's rooming-in plan is about to be instituted. How would you go about preparing your team for the advent of the mothers?

8. The health committee of a club in the community of which you are now a resident has the responsibility of preparing the program of a two-hour meeting of the club. (a) List three topics that you, if you were a member of this committee, would suggest as suitable — either because they are currently under debate, or because they are health problems of which the members of the club should be aware. (b) Take one of these topics and prepare a specific program — that is, indicate what film, if any, might be shown; from what source a speaker might be obtained; and the ways in which the club members might be encouraged in the program.

9. Prepare a statement of your own philosophy of nursing in the form of "This I Believe." In preparing your statement, review chapters 1, 2, 3, 4, 7 and 28. Include in your statement the reasoning behind your philosophy.

10. Study the lives of some leaders (nursing and other) who have influenced modern nursing, such as: R. Louise McManus, Helen Bunge, Elizabeth Hagen, Mildred Montag, Kenneth Herrold and Robert Merton.

SUGGESTED REFERENCES*

LEADERSHIP: GENERAL

Clemence, Sister Madeleine. "Existentialism: A Philosophy of Committment." *American Journal of Nursing,* **66:**500-505, Mar. 1966.
Eisenhower, D. D. *At Ease, Stories I Tell to Friends.* New York, Doubleday, 1967.
Gardner, J. W. *Excellence.* New York, Harper, 1961.
Leone, L. P. "Accent on Leadership." *American Journal of Nursing,* **58:**1419-1421, Oct. 1958.

---

* In each chapter all citations are footnoted and are not included here. All starred references are recommended for additional reading.

* McGregor, D. "Analysis of Leadership." In *The Human Side of Enterprise*. New York, McGraw-Hill, 1960. pp. 179-189.

LEADERSHIP ON THE JOB

* Brown, E. L. *Newer Dimensions of Patient Care*. New York, Russel Sage Foundation. Part I, 1961; Part II, 1962; Part III, 1964.
* Christman, L. B. "Nursing Leadership – Style and Substance." *American Journal of Nursing*, **67:**2091-2093, Oct. 1967.
Crawford, N. "You Can Help Your Profession by Writing." *Nursing Outlook*, **8:**513-516, Sept. 1960.
Davidson, L. C. "Students' Perception of Leadership in Nursing Care." *Nursing Outlook*, **16:**30-31, Dec. 1968.
* Hagen, E. and Wolff, L. *Nursing Leadership Behavior in General Hospitals*. New York, Bureau of Publications, Teachers College, Columbia University, 1961.
Ingmire, A. E. *A Leadership Program in Nursing, 1964-1966*. San Francisco, University of California, San Francisco Medical Center, 1967.
Kneisl, C. R. "Increasing Interpersonal Understanding Through Sociodrama." *Perspectives in Psychiatric Care*, **6(3):**104-109, 1968.
Leadership in Nursing Series. Washington, D.C., Leadership Resources, Inc., 1966.
McKinley, J. E. "Inservice Education for Leadership." *Nursing Outlook*, **16:**47-49, Sept. 1968.
* Olson, M. "Social Influence on Decision Making." *Journal of Nursing Education*, **7:**11-16, Jan. 1968.
Peeples, E. H., *et al.* "Social-Psychological Obstacles to Effective Health Team Practice." *Nursing Forum*, **7:**28-37, Winter 1968.
* Sigma Theta Tau. *The Assessment of Leader Behaviors*. 20 Hillside Circle, Storrs, Connecticut, Sigma Theta Tau Headquarters, Feb. 1969.

See also references in Chapter 7 on "Relationships and Personal Growth."

CITIZEN LEADERSHIP

* Albrecht, J. J. "The Nurse as a Citizen or Politics is the Art of the Impossible." *Maryland Nursing News*, **37:**9-21, Spring 1969.
* The American Heritage Foundation. *Good Citizen: The Rights and Duties of an American*. New York, The Foundation, 1965.
Broe, E. "The Nurse – A World Citizen." *Nursing Outlook*, **11:**905-908, Dec. 1963.
"Every Nurse Is a World Citizen." *Nursing Outlook*, **11:**873, Dec. 1963.
* Interdepartmental Committee on the Status of Women. *American Women, 1963-1968*. Washington, D.C., Government Printing Office. 1968.
* Rockefeller, M. C. "The Why of Citizen Involvement in Patient Care." *Nursing Outlook*, **11:**580-581, Aug. 1963.

Organizations and
Related Activities

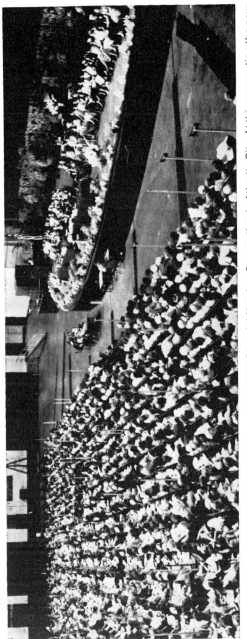

Fig. A. The assembled House of Delegates at the 1952 Biennial Nursing Convention in Atlantic City. At this convention the new structure of the national nursing organizations was voted on. It resulted in the creation of the National League for Nursing and the restructuring of the American Nurses' Association. (American Journal of Nursing)

PREVIEW

Why are there so many nursing organizations? This is a natural question for you to ask when you study this part, which begins with your organization, the National Student Nurses' Association, and then proceeds to tell about several others in this country including the ANA, the NLN, the American Association of Industrial Nurses, the American Association of Nurse Anesthetists, the American College of Midwifery, the Association of Operating Room Nurses, the Committee on Nursing of the American Medical Association, the Conference of Catholic Schools of Nursing, the Guild of Saint Barnabas, the National Association for Practical Nurse Education and Service, the National Council of Catholic Nurses of the United States of America,[1] the National Federation of Licensed Practical Nurses, and the Nurses Christian Fellowship. It does seem like a large number of organizations for you to learn about now, and it includes certain ones that you will want to join when you graduate.

However, had you been a student of nursing in 1951, your task would have been much greater. There were several more national organizations then, as well as a group of interorganizational or "joint" committees and services. Each of these associations, leagues, organizations, committees and services had been formed to meet real needs and was engaged in a variety of activities to meet these needs. Yet some important needs were not being met. Nurses began to question whether restructuring of the national organizations concerned with nursing was in order which would enable them best to serve society and their members.

Accordingly, a study of the structure of 6 nursing organizations was undertaken in the early 1940's—the ANA, the American Association of Industrial Nurses (AAIN), the Association of Collegiate Schools of Nursing (ACSN), the National Association of Colored Graduate Nurses (NACGN), the National League of Nursing Education (NLNE) and the National Organization for Public Health Nursing (NOPHN). This study was a lengthy undertaking and an expensive one. The treasuries of the organizations and the pocketbooks of their members were strained for over 10 years. During this time a research organization, the Raymond Rich Associates, was employed to make a study,[2] a committee composed of representatives of all 6 organizations was appointed and supplied with a staff, quantities of study materials were prepared and sent to the organizations' constituents, meetings were held, and opinionnaires and ballots were sent to the voting memberships.

In the course of this study it became apparent that the functions which the 6 organizations were or should be performing were of 2 kinds—those

[1] The National Council of Catholic Nurses of the USA was disbanded as of December 31, 1969.

[2] "R. Rich Associates Report on the Structure of Organized Nursing," *American Journal of Nursing,* **46:**648-661, Oct. 1946.

which are the responsibility of the profession only, and those which can be carried out best by nurses and others. Essentially, the 1st question to be answered was: Can these 2 kinds of functions be undertaken best by 1 organization, by 2 organizations, or by the 6 existing organizations? The 2nd problem was to sort out the functions according to the 2 categories.

The majority of the memberships decided on 2 organizations: (1) a reorganized ANA in which registered nurses could work for the continuing improvement of professional practice, the economic and general welfare of nurses, and the health needs of the American public, and (2) a new NLN in which all members of the health team, agencies supplying nursing service and education, and lay members of the community could act together to provide the best possible nursing services and to assure good nursing education.

Technically, this reorganization was brought about by the absorption of the NACGN into the ANA and the merging of the ACSN, the NLNE and the NOPHN into the NLN.[3] Actually, however, much more was involved in the reorganization. The functions and the activities of the reorganized ANA and the new NLN, taken together, far exceeded those of the 5 organizations from which they grew. Moreover, the constitutions and the bylaws of the ANA and the NLN were drawn up in such a way that the functions and the activities of the 2 organizations would complement each other. This meant that the ANA took over some of the work formerly carried by the NLNE and NOPHN, and the NLN was given responsibility for some of the "joint" activities which had been carried out by all 6 of the former organizations. A Coordinating Council, composed of the boards of directors of the ANA and the NLN, was established so that programs of common concern could be coordinated. In addition, some common services have been established, such as the ANA-NLN Film Service and others.

Thus, you will see that the 2 largest national organizations concerned with nurses and nursing are not the result of haphazard growth. They have been planned so that their functions and activities would mesh but not overlap. It is important that you realize this as you study the ANA and the NLN. If you wish to see their common purpose — the best possible nursing care for the American people — fully realized, you will be vitally concerned with the programs of both the ANA and the NLN.

---

[3] The AAIN chose not to participate in the reorganization.

Program and Activities
Membership
Official Publications
Conventions
Governing Bodies
Committees
Spokesman for Students
Headquarters

CHAPTER

18

National Student Nurses' Association of the USA

There is ferment among students today, characterized by their growing awareness that they can and should assume more of the responsibility for their own education and social development and for that of future generations of students. Ideas like "student power" demonstrate the interest that students have in taking a responsible part in decision making with regard to their own education. Also, the increasing dedication of student groups to important social and civic causes is indicative of their increasing social responsiveness and political alertness.

The program of the National Student Nurses' Association (NSNA) reflects this same civic and social responsiveness. Focusing on the future, it embraces broad health and welfare interests and activities.

Organized in 1953, NSNA is a national preprofessional organization, established by and for nursing students under the aegis of the ANA and the NLN.[1] Its stated purpose is "... to aid in the preparation of student nurses for the assumption of professional responsibilities." Membership

[1] Either "nursing student" or "student of nursing" is acceptable today. However, when this organization was formed, the term "student nurse" was used, and it has not been changed.

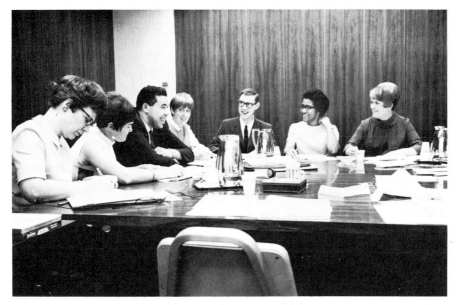

Fig. 18-1. NSNA officers and National Urban League representative plan cooperative efforts in nursing recruitment. (National Student Nurses' Association of the USA)

in this extracurricular association is individual and voluntary. The program is designed to supplement the educational program of the school of nursing and to provide field experience in all phases of organization work.

Article II, Section 2 of the current NSNA bylaws (1970) enunciates an important professional objective: "to prepare for membership and participation in the American Nurses' Association, the professional membership organization of nurses."

Other functions include serving as a channel of communications and providing a close bond among nursing students here and abroad; fostering good citizenship and encouraging participation in community affairs; and stimulating understanding of the programs of the NLN.

NSNA is related to the parent organizations (ANA and NLN) through the appointment of advisors and through close-working relationships of the staffs at national headquarters.

PROGRAM AND ACTIVITIES

The activities of the NSNA, as indicated in the introduction to this chapter, reflect a growing social concern for others. Programs involve interaction with other national student and health groups, as well as cooperative endeavors with state and local student nurses associations.

Nursing Recruitment

Recruitment of nursing students has always been a major interest of the NSNA. There is representation on careers in nursing committees at national, state and local levels. Work with future nurses clubs is encouraged and many recruitment activities are carried out at state and local levels. Nursing recruitment efforts are shown in Figure 18-1.

In November 1968, an NSNA news release reported that work had begun "...in eleven specially selected areas throughout the USA, to increase the number of black, Indian, and Spanish-speaking Americans who enter schools preparing registered nurses." Called "Breakthrough to Nursing," this exciting project was initiated in 3 target cities, Omaha, Minneapolis and Pittsburgh, in 1967 to 1968. As a demonstration project with the aim of placing 15 students in schools of nursing by September 1968, it was successful. The 3 original target cities plus 14 new target areas will carry the project forward into its next stage. The goal is cooperative action on the project across the country. Figure 18-2 shows work in relation to this program.

Working closely with other interested groups like the Urban League and various centers, the demonstration projects have focused upon working in a 1 to 1 relationship with interested high school students, although other activities such as working with counselors and speaking to groups of students have been continued. Tutorial work has been carried on with students needing extra help in preparing for admission to nursing school. Figure 18-3 shows nursing students engaged in tutorial activities. Various civic groups and industries have been approached for financial aid for

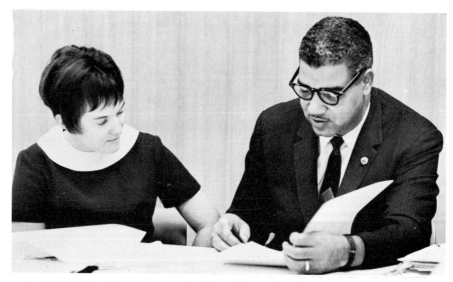

Fig. 18-2. NSNA officer confers about Breakthrough to Nursing Project with National Urban League executive, Whitney M. Young, Jr. (National Student Nurses' Association of the USA)

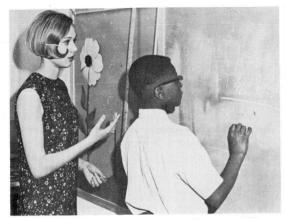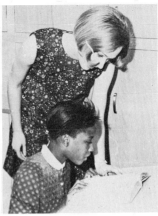

Fig. 18-3. Tutoring is one phase of the "Breakthrough" project. The above pictures show nursing students tutoring young students interested in entering schools of nursing. (National Student Nurses' Association of the USA)

economically disadvantaged students, since this was found to be a major need of the group.

All of the projects have had great success in obtaining the cooperation of faculties of the schools of nursing in their communities. Also, good publicity has been forthcoming via the local news media. Started in a small way as a practical demonstration of ways to stimulate the recruitment of minority groups into nursing (for example, Negroes represent 11 per cent of the total population, but only 2.9 per cent of the total of nursing students), this project is a dynamic expression of NSNA's commitment to civil rights.[2]

Interaction With Other Groups

In addition to its own program, the NSNA participates in programs of several other important groups. For example, it is an affiliate member of the National Interagency Council on Smoking and Health, a participating member of the 1970 White House Conference on Children and Youth, and an active participant in the National Coalition of Student Professionals. NSNA is represented at conferences such as those of the U.S. National Student Association (USNSA).

In cooperation with USNSA, the NSNA has supported action to help in decreasing the use of drugs on campuses and has participated in conferences such as the one on causes of student suicide, a conference supported by a grant from the National Institutes of Mental Health.

NSNA also cooperates with the Student American Medical Association (SAMA). This group planned a joint project for the summer of 1969 and 1970, in which medical and nursing students worked with health problems of

[2] B. Michelson, "Breakthrough to Nursing—Students Pave the Way for Minority Groups," *International Nursing Review,* **15:**61-66, Apr. 1968.

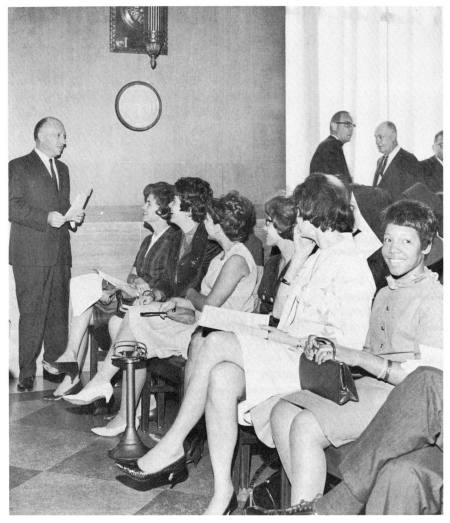

Fig. 18-4. Nursing students attend legislative hearing in Washington and speak with Senator Javits. (National Student Nurses' Association of the USA)

people in Appalachia. Interdisciplinary symposia, sponsored by the Student American Pharmaceutical Association in cooperation with NSNA and SAMA, were held during the 1969-1970 school year. These students are coming together to learn how to begin working together for comprehensive patient care.

NSNA is one of the charter members of the National Coalition of Student Professionals, consisting of the student organizations in dentistry, law, pharmacy, medicine, and architecture, as well as nursing. The purpose of the National Coalition of Student Professionals is to develop a system for responding to health issues and for collaboration on joint projects.

International Activities

Meetings for students are planned in connection with the Quadrennial Congresses of the International Council of Nurses. Attendance at these meetings is limited to the members of the nursing student organizations of their respective countries. Students may attend the business and program meetings of the Congress. In addition, a professional meeting and social event are planned for them.

One of the long-term projects of the NSNA involved the provision of funds for building and equipping a dormitory for nursing students at the National Defense Medical Center in Taiwan. Carried out over a 5-year period, in cooperation with the American Bureau for Medical Aid to China, this project was completed in 1966.

Other Program Activities

Program and business meetings at NSNA annual conventions reflect the interests of the association in current issues of concern to nursing students as professionals and as citizens. Figure 18-4 shows nursing students attending a legislative hearing in Washington, D.C.

A scholarship for a graduate nurse, as a former NSNA member, is awarded annually. It is administered by Nurses' Educational Funds, Inc.

MEMBERSHIP

Membership in 1970 was over 62,000 individual members in 51 constituent state student nurses' associations (49 states, the District of Columbia and Puerto Rico). One school of nursing has been opened in Alaska, and, as of early 1970, there has not been time for the students to form an association. There are in addition, approximately 270 district or local associations.

Who is Eligible?

All students of preservice schools for the preparation of registered nurses are eligible for membership, whether they are enrolled in diploma, baccalaureate, or associate degree programs. Advisors are designated as associate members.

How to Join

In 36 states, members may join and participate through district associations. Every member is automatically a national member and receives an NSNA membership card on payment of district, state and national dues. In the 15 states without district associations, the student joins NSNA through the state association and also, of course, receives a national membership card.

Dues, Finances

National dues, in 1970, were $5.00 per capita. National, state and district dues range from $1.00 to $3.75 or more, varying according to the decision of the membership in each state and district association.

OFFICIAL PUBLICATIONS

Imprint and the *American Journal of Nursing* are NSNA's official publications. *Imprint,* the successor of the *NSNA News Letter,* is an attractive, lively quarterly initiated in 1968, which is mailed to each individual member. It carries news of the important activities of the association as well as timely articles. The Corresponding Secretary of NSNA serves as student editor of *Imprint.*

The *American Journal of Nursing,* a monthly publication of the American Journal of Nursing Company (AJN Co.), was voted by NSNA, in 1964, to be the official magazine of the Association. Space is made available in each issue of the Journal for student news, including the annual convention program. Members of the NSNA may subscribe for the Journal at a special reduced rate.

CONVENTIONS

A national convention is held each year in conjunction with the alternating biennial conventions of the ANA and the NLN. NSNA and state organization officers, meeting at a national convention, are shown in Figure 18-5.

Conventions are financed from registration fees, and there is a separate convention budget. Convention management and various other kinds of services are provided by ANA and NLN in alternate years,[3] and reimbursement is made for certain items. The AJN Co. underwrites the expenses of the daily convention paper, with editing and production provided by the ANA or the NLN pressroom staff working with student reporters.

Attendance at NSNA conventions is generally over 4,000. Meetings at NSNA conventions range from small workshop-type sessions to large general programs on issues facing the profession and society. Sessions are lively, with much discussion and debate. Stands taken on major health and social issues, as well as on program planning, guide the association's efforts following the convention.

[3] The ANA holds its conventions in the even-numbered years, the NLN in odd-numbered years. Because NSNA annual conventions are held in conjunction with these it is possible for the parent organization, which is meeting at the time, to provide various convention services.

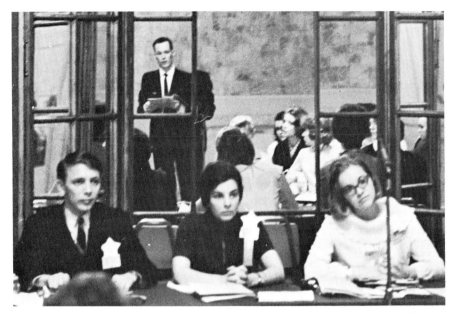

Fig. 18-5. National and state officers meet at convention. (National Student Nurses' Association of the USA)

GOVERNING BODIES

Voting Body

The voting body consists of delegates selected by the constituent associations to represent the membership of the Association as a whole. Delegates are allocated according to the number of members in good standing in each constituent association on a date 8 weeks before the annual convention. Representation is, in general, based on 1 delegate for each 500 members or less, each state therefore being entitled to at least 1 delegate. This voting body elects the national officers, 1 advisor and the 5 members of the Committee on Nominations, all of whom serve a 1-year term. The delegates adopt policies, programs and resolutions for the Association on current social and health issues, at business meetings during the annual conventions.

Board of Directors

The NSNA Board of Directors is delegated to transact the business of the Association between the annual conventions; to devise a program to carry out the purposes of the Association; to provide a national headquarters, and to appoint an executive director; to be responsible for the finances and safekeeping of records; and to carry out the other functions as specified in the bylaws.

The board consists of 6 officers and 2 directors who are elected for 1-year terms. Board meetings are attended by 3 advisors. The ANA and NLN each appoint an advisor for a 2-year term beginning in alternate years. The third advisor is a former NSNA member with experience on the NSNA board of directors or on a national committee, who is elected to serve for 1 year.

COMMITTEES

Nominations

The 5 members of the Committee on Nominations are elected annually by the delegates. Constituent associations nominate members and submit biographic data, listing their nominees' qualifications and experience. The committee meets, preceding the midterm board meeting, and selects the slate of candidates from this pool of names. The bylaws describe the essential procedure for nominations and elections.

Program

The Committee on Program, chaired by the first vice-president, plans educational and social programs for the convention and for the Association.

Bylaws

The second vice-president serves as chairman of the Committee on Bylaws. The Committee receives and reviews all proposed amendments to the NSNA bylaws; periodically reviews state bylaws to ensure harmony with national bylaws on certain essential provisions; and prepares model forms for state and district bylaws to assist constituents.

Finance

The Committee on Finance, chaired by the treasurer, reviews the budget for the year and presents it for Board approval.

Policies

The Committee on Policies, chaired by the recording secretary, reviews policies annually and suggests revisions of the policy book for Board action.

SPOKESMAN FOR STUDENTS

The following quotation indicates how the NSNA has acted as the "spokesman" for nursing students in the USA:

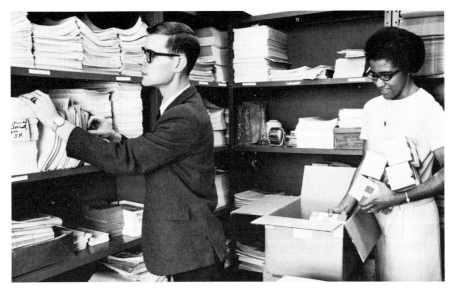

Fig. 18-6. National officers select publications from NSNA stock room at headquarters. (National Student Nurses' Association of the USA)

By taking a stand on issues of importance to nursing students, the NSNA serves as a voice for students and as a source of direction and information. NSNA has taken official action in recent years in support of economic security, changes in education for nurses, a broad range of legislation, American Nurses' Association Code for Nurses, and the student's right to educational experience rather than being expected to provide nursing service.[4]

HEADQUARTERS

NSNA has had a national headquarters since 1958. In 1969, the head-quarters staff consisted of the executive director, a staff editor, an administrative assistant, 2 staff secretaries and membership and order clerk. Miss Frances Tompkins, the first executive director, retired as of December 31, 1969. Miss Mary Ann Tuft is the present executive director. The headquarters is located at 10 Columbus Circle, New York, New York 10019. National officers of the NSNA are shown working in the National headquarters, in Figure 18-6.

PROBLEMS

1. (a) What are some of the activities and projects of your state student nurses' association? (b) Which of them are also national programs? (c) How

[4] The quotation, "Spokesman for Students" was taken from the final statement in the leaflet, *Facts About NSNA*, published in 1967 by the National Student Nurses' Association, 10 Columbus Circle, New York, New York 10019.

many does your district association participate in? (d) Discuss some of the kinds of activities you think your local group should be carrying on. (e) Discuss some of the current social issues in which you believe the NSNA or your local group should be involved.

2. (a) How are delegates to national conventions selected in your state? (b) How many delegates represented your state at the last NSNA convention? Who were they? (c) When and where is the next convention to be held?

3. Discuss ways you think the NSNA and state and local student groups can assist nursing students to participate on curriculum committees in their schools.

4. (a) With what organizations is the NSNA most closely related? (b) How are these relationships maintained? (c) Is your state association involved in any joint activities with other student groups preparing for the health professions? If yes, what is their current major interest?

SUGGESTED REFERENCES*

Corcoran, J. "NSNA's First Six Years." *American Journal of Nursing,* **59:**695, May 1959.
* Gilhooley, M. A. N. and Elliot, F. E. "The Status of Organizations in Schools of Nursing." *American Journal of Nursing,* **58:**703-705, May 1958.
* McGarvey, M. R., *et al.* "A Study in Medical Action—The Student Health Organizations." *New England Journal of Medicine,* **279:**74-80, July 11, 1968.
Mickelson, B. "NSNA: Adolescent or Adult." *Imprint,* **15:**8, Jan. 1968.
"National Student Nurse Association." *American Journal of Nursing,* **53:**978-983, Aug. 1953.
National Student Nurses' Association. *Book of Reports.* New York, The Association. Published annually.
———. List of Publications. New York, The Association. Published annually. Mimeographed.
———. "Convention, National Student Nurses' Association." *American Journal of Nursing,* **68:**1293-1928. June 1968. See also, reports in the *American Journal of Nursing* for each year since 1958.
———. *Bylaws.* New York, The Association, May 1968.
———. *Facts About NSNA.* New York, The Association, 1965.
* ———. *NSNA's Ten Tall Years.* New York, The Association, Aug. 1963.
* ———. *Highlights from the 1962-1963 Annual Reports of the State Student Nurses' Associations Submitted at 1963 Convention, Summarized, August, 1963.* New York, The Association, 1963, p. 9. Mimeographed.
"NSNA Meets." *American Journal of Nursing,* **69:**1267-1272, June 1969.
Price, G. "The Adviser to Students and Her Advice." *American Journal of Nursing,* **64:**130-132, Apr. 1964.
Schutt, B. G. (editorial) "Those Ten Tall Years." *American Journal of Nursing,* **63:**65, May 1963.
* Steinke, M. L., *et al.* "National Student Nurses' Association." *The Yearbook of Modern Nursing, 1957-58.* Ed. by M. C. Cowan. New York, Putnam, 1958. p. 388.

* In each chapter all citations are footnoted and are not included here. All starred references are recommended for additional reading.

"Students at the ICN Congress." *American Journal of Nursing,* **61:**92-93, July 1961.
"Things Are Happening in Appalachia." *Imprint,* **16:**3-5, Nov. 1969.

For further references, consult NSNA's current *List of Publications,* available from the NSNA, 10 Columbus Circle, New York, New York, 10019.

See also current issues of the *American Journal of Nursing,* which carries many items about NSNA or references to NSNA, as well as its NSNA Student Page, and see current issues of *Imprint* published quarterly by NSNA.

CHAPTER

19

The Alumni Association

After you have been in school for some time, and particularly as your commencement nears, you will begin to realize that the relationship between you and your school is one that never really will be severed. Your teachers and fellow-students have become like members of your family; even though you may be separated from them for long periods of time, there will always be a bond between you and them. You will continue to be interested in your school and want to help it grow, just as you will want to keep in touch with your parents' home and its activities after you establish a life and home of your own. You will wish for, and appreciate, ways in which your school will show continued interest in you.

It is to meet this need of yours, and of other graduates, that alumni associations exist.

MEANING

An alumni association is an organized group of graduates from an educational institution. When the group is composed of men only, or of both men and women, the term *alumni association* is generally used. When the graduates are all women, the term *alumnae association* is employed. (Those of you who have studied Latin will recognize the reason for this.) Because many schools of nursing were originally limited to women students, their graduates' organizations were called *alumnae associations,* and this term has often persisted even after the addition of men students and graduates. However, when we speak of these associations as a group, we call them *alumni associations.* Your own association may use the feminine form in its title.

HISTORICAL SIGNIFICANCE

We all know from our nursing history that alumni associations of nursing schools were practically the first form of nursing organization in this country. Several years before any action was taken by nurses in this country to form a nursing organization of national scope, some alumni associations had developed in connection with a few nursing schools. At the third annual meeting of the American Society of Superintendents of Training Schools in 1896, a constitution and bylaws were prepared for an organization of all nursing school alumni. In the following year they were adopted and the organization became known as the National Associated Alumnae of the United States and Canada. Afterward the name was changed to American Nurses' Association (ANA) when the USA and Canada each decided to have its own organization.

When the ANA was reorganized and the state nurses association became its unit of organization, the district association became the unit in the state and the alumni association became the unit in the district. The alumni association then became the link between the profession of nursing, the individual nurse and her alma mater, the nursing school. Later, having the alumni as a basic unit in the ANA was discontinued.

The latest development in the history of school of nursing alumni associations is their adaptation to changing patterns in nursing education. As educational programs in nursing have been established in institutions of higher learning, graduates from these programs have, of course, become members of the college or university alumni associations. Often, the over-all alumni association has a section for each of the groups of the various schools. In such instances, of course, there is a section or constituent group of nurse graduates.

OBJECTIVES

Each nursing school alumni association establishes its own objectives. When the nurse alumni constitute a section of a college or university association, the objectives of the section are, in general, based on those of the entire association.

When we study the reasons for the formation of alumni associations of either kind, we find that some of the important ones are to provide graduates of the institution with opportunities for:

1. Keeping abreast of the school's activities.
2. Assisting the school to develop along sound lines.
3. Helping the present generation of students with their problems.
4. Becoming interested, well-informed and active members of their professions or other fields of endeavor and increasingly useful and helpful members of society; planning for study groups, institutes and programs to discuss trends in nursing education, research and practice.
5. Keeping alive school friendships.
6. Helping individual members of the association.
7. Assisting in securing endowment funds or money for a variety of purposes, such as to establish scholarship and loan funds.
8. Recognizing outstanding alumni through an achievement awards program.
9. Becoming part of an organization through which your alma mater continues to be of service to you after graduation through a cooperative program of continuing education.
10. Helping to interpret the program of the school and to recruit able students.

ACTIVITIES

It would be inappropriate to discuss here all the specific ways in which the university or college alumni associations achieve their objectives. Rather, it may be helpful to describe some of the activities of nursing school alumni associations or the nursing sections of university alumni associations.

For the School

The alumni association's relationship to the school should be a very close and vital one, but its officers and members should realize that they have no power to dictate the details of administration or curriculum to the officers of administration and the faculty of the school. However, they may find ways in which their members can do real work for the school, particularly in connection with its public relations and recruitment programs. An alumni association often contributes to the school's financial support and helps to raise money for new buildings and for endowment funds. It may support a special professorship.

To be of most assistance in interpreting the program of the school, effective channels of communication between the faculty and the alumni need to be maintained. Alumni can be of special assistance in interpreting the educational program during times of change, as when a diploma school is discontinued and the hospital becomes an experience field for an institution of higher education, or as when there are major curriculum changes.

For the Students

The provision of scholarships is one way the alumni association can assist students with their problems. However, there are other, more personal ways in which help can be given.

To have the type of member that is desirable, the alumni association needs to give careful thought to its relationships with students of nursing in the school, its potential members, so that they will begin early to learn their professional responsibilities. This should not be left until the day of graduation but should be started in the first school term, when the students can be informed about what the association is and what it is attempting to do. Today's students are vitally interested in their own program of education and in social movements such as ensuring civil rights and assisting minority groups. Students can expect that their alumni association will be interested in assisting them to promote such socially useful activities, as well as in helping to initiate them into the profession as graduates. Liaison committees between students and the school's alumni association are one way of promoting shared activities.

For Its Members

For its own members the association should supply purposes and activities that will give true spiritual as well as professional and personal vision in daily life. Among alumni activities designed for the benefit of members we find many interesting and practical ones. Some alumni have raised money to endow a room or a bed in a hospital for the use of its members. Others have established benefit and pension funds for sick members. Some are raising money for scholarships, fellowships and loan funds for members who wish to continue their education. Others are providing funds to furnish rest and recreation rooms for nurses in hospitals, while others are attempting to establish club houses and convalescent homes for nurses.

The alumni program can be varied, personal, and most helpful. It need not duplicate the district nursing association activities, but a close relationship to these activities is advisable.

Discussions at alumni meetings are vital if the members themselves participate. Topics may vary, covering the history of the school or current trends and events in nursing or in the world of today. Social legislation, changes in nursing education and nursing practice, accreditation activities, advances in medical practice affecting nursing, and other equally important topics are worthy of consideration.

Other activities and topics in which alumni groups are becoming increasingly interested are student recruitment; international affairs, such as those in connection with the ICN, the UN, the WHO, and programs for students to study abroad in different countries; collection of artifacts and preservation of historical materials related to the school of nursing; nursing needs and resources with emphasis on the balancing of civil and military needs; planning for civil defense and consideration of what the nurse should know about Medicare and Medicaid programs.

Some alumni associations publish magazines or newsletters. These are particularly welcome to far-distant members who wish to keep abreast of the activities of the school and the friends of their student days. As an active member, remember that it will be important to keep your address and marital status current and up-to-date in the alumni office.

Some alumni groups also present awards and citations to alumni or other persons for outstanding contributions to the school, the profession, or the community.

For the Community

To serve the real purpose for which nurses have existed down through the ages, the alumni must give consideration to the needs of the community. This can be done in many ways, but certainly the aim should be to do all in our power to promote civic, health and other projects. To accomplish this aim the alumni should send delegates and active participants not only to nursing conventions, but also to hospital, medical and civic meetings where discussions on health and disease are conducted. Alumni also should consider it important to cooperate very closely with all health and social organizations in securing the finest preparation possible for nurses and the best mode of distribution of nursing service to the community.

To do the best job possible in planning a program of activities, it is suggested that alumni officers consult with the officers of district nurses associations and local leagues for nursing. At least the current objectives of these organizations might be obtained and used as a guide. Membership in your alumni, important as it is, does not take the place of membership in your professional association. Both kinds of membership are important but for different reasons.

REASONS FOR HOLDING MEMBERSHIP

Regardless of what changes may take place, the alumni association always will be an important link in the chain of your professional relationships. Reasons for becoming active in your alumni association are many, but only a few of the important ones will be mentioned here.

If you do not belong to and participate actively in the affairs of your alumni association, you probably will drift gradually from contact with your school and professional colleagues and become a lone and lonesome worker. Your alumni association obviously needs you to carry out its purposes, but before you go very far in the profession you will realize that you stand as much in need of it as it does of you.

Each individual graduate should have real faith in what the alumni association is trying to do, and this is best shown by joining and participating in its activities. As each spoke in a wheel is necessary to make it go, each individual member counts to make his association go. You can act as an important agent of change if there appears to be a need for taking new directions in the association. The question you should ask yourself should not be, "Can I afford to belong to my alumni?" but rather, "Can I afford not to belong?"

PROBLEMS

1. (a) Who are the present officers of the alumni association of your school? (b) How do you expect to participate in its activities after you are graduated?

2. (a) What kind of program is the alumni association of your school conducting this year? (b) What type of program would you suggest to maintain a vital association in tune with the needs of the times? (c) How many times have you attended a meeting of the alumni association of your school? (d) Tell what you enjoyed about it.

3. (a) Which alumni have received honors or awards from the alumni association of the school of nursing in which you are enrolled? (b) Why were these honors or awards bestowed upon each of these nurses?

4. Suppose you belong to an alumni association of a hospital school of nursing that has been phased out and the nursing service of the hospital is now being used as an experience field in nursing for a local collegiate school of nursing. (a) How would you revise the objectives of the alumni association? (b) What should be the relationship of the association to the hospital?

CHAPTER

20

American Nurses' Association

The American Nurses' Association (ANA) is the national professional organization of registered nurses in the USA and its territorial possessions. It is composed of the nurses associations of the 50 states, the District of Columbia, Puerto Rico, the USA Virgin Islands, the Panama Canal Zone and Guam. The state nurses associations are in turn composed of more than 800 district nurses associations. The ANA has been one of the constituent members of the International Council of Nurses (ICN) since the Council's organization in 1899.

Because the ANA plays such an important part in the professional life of the nurse, whose interest and active participation determine the successful accomplishment of the objectives of the ANA, this chapter discusses some of the various phases relating to the ANA that will be of concern to you on graduation.

While many of the current objectives and programs of the ANA are presented here, it must be remembered that such an organization restates its aims from time to time, depending upon the issues and problems it faces.

You can keep in touch with the general activities of this Association by reading current issues of the *American Journal of Nursing* and literature distributed by the Association to its members, by attendance at meetings of the Association and by active participation in its many activities.

ORIGIN AND CHRONOLOGICAL REVIEW

Several years before any action was taken by nurses in this country to form a nursing organization of national scope, some alumni associations had developed in connection with a few nursing schools. Among them were the Bellevue alumni group, which was organized in 1889, that of the Illinois Training School, which started in 1891, and that of Johns Hopkins, which followed in 1892. It is interesting to note that Johns Hopkins had the first alumni society into which successive classes entered in a body.

At the 3rd annual meeting of the American Society of Superintendents of Training Schools[1] in 1896, a committee was appointed to prepare a constitution and bylaws for a proposed national nurses' association. This committee included representatives from the oldest alumni associations of nursing schools. The following schools sent delegates to the committee meeting which was held in 1896 to organize the national nurses' association.

Massachusetts General Training School, Boston
University of Pennsylvania Training School, Philadelphia
New York Training School, New York
New Haven Training School, New Haven, Conn.
Orange Memorial Training School, Orange, N.J.
Johns Hopkins Training School, Baltimore
Philadelphia Training School, Philadelphia
Garfield Training School, Washington, D.C.
Illinois Training School, Chicago
Farrand Training School, Detroit

The constitution and the bylaws which were prepared by this group were adopted in 1897 at Manhattan Beach, N.Y., and the organization then became known as the National Associated Alumnae of the United States and Canada.

OBJECTIVES

The purposes of the ANA are to foster high standards of nursing practice and to promote the welfare and the professional and educational advancement of nurses, to the end that all people may have better nursing care. These purposes are unrestricted by considerations of nationality, race, creed, or color. ANA represents nurses, serving as their spokesman, with allied national and international organizations, governmental bodies, and the public.

Platform

To help its constituents work toward these broad objectives, the ANA adopts a platform at its biennial conventions. The platform as adopted in May 1968 follows:

[1] This organization was the forerunner of the National League of Nursing Education, which was merged with the National League for Nursing in 1952.

1. Advance the practice of nursing by establishing standards of practice for the major clinical areas, by promoting implementation of these standards, and by providing recognition of excellence through certification of qualified practitioners.

2. Work toward implementing the Academy of Nursing for the advancement of knowledge, education and nursing practice.

3. Promote research which will enlarge the scientific bases of nursing, foster dissemination of new knowledge, and assist in its application in nursing practice.

4. Promote study and reform of licensing legislation for the practice of nursing.

5. Promote continuing education for the purposes of improving nursing practice and developing nursing as a lifelong career.

6. Foster study and improvement of education for nursing, and provide leadership and support for community planning for the sound and orderly transition of nursing education into institutions of higher learning.

7. Promote increasing public support for students, and for educational programs that meet standards acceptable to the profession.

8. Promote participation by the nursing profession in comprehensive community planning for health care.

9. Foster study of health care needs and advance sound utilization of the health manpower required to insure a high quality of nursing care of all people.

10. Recruit students into nursing education programs which will prepare them for the greatest possible contribution to meeting the nursing needs of people.

11. Promote studies and programs designed to improve health care systems and thus improve the delivery of nursing services to people.

12. Improve standards for nursing services in health care facilities; and work with government, health care organizations and agencies toward the achievement of quality health services for all people.

13. Promote equal opportunities in education, employment and advancement in nursing, and support and assist in the implementation of civil rights legislation so that all people have access to health care.

14. Assist nurses to improve their employment conditions through expanding and strengthening economic security programs using techniques such as collective bargaining.

15. Promote desirable social, economic and health legislation.

16. Promote sound planning, including the preparation of nursing personnel, for meeting the health needs of people in times of emergency.

17. Strengthen the functioning of the professional association so that it can better discharge its responsibilities to nurses and the public.

18. Promote collaborative efforts by nurses and others to meet health needs throughout the world.[2]

[2] American Nurses' Association, *Platform*, New York, The Association, May 1968.

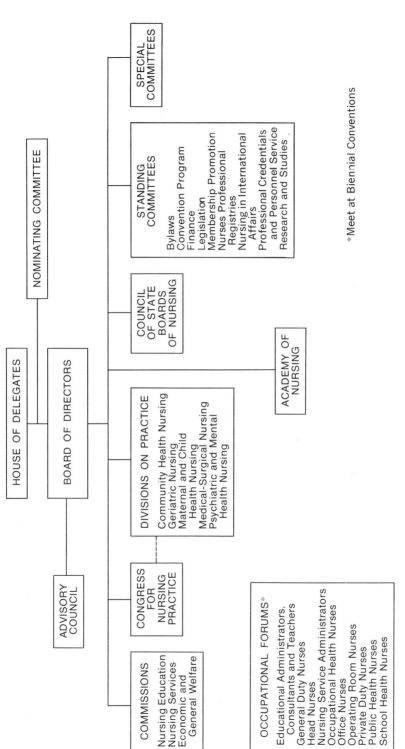

HOUSE OF DELEGATES

NOMINATING COMMITTEE

ADVISORY COUNCIL

BOARD OF DIRECTORS

SPECIAL COMMITTEES

STANDING COMMITTEES
Bylaws
Convention Program
Finance
Legislation
Membership Promotion
Nurses Professional
    Registries
Nursing in International
    Affairs
Professional Credentials
    and Personnel Service
Research and Studies

COUNCIL OF STATE BOARDS OF NURSING

ACADEMY OF NURSING

DIVISIONS ON PRACTICE
Community Health Nursing
Geriatric Nursing
Maternal and Child
    Health Nursing
Medical-Surgical Nursing
Psychiatric and Mental
    Health Nursing

CONGRESS FOR NURSING PRACTICE

COMMISSIONS
Nursing Education
Nursing Services
Economic and
    General Welfare

OCCUPATIONAL FORUMS*
Educational Administrators,
    Consultants and Teachers
General Duty Nurses
Head Nurses
Nursing Service Administrators
Occupational Health Nurses
Office Nurses
Operating Room Nurses
Private Duty Nurses
Public Health Nurses
School Health Nurses

*Meet at Biennial Conventions

Fig. 20-1. Membership organization chart of the American Nurses' Association as of June 1968.

ORGANIZATION PLAN AND RELATIONSHIPS

General Plan of Organization

The general organizational plan of the ANA is directly related to the purposes and functions of the Association and to the various programs established to implement these purposes and functions. As we have indicated, objectives and programs may be changed from time to time as new issues and problems arise. The present (1970) functions of the Association are:

1. To establish functions, standards, and qualifications for nursing practice.

2. To enunciate standards of nursing education and implement them through appropriate channels.

3. To enunciate standards of nursing service and implement them through appropriate channels.

4. To establish a code of ethical conduct for practitioners.

5. To stimulate and promote research designed to enlarge the knowledge on which the practice of nursing is based.

6. To promote legislation and to speak for nurses in regard to legislative action.

7. To promote and protect the economic and general welfare of nurses.

8. To provide professional record service and assist states with counseling and placement activity.

9. To provide for the continuing professional development of practitioners.

10. To represent nurses and serve as their spokesman with allied national and international organizations, governmental bodies, and the public.

11. To serve as the official representative of the United States nurses as a member of the International Council of Nurses.

12. To promote the general health and welfare of the public through all association programs, relationships, and activities.

13. To promote relationships with the National Student Nurses' Association.[3]

The organization plan of the ANA now in effect, following the action taken at the 1968 ANA biennial convention, is shown in Figure 20-1.

The business of the Association is carried on through its House of Delegates and its Board of Directors. The House of Delegates, ANA's top policy making body, meets every other year in the even numbered years. It is composed of representatives, elected by all of the constituent associations, who come together to discuss the issues and problems brought

[3] American Nurses' Association, *Bylaws,* New York, The Association, 1968, pp. 5-6.

to them, to decide upon program and policy, and to conduct the general business of the Association. For example, among the issues discussed at the 1968 convention were 2 health issues, smoking and abortion laws, and 3 resolutions having to do with the nurse's responsibility for quality care and for involvement in comprehensive health planning and in regional medical programs. As a result of the discussions, statements were adopted enunciating the position of the ANA on these important issues.[4]

The House of Delegates also elects the officers and Board of Directors of the Association. The officers consist of the president, the 1st, 2nd, and 3rd vice-president, a secretary and a treasurer. The Board of Directors consists of the officers of the Association and 10 directors. Among its many functions, the Board of Directors is responsible for transacting the general business of the Association in the interim between biennial conventions and for establishing major administrative policies governing the affairs of the Association.

Commissions

One of the major changes in structure adopted by the ANA at its 1966 biennial convention was the establishment of commissions. The 3 commissions are concerned with: (1) nursing education, (2) nursing services and (3) economic and general welfare.[5] Each commission consists of 9 members who serve 4-year terms; 3 members elected biennially by the House of Delegates; and 1 appointed by the Board of Directors biennially, except that every fourth year 2 members are appointed. The commissions are responsible for developing and implementing a broad program of action in their respective areas of responsibility. It is through these that ANA provides for standards for nursing education and nursing services and promotes and protects the economic and general welfare of nurses. Each is accountable to the Board of Directors and the House of Delegates.

Divisions on Practice and Congress for Nursing Practice

In 1966, the ANA established divisions on practice for the purpose of advancing the practice of nursing. There are 5 divisions: (1) Community Health Nursing, (2) Geriatric Nursing, (3) Maternal and Child Health Nursing, (4) Medical-Surgical Nursing and (5) Psychiatric and Mental Health Nursing.

The overall purpose of the divisions is the advancement of nursing practice. They provide an arrangement whereby nurses interested in the same area of nursing can come together for the purpose of improving their

---

[4] See "For 1968 Delegate Action," *American Journal of Nursing*, **68**:787-791, Apr. 1968, and "ANA Convention—A Week of Firsts," *American Journal of Nursing*, **68**:1258-1277, June 1968, for the action taken on these issues.

[5] A fourth commission on research was established at the 1970 ANA Convention. See "ANA Convention Report," *American Journal of Nursing*, **70**:1268-1287, June, 1970.

practice. This goal of improvement is accomplished in each division mainly through the enunciation of standards of nursing practice, by provision for recognition of professional achievement and excellence and by holding clinical and scientific sessions. Membership in a division of one's choice is open to the members and associates of the association.

In 1968, delegates to the ANA convention provided for a Congress for Nursing Practice. The congress consists of 9 members—the elected chairmen of the 5 practice divisions and 4 members appointed by the Board of Directors. It carries the same kind of broad responsibility as the commissions.

Academy of Nursing

Because of the ANA's strong belief that professional achievement and excellence should be recognized, when the 1966 House of Delegates voted for major changes in the ANA organization, it made provision for this recognition by providing for an Academy of Nursing. Since that time, work basic to the initiation of the Academy has been underway. For example, the various divisions are developing standards of practice. Once these standards are agreed upon, the divisions will be responsible for establishing Certification Boards.

The broad purpose of the Academy of Nursing will be the advancement of knowledge, education and practice. Its members will be certified by division Certification Boards for fellowship in the Academy. They will be selected for their outstanding contribution to nursing. You will be interested in following the development of this very significant body within the ANA.

Occupational Forums

Occupational forums have been set up for the general purpose of providing a place where representatives of the major occupational areas in nursing can come together to discuss matters of concern related to their roles and conditions of work. At the present time (1970) there are 10 forums representative of the various state sections, for example, general duty nurses, head nurses, office nurses, private duty nurses and others as listed in Figure 20-1. The forums are held at the time of the biennial conventions.

What Is the Relationship of the ANA to the ICN?

The ANA is one of the 3 nursing associations, along with those of Great Britain and Germany, that became charter members of the ICN in which 73 national nursing associations now (1970) have active membership. Through this relationship every individual nurse belonging to the ANA is privileged to have representation in the ICN.

Relationship to the American Nurses' Foundation

The American Nurses' Foundation was established by the ANA in 1955 as the research arm of the Association. See Chapter 23 for a full discussion of its purposes and activities.

Relationship to Other Organizations

The ANA works closely with the NLN through the ANA-NLN Coordinating Council composed of the membership of the Boards of Directors of the 2 organizations. The purpose of this Council is the coordination of those programs that are of common concern to the 2 organizations. The staffs of the 2 organizations also cooperate closely. Examples of joint program efforts are the ANA-NLN Committee on Nursing Careers and the former ANA-NLN Film Service.[6] The latter service operates a film library and stimulates the production of needed films on nursing.

The ANA works with many related health organizations in the interest of improved nursing service and effective delivery of health care. The ANA also maintains a liaison with other allied health groups such as the American Hospital Association and the American Society of Hospital Pharmacists. Relationships are also maintained with a number of governmental agencies, particularly with the Division of Nursing, Bureau of Health Professions Education and Manpower Training, National Institutes of Health, U.S. Department of Health, Education, and Welfare.

It goes without saying that the ANA works especially closely with the National Student Nurses' Association. One example of the various formal ways these 2 associations work together is the ANA-NSNA Committee on Common Interests and Goals. There are also many informal ways in which they both cooperate.

These represent only some of the numerous working relationships maintained by the ANA with other groups whose interests are similar to those of the Association.

PROGRAMS

In their professional organization, nurses have an instrument that, if properly used, will improve every phase of their working and professional lives.

Through the work of its commissions and divisions, the ANA provides a coordinated program aimed at the continuing improvement of the quality of nursing care. As mentioned earlier, the 5 divisions on practice and the Congress for Nursing Practice are responsible for determining the scope of

[6] The ANA-NLN Film Service was taken over by the American Journal of Nursing Company as of January 1, 1970.

nursing practice and advancing the standards, knowledge and skills in their respective areas of service. Some of their activities, in addition to developing and implementing standards for practice, include educational conferences, such as the regional clinical conferences; the encouragement of needed research; and taking action on legislation related to nursing.

One of the most significant and far-reaching actions of the ANA in recent years was the position taken on education for those who work in nursing. Basic to the quality of nursing practice is the quality of nursing education, which assures the public that those who practice are competent to do so. Simply, the ANA position is that "Education for those who work in nursing should take place in institutions of learning within the general system of education."[7] It is suggested that you discuss the ANA position paper on education with reference to its contribution to the goal of improved nursing practice. Also, refer to chapters 3 and 10 of this book. "Nursing as a Profession" and "Nurses in Education . . . ," for a discussion of the implications of this statement for nursing education.

The ANA has issued a joint statement with the NLN on community planning for nursing education, with which you should be familiar, and has encouraged state nurses associations to develop state and regional plans for nursing education within their respective states.

Through the Council of State Boards of Nursing, uniform licensing practices and standards are encouraged. The ANA works closely with state boards through this Council. The ANA provides professional resources to state boards in matters relating to interpretation of nursing practice acts, developing standards for programs in preservice nursing education, and providing the means whereby policy and content of the State Board Test Pool Examination are developed.

Improving the quality of nursing services is the focus of the Commission on Nursing Services. Major health needs are studied for their implications for nursing services and recommendations are made regarding requirements for personnel and resources. The ANA Committee of Emergency Health Preparedness and National Defense has developed criteria and guidelines to use in the event of disaster or national emergency.

A broad program on the economic and general welfare of nurses is carried out on all levels—local, state and national. The ANA advises and assists the constituent state nurses associations which, in turn, represent nurses in their individual places of employment.

Within all of its programs and activities, the ANA has consistently worked for full integration of all qualified nurses into the profession. Equal opportunities in education, employment and participation in Association activities have been promoted. The ANA's concern for civil rights—to the end that all people will have equal access to health care—is well known.

The ANA activities are so broad that they permeate all phases of nursing.

[7] "ANA Position on Education for Nursing," *American Journal of Nursing,* **65:**106-111, Dec. 1965.

It is not possible to cover them completely in a few paragraphs. Some are treated in other chapters. The Professional Credentials and Personnel Service has been discussed in Chapter 14, "Obtaining, Filling, and Resigning From a Position." The activities of the ANA Department of International Affairs are indicated in Chapter 25, "International Nursing and Allied Organizations." Some of the ways in which the ANA promotes the passage of legislation which is beneficial to nurses are discussed in Chapter 27, "Legislation Affecting Nursing." The economic security program is discussed in Chapter 15, "Planning Economic Security." Some of the many other activities of the ANA will be described here.

Research and Statistics

The ANA Department of Research and Statistics conducts research relating to the program interest and needs of the Association. Activities include the development of current and comprehensive nurse manpower data, information about ANA and its membership, the provision of information support for other ANA programs, and the dissemination of information to nurses and the public through *Facts About Nursing* and other reports.

Publications

The ANA issues many publications in connection with its program. An important one with which you should be familiar is *ANA in Action.*

Public Relations

The Department of Public Relations of the ANA functions as a publishing and information service for the profession. It interprets ANA programs, activities and goals for nurses, allied professional and health groups, the government and the public. This Department also publishes newsletters, clinical papers, proceedings of conferences, institutes, and conventions, and other material pertinent to nurses and the profession.

How Can You Become Familiar With the ANA Program?

Since the program of activities is changed from year to year, depending on the needs and the problems of the individual nurse, the profession, and the users of nursing services (the public), it is suggested that you try to make a list of the activities in which this association now is engaged by reviewing this year's issues of the *American Journal of Nursing* and by consulting the proceedings of biennial conventions. Your class might also study the *Platform of the American Nurses' Association* and recent issues of *ANA in Action.*

MEMBERSHIP

Reasons for Membership

You should become a member of the ANA because it is the national professional membership association of registered nurses organized for the benefit of nurses and the public whom they serve. By joining it, you will express publicly your belief in the nursing profession. Membership in this organization also gives you the opportunity to make new friends not only in your own country, but also through association representation in the ICN; to get stimulating and fresh points of view on nursing, its objectives, problems, and ideals; and to share in the best thinking of the profession. It offers you a chance to make your contribution toward the general welfare of all nurses, the advancement of nursing practice, nursing service and nursing education, and the formulation of policies in connection with national nursing affairs. In so doing you obviously further your own professional development and growth as well as make a contribution to society as a registered nurse.

How Do You Become a Member of the ANA?

ANA membership is open to any registered nurse who is licensed in at least 1 jurisdiction of the USA. If the state nurses association in the state in which you live and practice is divided into districts, you apply for membership in the district association. The acceptance of your completed application blank and your payment of membership dues make you a member also of the state and the national organization.

USA nurses who are engaged in nursing in foreign countries may maintain their ANA membership through the state nurses association of the state in which they last lived or worked or may apply to the ANA for direct membership.

If you are ever in doubt as to what you should do to become a member of the ANA or to continue as such, consult either the executive director of the nurses association of the state where you reside or the headquarters of the ANA.

Some of the most important reasons for membership in the ANA are reviewed in Chapter 17, "Leadership Role of the Professional Nurse." As individuals we cannot perform the full range of responsibilities we have as professional persons; only as participating members of our professional association can we fulfill these responsibilities. Other reasons for membership are given at the end of this chapter.

In What Way Is the ANA Membership Card of Practical Value?

The following purposes are only a few among the many for which a membership card in the ANA is of value. A member finds that her card is useful for presentation to prospective employers and when registering with a nurse placement service or when demonstrating professional status to a patient or others. When you study Chapter 25, "International Nursing and Allied Organizations," you will see how important it will be for you to be an ANA member if you want to go abroad for study, observation, or work experience.

An ANA membership card is also employed for voting purposes at state nursing conventions. As a means of identification it can be shown in opening bank and credit accounts, in traveling, in cashing checks, and for presentation when seeking accommodations at nursing clubs and at hotels at home and abroad.

Membership Dues

At the present writing, 1970, the annual national dues for active membership are $12.50 per capita; for associate membership, the dues are $3.50. A special provision has been made for the new graduate and, for the first full year following graduation and licensure to practice, the dues are one-half the annual dues in effect for the membership. Nurses who do not anticipate employment in nursing during the current year may be associates. Further information about membership categories can be found in the current bylaws of the ANA.

The amount of membership dues levied by the district and the state nurses associations varies with state and district and is determined by the respective memberships.

OFFICIAL MAGAZINE

The *American Journal of Nursing,* a monthly periodical edited by professional nurses, is the official journal of the ANA. It is discussed fully in Chapter 24, "Nursing Journals in the USA."

HEADQUARTERS

You are always welcome at ANA headquarters—the clearing center for all activities of the ANA—which is located at 10 Columbus Circle, New York, New York, 10019, together with the offices of the NLN, the NSNA, the ANF and the AJN Co. The headquarters staff is over 100 people.

PROBLEMS

1. Review material in the *American Journal of Nursing* for the past 3 years which reflects the ANA's interest in health care for the public. Discuss

this in terms of the role of the Association in national health legislation.

2. Discuss the Association's concern for the provision of adequate numbers of qualified nursing personnel and its activities for the past 5 years toward this end.

3. (a) Where and when was the last biennial convention of the ANA? (b) What was the general theme of the program? (c) Where and when is the next biennial convention to be held?

4. (a) How can you become a member of the ANA? (b) What are the advantages of membership? (c) Describe the functions of the different commissions and divisions of the ANA.

5. (a) What sections exist in the state nurses association of your state? (b) Who are their officers? (c) What are their functions?

6. (a) Identify and give information about the following: Dorothy A. Cornelius, Sister Delphine, Margaret B. Dolan, Jo Eleanor Elliott, Audrey Logsdon, Jessie M. Scott. (b) Who are the current chairmen of committees and commissions of the ANA? (c) Determine from the current official directory of the *American Journal of Nursing* the staff personnel responsible for ANA programs.

7. It is suggested that reports on the following subjects be presented before the entire class group as a basis for discussion: (a) current platform of the ANA, (b) economic security program of the ANA, (c) recent legislative activities of the ANA, (d) research and statistical activities, (e) activities of your state and special interest groups.

8. (a) Differentiate between the functions that a professional association should carry for the benefit of individual practitioners, the profession as a whole and society. (b) What is the relationship of a voluntary professional association to government?

9. (a) Study current reports of the ANA concerning its structure and its relationship to the NLN. (b) Decide whether you believe these 2 organizations should dissolve and a single new association be formed that would encompass and unify their objectives and programs. (c) What would be the advantages and disadvantages of such an association? In this connection, you might survey the opinions of a selected group of graduate nurses who are practicing in the various fields of nursing.

10. (a) What nurses have received special awards, or honors at the ANA conventions since 1965? (b) For what were these awards and honors given to each nurse?

SUGGESTED REFERENCES*

"Abstracts of ANA Clinical Papers." *American Journal of Nursing,* **67**:2578-2586, Dec. 1967.

---

* In each chapter all citations are footnoted and are not included here. All starred references are recommended for additional readings.

American Nurses' Association. *ANA in Action.* New York, The Association. Issued quarterly.

————. *List of Publications.* New York, The Association. Revised annually.

* ————. *Facts About Nursing: A Statistical Summary.* New York, The Association. Issued annually.

* ————. *American Nurses' Association Platform.* New York, The Association. Current issue.

A Blueprint to Build On: A Report to Members 1966-1968. New York, The Association, 1968.

* ————. *Interpretation of the Statements of the Code for Professional Nurses.* New York, The Association, 1968.

————. *The Nation's Nurses.* New York, The Association, 1968.

* ————. *Report to the Members.* New York, The Association. Current issue.

* ————. *1896-1946: Tomorrows and Yesterdays, as Told on the Fiftieth Anniversary of the Association's Founding.* New York, The Association, 1946.

"The American Nurses' Foundation Builds a Program." *American Journal of Nursing,* **57:**310-311, Mar. 1957.

* "ANA Helps You Measure Up Professionally." *American Journal of Nursing,* **63:**95, Jan. 1963.

* "A Conversation With the ANA President and Chairmen of the Three ANA Commissions." *American Journal of Nursing,* **68:**792-799, Apr. 1968.

* "The Differences Between Professional Organizations and Labor Unions." *Weather Vane,* **37:**5-6, Jan. 1968.

Dolan, M. "Putting Our Own House in Order." *American Journal of Nursing,* **62:**76-79, Dec. 1962.

Lewis, E. P. "The Fairview Story." *American Journal of Nursing,* **66:**64-70, Jan. 1966.

* Merton, R. K. "Dilemmas of Democracy in the Voluntary Organizations." *American Journal of Nursing,* **66:**1055-1061, May 1966.

"The Nurse in Research—ANA Guidelines on Ethical Values." *American Journal of Nursing,* **68:**1504-1507, July 1968.

"Nurses Work Together in ANA." *American Journal of Nursing,* **65:**104-106, Oct. 1965.

"The Profession Prepares for the Future." *American Journal of Nursing.* **66:**1549-1567, July 1966.

See also recent ANA Convention Reports and recent reports of ANA clinical conferences.

CHAPTER

21

National League
for Nursing

The National League for Nursing (NLN), a membership organization of individuals and agencies, was established in 1952 through the amalgamation of several organizations and committees.[1] The forerunners of the NLN and their founding dates are: the National League of Nursing Education (NLNE) — 1893; the National Organization for Public Health Nursing (NOPHN) — 1912; the Association of Collegiate Schools of Nursing (ACSN) — 1933; the Joint Committee on Practical Nurses and Auxiliary Workers in Nursing Services — 1945; the Joint Committee on Careers in Nursing — 1948; the National Committee for the Improvement of Nursing Services — 1949; and the National Nursing Accrediting Service — 1949.

PURPOSE AND PHILOSOPHY

The object of the NLN is "to foster the development and improvement of hospital, industrial, public health, and other organized nursing service and of

[1] For an account of the events leading to the formation of the NLN, see the Preview of this unit.

nursing education through the coordinated action of nurses, allied professional groups, citizens, agencies, and schools to the end that the nursing needs of the people will be met."[2]

The philosophy of the NLN is a realistic one. It is based on the recognition that many groups and people in our society have a stake in and a contribution to make toward the development and improvement of organized nursing services and educational programs in nursing.

This philosophy has been elaborated by Ruth Freeman, president of the NLN from 1955 to 1959. In an editorial in *Nursing Outlook,* the official organ of the NLN, Miss Freeman has described some of the ways that people other than nurses are involved in and can participate in the activities of the NLN.

... Nursing education, for example, is just as much the responsibility and concern of university administrators and educators as it is of nurses; it must meet the objectives and fit the patterns and standards of higher education even while it prepares workers to carry out the functions and responsibilities defined by nursing.

... A young newspaperman might see intriguing possibilities for interpreting nursing to the public; a high school counselor might learn new ways to guide students or student activities; a personnel manager in industry might gain great satisfaction from using his special skills in an important social service.[3]

You can doubtless add many more people to these examples mentioned by Miss Freeman: hospital administrators, public health officers, allied nursing personnel, members of the governing boards of hospitals and visiting nurse associations, patients – the list is endless.

MEMBERSHIP

How can the full force of all this "talent unlimited" be harnessed? According to the NLN philosophy, the answer is, "Through nurses and non-nurses working together in full partnership." Accordingly, the NLN bylaws make provision for 2 kinds of members – individual and agency. An individual member may be a registered or a licensed practical nurse, a nurse's aide, a member of an allied profession, or an interested layman. Agency membership is open to organizations or groups that provide nursing service, and to schools, divisions, or departments that conduct educational programs in nursing. Other organizations may become allied agency members.

As has been pointed out in the Preview of this unit, nurses all over the country did some hard and sober thinking before they provided for non-nurse membership in one of the large national nursing organizations. It was a truly pioneering venture to bring together the professional worker and others, including the consumer, to work together toward improving nursing service and nursing education.

[2] From the *Certificate of Incorporation* of the National League for Nursing.
[3] R. Freeman, "Talent Unlimited," *Nursing Outlook,* **6:**315, June 1958.

It was also a demonstration of the "grown-upness" of nursing. As you know, social scientists have evolved a theory that to reach maturity a person passes through several stages: dependence on others, independence of others, and interdependence with others. In designing the NLN, the nursing profession recognized its interdependence with all members of society and demonstrated the trust and confidence in society that is characteristic of maturity.

This partnership with non-nurses has also broadened the resources that can be brought to bear on the study and solution of the problems confronting nursing service and nursing education. Just consider the potentialities inherent in such a diverse membership group!

... On one NLN committee [as far back as 1958] ... there [were] representatives of seven different professional fields as well as a nursing student and a patient. It would take one person a total of 38 years of academic training, excluding any specialty or advanced training, to get the various basic professional trainings represented in this committee. The potential impact of such a sum of talent and wisdom turned on a problem is enormous.[4]

ORGANIZATION

The way in which the NLN membership is organized is pictured in Figure 21-1. When you graduate you will have an opportunity to become a vital part of the organization, either as an individual or through your connection with a member agency.

Individual members join the NLN through the nearest-to-home local leagues. As a member of a local unit, the nurse automatically becomes a member of the constituent league in that area and a member of the NLN. The term "constituent league" may mean a city, a state, a region, a district, or one or more states – any area approved by the NLN Board of Directors as meeting certain criteria for the purpose of program and finances.

Presidents of constituent leagues meet at least once a year, at an annual conference of the National Assembly of Constituent Leagues, for discussion of program and other matters that have to do with activities of members at the grass roots level in relation to the national NLN program. The constituent leagues also band together into regional assemblies for regional planning, implementation of national programs and sharing of ideas. There are now (1970) 6 regional assemblies, which encompass all of the continental USA and Hawaii. These assemblies may meet in-between the meetings of the national assembly, thus providing for interchange of ideas among the local leagues in a region.

At its biennial convention in 1967, changes were made in the structure of the NLN.[5] Two divisions were created, a Division of Individual Members and a Division of Agency Members. As shown in Figure 21-1, Chart A, these

[4] *Loc. Cit.*
[5] See NLN *Bylaws.* Amended May 1967. New York, The Association, 1967.

NATIONAL LEAGUE FOR NURSING
Chart A

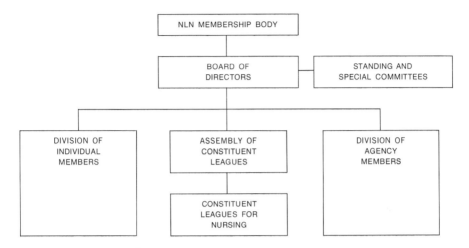

NATIONAL LEAGUE FOR NURSING
Chart B

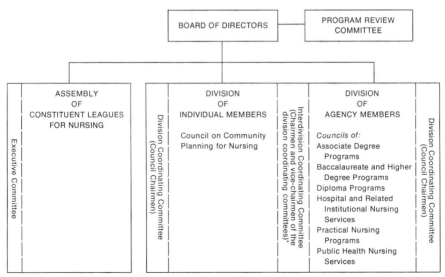

* Also the chairman and vice chairman of the Assembly of Constituent Leagues for Nursing by vote of the NLN Board of Directors, January 1968.

Fig. 21-1. Organization of the National League for Nursing. Chart A shows the overall organization; Chart B shows in more detail the organization plan for the Assembly of Constituent Leagues and the Divisions.

divisions function to further the development and improvement of nursing services and nursing education. Each division works through its respective councils.

Presently (1970), the Division of Individual Members has 1 council, the Council on Community Planning for Nursing, which is composed of all individual members of the League. There are 6 councils within the Division of Agency Members: (1) Council of Associate Degree Programs, (2) Council of Baccalaureate and Higher Degree Programs, (3) Council of Diploma Programs, (4) Council of Practical Nurse Programs, (5) Council of Hospital and Related Institutional Nursing Services, and (6) Council of Public Health Nursing Services.

The NLN Board of Directors is composed of the elected officers, the chairman of the executive committee of each council, the members of the executive committee of the Assembly of Constituent Leagues for Nursing, and such additional directors as are required to make a total of 33 voting members. The bylaws, as amended in 1969, also provide for a president-elect to serve for a 2-year period (prior to assuming the presidency) as one of the elected officers.

Each division within the League has a Division Coordinating Committee responsible for coordinating the work of its councils as well as that of the 2 divisions. There is also an Interdivision Coordinating Committee composed of the chairman and vice-chairman of each division coordinating committee, and of the Executive Committee of the Assembly of Constituent Leagues for Nursing. This committee not only effects coordination between divisions but maintains a relationship with the Program Review Committee.

It is suggested that you study the *Bylaws* of the NLN as amended May 1967 to determine the specific functions of the new divisions and councils, of the Assembly of Constituent Leagues, and of the various national committees, including the important Program Review Committee.

There are other elected and appointed national committees through which members work on special problems. In 1970, for example, there were more than 75 such committees with more than 500 persons from all over the country working on them. In addition, constituent leagues have committees through which many NLN members channel their contributions.

From this you can see that there is not only one place for you in the NLN when you become a nurse; there are many places where you can contribute the knowledge gained from your experiences and draw upon the information and wisdom of other NLN members.

ACTIVITIES

Fact Finding and Research

As a student in a school of nursing and through your observations in the hospitals and public health nursing agencies in which you are having your

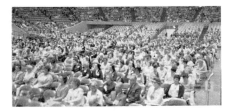
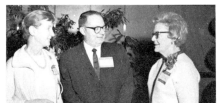

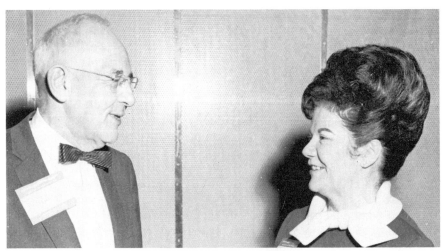

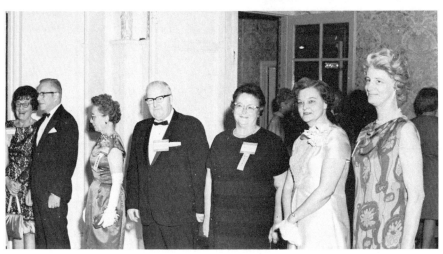

Fig. 21-2. *(Top left)* Activities at the NLN 1969 Biennial Convention in Detroit. (Nursing Outlook) a business session. *(Top right)* Anne Kibrick, first vice president, NLN; Philip M. Hauser, Professor of Sociology, University of Chicago; and L. Ann Conley, Retiring NLN President at the opening general session of the convention. *(Center)* John S. Millis, Chancellor, Case-Western Reserve University, Cleveland, and Margaret Walsh, newly appointed general director of NLN. *(Bottom)* The Convention reception to meet NLN Board of Directors with Miss Gwendolyn MacDonald, newly elected NLN president, second from the right.

field experience, you know that the problems of these institutions and agencies are myriad. You probably also have a vivid idea of what many of these problems are.

Everywhere you see the need for more nursing personnel of all categories. The faculty in your school is probably shorthanded. You see that patients are sometimes deprived of good nursing care because of the shortage of nursing service personnel; certainly they would be getting better care if there were more nurses. There are other needs of this kind that you may not be aware of. School health services, occupational health services, nursing homes—all are expanding rapidly, and all need nurses.

Perhaps you and your classmates have had to travel considerable distances for field experience in public health nursing, because your community has no public health nursing agencies. This is hard on you, but think what it means to the people in the community who need this kind of service.

Your teachers and the nurses in service agencies could tell you of many more problems. They know that nursing concepts and practices are changing rapidly. How are they to keep abreast of these advances, so that their patients will have the benefits of modern nursing care and you will be prepared to give that kind of care?

New categories of workers have been added to the nursing services of hospitals and other health agencies—workers that were perhaps scarcely known when many supervisors and nursing service directors were preparing for their positions. Nursing administrators want to find out how to include these workers in their staffing patterns, how to teach them, how to orient them to their jobs.

Your teachers want you to have the best kind of education—education that is based on the most recently discovered knowledge about how people learn. How are they to keep up to date?

Financing ranks high in the problems of nursing education. The dean or director of your school is probably worrying about where the money is coming from for new teachers and badly needed student residences, classrooms, and library and laboratory facilities. The question of money may be bothering you, too. Perhaps you are planning on continuing your education after you become a nurse. Certainly, many nurses want to do this so that they can give patients the very best that is in them. But plans to continue studies often have to be postponed, sometimes forever, for economic reasons.

How does the NLN go about helping those in nursing services and schools of nursing solve these problems? As you have seen in Chapter 5, the first steps in problem solving are identifying and defining the problem and collecting data about it.

The NLN does just that. As an example, let us take one outstanding problem—the shortage of nurses. Through research studies of its own and those it encourages constituent leagues to undertake, NLN assesses nursing's personnel and educational needs. If you will turn to the current issue of *Facts About Nursing,* published by the American Nurses' Association

(ANA), you will find the statistical data, compiled by the NLN, which shows the extent to which these needs are being met.

Perhaps one of the things that has concerned you is what happens to patients once they leave the hospital and go home. NLN is concerned about this, too. Several years ago it undertook a study to find out how extensively continuing nursing care from hospital to home is available to patients and what some of the blocks are to starting or strengthening referral plans between hospitals and community nursing agencies. Then it recast the study findings into a popular vein, gathered original material about actual community experience in setting up continuity of nursing-care programs, and published a guide to community action on this problem. The guide is titled *Nursing Service Without Walls*. NLN also publishes reports of actual experiences, such as *Continuity of Nursing Care from Hospitals to Home*, a project undertaken by a local league and a county health department in California.

Again, while many people realize that the absence of money is the root of many problems of nursing education, there is very little information on how much it costs to prepare a nurse. Through a series of research projects the NLN has helped schools of nursing to collect the data necessary for approaching this problem and has supported Federal legislation channeling money to nursing schools.

Recruitment of Students

To overcome that pressing problem, the shortage of nurses, more people like you must be encouraged to enter nursing. How did you become interested in nursing? Perhaps you saw a poster entitled "Be a Nurse – and Walk with Pride." Possibly your interest was strengthened by membership in the Future Nurses Club or Health Careers Club in your high school. Maybe your mind was finally made up by the information which your high school counselor gave you on careers in nursing and schools of nursing.

In back of all these "stimulants" to select a career in nursing is the ANA-NLN careers program. Through it, posters and exhibits are provided and informational literature is prepared and disseminated. In sponsoring this program, the ANA and NLN are cooperating in performing a service not only for nursing but for young people who need help in selecting useful and satisfying careers.

Of particular service to young people in selecting a school of nursing are NLN's series of pamphlets listing schools of nursing, their admission requirements, financial control and other information, such as living arrangements and description of the type of education program offered. Among those updated annually are: *Education for Nursing: The Diploma Way*, which lists NLN-accredited schools granting a diploma in nursing; *Associate Degree Education for Nursing*, which lists state-approved and NLN-accredited associate degree programs in nursing; and *College Education: Key to a Professional Career in Nursing,* which lists programs of nursing education giving a baccalaureate degree.

There are also other pamphlets published from time to time. NLN's *Husband/Father/Humanitarian/Specialist — Nurse* highlights some of the opportunities for men in nursing, and its lists of sources of financial aid are invaluable to both preservice and graduate nurse students.

Testing Services

Attracting people to nursing is as important as selecting those who have a reasonable chance of completing their preparation for it. As an aid in evaluating applicants to their programs, many schools use selection examinations. Three such examinations are offered by the NLN: 1 for applicants to schools of practical nursing; 1 for applicants to programs preparing registered nurses; and 1 for graduate nurses who wish to continue their education in a college or university.

The NLN also provides 3 kinds of achievement tests: 1 kind for students of practical nursing; 1 kind for students in schools preparing registered nurses; and 1 for aides in preservice and inservice training programs. Possibly you have taken some of these tests. If so, your teacher has probably explained to you what they are for: to help her compare your progress with that of students in similar educational programs throughout the country. The results of the test may help her to improve the course so that it is more in line with the courses given in other schools. NLN achievement tests, then, are one means by which the NLN helps schools of nursing to improve their educational programs.

As you will find when you read Chapter 27, the NLN, with the cooperation of the boards of nursing, also develops and scores the licensing examinations for registered and practical nurses.

Institutes, Workshops, Conferences, Seminars

To help those in service agencies and schools of nursing to keep pace with the growing and changing needs and concepts in nursing, the NLN and its constituent leagues arrange for meetings of many kinds. In some of these meetings, such as those conducted for the councils of member agencies, the members themselves constitute the main resource for identifying and solving their problems. In other meetings NLN staff members and other experts serve as resource personnel.

Representative of these meetings are the regional workshops of the Council of Public Health Nursing Services and of the Council of Diploma Programs; the workshops on hospital staffing and staff development of the NLN's Department of Hospital Nursing Services; and the Nursing Advisory Service of NLN and the National Tuberculosis and Respiratory Disease Association.

Consultation Services

To help strengthen existing nursing services and educational programs in nursing and to aid in the sound development of new programs, the NLN offers a wide variety of consultation services. NLN consultants in public health nursing, for example, help communities to establish the kind of public health agencies that they need or to combine existing services so that coverage of the community will be expanded. An illustration is the consultation available to junior and senior colleges which are conducting or are considering the establishment of educational programs in nursing.

NLN, with the help of a grant from the Sealantic Fund, held special conferences for junior and community college administrators in the days when nursing programs were beginning to emerge in these schools. In the year 1967-68, 2 conferences were conducted jointly by the Council of Associate Degree Programs and the Council of Baccalaureate and Higher Degree Programs for colleges and universities involved in or planning the establishment of new nursing education programs. More than 500 (547) administrators and nurse educators from every section of the country attended these conferences.

Accreditation

Accreditation is another means through which the NLN is helping schools of nursing to improve the quality of education they offer their students. Very possibly your school is accredited by the NLN and has been visited by NLN accrediting representatives. If so, these visitors may have told you something about the NLN accrediting program. The NLN now also accredits practical nursing education programs and public health nursing services.

What you may not know is that accreditation is not unique to nursing education. Practically every institution of higher learning in this country belongs to a regional association which periodically evaluates it as a whole in terms of certain standards; if the institution meets these standards it is accredited. However, the regional associations do not accredit the programs in these or other institutions that prepare for the professions. The agencies that accredit professional programs are recognized by the National Commission on Accreditation. This commission has designated the NLN as the accrediting body for nursing programs in institutions of higher education. NLN is recognized also as the accrediting agency for nursing education by the ANA, the Office of Education, U.S. Department of Health, Education, and Welfare, and the National Federation of Licensed Practical Nurses.

There are several reasons for accrediting educational institutions and programs. Among them are: (1) to guide students in the choice of a program that will meet their needs, (2) to serve as a guide to other schools in the transfer of students and (3) to stimulate continued improvement of schools.

The NLN accreditation program has been directed chiefly toward this last objective; in fact, it is sometimes referred to as the "school improvement program." Through it schools of nursing have been encouraged to evaluate themselves and to work toward eliminating the weak points which they have identified in this self-evaluation. It is a voluntary program — that is, no school is compelled to participate in it — and some good schools, particularly in days gone by, have not applied for NLN accreditation. Increasingly, however, schools have recognized the values that are derived from participation in this program, and a substantial majority of them will have applied for and received NLN accreditation. As of January 1, 1969, of 1,293 nursing education programs preparing students for licensure as RN's, 791 were NLN accredited and this number is increasing steadily.[6]

Educational Aid

It is important for nursing services and nursing education that future administrators, supervisors, and teachers, as well as consultants, research workers and expert practitioners, be prepared in graduate programs — that is, programs that lead to a master's or higher degree. Of all categories of nursing personnel, those who are qualified for these leadership positions are in shortest supply.

As has been pointed out, the stumbling-block in many instances is money. Again, the NLN found a partial solution. In the past several years the Federal Government has been a major source of funds to encourage recruitment of students into nursing and to enable nurses to continue their education in programs preparing them for positions as administrators, supervisors, teachers and nursing specialists at the post-baccalaureate and post-masters levels. NLN cooperates actively with the PHS, U.S. Department of Health, Education, and Welfare, which administers the programs, undertaking needed studies and advising its agency members about provisions of the Federal statute. NLN also publishes lists of sources of support in *Scholarships, Fellowships, Educational Grants and Loans for Registered Nurses* and *Scholarships and Loans — Beginning Education in Nursing*.

In addition, the League administers Nurses' Educational Funds, Inc., a program supported by individuals, nursing organizations, foundations, business firms and others, that provides grants ranging from $1,000 to $6,000 annually to enable nurses to complete baccalaureate or graduate study in nursing.

Publications and Films

The written word as well as the spoken one is utilized to help those in nursing services and schools of nursing solve the many problems that con-

[6] American Nurses' Association, *Facts About Nursing: A Statistical Summary,* New York, The Association, 1969, p. 101.

front them. One important medium for this kind of communication is *Nursing Outlook,* the official organ of the NLN, which is published by the AJN Co. Information about this magazine is contained in Chapter 24.

The NLN also arranges for the preparation of and publishes a considerable number of books, pamphlets, and leaflets. These include self-evaluation guides, research studies, criteria for evaluating nursing services and nursing education, bibliographies, reports of the information and opinions exchanged at meetings, and technical materials prepared by specialists on such subjects as integrating psychiatric nursing in the preservice curriculum, and inservice education. Through the *League Exchange* series of publications, NLN members can make available to each other useful materials that are too long or are otherwise unsuitable for publication elsewhere.

The NLN also publishes record forms that can be used in schools of nursing and public health nursing agencies, and reservoirs of test questions for use in evaluating nurse aides.

An annually updated list of current publications distributed by the NLN is available from NLN headquarters.

RELATIONSHIPS WITH OTHER ORGANIZATIONS

The NLN and the ANA functions and activities were planned to complement each other. Programs of common concern are promoted through the ANA-NLN Coordinating Council, which is composed of the boards of directors of the 2 organizations. Constituent and local leagues and state and district nurses associations also have councils through which they coordinate their endeavors.

The NLN also has cooperative relationships with non-nursing organizations whose interests intersect those of the NLN at various points. These organizations often cosponsor NLN activities. For example, the nation's first accreditation program for community nursing services was established by NLN with the cosponsorship of the American Public Health Association. The school-cost analysis study was also the result of cooperation with the PHS of the U.S. Department of Health, Education, and Welfare.

The NLN also encourages the trend toward interorganizational planning for health, education, and welfare through participation in a number of interorganization committees. These are with such national agencies as the National Federation of Licensed Practical Nurses, the American Public Health Association, the National Tuberculosis and Respiratory Disease Association, the American Association of Junior Colleges and the American Hospital Association. The NLN holds membership in the National Health Council, the National Social Welfare Assembly and the American Council on Education.

HEADQUARTERS

The national headquarters is located at 10 Columbus Circle, New York, New York, 10019. The headquarters staff consists of over 200 executive, professional and clerical workers. On the staff are experts in nursing service and in nursing education, as well as specialists in such fields as inservice education, public health nursing education, psychiatric nursing, nursing in tuberculosis and respiratory diseases, and maternal and child health nursing. The staff also includes business administrators, consultants on college and junior college administration, psychologists, statisticians, editors and public-relations experts.

Anna Fillmore was general director of the NLN from the time the organization came into being in 1952 until 1959. In 1959 Inez Haynes became the general director. Miss Haynes retired in 1969 and was succeeded by Mrs. Margaret E. Walsh.

FINANCIAL SUPPORT

The NLN is supported by membership dues, income from its services, and grants. NLN's first 5 years, were made possible by grants from the Commonwealth Fund, the National Foundation (then the National Foundation for Infantile Paralysis), and the Rockefeller Foundation; and the Commonwealth Fund contributed hundreds of thousands of dollars to an NLN fellowship program.

Other grantors include the American Hospital Association, the American Medical Association, the American Nurses' Association, the Avalon Foundation, the National Institutes of Health, the Sealantic Fund, the PHS of the U.S. Department of Health, Education, and Welfare, the U.S. Vocational and Rehabilitation Administration.

YOUR MEMBERSHIP IN THE NLN

After you graduate, you may join the NLN through the local league for nursing in your community, if there is a local league; otherwise you would join through your nearest constituent league. Application forms are available from these organizations or may be requested from national headquarters.

As an individual member you will join the Division of Individual Members and become a member of that division's Council on Community Planning for Nursing. This council, concerned with trends in the health field as these affect nursing service and nursing education, may have various national committees. You may soon find yourself involved in the work of similar committees in your own state or community, for example, a committee on nursing manpower. As a member of a hospital or agency staff or a school of nursing faculty, you may also be involved in the work of one of the councils of the Division of Agency Members.

When you are a recent graduate from a school of nursing, your local or state league may be able to arrange for you to hold a courtesy membership (without dues) from the date of your graduation until January 1st of the next year. Even before your graduation date, however, you will want to explore ways in which you, as a nurse, will want to participate in NLN activities. By joining the NLN you will make friends with whom you share a vital interest — the improvement of nursing services and nursing education.

PROBLEMS

1. (a) Is there a local league for nursing in your community? (b) What are its purposes? (c) Who is its president? (d) When will its next meeting be held? (e) What is its current program?

2. (a) When and where will the next convention of the NLN be held? (b) Pretend you are on the Committee on Program for this convention: (1) Name 2 topics that you think should be on the program. (2) Whom would you suggest to discuss these topics?

3. (a) Decide what you consider are the 2 outstanding problems facing: (1) your school of nursing and (2) one of the hospitals in which you receive your clinical experience. (b) Find out in what ways, if any, your local or state league for nursing is trying to help find solutions to these problems.

4. (a) Make a list of 6 non-nurses of your acquaintance who could be of assistance to the schools of nursing and the nursing services in the hospitals and other health agencies in your community. (b) How would you go about "unleashing the talents" of these people, so that they can contribute to the improvement of nursing services and nursing education?

5. What are the major recommendations of the League's Committee on Perspectives?

6. What role does a council of member agencies have in the national accreditation process?

7. List the contributions of the following to NLN: Lois M. Austin, L. Ann Conley, Alice M. Dempsey, Gwendolyn MacDonald, Fr. Edward J. Drummond, S.J., Ruth B. Freeman, Lucile Petry Leone, John S. Millis, Henry C. Mills, Helen Nahm, F. Robert Paulsen, Mary C. Rockefeller, Sister M. Cornile Dulohery, Ruth Sleeper.

8. (a) Who are the current chairmen of the executive and other committees of the divisions and councils of the NLN? (b) Determine from the current official directory of *Nursing Outlook* the staff personnel responsible for the NLN programs.

SUGGESTED REFERENCES*

Conley, L. A. "The League and Community Planning." *Nursing Outlook,* **16:**29, Apr. 1968.

* Editorial. "The League Idea at Work for Nursing." *Nursing Outlook,* **11:**251, Apr. 1963.

* Fillmore, A. "Our First Five Years." *Nursing Outlook,* **6:**14-17, Jan. 1958.

* Haynes, I. "NLN at Ten." *Nursing Outlook,* **10:**372-377, June 1962.

"League Exchange." *Nursing Outlook,* **8:**494, Sept. 1960.

"Messages from Three Presidents." *Nursing Outlook,* **10:**378-381, June 1962.

Mitchell, T. L. "The 'Big Bad League' Becomes a Friend." *Nursing Outlook,* **11:**350-351. May 1963.

National League for Nursing News. New York, The League, 1952—.

National League for Nursing. *Biennial Reports,* 1967/1968, New York, The League, 1969.

———. *The NLN Evaluation Service.* New York, The League, 1968.

———. *The Nursing Advisory Service of NLN and NTRDA.* New York, The League, 1968.

———. *NLN...Who We Are...What We Do.* New York, The League, 1967.

———. *Nursing Education Accreditation—A Service of the National League for Nursing.* New York, The League, 1967.

———. *In League for Nursing.* New York, The League, 1967.

———. *This is a Cam...An NLN Cam is a Council of Agency Members.* New York, The League, 1967.

———. *Perspectives for Nursing.* New York, The League, 1965. Augmented 1967.

———. *The School Improvement Program of the National League for Nursing.* New York, The League, 1963.

———. *Facts About the National League for Nursing.* New York, The League. Current edition.

———. *NLN Publications Catalog.* New York, The League. Current edition.

* "National League for Nursing Convention: Detroit, May 19-23." *Nursing Outlook,* **17:**42-64, 1969.

Newton, M. "What's Ahead for Nursing and NLN?" *Nursing Outlook,* **9:**600-604, Oct. 1961.

* Novello, D. J. "Regionalization: The Core of the Revamped NLN Structure." *Nursing Outlook,* **17:**16-19, Feb. 1969.

"Q and A on NLN Structure Revisions." *Nursing Outlook,* **15:**37, Mar. 1967.

Stevenson, N. L. "Perspective on Developments in Practical Nursing." *Nursing Outlook,* **8:**34-37, Jan. 1960.

* "The Why of Lay Participation in NLN." *Nursing Outlook,* **12:**582-585, Aug. 1963.

See reports on most recent conventions. These appear in *Nursing Outlook* shortly after each convention. See also the *Biennial Reports* and the various departmental *News Letters* and *Memos to* agency members of the NLN.

———

* In each chapter all citations are footnoted and are not included here. All starred references are recommended for additional reading.

American Association of Industrial Nurses

American Association of Nurse Anesthetists

American College of Nurse-Midwifery

Association of Operating Room Nurses

Committee on Nursing of the American Medical Association

Conference of Catholic Schools of Nursing

Guild of Saint Barnabas

National Association for Practical Nurse Education and Service

National Federation of Licensed Practical Nurses

Nurses Christian Fellowship

CHAPTER

22

Other National Nursing and Allied Organizations

Two national nursing organizations concerned with the broad problems of nursing practice and the individual nurse, and with nursing services and nursing education have been described in the immediately preceding chapters. Others, listed above, will be described briefly in his chapter.[1]

AMERICAN ASSOCIATION OF INDUSTRIAL NURSES

Origin

Many years before the American Association of Industrial Nurses (AAIN) was organized, several small groups of industrial nurses (now called occupational health nurses) met frequently to resolve mutual problems and to plan for the development and advancement of standards for industrial nursing.

---

[1] Among the other organizations that have committees concerned with nursing are the American Hospital Association and the American Psychiatric Association.

The National Organization for Public Health Nursing (NOPHN) had a section for industrial nurses, and the ANA had concerned itself with industrial nursing. In spite of these efforts to assist the industrial nurse, small clubs were springing up all over the country, because the nurses desired to work out together the specific problems in industrial nursing.

For some time, it was debated whether industrial nurses should be a permanent section of the NOPHN or maintain their own organization. It was argued that the functions of the industrial nurse are similar in many respects to those of nurses in public health. It was agreed further that this is true of all nurses. Finally, it was conceded and is now well established that industrial nursing is a specialized branch of nursing concerned with meeting the needs of workers for the purpose of developing and maintaining the highest level of health and efficiency.

As the common problems of the industrial nurse group began to emerge, the following eastern clubs held a series of 4 joint annual meetings:

New England Industrial Nurses Club, organized 1915
Detroit Industrial Nurses Club, organized 1920
New York Industrial Nurses Club, organized 1921
Philadelphia Industrial Nurses Club, organized 1924
New Jersey Industrial Nurses Club, organized 1930

The discussions of these groups resulted in the decision that industrial nurses should unite into an autonomous organization and work out their own problems.

The AAIN was organized April 19, 1942, and became incorporated January 24, 1944. By April 1968, it was composed of 24 state, 74 local, and 2 regional associations. The programs of the Assocation include: professional exchange, information dissemination, education, nurse-physician-management relations, legislation and creation of professional standards.

Purposes

According to the current (1970) *Articles of Incorporation and By-Laws*, the purposes are:

... To constitute the professional association of nurses engaged in the practice of industrial nursing; to maintain the honor and character of the nursing profession; to improve community health by bettering nursing service to workers; to develop and promote standards for industrial nurses and industrial nursing services; to stimulate interest in and provide a forum for the discussion of problems in the field of industrial nursing; to stimulate industrial nurse participation in all nursing activities local, state, and national and to do within the limits of the law all things necessary, proper, incidental, suitable, useful, and conducive to the complete accomplishment of the foregoing purposes.[2]

[2] American Association of Industrial Nurses, Inc., *By-Laws*, New York, The Association, n.d., p. 1.

Relationships with Other Organizations

One of the chief objectives of the AAIN is to work in direct cooperation with all allied groups. It has worked actively with the other national nursing organizations on structure study, recruitment, and similar activities of concern to all nurses. One of its activities was the preparation of *Criteria for Evaluation of Programs of Study in Industrial Nursing.* A conference committee of the AAIN and the NLN has prepared the *Guide for Evaluating and Teaching Occupational Health Nursing Concepts.* The association works closely with medical, industrial and other groups concerned with health in industry.

Official Journal

Occupational Health Nursing, which replaced the *American Association of Industrial Nurses Journal* as the official publication in January 1969, will give you the news of the organization. It will keep you in touch with the advancing frontier in industrial nursing.

Headquarters

The American Association of Industrial Nurses, Inc., is located at 79 Madison Avenue, New York, New York, 10016.

AMERICAN ASSOCIATION OF NURSE ANESTHETISTS

The American Association of Nurse Anesthetists (AANA) is an independent organization of nurses who are specialists in giving anesthesia.

Origin and Objectives

The AANA was founded in 1931, although graduate nurses have been administering anesthesia since the 1880's. From the beginning its objectives have been: (1) to restrict membership to nurses qualified by training and experience to administer anesthesia and (2) to raise standards of education and service for nurse anesthetists.

Membership

Membership is open to all qualified nurse anesthetists, regardless of sex or color, who pass the admission examination and meet the following requirements:

1. High school graduation or its equivalent
2. Graduation from a state-approved nursing school

3. Registration as a professional nurse with a state license to practice

4. Graduation from a school of anesthesia offering a program of not less than 18 months

At present, the AANA's instrument for measuring the competency of candidates for membership is a qualifying examination. This examination first was administered in 1945.

The instrument for raising standards of education is its accrediting program, which was established in January 1952. Only graduates of recognized schools of anesthesia are eligible to take the qualifying examination.

In 1968 there were 13,406 members in the AANA.

Activities

The AANA, in conjunction with the American Hospital Association, holds an annual meeting each year for the benefit of nurse anesthetists. It publishes materials of value to nurse anesthetists, such as its *Statement of Principles Regarding Personnel Policies for Nurse Anesthetists, Adopted September 1952.* The AANA also carries out a rather extensive program of workshops and conferences in connection with its 52 affiliated associations. It is recognized by the U.S. Department of Health, Education, and Welfare as the accrediting agency for schools of anesthesia for nurses and it carries on any activity which will benefit the nurse anesthetist.

Official Publication

The Association publishes a bimonthly magazine, the *Journal of the American Association of Nurse Anesthetists.* In alternate months it publishes the *AANA News Bulletin.*

Headquarters

If you write to the Executive Director, American Association of Nurse Anesthetists, Suite 3010, Prudential Plaza, Chicago, Ill., 60601, you can secure answers to your questions.

AMERICAN COLLEGE OF NURSE-MIDWIFERY

On November 12-13, 1955, the American College of Nurse-Midwifery was organized formally in Kansas City, Missouri. This organization replaced the Section on Nurse-Midwifery that previously existed in the NOPHN. The new national structure in nursing had no provision for this special-interest group. Nurse-midwives from 8 states attended the meeting in 1955.

Miss Hattie Hemschemeyer was elected president. In 1956 the College became a member of the International Confederation of Midwives.

Objectives and Activities

The following are objectives of the College:

1. To enable nurse-midwives to concentrate their efforts in the improvement of services for mothers and newborn babies, in cooperation with other allied groups

2. To identify the areas of nurse-midwifery practices as they relate to the total service and educational aspects of maternal and newborn care

3. To study and evaluate the activities of the nurse-midwife in order that qualifications for these activities may be established

4. To plan and develop, with the assistance of allied professional groups, educational programs in nurse-midwifery that will meet the qualifications of the profession

5. To establish channels for communication and interpretation of nurse-midwifery to allied professional and nonprofessional groups on a regional, national and international basis

6. To sponsor research and develop a literature in the field of nurse-midwifery[3]

Activities in carrying out these objectives include annual meetings of the membership (usually held immediately before the biennial meetings of the ANA and the NLN); committee work, scientific workshops and conferences; cooperation with the International Confederation of Midwives and with allied national groups interested in maternal and infant care; interpretation of nurse-midwifery to allied professions and the community; surveys and studies; development of standards of education and practice in nurse-midwifery; and guidance of new schools of nurse-midwifery. Nurse-midwifery is considered a clinical nursing specialty. There are now (1970) 7 programs leading to a masters degree and a certificate in nurse-midwifery and 2 that lead to a certificate in nurse-midwifery alone.

Official Journal

The *Bulletin of the American College of Nurse-Midwifery* is published quarterly. It includes scientific articles, reports of studies and surveys, announcements of the College and other pertinent information.

Organization

The College is governed by an Executive Board composed of the president, past-president, president-elect, vice president, secretary, treasurer and 2 members-at-large elected by mailed ballot from the membership. All of the work of the College is carried on through the volunteer efforts of the Board and its committees and the individual members of the College. Lucille Woodville, assistant chief, Maternal and Child Health Branch of the PHS, U.S.

[3] "Message from Our President," *Bulletin of the American College of Nurse-Midwifery,* 4:69-72. Sept./Oct. 1959.

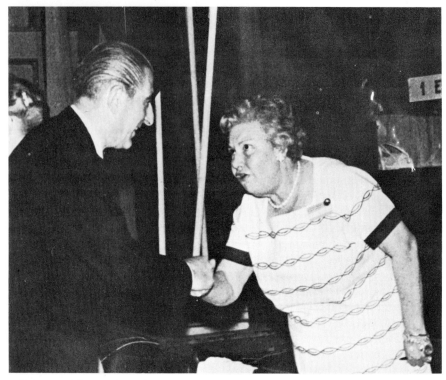

Fig. 22-1. Miss Lucille Woodville, Assistant Chief, Maternal and Child Health Branch, Indian Health Service, Health Services and Mental Health Administration, U.S. Health, Education, and Welfare, and President, American College of Nurse-Midwives, was elected President of the International Confederation of Midwives in November 1969 at the first Congress of the Confederation held in this hemisphere in Santiago, Chile. Miss Woodville is shown being congratulated by Sr. Eduardo Frei Montalva, President of the Republic of Chile. (Gastone Franco Campos, Santiago, Chile).

Department of Health, Education, and Welfare, is the current (1970) president of the ACNM. Miss Woodville has recently also been elected president of the International Confederation of Midwives (see Figure 22-1).

Information

For further information you may write to the American College of Nurse-Midwifery at 50 East 92nd Street, New York, New York, 10028.

ASSOCIATION OF OPERATING ROOM NURSES

The Association of Operating Room Nurses (AORN), a national organization for registered professional nurses engaged in operating room nursing, was formally organized and incorporated in 1957. However, the organization had its origin in local groups, the first of which began meeting in New York City as early as 1949 under the leadership of Miss Edith Dee Hall.[4]

The first national meeting of the AORN was held in New York City in 1954 with an attendance of 1,791. This was the first of the National Congresses that are held annually by the Association in major cities throughout the country. Regional educational 2-day institutes are held several times yearly throughout the USA.

The Association has been responsible for the development of teaching films on topics related to the operating room suite, personnel and patient care. Also, conferences are held at national meetings for clinical and inservice education instructors with regard to the education of nursing students.

Philosophy, Aim, Objectives, Activities

The AORN believes it is the responsibility of the operating room nurse to assure high quality nursing care to patients undergoing surgery, to guide the essential and continuing education of operating room nursing personnel and to contribute to general nursing education through a board program of educational activities.

The aim of the association is to improve standards of operating room nursing care. Its objectives are:

1. To motivate and encourage operating room personnel to accept responsibility for continued education in order to attain and maintain competency in the comprehensive care of the patient undergoing surgery.

2. To increase understanding, knowledge and skills of personnel engaged in operating room nursing.

3. To foster leadership qualities in the registered professional nurse.

4. To promote and encourage effective communications and interpersonal relations.

5. To promote increased interest and participation of nurses in professional relations.

6. To maintain cooperative relations with other professional organizations and allied groups.

7. To study existing practices and new developments in the field of operating room nursing education.

By 1968 AORN had 135 local chapters in 41 states (including Alaska, Hawaii and the Canal Zone). Individual members are also located in over 26 foreign countries and territories.[5] The official publication of the Association, *AORN Journal,* provides personnel in the operating room and related services with original, practical information based on scientific fact and principle.

---

[4] *The AORN Story.* New York. The Association of Operating Room Nurses, 1967, pp. 6-10.
[5] Membership in ANA and/or NLN is encouraged for all members. However, it is mandatory for those serving as national officers or directors to belong to at least one of these organizations.

In addition, selected material from the annual AORN congress and regional institutes on operating room nursing is presented.[6]

The first joint meeting was held with representatives of the ANA, NLN, and the American Nurses' Foundation (ANF) in 1964 for the purpose of exploring problems inherent in operating room nursing. The Association also is working cooperatively with the American College of Surgeons on programs for nurses at regional meetings of the American College of Surgeons.

In 1965, the Board of Directors issued a statement on "Standards for Administrative and Clinical Practice in the Operating Room" which was published in the March-April 1965 issue of the *AORN Journal.* In 1967, the Association published an instructor's manual entitled *Teaching the Operating Room Technician,* which should provide a more standardized approach to the training of nonprofessional personnel for use in the operating room. A companion piece entitled *O.R. Topics, An Anthology of Selected Articles,* was published in 1968 and contains articles pertinent to the nursing care of patients undergoing surgical intervention.

Information

For further information you may write to the Association of Operating Room Nurses, 8085 East Prentice, Englewood, Colorado 80110.

COMMITTEE ON NURSING OF
THE AMERICAN MEDICAL ASSOCIATION

In 1955, the House of Delegates of the AMA approved the action of the Board of Trustees in combining several autonomous groups on nursing into an over-all committee on nursing. At that time the AMA members of the National Joint Commission for the Improvement of Patient Care were constituted as the Committee on Nursing, which was later named the Committee for Liaison with national nursing organizations.

As the interests and the activities of the Committee were broadened, a need for a central coordinator of affairs pertaining to nursing was identified. Therefore, in July of 1960, the Department of Nursing of the AMA was created and categorized with Drugs, Foods and Nutrition, Medical Education, and others, under the Division of Scientific Activities.

The Committee on Nursing

The Committee on Nursing is comprised of 8 physicians, including the chairman and cochairman, appointed annually by the Board of Trustees. The Director of the Section on Nursing serves as the Secretary of this Committee. The group meets at least 4 times a year and when necessary, more

[6] "General Information," *AORN Journal,* **1:**5, Jan./Feb. 1963.

frequently. The Committee reports annually to the Board of Trustees, which report is published with other Committee and Council reports in the *Journal of the American Medical Association (JAMA)*.

The members of the Committee are continuously concerned with high standards of patient care and view achievement of quality patient care as a joint effort of nurses and physicians. The members of AMA must be informed on trends, problems and standards in nursing service and education.

Purpose and Programs

A statement of objectives and program was published in the August 4, 1962 issue of *JAMA* and states intentions, purposes and directions for the future. The statement clearly announces the belief that: "(1) nurses have a separate and distinct professional status and their contributions are those of coworkers; (2) nursing should expect the medical profession to support and endorse high standards of nursing education and service; and (3) each of the various levels of academic and technical accomplishment in nursing makes its own unique contribution to the total health care of the public."[7]

Current Activities

The objectives are implemented by the Committee in several ways, some of which are:

1. The committee and its secretary maintain liaison with such nursing organizations as the ANA, NLN, National Federation of Licensed Practical Nurses and National Association for Practical Nurse Education and Service, as well as with other allied groups.

2. Three AMA-ANA conferences have been held, each on a different topic: (a) "Medical and Nursing Practice in a Changing World;" (b) "Nurse-Physicians Collaboration Toward Improved Patient Care;" and (c) "The Sick Person Needs. . . ."

3. The exhibit, "Physician-Nurse Communications," has been shown at a number of national and allied medical conventions, as well as at the AMA annual convention and several state medical society meetings.

4. Nineteen reports sponsored by the Committee on Nursing have been published.

5. A 1963 survey showed that 43 state medical societies were maintaining direct liaison with nursing representatives in their states.

6. Encouragement of meetings of state medical society committees on nursing.

7. Preparation of a brochure entitled "Guide for the Organization of State and County Committees on Nursing with Suggested Activities."

8. Committee sponsored programs at ANA annual conventions.

[7] "Objectives and Program of the AMA Committee on Nursing." *Journal of the American Medical Association,* **181**:430, Aug. 4, 1962.

9. Development of a Panel of Nurse Consultants that meets annually with the Committee on Nursing.

Information

For further information write to the Secretary, Committee on Nursing, American Medical Association, 535 North Dearborn Street, Chicago, Ill., 60610.

CONFERENCE OF CATHOLIC SCHOOLS OF NURSING

The Conference of Catholic Schools of Nursing (CCSN) is administered through the Division of Nursing Education of the Catholic Hospital Association of the USA and is a constituent member (Group B) of the American Council on Education.

Formation

In February, 1948, the Catholic Hospital Association sponsored a special meeting on nursing education for Catholic nursing schools. One of the recommendations from the group present at this meeting was for the organization of the CCSN. A suggested plan for the development of the proposed Conference was approved by the Council on Nursing Education, a unit of the Catholic Hospital Association, and by those attending the special meeting in February. The CCSN was organized formally at a meeting held in Cleveland, Ohio, in May, 1948.

Office space was made available in the national headquarters office of the Catholic Hospital Association in St. Louis during February, 1948. Headquarters office has been maintained there since that time.

Membership

The CCSN is a voluntary association of educational units in nursing under the control of Catholic institutions in the USA. Institutional membership includes schools operated by Catholic institutions, schools of practical nursing operated by Catholic hospitals, associate degree programs operated by a junior college or senior college, diploma programs operated by a hospital or independent corporation, degree programs operated by Catholic colleges or universities and programs for graduate nurses in Catholic universities.

There is also provision for associate membership open to individuals who are interested in educational programs in nursing in Catholic institutions, and to agencies not eligible for institutional membership.

Functions and Activities

The CCSN has a broad program of activities which benefit schools of nursing:

1. It suggests desirable goals for Catholic nursing education through recommendations initiated by the Council and approved by the delegates at annual meetings of the Conference.

2. It sponsors, when appropriate, workshops and institutes on current problems on a national, regional and sisterhood basis.

3. It furnishes consultation service on request.

4. It conducts studies in areas of interest to Catholic nursing schools.

5. It circulates frequent reports to members on current developments in nursing education and on studies made by the headquarters staff. A special report prepared by the Council of CCSN, *Nursing Education and Catholic Institutions*, was published in March, 1963.

6. It attempts to stimulate the personnel in Catholic schools to participate actively in other nursing organizations and supplements the activities of other nursing organizations so as to meet the particular needs of Catholic schools.

The CCSN also gives information to individual nurses and others. The general type of information requested and provided includes such items as a roster of names of Catholic nursing schools and their location and accreditation status for the use of prospective students; statistical information regarding the number of Catholic nursing schools and their annual enrollments, admissions, and graduations; and descriptions of current practices in Catholic schools in relation to various arrangements common to educational programs.

Financial Support

The CCSN is financed through annual dues of members, in addition to a subsidy from the Catholic Hospital Association.

Official Journal

Hospital Progress, the official magazine of the Catholic Hospital Association, serves as the official organ of the CCSN. It can be secured by writing the editor, 1438 South Grand Blvd., St. Louis, Mo., 63104.

Information

For further information write to the Executive Secretary, Division of Nursing Education, Catholic Hospital Association, 1438 South Grand Blvd., St. Louis, Mo., 63104.

GUILD OF SAINT BARNABAS FOR NURSES

The Guild of Saint Barnabas for Nurses is an organization which encourages nurses and students of nursing to put their Christian powers to work.

Origin

Preliminary plans for forming the American Guild were discussed by 3 nurses on St. Barnabas Day (June 11), 1886. The Guild was organized in Boston in October of that year following meetings in Boston, New York, Philadelphia and Chicago. An organization of the same name, with similar purposes, had been established 10 years earlier in England.

Membership and Organization

Although the Guild is sponsored nationally by the Protestant Episcopal Church, it is nonsectarian. Membership consists of nurses, qualified persons in associated disciplines, members-at-large and associate members. It finds expression in local chapters, each of which is free to establish its own program. In 1968 there were 27 of these chapters with a total membership of 2,000.

Purposes and Activities

The objectives of the Guild are to provide members with personal advantages resulting from professional activities, to stimulate cultural pursuits and to help members realize the Christian aspects of life and work. They include provisions of scholarships for graduate nurses and students of nursing, and interest in education and research. Guild chapters also participate in community projects, supplying wheel chairs, clothes and missionary bundles for those in need.

Biennial conventions are held and a newsletter is published 4 times a year.

Information

Information about the Guild and suggestions for organizing a chapter may be obtained by writing to the Chairman, Committee on Nursing Relations, Miss Phyllis Andrews, R. N., 38 Rockingham Street, East Lynn, Massachusetts. Mrs. Daisy W. Phinney, R. N., is the national president (1969).

NATIONAL ASSOCIATION FOR PRACTICAL NURSE EDUCATION AND SERVICE

The National Association for Practical Nurse Education and Service (NAPNES) is a nonprofit organization established in 1941 to:

1. Inform the public about the role and functions of the licensed practical/vocational nurse.

2. Develop and promote the use of sound standards for practical nursing education.

3. Promote effective liaison between practical/vocational nursing organizations and groups allied in function and interest.

Membership

All persons and groups interested in supporting and promoting practical/vocational nursing are eligible for membership in NAPNES. Currently (1970), NAPNES has about 30,000 members. Categories of membership are: "Per Capita," which pertains to members of state licensed practical/vocational nurse associations that are affiliated with NAPNES; "Group," which includes other state practical nurse associations, hospitals and other health agencies, and schools of practical/vocational nursing; "Individual" and "Life," which include licensed practical/vocational nurses, practical/vocational nursing educators and professional nurses, physicians, hospital administrators and others concerned with the advancement of practical/vocational nursing; and "Student," which includes students of practical/vocational nursing.

Organization

The voting body of NAPNES, which establishes its bylaws, determines its basic policies and conducts its other important business, consists of its individual and life members and delegates representing state associations. Between annual conventions, the business and funds of the Association are administered by the 26-member Board of Directors, which is made up of representatives from nursing, practical/vocational nursing education, medicine, hospital and nursing home administration, and other fields allied with nursing. Policies and activities are implemented by the Association's councils and committees.

Activities

To achieve its purposes NAPNES:

1. Serves as a clearing house for information about practical/vocational nursing.

2. Sponsors workshops and seminars in conjunction with universities, national organizations, and state LPN (licensed practical nurse)/LVN (licensed vocational nurse) associations.

3. Conducts an annual convention for the exchange of ideas and experiences among those concerned with practical/vocational nursing.

4. Maintains a national accreditation service for educational programs

in practical/vocational nursing, established in 1945 and recognized by the Office of Education of the U.S. Department of Health, Education, and Welfare.

5. Maintains a consultation service for those conducting or contemplating the establishment of educational programs in practical/vocational nursing.

6. Prepares publications that are useful to faculties in schools of practical/vocational nursing.

7. Provides scholarships to students of practical/vocational nursing for both preservice programs and continuing education for LPN's and LVN's.

8. Disseminates information about practical/vocational nursing careers and schools of practical/vocational nursing to prospective students of these schools and career counselors.

9. Engages in activities aimed at protecting and strengthening the position of LPN's and LVN's and cooperates with state LPN/LVN associations in activities of this kind.

10. Provides consultation to state LPN/LVN associations on matters relating to their organization and programs.

Official Journal

The Journal of Practical Nursing, published monthly, has a circulation of more than 42,000. Included among its educational features are nursing-care studies, nursing and medical news items, book reviews and reports on new drugs.

Information

Further information may be obtained by writing to the Executive Director, National Association for Practical Nurse Education and Service, Inc., 535 Fifth Avenue, New York, New York, 10017.

NATIONAL FEDERATION OF LICENSED PRACTICAL NURSES

The National Federation of Licensed Practical Nurses (NFLPN), the national membership organization of licensed practical nurses, was organized in 1949.

Membership

The organization is a federation of state and territorial associations of licensed practical or vocational nurses. The state associations are composed of districts, county divisions, areas, or chapters. The members of the state associations are licensed practical nurses or licensed nurses with equivalent titles. Students of state-approved schools of practical nursing may be affiliates, but not members, of the state and national associations.

In 1968, there were 30,000 members from all states in the country, including the District of Columbia.

Organization

The business of the NFLPN is carried on through: (1) the House of Delegates, composed of representatives of the constituent state associations, which meets annually to elect the officers and members of the Executive Board, and (2) the Executive Board, which administers the affairs and funds of the NFLPN between annual conventions, admits state associations to membership, maintains a headquarters office and staff, creates standing committees and performs other duties that are specified in the bylaws of the organization.

There is also an interorganization council which is composed of representatives of national organizations related to nursing. The purpose of the council is to provide a forum for discussion of mutual areas of concern in practical nursing.

Objectives and Functions

The objectives and functions of the NFLPN are:

1. To preserve and foster the nursing ideal of comprehensive care for the ill and aged.

2. To associate together all licensed practical/vocational nurses and licensed nurses having an equivalent title.

3. To promote the economic and general welfare of all licensed practical/vocational nurses.

4. To secure continued recognition of all licensed practical/vocational nurses.

5. To uphold the standards and ethics of all licensed practical nurses and to interpret them to the public.

6. To promote the continued effective use of all licensed practical/vocational nurses.

7. To promote the efficient functioning of constituent state licensed practical/vocational nurse associations.

8. To cooperate with all members of health groups and with organizations interested in better patient care.

9. To collect and distribute information on practical/vocational nursing.

10. To further the continuing nursing education of all licensed practical/vocational nurses.

11. To promote, support and speak for all licensed practical/vocational nurses in regard to legislative action.

12. To represent and serve as the spokesman for licensed practical/ vocational nurses with allied health and governmental groups and the public.[8]

Publications

The NFLPN publishes a bimonthly magazine, *Bedside Nurse,* which contains information concerning the activities of the national and state organizations, timely articles on nursing procedures, drugs, legislation and new developments in practical nurse education, and book reviews.

Interorganizational Relationships

In 1967, the following organizations were represented on the interorganizational Council of the NFLPN: the AAIN, the AHA, ANHA (American Nursing Home Association), the AMA, the ANA, the NLN, and the Office of Education of the U.S. Department of Health, Education, and Welfare. The NFLPN Executive Board is authorized to invite representatives of other groups or agencies to provide comprehensive representation for discussion of current issues.

The NFLPN and the ANA maintain a liaison. In June 1964, the ANA authorized a liaison arrangement through a committee composed of representatives of the Boards of the 2 organizations. In 1957, the NFLPN House of Delegates adopted the *Statement of Functions of the Licensed Practical Nurse,* which had been approved by the ANA Board of Directors and the Executive Board of the NFLPN. An elaboration of this statement was approved by the Executive Board of the NFLPN and the Board of Directors of the ANA in January 1964. This version of the statement of functions is distributed by both organizations.

Soon thereafter, the NFLPN and the NLN established an interorganizational committee. The objectives of this committee are:

1. To enable NFLPN and NLN to work closely on questions of mutual interest—(a) to clarify understandings through discussion and interpretation; and (b) to provide a forum in which the representatives of each organization may interpret problems or needs regarding practical nursing which are of mutual interest and assistance to each board of directors.

2. To act as a medium through which joint official statements could be made after clearance with the respective boards of directors.

3. To coordinate efforts in developing sound standards of practical nursing education and service.

4. To promote interpretation of practical nurse education and service—their objectives and values—to the participating organizations and the consumers of nursing service.

[8] NFLPN, *Bylaws,* New York, The Federation, 1967, p. 1.

5. To recommend to both boards of directors immediate and long-term plans for practical nurse education and service.[9]

The NFLPN works closely with the Office of Education and has representatives on many committees concerned with the preparation and the practice of practical nurses. Two licensed practical nurses served on the Surgeon General's Consultant Group on Nursing, which produced the report, *Toward Quality in Nursing: Needs and Goals* in 1963. A licensed practical nurse also was appointed by the U.S. Commission on Education to serve on the Advisory Committee on Health Occupations Education, 1964-1967. In 1968, a government relations representative was appointed to serve the interests of NFLPN in Washington, D.C.

Headquarters

The headquarters activities, under the direction of an executive director, are carried on at 250 West 57th Street, New York, New York, 10019.

NURSES CHRISTIAN FELLOWSHIP

In Chicago, in 1936, a few nurses began monthly meetings. The purpose of these meetings was primarily to strengthen the Christian beliefs of the members, and to give assistance in facing personal and professional problems with a conscious Christian attitude. Soon other nurses became interested in this group and, in 1948, the Christian Nurses Fellowship was formally organized on a national level. In 1952, the name was changed to Nurses Christian Fellowship. It affiliated with the Inter-Varsity Christian Fellowship, a world-wide interdenominational student organization that seeks to meet the spiritual needs of college and university students in the same way that the Nurses Christian Fellowship endeavors to help nurses.

Purpose and Activities

The aim of the Nurses Christian Fellowship is to aid both nursing students and graduates in their spiritual lives. This purpose is based in the belief that total patient care involves the spiritual as well as the physical and mental needs of the patient. Members of the group believe that unless the nurse is alert to her own spiritual needs, she is unlikely to be sensitive to such needs in her patients.

Miss Grace Wallace, the national director, (1970) works with a staff of 9 graduate nurses who serve by visiting nursing schools interested in help and direction. However, each local group is autonomous. Programs are designed to meet the needs of the nurses in the particular school or hospital with the consent of the nursing school authorities.

[9] *Rules of Procedure for NFLPN-NLN Interorganization Committee,* New York, The Associations, September 1963. Reaffirmed in 1964. Mimeographed.

Periodical

A bulletin, *The Nurses Lamp*, is issued bimonthly. It includes articles of special interest to nurses, as well as pertinent information concerning nursing activities throughout the USA.

Information

Information about Nurses Christian Fellowship may be obtained by writing to Miss Grace Wallace, R.N., Director, Nurses Christian Fellowship, 130 North Wells Street, Chicago, Ill., 60606.

PROBLEMS

1. What are the objectives of the following organizations and how does the profession of nursing cooperate with them: American Academy of Medical Administrators, American Dental Association, American Hospital Association, AMA, American Nursing Homes Association, Joint Commission on Accreditation of Hospitals, American Public Health Association, American Public Welfare Association, National Health Council, American Council on Education, American Dietetic Association, American Psychiatric Association, American Association of Junior Colleges, Council of Social Work Education, National Tuberculosis and Respiratory Disease Association, Association of American Universities, National Social Welfare Assembly, National Retired Teachers Association, American Association of Retired Persons.

2. A student could describe the work of the American Protestant Hospital Association in respect to objectives, activities, membership, affiliations, accomplishments, publications.

3. Describe the influence of the Catholic Hospital Association of the USA on the following: religious and ethical objectives in health plans, medical education, nursing education, hospital management and practices, social legislation.

4. What is the relationship of the AAIN to: (a) the ANA, (b) the International Congress on Occupational Health.

5. Discuss the significance of the ANA and AMA holding joint conferences. Review the proceedings of the last joint conference and discuss its specific significance.

6. (a) What is the relationship of the AORN to the ANA? (b) To the AMA? (c) To the American College of Surgeons?

7. (a) Compare the NFLPN with the ANA in respect to: (1) membership requirements, (2) purposes or objectives, (3) functions. (b) What is the difference between the NFLPN and NAPNES?

8. Identify the following: Viola C. Bredenberg, Ella G. Casey, Veronica L. Conley, Margery E. Drake, Daisy Wright Finney, Marion L. Fox, Hattie

Hemschemeyer, Eileen I. Hogan, Lucille Woodville, Lillian E. Kuster, Florence A. McQuillen, Alice C. Sanne, Mrs. Etta Schmidt, Mrs. D. Ann Sparmacher, Grace Wallace.

SUGGESTED REFERENCES*

GENERAL

Encyclopedia of Assocations: National Associations of the United States, vol. 1. Detroit, Gale Research Co., 1968.

AMERICAN ASSOCIATION OF INDUSTRIAL NURSES

Coates, H. M. "The American Association of Industrial Nurses: Past and Present." *American Association of Industrial Nurses Journal,* **9:**8, Dec. 1961.
"Committee on Education, 1943-1968." *American Association of Industrial Nurses Journal,* **16:**10-11, Jan. 1968.
"Views and Profile of AAIN Membership." *Occupational Health Nursing,* **17:**11-17, Feb. 1969.
Wagner, S. P. "Enhancing Our Effectiveness." *American Association of Industrial Nurses Journal,* **11:**7-13, Apr. 1963.
Williams, E. V. "The 1st AAIN." *American Association of Industrial Nurses Journal,* **16:**7-9, Jan. 1968.

See reports of the President published in *Occupational Health Nursing.*

AMERICAN ASSOCIATION OF NURSE ANESTHETISTS

American Association of Nurse Anesthetists. *List of Schools that Have Been Accepted for the Qualifying Examination of the AANA,* Chicago, The Association. Revised semiannually — February and August.
————. *Approved Schools for Nurse Anesthetists.* Chicago, American Association of Nurse Anesthetists. Revised semiannually — February and August.
Bunch, J. B. "Nurse Anesthetists: Conditions of Employment." *Journal of the American Association of Nurse Anesthetists,* **35:**353-361, Oct. 1967.

See also current issues of the *Journal of the American Association of Nurse Anesthetists.*

AMERICAN COLLEGE OF NURSE-MIDWIFERY

Descriptive Data . . . Nurse-Midwives USA. New York, American College of Nurse-Midwifery, 1968.
Editorial. *Bulletin of the American College of Nurse-Midwifery,* **8:**42-43, Summer 1963.
Editorial. "Time of Decision." *Bulletin of the American College of Nurse-Midwifery,* **7:**3-4, Mar. 1962.
"Message from Our President." *Bulletin of the American College of Nurse-Midwifery,* **4:**69-72, Sept./Dec. 1959.
1968 Report on the Second Work Conference for Nurse-Midwifery. (Held in Milwaukee, May 1968.) New York, American College of Nurse-Midwifery, 1968.

* In each chapter all citations are footnoted and are not included here. All starred references are recommended for additional reading.

* *Nurse-Midwifery. A Clinical Nursing Specialty.* New York, Maternity Center Association, n.d.
* *Twenty Years of Nurse-Midwifery, 1933-1953.* New York, Maternity Center Association, 1955.

ASSOCIATION OF OPERATING ROOM NURSES

* *Aims, Philosophies, and Objectives.* New York, The Association of Operating Room Nurses, 1967.
"AORN Proceedings." *AORN Journal,* **2**:82-90, July/Aug. 1964.
Bylaws of the Association of Operating Room Nurses. New York, The Association, 1967.
"Eleventh Annual AORN Congress." *AORN Journal,* **2**:78-99, Mar.-Apr. 1964.
"Regional Institutes." *AORN Journal,* **1**:72-73. Jan./Feb. 1963.
*"A Report on the Sixteenth National Congress, Cincinnati 1969." *AORN Journal,* **9**:37-52, Mar. 1969.
* "Standards for Administrative and Clinical Practice in the Operating Room." *AORN Journal,* **8**:80-82, Aug. 1968.
West, E. I. (editorial) *AORN Journal,* **1**:14, Jan./Feb. 1963.

CONFERENCE OF CATHOLIC SCHOOLS OF NURSING

"C.C.S.N. Observes 10th Anniversary." *Hospital Progress,* **38**:78-79, 94, 108, July 1957.
Nursing Education and Catholic Institutions: A Report of the Council of the Conference of Catholic Schools of Nursing. St. Louis, the Conference, Mar. 1963.

GUILD OF ST. BARNABAS FOR NURSES

The Guild of St. Barnabas for Nurses. *The Guild Prayer.* 38 Rockingham St., East Lynn, Mass., The Guild, n.d.
————. *Rule of Life.* Lynn, Mass., The Guild, n.d.
————. *Suggestions for Organizing a Chapter.* Lynn, Mass., The Guild, n.d.
* *Newsletter.* Lynn, Mass., The Guild of St. Barnabas for Nurses. Published 4 times a year.

NATIONAL ASSOCIATION FOR PRACTICAL NURSE EDUCATION AND SERVICE

Martin, R. G. "Our Accrediting Program — Yesterday, Today and Tomorrow." *Journal of Practical Nursing,* **18**:22-23, June 1968.
"NAPNES and Its Accrediting Program." *Journal of Practical Nursing,* **17**:29, Nov. 1967.
National Association for Practical Nurse Education and Service. *Career Opportunities as a Licensed Practical Nurse Including a Directory of State-Approved Schools and Programs of Practical Nursing.* New York, The Association. Issued annually.
————. *Guidelines for Seminars and Workshops Conducted by State LPN/LVN Associations.* New York, The Association, 1968.

NATIONAL FEDERATION OF LICENSED PRACTICAL NURSES

* American Nurses' Association. *Facts About Nursing: A Statistical Summary.* New York, The Association, 1968, pp. 238-239.

* Day, F. G. "NFLPN Must Close Door to NAPNES." *Bedside Nurse,* 1:8-9, Jan.-Feb. 1968.
* See also issues of *Bedside Nurse.* 250 W. 57th St., New York, National Federation of Licensed Practical Nurses.

NURSES CHRISTIAN FELLOWSHIP

* *Nurses Christian Fellowship.* Chicago, Nurses Christian Fellowship, n.d.
The Role of Nurses Christian Fellowship in Total Patient Care. Chicago, Nurses Christian Fellowship, n.d.
The Nurses Lamp. Bulletin of the Nurses Christian Fellowship. 1519 North Astor St., Chicago. Published bimonthly.

CHAPTER

23

American Nurses' Foundation

The American Nurses' Foundation (ANF), an independent, voluntary, nonprofit organization, was established by the ANA in 1955. It serves the nursing profession through its program of conducting, supporting and promoting nursing research, as well as by disseminating the findings of research.

ORIGIN AND DEVELOPMENT

In 1950, recognizing the need to study nursing functions because of the growing shortage of nurses, the ANA House of Delegates approved a plan for a 5-year program of research. During the next 5 years, nurses invested a total of $400,000 in this program which resulted in a number of valuable studies.[1] These studies demonstrated the need for a continuing coordinated program focused upon research and the dissemination of research findings.

In 1954 at the closing business session of the ANA House of Delegates meeting, the ANA Board of Directors was authorized to "secure information and to develop a foundation or trust for receiving tax-free funds for

[1] American Nurses' Association, *Nurses Invest in Patient Care*, New York, The Association, May 1956.

desirable charitable, scientific, literary or educational projects in line with the aims and purposes of the American Nurses' Association."[2] The following year, the ANA created the ANF.

The first grant received by the newly formed Foundation was a PHS grant for the purpose of studying public health nursing. The investigation was "concerned with nurse-patient relationships and factors affecting the public health staff nurse in carrying out her duties."[3] The grant became effective April 1, 1956. In 1962 the ANF published the first report of this study in a publication entitled *Content and Dynamics of Home Visits of Public Health Nurses, Part I.*[4]

Clara A. Hardin, Ph.D., was the first executive director of the Foundation. Following her death in early 1964, Lucille E. Notter, editor of *Nursing Research*, served as acting director. She was succeeded in the Fall of 1964 by Wanda McDowell, Ph.D., R.N. Prior to coming to the ANF, Dr. McDowell had been associate professor, project director of *A study of Nurse Action in the Relief of Pain* and coprincipal investigator of the project, *The Nurse-Monitor in a Patient Care System*, all at The Ohio State University. She remained with the Foundation until December 1968. Mrs. Susan D. Taylor is currently (1970) serving as acting director.

OBJECTIVES

As stated in the original certificate of incorporation, the purpose of the ANF was "to increase the public knowledge and understanding of professional and practical nursing and of the science and arts upon which the health of the American people depends."[5] This was to be accomplished by means of research, grants, scholarships and fellowships, and by "all other proper means."

A 1967 publication of the ANF lists the objectives of the Foundation as follows:

1. To conduct and promote scientific nursing research in patient care with full utilization of basic and applied disciplines and to provide consultation service in the interest of scientific nursing approach

2. To provide financial support for research including support for the exploration of promising ideas

3. To provide interdisciplinary research experience

4. To disseminate and to promote the dissemination of research findings through publications, conferences, and other communication media

[2] *Ibid.*, p. 52.
[3] *Ibid.*, p. 53.
[4] C. A. Hardin and W. Johnson, *Content and Dynamics of Home Visits of Public Health Nurses, Part I.* New York. American Nurses' Foundation, 1962. Part II was published in 1969.
[5] American Nurses' Association. *Nurses Invest In Patient Care.* New York, The Association, May 1965, p. 52.

5. To conduct experimental investigations to discover methods of implementing research results[6]

PROGRAMS

In line with its objectives, the ANF has: (1) carried out research and supported research by others; (2) published the reports of its research as well as the reports of investigators whose work was supported by the ANF; (3) published a quarterly, *Nursing Research Report;* (4) promoted conferences on research (during the 1950's); and (5) carried responsibility for the production of abstracts of studies in nursing.

Research Program

The current (1970) program of the Foundation focuses on 2 major efforts. The first is the conduct and support of research in the area of nursing and long-term care, with initial emphasis on nursing and the aged patient. The second major, and equally important, project is the developmental-grant program.

The main area of research interest, nursing and long-term care, is based upon 2 broad hypotheses:

(1) that the professional nurse practitioner carries the primary load in the therapeutic regimes of patients with chronic and long-term illness; and (2) that research within the broad area of nursing and long-term care of the aged will identify nursing processes as related to a particular population in our society.[7]

The initial phase of this investigation consists of a review, critique and synthesis of the research literature in order to bring together the known facts, to delineate the researchable questions and to develop a base line for the investigation to follow. The principal investigator assigned to this study is Mrs. Alice J. Gifford, Sc.D., R.N., an associate professor in the Department of Public Health, The Johns Hopkins University School of Hygiene and Public Health. Her work began in October 1968.[8]

Under the second major area of interest, developmental grants in amounts up to $3,500 for a 1-year period are offered with the objective of encouraging and supporting promising research ideas related to the study of patient care. These grants may be used to carry out a pilot or exploratory study, to develop a method or tool needed for the research, or to perfect a research design.

Recent studies supported by the ANF under this program include:

[6] "Structure, Program and Financing of the American Nurses' Foundation," *Nursing Research Report,* **2:**1, Dec. 1967.
[7] "Foundation Participates in ANA Biennial Convention at Dallas," *Nursing Research Report,* **3:**5, June 1968.
[8] "Dr. Alice J. Gifford Initiates Pilot Project on Long-term Care," *Nursing Research Report,* **3:**3, Dec. 1968.

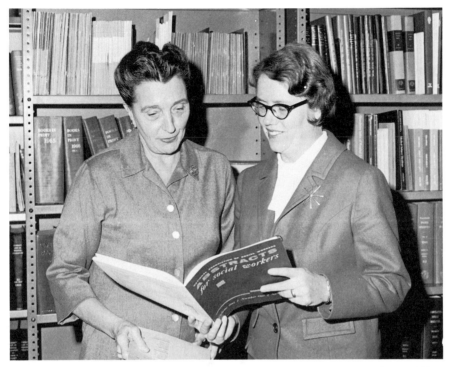

Fig. 23-1. Mrs. Lois Miller, Librarian, Sophia F. Palmer Library of the AJN Co., and Mrs. Susan D. Taylor, Assistant Executive Director of the ANF, discussing the abstracting service of the ANF. (American Nurses' Foundation)

The Effects of Family Goals on Family Task Performance and Utilization of Extrafamily Resources During Acute Illness Experience, by Betty J. Ruano. This study is designed to detect the effects of a 6-week illness and hospitalization of 50 families.
Social Involvement and Other Correlates of Psychological Health and Longevity: A Prospective Study of Older Subjects, by Frances J. Thomas. Miss Thomas is gathering, by interview, longitudinal data on a sample initially composed of 2,500 older noninstitutionalized subjects.

The importance of these developmental grants in encouraging nurses to undertake research cannot be overestimated. They have been, and should continue to be a crucial force in opening up new areas of research in nursing.

Abstracting Service

As a result of an abstracting project initiated in January 1957, supported by a grant from the PHS of the U.S. Department of Health, Education, and Welfare and carried out at the Institute of Research and Service in Nursing Education, Teachers College, Columbia University, an ongoing abstracting service was undertaken by the ANF in January 1962.[9] Under the direction of Mrs. Susan D. Taylor, abstracts of hundreds of studies in nursing or related to nursing are produced each year. Volunteer abstractors, nurses competent in the various areas and specialties in nursing, prepare the abstracts which are then published in the journal, *Nursing Research*. Figure 23-1 shows Mrs. Taylor conferring about the abstracting service.

Dissemination of Research Findings

A major program of the ANF is the dissemination of research findings through its various publications that are chiefly reports of studies supported or conducted by the Foundation; through its participation in and support of conferences; and through its operation of the abstracting service.

As part of this program, the ANF publishes a newsletter. *Nursing Research Report* is a quarterly report of activities in which the Foundation is involved or interested. Each issue, in addition to presenting news items about the ANF and its staff, commonly carries a report by one of the investigators whose research is supported.

ORGANIZATIONAL STRUCTURE

The ANA's Board of Directors comprise the members of the ANF. They are responsible for electing the ANF Board of Directors which in turn carries the overall responsibility for the policies and program of the Foundation. Each year at its annual meeting, the ANA Board of Directors receives a report from the Foundation regarding its program activities and its financial status.

Two important committees assist the ANF Board of Directors in guiding and developing its programs: the Research Advisory Committee and the Committee on Scientific Publications and Communications.

Research Advisory Committee

The membership of the Research Advisory Committee consists of nurse and other experts in the various areas of research. They meet semi-annually to review the applications for grant support submitted to the Foundation and to assist the Foundation in the development of plans for initiating and carrying out its own research program. This committee also advises the ANF Board of Directors about important trends and developments in nursing research.

Committee on Scientific Publications and Communications

The primary concern of the Committee on Scientific Publications and Communications is the dissemination of the findings of research under-

[9] H. Hilbert, "A Trial Plan for Abstracting Reports of Studies in Nursing—A Project Report," *Nursing Research*, 11:172-175, Summer 1962.

taken or supported by the Foundation. This committee meets periodically to review the reports of researchers and to make recommendations with respect to their publication by the Foundation. The committee also considers and recommends other possible means of dissemination of research findings, such as conferences, workshops, or audio-visual media.

RELATIONSHIP WITH THE ANA

As stated at the beginning of this chapter, the ANF was established through action of the ANA and a close relationship has been maintained over the years. This relationship is established in the bylaws of the Foundation which specify that at least one-third of the ANF Board of Directors shall be members of the ANA Board of Directors.

To further ensure coordination of the activities of the 2 organizations, the executive director of the ANA also serves as executive vice-president of the ANF, and the ANA business manager is also the ANF assistant secretary-treasurer. In addition, the ANA provides many services and facilities to the ANF such as the stenographic pool, the mailroom and the order department. This cooperation is possible because the offices of the ANF are located within the same building as those of the ANA. The proximity of offices also provides for the exchange of information between staffs of each organization on both a formal and an informal basis.

FINANCIAL SUPPORT

As already mentioned the ANF is a nonprofit, voluntary organization. All members of the ANA contribute to its support since the ANA allocates some of its money each year to the ANF. Groups of nurses have conducted fund raising projects for the benefit of the Foundation; for example, the Pennsylvania Nurses Association contributes the revenue from its sale of iris rhizomes.[10] Nurses also contribute as individuals. And, of course, the provision of services and facilities by the ANA also helps to support the Foundation.

Over the years, the ANF has been the recipient of grants for the financing of such specific research projects as the one entitled *Development of a Continuing Education Program for Nurse Practitioners in Upper New England on the Utilization of Research Findings in the Improvement of Patient Care.* This was supported by the Irene Heinz Given and John LaPorte Given Foundation. Other grants have been received from the PHS and private foundations.

[10] See "American Nurse Iris: Pennsylvania Nurses Association," *Nursing Research Report* 2:8, Dec. 1967.

PROBLEMS

1. Select 1 of the projects reported in ANF's *Nursing Research Report* and prepare to discuss the research in class, placing emphasis on the implications of the research for the improvement of nursing care and for further research needed in the specific area under study.

2. Prepare a list of 5 nursing-care problems which you think should be studied and which you think the ANF might consider for support under their developmental-grant program.

3. Describe how you would go about developing a fund-raising plan if you were the executive responsible for the ANF.

SUGGESTED REFERENCES*

* "American Nurses' Foundation." *International Nursing Review,* **15:**152-156, Apr. 1968.

Elms, R. R. "Search or Research? Nursing Approaches to Patients on Admission to Hospital." *Nursing Outlook,* **13:**55, July 1965.

Elwood, E. "Nurse Researcher Tests Effects of Breathing Exercises on Patients with Emphysema." *Nursing Research Report,* **2:**1, 3-5, June 1967.

Hardin, C. "American Nurses' Foundation, Inc." *American Journal of Nurses,* **60:**1629-1630, Nov. 1960.

————. "The American Nurses' Foundation Builds a Program." *American Journal of Nursing,* **57:**301-311, Mar. 1957.

Hughes, E. C., *et al. Twenty Thousand Nurses Tell Their Story.* Philadelphia, Lippincott, 1958.

* Lambertsen, E. C. *Nursing and Long-term Care — The Research Program of the American Nurses' Foundation.* New York, The American Nurses' Foundation, 1968.

Macgregor, F. C. "Talent Salvage in Nursing." *Nursing Outlook,* **16:**33-37, Aug. 1968.

McBride, M. A. "Nurse Researcher at Yale University Tests Three Approaches to Relieve Pain." *Nursing Research Report,* **2:**1, 4, 6, Mar. 1967.

McDowell, W. "ANF Symbol: ANF Research Program." (editorial) *Nursing Research Report,* **2:**2, Dec. 1967.

Neal, M. V. "Vestibular Stimulation and Developmental Behavior of the Small Premature Infant." *Nursing Research Report,* **3:**1, 3-5, Mar. 1968.

* Notter, L. E. "Developmental Grants for Nursing Research." (editorial) *Nursing Research,* **17:**387, Sept./Oct. 1968.

"Research — Pathway to Future Progress in Nursing Care." *Nursing Research,* **9:**4-7, Winter 1960.

* Taylor, S. D. "How to Prepare an Abstract." *Nursing Outlook,* **15:**61-63, Sept. 1967.

See also *Nursing Research Report,* published quarterly by the ANF.

---

* In each chapter all citations are footnoted and are not included here. All starred references are recommended for additional reading.

CHAPTER

24

Nursing Journals in the USA

When you wish to acquire information for a paper that you are writing or about a nursing problem that you are trying to solve, you probably "make a beeline" for the *American Journal of Nursing, Nursing Outlook, Nursing Research,* or one of the many new nursing journals that have come into being in recent years. It is probable, also, that you make it a practice to read each copy of some of these magazines as it is issued. The nurse who is a constant reader of these periodicals can be sure that she will be well informed about her profession.

The *American Journal of Nursing, Nursing Outlook, Nursing Research* and the *International Nursing Index* are sponsored, or designated as official, by the professional nursing associations and are published by the American Journal of Nursing Company (AJN Co.), a non-profit organization, set up by the ANA (then, in 1900, the Associated Alumnae of Trained Nurses of the United States and Canada, also known as the Nurses' Associated Alumnae of the United States and Canada) to publish the *American Journal of Nursing.* The Company conducts its business under the general direction of a Board of Directors consisting of 11 members, 2 of whom are designated by the NLN. The members of this board are elected by the ANA Board of Directors, inasmuch as the ANA is the sole stockholder for the Company. General policies are determined by the Board of Directors of the Company. The editorial policies of each of the 4 publications are determined, within the framework of the general policies, by the chief editors of each magazine. Editorial freedom regarding content selected for publication is preserved as the right of the chief editors.

The term "official magazine" refers to the fact that the magazine is so designated by an association. It is not necessarily owned by the association. It will carry material representing the point of view of the association. However, as a professional journal it will concentrate on reader interest and the needs of the profession. The *American Journal of Nursing* has been designated as the official journal of the American Nurses' Association and the National Student Nurses' Association; *Nursing Outlook* has been designated as the official journal of the National League for Nursing; and *Nursing Research* and the *International Nursing Index* are sponsored by both the ANA and the NLN.

AMERICAN JOURNAL OF NURSING

The *American Journal of Nursing*, a monthly periodical, is the official journal of the ANA. Until January 1953, after the National League of Nursing Education (NLNE) merged with other organizations to form the NLN, the *Journal* served also as the official journal of the NLNE. It was the first official professional nursing journal established in the USA and now has served the profession for over 69 years. Its circulation numbers more than 250,000 — larger than that of any other official professionally sponsored magazine to which subscription is voluntary and independent of organization membership.

ANA members may subscribe to the *Journal* at reduced rates through their district nurses associations. Thus, the *Journal* is available to every ANA member at a smaller cost than that paid by any other subscriber.

How Did The *Journal* Begin?

In 1895 there were magazines for nurses, but they were not published by nurses. A member of the American Society of Superintendents of Training Schools for Nurses, an organization which eventually became the NLNE, suggested in 1895 that nurses needed "a journal managed, edited, and owned by the women of the profession." Shortly after this date, the Associated Alumnæ of Trained Nurses of the United States and Canada, the forerunner of the ANA, was formed and, in 1899, appointed a Committee on Periodicals, with Mary E. P. Davis as chairman. As a result of the Committee's work, the AJN Co. was established. The first issue of the *American Journal of Nursing* appeared in October 1900. The *Journal* has been published monthly ever since.

The *Journal* was financed originally by individual nurses and alumni groups. However, in 1915 the ANA by purchasing all the outstanding stock became the sole owner of the Journal Co., with the ANA Board of Directors acting as stockholder.

Briefly, What Is the *Journal*'s History?

In its early years the *Journal* employed the J. B. Lippincott Co. to take care of the details of publication, but in 1917 the *Journal* became its own publisher. Sophia Palmer, a member of the original Committee on Periodicals, was the first *Journal* editor, serving until her death in 1920. Mary M. Roberts was appointed to succeed Miss Palmer in 1921, and continued in this position until 1949, when she retired with the title of editor emeritus. It is to these 2 women who guided the *Journal* through almost the entire first 50 years of its existence that a great share of the credit must go for developing the *Journal* into the fine and respected professional magazine it is today.

In 1949 Nell V. Beeby became editor of the *Journal*. In 1950, the *Journal* Company began plans for a national library. It was formally named the Sophia F. Palmer Library in 1953. After AJN Co. had been expanded, in 1952, to assume the responsibility of publishing *Nursing Research* and *Nursing Outlook,* Miss Beeby was named executive editor of the company (1956), which now demanded full-time direction. Upon Miss Beeby's death in 1957, Miss Pearl McIver was appointed to this position. Miss McIver was succeeded by Miss Lucy D. Germain in 1959 and by Mr. Philip E. Day in 1964. Mr. Day became the first to hold the title of publising director.

Jeanette V. White became the *Journal* editor in 1956. When she died in 1957, Edith P. Lewis, who had been on the *American Journal of Nursing* editorial staff, became acting editor. She served in this capacity until Barbara G. Schutt was appointed editor in December 1958.

You can learn more about the *Journal*'s history by reading the material referred to at the end of this chapter listed under the heading "American Journal of Nursing," and by reading current issues of the *Journal*.

Who Edits the *Journal*?

The editor of the *Journal* and her staff select and edit the material appearing in the magazine in accordance with the broad general policies determined by the company's board of directors. In the beginning, the *Journal*'s editorial staff was made up exclusively of professional nurses drawn from a wide variety of fields of nursing to assure representation of all nursing areas in the magazine. In 1953, a layman was added to the staff as news editor, and in 1962 a professional journalist was appointed managing editor. As the publishing company has grown, it has become necessary and desirable to add business and technical personnel to the company staff, but editorial policy remains the exclusive province of the editorial staff, a majority of whom are professional nurses.

What Are the *Journal*'s Objectives?

In the first issue of the *Journal,* we read: "It will be the aim of the editors to present month by month the most useful facts, the most progressive thought, and the latest news that the profession has to offer . . . ." No better statement could be formulated even now, over 69 years later, to describe the *Journal*'s objectives. Throughout its entire existence, it has served as a chronicle of nursing events, as a reporter of the newest developments, as an interpreter of nursing to nurses and the public, and as a means of communication between nurses in this country and abroad.

The *Journal* has carried out its objectives well and has played a significant part in the development of the nursing profession. It has stimulated and encouraged new movements and has been instrumental in raising the standards of the profession and acquainting widely separated groups of nurses with these common standards. It has served as a clearing-house for nursing problems, for all nurses have a voice in the *Journal.* Finally, it has remained, as it originally was intended, "a journal managed, edited, and owned by women and men of the profession."

What Kind of Articles Appear in the *Journal*?

With the establishment of the other 2 professional nursing magazines, the *Journal* now is enabled to devote its pages mainly to the needs and the problems of the individual nurse in her professional practice. As the official journal of the ANA, the *Journal* carries materials that may be classified under 5 major headings: (1) material that promotes the program of the ANA, (2) material of a general nature relating to nursing and allied fields that promotes understanding of current developments in the profession, (3) clinical material of a breadth and scope to interest both the general practitioner and the clinical specialist of the profession, (4) information about international affairs and the programs of government and voluntary agencies in this country that directly or indirectly influence the employment of nurses and the development of the profession and (5) material of interest to students enrolled in schools of nursing.

A typical issue of the *Journal* might feature the most recent developments in the care of patients in coronary care units, a report on nurses' activities in the ANA's economic security program, an overview of drugs being used in cancer research, an article on helping the nurse to deal with the dying patient, and a report on participation of nurses in planning for future health care. The *Journal* also carries news about nurses, reports what nurses are doing in other countries and publishes many other articles of general interest to the nurse.

In short, the *Journal* is intended not for any 1 group of nurses, but for all nurses who are interested in what is going on in their profession. It is intended to serve as their monthly guide to contemporary events and to progress being made in every area of nursing practice. Today these events and improvements are moving forward at an ever-accelerating pace. To keep up with these changes is a "must" in every nurse's life if she is to fulfill her obligations to patients, to those with whom she cooperates in the other health professions, and to herself.

NURSING OUTLOOK

Nursing Outlook is a monthly periodical with a circulation of about 30,000. As the official journal of the NLN it is responsible for interpreting nursing service and nursing education to the NLN membership. Included within the NLN membership are registered and licensed practical nurses, educators, social workers, physicians, public health and hospital administrators, lay people who are concerned with providing nursing service within their communities or who are interested in nursing service and nursing education because they are the consumers of nursing service and various types of allied nursing personnel.

When and How Did *Nursing Outlook* Begin?

In June, 1952, when the NLN was organized, it requested the AJN Co. to undertake publication of *Nursing Outlook* as its official journal. In a contract, dated September 22, 1952, between the AJN Co., and NLN, *Nursing Outlook* was designated the official publication of NLN. The first issue of this magazine appeared in January, 1953. Mildred Gaynor was the first editor and remained in this position until her retirement in 1967. Under her guidance, the *Journal* grew in stature and at her retirement, its subscribers numbered approximately 28,000.

Of the organizations which merged to form the NLN, the National Organization for Public Health Nursing (NOPHN) was the only one which published a monthly magazine devoted to the interests of its members. In December, 1952, the final issue of this magazine, *Public Health Nursing,* was published; its assets and responsibilities were transferred to the AJN Co. when *Nursing Outlook* was initiated. The story of *Public Health Nursing* is an exciting one and may be found in the March 1933 issue of that magazine.

Who Controls and Edits *Nursing Outlook*?

Nursing Outlook is at present both owned and published by the AJN Co. The latter's board of directors, which includes 2 members designated by the

NLN, determines the broad over-all policies of the magazine. The editorial staff, consisting of professional nurses and one professional editor, select and edit the articles to be published in the magazine, with Alice M. Robinson as editor. Final responsibility for all content rests with the editor.

What Are the Objectives of *Nursing Outlook*?

The editorial in the first issue of the magazine states, *"Nursing Outlook* is designed to assist all nurses, and others who are interested, in fostering the development and improvement of nursing services and nursing education."

What Kind of Material Does *Nursing Outlook* Publish?

The content of *Nursing Outlook* includes: (a) material that promotes the programs of NLN; (2) materials in all the areas of public health nursing; (3) articles, reports and service columns covering all types and areas of nursing education programs; (4) articles and service pages presenting methods and ideas useful in developing and improving the administration of institutional nursing service.

NURSING RESEARCH

Nursing Research is a specialized journal sponsored by the NLN and the ANA. It is published 6 times a year; the first issue appeared in June 1952.

How Did *Nursing Research* Begin?

For a number of years the former Association of Collegiate Schools of Nursing (ACSN) believed that there was a need for a magazine devoted primarily to nursing research. Accordingly, in June 1951, it requested the AJN Co. to undertake the publication of such a magazine. The appearance of the first issue of *Nursing Research* in June, 1952, coincided with the merging of the ACSN into the NLN, and it was agreed that *Nursing Research* would be sponsored by the NLN but would continue to be published by the AJN Co.

To get the magazine started, the ACSN contributed $900, individuals donated $500, and the ANA pledged $500. The AJN Co. agreed to underwrite all publishing costs. The number of subscribers in 1952 was much greater than had been anticipated (approximately 10,000), so the ANA contribution was not needed at that time. The number of subscribers has decreased since 1952; by 1970 there were approximately 7,400.

At first, 3 issues of *Nursing Research* were published a year. In 1959, this was increased to 4 issues, and in 1968, *Nursing Research* became bi-monthly.

Who Controls *Nursing Research*?

In the beginning, editorial policies were determined by an editorial board of 20 persons. The members of this board were nominated by the NLN and elected by the AJN Board of Directors. The first chairman of the editorial board was Helen L. Bunge. She was succeeded in 1957 by Hortense Hilbert. This board carried much of the responsibility for the content of *Nursing Research*. Edith P. Lewis served as managing editor from 1953 until 1959 when, because of growth in the journal, Barbara L. Tate was appointed as the first editor on a part-time basis. Lucille E. Notter became the first full-time editor in September 1961. In 1967, a part-time associate editor was added to the staff.

With the acquisition of a part-time editor, and later a full-time editor, the functions of the editorial board changed, and the editor became responsible for the content of the journal. In 1962, the editorial board was changed to a 9-member editorial advisory committee responsible for acting in an advisory capacity to the editor. This committee meets about once each year at the call of the editor.

In addition to an editorial advisory committee, the editor makes use of a panel of experts to assist in the review of manuscripts. This panel is composed of approximately 40 to 50 persons expert in the various fields of nursing and research. Final responsibility for the selection of all content resides in the editor.

What is *Nursing Research*'s Purpose?

Nursing Research was created to serve the purposes described in an editorial in the first issue: "to inform members of the nursing profession and allied professions of the results of scientific studies in nursing; and to stimulate research in nursing."

It carries original reports of research in nursing problems, and it endeavors to keep nurses informed about research activities in the profession. It carries articles on scientific and research methods, items of news in the field of nursing research, abstracts, and book reviews.

INTERNATIONAL NURSING INDEX

The first issue of the *International Nursing Index (INI)* was published in 1966. The *INI* is a cumulative quarterly, i.e., each new issue cumulates the material in the previous issues for that year. The first 3 issues each year are paperbound; the fourth issue is a clothbound annual cumulation for the

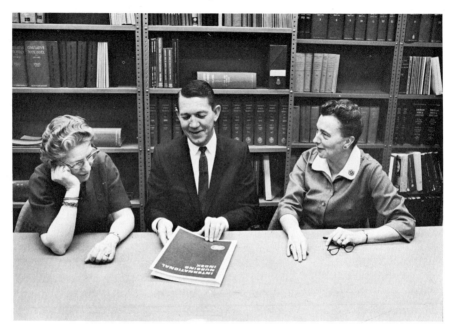

Fig. 24-1. Working with proofs of the first issue (1966) of the *International Nursing Index*, Lucille Notter, editor; Philip Day, publishing director; and Lois Miller, librarian and assistant editor. (American Journal of Nursing)

entire year. A *"Nursing Thesaurus,"* a guide to headings under which specific subjects may be found in the *Index*, is issued with the first issue each year and is included in the annual cumulation. Figure 24-1 shows the editor with other AJN Co. officials looking over the first edition of the *INI*.

Why Was Publication of *INI* Undertaken?

The need for a comprehensive index to nursing literature had been recognized for many years. As far back as 1922, Katherine DeWitt, the *American Journal of Nursing*'s first editor, spoke of the need for an index which would help nurses to locate articles on the subjects in which they were interested. The need was occasionally expressed during the years following 1922; however, the work of preparing a comprehensive index was considered too complex and costly to be undertaken.[1]

In 1964, the ANF, under a grant from the AJN Co., conducted a study to develop a plan for an index to nursing periodical literature.[2] Impetus for this study came from strong urging by the Interagency Council on Library Tools for Nursing, an advisory group composed of representatives of

[1] P. E. Day, "The International Nursing Index," *American Journal of Nursing*, **66:**783-786, Apr. 1966.

[2] V. M. Pings, *A Plan for Indexing the Periodical Literature of Nursing*, New York, American Nurses' Foundation, 1966.

agencies and organizations interested in the preparation of library aids for nurses (organized in 1960).

Also in early 1964, the National Library of Medicine (NLM) in Washington, D.C. began using MEDLARS (Medical Literature Analysis and Retrieval System), an electronic, computerized system, to prepare *Index Medicus.* NLM indicated a willingness to include nursing among the subjects considered as bibliographic by-products of MEDLARS.

As a result of the ANF study made by Vern Pings, Ph.D., R.N., medical librarian, College of Medicine, Wayne State University (Detroit, Michigan), the AJN Co. decided to publish the *Index* in cooperation with the NLM and utilizing their computerized system. The staff of the new index consisted of an editor, Lucille E. Notter, editor of *Nursing Research;* a librarian, Mrs. Lois B. Miller, AJN Co. librarian; and 2 indexers, Rosalie Bruning, R.N., and Fred Pattison, AJN Co. assistant librarian. An editorial advisory committee serves to assist in the development of the broad policies guiding the publication of *INI.* The index is officially sponsored by the ANA, and the NLN.

What is the Scope of the *INI*?

Today (1970), the *INI* is in its fifth year of publication. It currently indexes the nursing content of over 180 nursing periodicals from this country and from other countries of the world, as well as nursing content found in the more than 2,000 journals of medicine and related health fields indexed in *Index Medicus.*

The material in the *INI* is arranged under both a subject and a name (author) section. The *Index* also carries lists of nursing publications of various nursing organizations and the agencies interested in nursing. In addition, the annual cumulation includes lists of nursing books received by the AJN Co. Library during that year. There is also a list of doctoral dissertations completed. You will find the *INI* in your school of nursing library and will no doubt use it frequently in your classwork. When you graduate, it will be a very useful tool to use in looking up articles of interest to you in your work, whether clinical nursing or other areas, writing an article, or preparing a book for publication.

OTHER SERVICES OF THE AMERICAN JOURNAL OF NURSING COMPANY

Other services which the AJN Co. provides for nurses include:

1. Preparation of annual and cumulative indexes of the 3 magazines.

2. Sponsoring of the Mary Roberts Writing Awards for nurses. Usually 8 are offered each year, 6 to registered nurses and 2 to nursing students.

3. Publishing of a daily paper at the biennial conventions of the ANA and the NLN.

4. Sponsoring of the "State Bulletin Awards Contest," which is conducted biennially to stimulate improvement in the publications of state nurses associations.

5. Provision of the Sophia F. Palmer Library, serving the staffs of AJN Co., ANA, ANF and NLN, as well as nurses doing graduate work in nearby universities.

6. Provision of a Reader Service to assist readers in locating information about articles, book reviews and so forth.

7. An Educational Services Division which provides a film service and printed material including programmed instruction units and other reprint services.[3]

OTHER JOURNALS SERVING NURSES

Within the past few years a number of new nursing journals have appeared. You will want to familiarize yourself with most of these. There are also several journals of note which appeared in the past but are no longer published. The most recent of these is *Tomorrow's Nurse*, (1960-1963), a journal for nursing students. Three others are *Nursing World* (formerly, *Trained Nurse and Hospital Review*), which was published from 1888 to August 1960; *Public Health Nursing*, 1909-1952, the official journal of the NOPHN, discontinued in 1952 when the NOPHN merged with the NLN; and *Nursing Science*, published from 1963 to 1965.

Journal of Nursing Education

First appearing in January 1962, *The Journal of Nursing Education* has continued as a quarterly. It is published as a service to nursing education by the McGraw-Hill Book Company, New York, New York. An editorial board composed of leading nurse educators representing each type of educational program serve as professional advisors in the selection of articles published in each issue and as guest editors for special theme issues. Devoted exclusively to nursing education, this journal is designed to provide for the dissemination of new and pertinent information for nurse educators, as well as opportunity for new and still unpublished authors in nursing to share their knowledge and experience.

Journal of Psychiatric Nursing and Mental Health Services

Published bimonthly by the Stuart James Company, Bordentown, New Jersey, volume 1 of the *Journal of Psychiatric Nursing and Mental Health*

[3] In January 1970, the AJN Co. took over the ANA-NLN Film Service.

Services appeared in 1963. Alphonse C. Sootkoos, the editor-in-chief, is assisted by an editorial staff of well-known psychiatric nurses. This is an interdisciplinary journal of interest to psychiatrists, psychologists, social workers, nursing personnel and others working in the fields of mental health and mental retardation.

Nursing Forum

First issued in 1961, *Nursing Forum* is published quarterly by Nursing Publications, Inc., Hillside, New Jersey, with Alice R. Clarke, R.N., as editor and publisher. In its first issue the editorial purpose was stated to provide a new outlet for the expression of original and stimulating ideas, concepts and thoughts. Book reviews, analytic editorials, and letters to the editor are included.

Perspectives in Psychiatric Care

This magazine is a publication of Nursing Publications, Inc. (which also publishes *Nursing Forum*), with Alice R. Clarke, R.N., as editorial director. Volume 1 was published in 1963. As its title indicates, it aims to present, in depth and perspective, clinical material of interest to all who are responsible for the care of the mentally ill. It is guided by an editorial board of well-known, qualified psychiatric nurses.

RN

RN, founded in 1937, is an independent monthly journal for registered nurses. Contents include all subjects of interest to the profession, in both clinical and nonclinical areas. The journal also sponsors an annual writing contest for senior nursing students. It is published by *RN* Publications, Oradel, New Jersey, a division of Litton Publications, Inc., with Richard F. Newcomb as editor.

Cardiovascular Nursing

Cardiovascular Nursing is a bimonthly scientific publication of the American Heart Association, New York, New York. First appearing in 1965, the purpose of this periodical has been to keep nurses up-to-date on new knowledge about cardiovascular diseases. It is distributed through local heart associations. The editors are Marie S. Andrews, R.N., and Maurice R. Chassin, M.D.

Geriatric Nursing

A monthly journal that began publication in November 1965, *Geriatric Nursing* contains articles of interest to nurses working with patients of the older age group. It is of particular interest to those nurses working in nursing homes. The editor, Ken Eymann, is assisted by an editorial staff of 3 senior editors who are registered nurses and 2 nurse-consultant editors. The journal is published by Miller Publishing Company, Minneapolis, Minnesota.

Special-Group Journals

A number of other journals are published by special groups in nursing. Some of these are: *Occupational Health Nursing,* formerly *American Association of Industrial Nurses Journal,* now in its 18th volume (1970); The *AORN Journal,* formerly *OR Nursing,* the official journal of the Association of Operating Room Nurses and first published in 1960. In addition, most state nurses associations and some of the state leagues for nursing publish an official journal or bulletin. See Chapter 22, "Other National Nursing and Allied Organizations," for more complete information on these publications.

OTHER INDEXES

Cumulative Index to Nursing Literature

Published by the Glendale Sanitarium and Hospital, Glendale, California, this index to nursing literature covers the period from 1956 to the present (1970). The first edition appeared in 1961 and covered the period 1956 to 1960. The Index is currently issued as 5 bimonthly supplements and an annual cumulation. It indexes major nursing journals published in the English language and selectively indexes other ancillary serials, including major medical journals. Mildred Grandbois, the first editor, continues to serve in this capacity.

Nursing Studies Index

The Nursing Studies Index, prepared under the direction of Virginia Henderson, R.N., with the assistance of the Yale University School of Nursing *Index* staff, is a retrospective index for the years 1900 to 1959. The index provides an annotated guide to reported studies, research in progress, research methods and historical materials in periodicals, books and pamphlets published in English. Volumes III and IV (1950 to 1956 and 1957 to 1959) have been published. Volumes I and II are still in preparation (as of 1970). The work of preparing the index has been supported by PHS grants to Yale University. J. B. Lippincott Company, Philadelphia, Pennsylvania, is the publisher.

PROBLEMS

1. (a) What do you consider the 5 best articles published in each of the following professional periodicals this year: *American Journal of Nursing, Nursing Outlook, Nursing Research*? (b) Why have you chosen these articles?

2. How do each of the following help you to keep up to date: *American Journal of Nursing, Nursing Outlook, Nursing Research*?

3. A number of nursing periodicals, other than those owned by the profession, have been started in recent years. What are the influences of this trend on nursing and nurses?

4. Analyse issues of *Nursing Outlook* and the *Journal of Nursing Education* for the past 3 years and identify the major trends in nursing education.

5. Using issues of the *American Journal of Nursing, R.N.* and *Nursing Forum* for the past 2 to 3 years, identify a current major issue in nursing and plan a class debate on the pros and cons of the issue.

SUGGESTED REFERENCES*

AMERICAN JOURNAL OF NURSING

"The American Journal of Nursing 1900-1940." *American Journal of Nursing,* **40:**1085-1091, Oct. 1940.

"But You Can't Print That!" (editorial) *American Journal of Nursing,* **67:**2065, Oct. 1967.

De Witt, K., and Munson, H. W. "The Journal's First Fifty Years." *American Journal of Nursing,* **50:**590-597, Oct. 1950.

Lewis, E. P. "Mary Roberts, Spokesman for Nursing." American Journal of Nursing, **59:**336-343, Mar. 1959.

"Might a Vote For Be a Vote Against?" (editorial) *American Journal of Nursing,* **68:**757, Apr. 1968.

* *The Story of the Journal, 1900-1960.* New York, The American Journal of Nursing Co., 1960.

"With the Journal Yesterday and Tomorrow" (editorial) *American Journal of Nursing,* **50:**457, Aug. 1950.

NURSING OUTLOOK

"The Continuity." (editorial) *Public Health Nursing,* **44:**657, Dec. 1952.

* Leahy, K. M. *"Nursing Outlook, 1953-1963." Nursing Outlook,* **11:**20-22, Jan. 1963.

———. "Introducing Your Editors." *Nursing Outlook,* **1:**49, Jan. 1953.

"A Mature Outlook at Ten." *Nursing Outlook,* **11:**40-51, Jan. 1963.

* In each chapter all citations are footnoted and are not included here. All starred references are recommended for additional reading.

"A New Magazine for Nursing" (editorial) *American Journal of Nursing*, **52**:1077, Sept. 1952.

"Presenting *Nursing Outlook*" (editorial) *Nursing Outlook*, **1**:21, Jan. 1953.

"The Story of Our Magazine." *Public Health Nursing*, **25**:162, Mar. 1933.

"To You Our Subscribers" (editorial) *Nursing Outlook*, **11**:19, Jan. 1963.

"What Happened to That Article You Wrote?" *Nursing Outlook*, **5**:220-221, Apr. 1957.

NURSING RESEARCH

* Bunge, H. L. "The First Decade of *Nursing Research.*" *Nursing Research*, **11**:132-137, Summer 1962.

"A Co-operative Venture." (editorial) *Nursing Research*, **1**:5, June 1952.

"Editor of Nursing Research." *Nursing Research*, **10**:195, Fall 1961.

Farrell, M. "H. L. Bunge — An Idealist and a Realist." *Nursing Research*, **11**:139, Summer 1962.

Heidgerken, L. E. *"Nursing Research—*Its Role in Research Activities in Nursing." *Nursing Research*, **11**:140-143, Summer 1962.

"Looking Ahead" (editorial) *Nursing Research*, **2**:3, June 1953.

"Lucille E. Notter, New Editor to Nursing Research." *Nursing Outlook*, **9**:441, July 1961.

"New Magazine for Nurses." *American Journal of Nursing*, **51**:664, Nov. 1951.

INTERNATIONAL NURSING INDEX

Cunningham, E. V. "A Critique of the Two Indexes to Nursing Literature." *Nursing Forum*, **6**:352-362, Fall 1967.

OTHER JOURNALS SERVING NURSING

"Editorial." *Nursing Science*, **1**:42-43, Apr. 1963.

"Editorial: Candidly Speaking on *Nursing Forum.*" *Nursing Forum*, **7**:10-13, 112, Winter 1968.

"Preface." *Nursing Forum*, **1**:6, Winter 1961-62.

CHAPTER
25

International Nursing
and Allied Organizations

The humanity which impels man to want to help out any human being who is sick is one of the greatest forces for the development of goodwill in the world. People of nations which are at political or economic odds can often make common cause against the universal enemy – disease. Moreover, since diseases are no respecters of the boundary lines between nations, it is often a matter of self-interest for one country to help others with their health problems.

The nursing profession is in the forefront of the groups that are participating in the development of international professional relationships and international health programs. Because of this participation nurses all over the world have drawn nearer together and nearer to other people who are working for international "good-health."

INTERNATIONAL COUNCIL OF NURSES

The International Council of Nurses (ICN) is the organization through which nurses throughout the world collaborate in strengthening and improving nursing service, nursing education and professional ethics. It is a federation of national nurses' associations in which one professional nurses' association from each country in the world can become a member, provided that it fulfills certain basic requirements. The member association of the ICN in the USA is the ANA.

Purposes

The Council's objectives, as stated in its *Constitution and Regulations,* are as follows:

The purpose of ICN is to provide a medium through which national nurses associations may share their common interests working together to develop the contribution of nursing to the promotion of the health of people and the care of the sick.[1]

In line with this objective, the functions of the ICN are stated as follows:

1. To promote the organization of national nurses associations and advise them in their continued development.

2. To assist national nurses associations to play their part in developing and improving.

   a. the health service for the public;

   b. the practice of nursing;

   c. the social and economic welfare of nurses.

3. To provide means of communication between nurses throughout the world for mutual understanding and cooperation.

4. To establish and maintain liaison and cooperation with other international organizations and to serve as representative and spokesman of nurses at international level.

5. To receive and manage funds and trusts which contribute to the advancement of nursing or for the benefit of nurses.

6. To do all such other things as may be incidental or conducive to the attainment of the objective of ICN.[2]

Origin

The International Council of Women met in London in 1899. Among the delegates were several nurses, including Mrs. Bedford Fenwick, who thought that the time was opportune for the formation of an international organization of nurses. Mrs. Fenwick therefore brought the matter before the members of the Matrons' Council of Great Britain and Ireland, an association corresponding to the American Society of Superintendents of Training Schools for Nurses in the USA and Canada. The Matrons' Council then called a meeting of nurses in London, and the ICN was organized July 1, 1899.[3]

Nurses from England, the USA, Canada, New Zealand, Australia, and Denmark are listed as founding members.[4]

A committee drafted a constitution which was sent later to constituent

[1] *International Council of Nurses: Constitution and Regulations, Rules and Procedure at Meetings,* adopted June 1965, Switzerland, The Council, May 1966, p. 8.

[2] *Ibid.*

[3] M. Breay and E. G. Fenwick, *History of the International Council of Nurses, 1899-1925,* London, International Council of Nurses, 1931.

[4] L. L. Dock, "The International Council of Nurses," *American Journal of Nursing,* 1:117-118, Nov. 1900.

members, and, interestingly enough, no revision was made in this original constitution until 1925, when changes were made to help to adapt the organization scheme to growing membership. The current (1970) *Constitution and Regulations: Rules and Procedure at Meetings* was adopted June 1965.

Membership Plan

The original plan was to have, ultimately, a membership composed of 1 national association from each country. However, in 1899 the national nurses associations were not organized sufficiently to make this possible, so the ICN at first included individual members. These "councilors," as they were called, acted as representative nurses from each country, and they returned home to work for the establishment of national nurses organizations.

In 1904, three countries had national organizations eligible for affiliation with the ICN and so became charter members. The USA became a member through the American Federation of Nurses, which was an association of the 2 national associations, the American Society of Superintendents of Training Schools of Nursing and the Associated Alumnae of Trained Nurses of the United States.[5] England entered through the Provisional Committee of Delegates of Leagues and Self-Governing Nursing Societies. Germany came in through the Nurses' Association of Germany. The national nursing associations of these countries are now the ANA, the Royal College of Nursing and National Council of Nurses of the United Kingdom, and the German Nurses' Federation.

Applications for membership in the ICN are considered by a membership committee and the Board of Directors and then presented to the Grand Council for final vote of acceptance.

The associations now (1970) affiliated with the ICN are:

Argentina—Federación Argentina de Enfermería
Australia—Royal Australian Nursing Federation
Austria—Trained Nurses' Association of Austria
Barbados—Barbados Registered Nurses' Association
Belgium—National Federation of Belgian Nurses
Bermuda—Bermuda Registered Nurses' Association
Bolivia—National Association of Professional Nurses of Bolivia
Brazil—Brazilian Nurses' Association
Burma—Burma Nurses' Association
Canada—Canadian Nurses' Association
Ceylon—Ceylon Nurses' Association
Chile—Colegio de Enfermeras de Chile
Columbia—Asociación Nacional de Enfermeras de Colombia
Costa Rica—Colegio de Enfermeras de Costa Rica
Denmark—The Danish Nurses' Organization
Ecuador—Asociación Ecuatoriana de Enfermeras
Egypt—Egyptian Nursing Association

[5] L. L. Dock, "International Relationships," in "Proceedings of the First Meeting of the American Federation of Nurses," *American Journal of Nursing,* **5:**680-688, July 1905.

El Salvador—Asociación Nacional de Enfermeras Salvadorenas
Ethiopia—Ethiopian Nurses' Association
Finland—The Finnish Federation of Nurses
France—Association Nationale Française des Infirmières et Infirmiers Diplômés
   d'Etat
Gambia—The Gambian Nurses' Association
Germany—German Nurses' Federation
Ghana—Ghana Registered Nurses' Association
Greece—Hellenic National Graduate Nurses' Association
Guyana—Guyana Nurses' Association
Haiti—Association Nationale des Infirmières Licenciées d'Haïti
Hong Kong—Hong Kong Nurses' Association
Iceland—Icelandic Nurses' Association
India—Trained Nurses' Association of India
Iran—Iranian Nurses' Association
Ireland—National Council of Nurses of Ireland
Israel—National Association of Nurses in Israel
Italy—Consociazione Nazionale della Associazioni Infermerie Professionali
   e Assistenti Sanitarie Visitatrici
Jamaica—Nurses' Association of Jamaica
Japan—Japanese Nursing Association
Jordan—Jordan Nurses' Association
Kenya—The National Nurses' Association of Kenya
Korea—Korean Nurses' Association
Lebanon—L'Ordre des Infirmières du Liban, Ecole d'Infirmières
Liberia—Liberian National Nurses' Association
Luxembourg—Association Nationale des Infirmières et Assistantes Sociales,
   Luxembourgeoises Diplomees
Malaya—Malayan Trained Nurses' Association
Mexico—Colegio Nacional de Enfermeras
Morocco—Association Nationale Marocaine des Infirmières et Infirmières Di-
   plômés d'Etat
Nepal—Trained Nurses' Association of Nepal
Netherlands—National Nurses' Association of the Netherlands
New Zealand—New Zealand Registered Nurses' Association
Nigeria—The Professional Association of Trained Nurses of Nigeria
Norway—Norwegian Nurses' Association
Pakistan—Trained Nurses' Association of Pakistan
Panama—Asociación Nacional de Enfermeras de Panamá
Peru—Federación Peruana de Professionales de Enfermeria
Philippines—Philippine Nurses' Association
Poland—Polskie Towarzystwo Pielegnarskie
Portugal—Associaçao das Enfermeiras e dos Enfermeiros Portugueses
Republic of China—Nurses' Association of the Republic of China
Rhodesia—Rhodesia Nurses' Association
Sierra Leone—Sierra Leone Nurses' Association
Singapore—Singapore Trained Nurses' Association
South Africa—South African Nursing Association
Spain—Consejo Nacional de Auxiliares Sanitarios—Sección Enfermeres
Sweden—Swedish Nurses' Association
Switzerland—Association Suisse des Infirmières et Infirmiers Diplômés
Thailand—Nurses' Association of Thailand
Trinidad—Trinidad and Tobago Registered Nurses' Association
Turkey—Turkish Nurses' Association

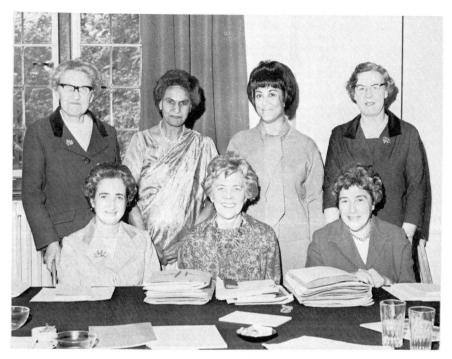

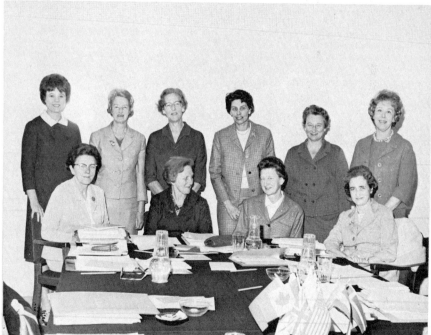

Fig. 25-1. *(Top)* ICN Professional Services Committee, Miss Virginia Arnold (seated center), USA, is chairman (1969) (ICN), *(Bottom)* ICN Membership Committee (1969), Miss Margrethe Kruse (seated second from left), Denmark, is chairman (ICN)

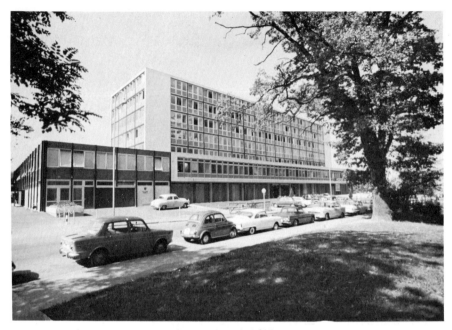

Fig. 25-2. ICN Headquarters in Geneva (1969). (ICN)

Uganda—Uganda National Association of Registered Nurses and Midwives
United Kingdom—Royal College of Nursing and National Council of Nurses of the
    United Kingdom
United States of America—American Nurses' Association
Uruguay—Asociación de Nurses del Uruguay
Venezuela—Asociación Venezolana de Enfermeras Professionales
Yugoslavia—Federation of Nurses' Associations of Yugoslavia
Zambia—Zambia Nurses' Association

Organizational Plan

The governing body of the ICN is the Council of National Representatives. The Council consists of the officers of the ICN and the presidents of member associations. The Board of Directors consists of the officers of the ICN and 11 elected members.

The Council usually meets every 4 years in connection with the Quadrennial Congress, and at such other times as the Board of Directors may decide. The Board of Directors meets at least once a year.

Besides the Council and the Board of Directors, the usual standing committees and special committees, as required, share in carrying on the work of the ICN. The members of these committees study various questions and issues pertaining to nurses, nursing and health. Some of the important current committees are those on Membership and on Professional Services (see Figure 25-1.

The programs of the ICN are further forwarded by a headquarters staff.

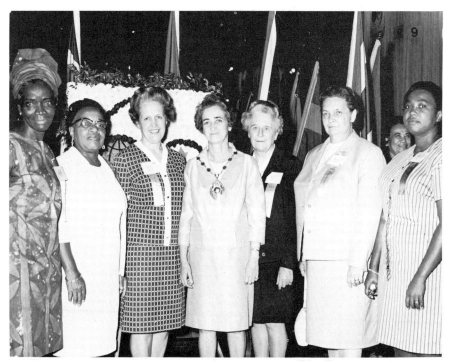

Fig. 25-3(a). ICN president (1965-1969) Alice Girard wearing the medallion of office with some of the representatives of other countries attending the Congress in 1969. Sheila Quinn, Executive Director of ICN is standing next to Miss Girard (second from the left). Miss Margrethe Kruse (Denmark) was elected president for the 1969-1973 period. (Gazette Photo Service, Montreal)

The headquarters office is currently located at: 37, rue de Vermont, 1202 Geneva, Switzerland. Mailing address is P.O. Box 42, 1211 Geneva 20, Switzerland (see Figure 25-2).

Quadrennial Congresses and Interim Conferences

The Quadrennial Congresses and interim conferences of the ICN afford opportunities for nurses from all over the world to meet and discuss professional problems. The 1969 Quadrennial Congress, held in Montreal, Canada, was attended by 10,000 nurses from 86 countries. Of this group, approximately 700 were nursing students. The decision was made to hold the 1973 Congress in Mexico. *Unity* was selected as the watchword by Alice Girard, the outgoing president. Figure 25-3 shows groups at ICN congresses.

You may wish to start making plans and saving for a trip to the next Quadrennial Congress.

Official Magazine

The *International Nursing Review*, published 4 times a year, is the official organ of the ICN. It started in 1923 as a multigraphed bulletin which was

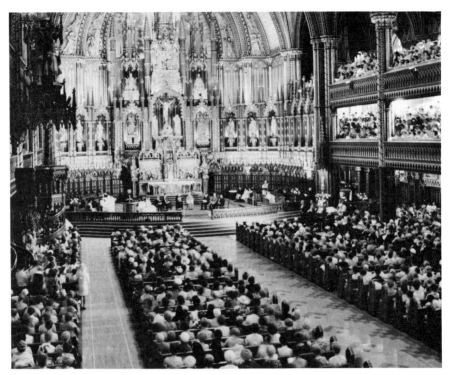

Fig. 25-3(b). Interfaith service in the Notre Dame church in Montreal during the Fourteenth Quadrennial Congress of the ICN, 1969. (Gazette Photo Service, Montreal)

circulated to affiliated associations and representative nurses everywhere. Christiane Reimann, who was then secretary to the Council, was instrumental in making its publication possible and continued as editor when it became a magazine in January 1926. Subsequent editors have been Anna Schwarzenberg, Daisy C. Bridges, Susan King-Hall, and Marjorie L. Wenger. The current (1970) editor is Alice M. C. Thompson.

The *International Nursing Review* gives news and includes articles on all phases of nursing in many countries, whether or not their nursing associations are affiliated with the ICN. *ICN Calling,* a monthly newsletter, was launched in 1968; it helps nurses to keep up-to-date on nursing around the world.

The ICN also makes available other publications that relate to its activities and objectives.

International Code of Nursing Ethics

The *International Code of Nursing Ethics,* first adopted by the ICN at São Paulo, Brazil, July 19, 1953, and revised in Frankfort, Germany in 1965, follows:

Nurses minister to the sick, assume responsibility for creating a physical, social and spiritual environment which will be conducive to recovery, and stress the prevention of illness and promotion of health by teaching and example. They render health-service to the individual, the family, and the community and coordinate their services with members of other health professions.

Service to mankind is the primary function of nurses and the reason for the existence of the nursing profession. Need for nursing service is universal. Professional nursing service is based on human need and is therefore unrestricted by considerations of nationality, race, creed, colour, politics or social status.

Inherent in the code is the fundamental concept that the nurse believes in the essential freedoms of mankind and in the preservation of human life. It is important that all nurses be aware of the Red Cross Principles and of their rights and obligations under the terms of the Geneva Conventions of 1949.

The profession recognises that an international code cannot cover in detail all the activities and relationships of nurses, some of which are conditioned by personal philosophies and beliefs.

1. The fundamental responsibility of the nurse is threefold: to conserve life, to alleviate suffering and to promote health.

2. The nurse must maintain at all times the highest standards of nursing care and of professional conduct.

3. The nurse must not only be well prepared to practise but shall maintain her knowledge and skill at a consistently high level.

4. The religious beliefs of a patient shall be respected.

5. Nurses hold in confidence all personal information entrusted to them.

6. Nurses recognise not only the responsibilities but the limitations of their professional functions; [they] do not recommend or give medical treatment without medical orders except in emergencies and report such action to a physician as soon as possible.

7. The nurse is under an obligation to carry out the physician's orders intelligently and loyally and to refuse to participate in unethical procedures.

8. The nurse sustains confidence in the physician and other members of the health team; incompetence or unethical conduct of associates should be exposed but only to the proper authority.

9. A nurse is entitled to just remuneration and accepts only such compensation as the contract, actual or implied, provides.

10. Nurses do not permit their names to be used in connection with the advertisement of products or with any other forms of self advertisement.

11. The nurse cooperates with and maintains harmonious relationships with members of other professions and with nursing colleagues.

12. The nurse adheres to standards of personal ethics which reflect credit upon the profession.

13. In personal conduct nurses should not knowingly disregard the accepted pattern of behaviour of the community in which they live and work.

14. The nurse participates and shares responsibility with other citizens and other health professions in promoting efforts to meet the health needs of the public — local, state, national and international.[6]

Nursing Abroad Through ICN Member Associations

At the 1969 ICN Congress, the Council of National Representatives approved a proposal from the Professional Services Committee that the Exchange of Privileges Programme be replaced by a service called "Nursing Abroad Through ICN Member Associations." "Nursing Abroad" was defined as, "a service offering nurses from ICN member associations arrangements for salaried employment and/or study abroad."[7] Under this service, arrangements will be made by mutual agreement between the member associations concerned. The purpose of "Nursing Abroad" is "to offer facilities for the promotion of international understanding among nurses by providing opportunities for professional experience and study abroad."[8]

Relationships with Other International Groups

The ICN has established relationships with the following organizations and programs of the United Nations (UN):

1. The Economic and Social Council. Through the fact that the ICN is on the consultative register of this council, all members of the ICN have a direct contact with the work of the UN and its specialized agencies.

2. The World Health Organization (WHO). The ICN is in official relationship with WHO, which enables it to cooperate in the programs of WHO by keeping closely in touch with the work of the Nursing Section.

3. The International Labor Organization (ILO). The ICN is on a special list of nongovernmental organizations maintained by the ILO for consultative purposes.

4. The UN Educational Scientific and Cultural Organization (UNESCO), and the UN International Children's Emergency Fund (UNICEF).

The ICN is also a member of 2 nongovernmental international organizations. These are:

1. The World Federation for Mental Health
2. The International Hospital Federation

The ICN also maintains close relationship with many international nongovernmental organizations, such as the International Committee of Catholic Nurses, the World Medical Association, the International Committee of

[6] "International Council of Nurses Code of Ethics," *American Journal of Nursing,* **65**:97, Aug. 1965.
[7] "CNR Adopts Proposal on Exchange Program." *ICN Bulletin* (ICN Congress in Montreal, Canada), Wednesday, June 24, 1969, no. 4, p. 7.
[8] *Ibid.*

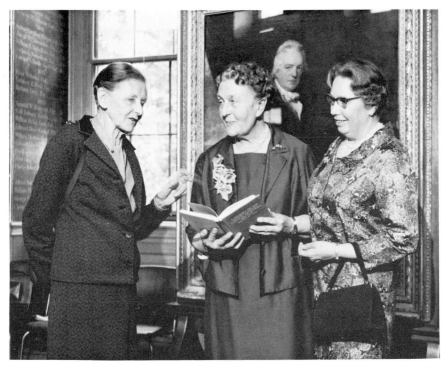

Fig. 25-4. Miss Daisy C. Bridges (center) former ICN General Secretary, on the occasion of the publication of her book, *A History of the International Council of Nurses, 1899-1964, the First 65 Years* (ICN)

the Red Cross, the International Council of Women, the International Confederation of Midwives, the League of Red Cross Societies and the Union of International Associations.

History of ICN

Miss Daisy C. Bridges, former ICN General Secretary, has compiled a history of the ICN entitled *A History of the International Council of Nurses, 1899-1964, the First 65 Years*. It was published in 1967.[9] (See Figure 25-4).

INTERNATIONAL COMMITTEE OF CATHOLIC NURSES

Another professional association which brings together nurses from all over the world is the International Committee of Catholic Nurses (CICIAMS).

[9] D. C. Bridges, *A History of the International Council of Nurses, 1899-1964, the First 65 Years*, London, Pitman Medical or Philadelphia, Lippincott, 1967.

History

At an international meeting in 1928, the presidents of associations of Catholic nurses decided to create an international organization through which they could coordinate their studies and endeavors. At the 1st Congress, which was held in 1933 at Lourdes, France, the International Committee officially was organized. Groups of nurses from 10 nations were at this first Congress. By 1954, the International Committee had 30 full members, and 16 countries were represented by participating members. As of 1969, the Association has affiliates in 68 countries.

Objectives

The objectives of the International Committee, as stated in its *Statutes,* are:

To encourage, in all countries, the organization and the development of Catholic professional associations capable of giving moral and spiritual support to Catholic nurses (and public health nurses) as well as helping them perfect their techniques.
To coordinate the efforts of Catholic professional associations while respecting their autonomy, in order to study and to represent christian thought in the profession in general.
To participate in the general development of the nursing profession and to promote health and social welfare measures along the lines of scientific progress and following christian principles, thereby ensuring the health and welfare to which every human being is entitled, and at the same time respecting the religious convictions of every individual.[10]

Membership Plan

Full members are professional Catholic associations constituted as such under the laws of their countries and fulfilling the conditions of their own regulations.

Participating members are: (1) professional Catholic associations which do not qualify as full members, (2) Catholic schools of nursing and social work giving instruction to students according to the regulations in use in their countries and (3) Catholic persons of high standing who represent the nursing profession in countries where Catholic associations do not yet exist.

Organization

The International Committee is directed by a General Council, which is composed of the presidents or the official delegate of the associations with full membership, and by an Executive Board, which is elected by the General Council.

The Headquarters of the International Council is in Brussels, Belgium. There are also 5 regional secretariats, 1 in each part of the world.

[10] International Committee of Catholic Nurses, *Statutes,* 32 rue Joseph II, Brussels 4, Belgium, The Committee, 1965.

Activities

The International Committee is interested in all areas of health and welfare work, particularly in maternal and child welfare, abandoned and maladjusted children, the social and economic condition of women, occupational health, mental health, rehabilitation of the physically handicapped, nutrition and dietetics, and basic education. It assists its members to communicate with each other through the organization of international conventions and sessions for study, through the publication of materials, through the organization of study trips, and through arranging for the exchange of students and nurses.

CICIAMS has official relations with WHO, is on a special list of nongovernmental organizations maintained by the International Labor Organization (ILO) and by UNICEF, and is a member of the International Conference of Catholic Organizations. In 1967, the Council of Europe was added to this list.

The *Code of Ethics,* adopted by the International Committee in 1954, is available from the headquarters office.

OTHER INTERNATIONAL HEALTH GROUPS AND ACTIVITIES

Disease, famine, and ignorance have been endured in many parts of the world by large numbers of people for many centuries.

The increased nearness of countries resulting from air travel, common political danger from abroad, the increased exchange of communications and people, and many other factors, during recent years, especially since World War II, have brought about a growing awareness that improvement of health, as well as of living conditions, is both imperative and possible for the entire world community. For example, this awareness is responsible for the whole idea of the Agency for International Development (AID) and the Peace Corps of the USA—the neighborly sharing of knowledge and re-sources—and practical expression in a variety of international technical assistance efforts.

In general, these efforts at improvement of people's living conditions have had 2 international approaches—multilateral and bilateral.

The *multilateral* approach to the solving of health problems utilizes the resources of many nations in mobilizing them for the common good. The UN uses this approach through the programs of its specialized and other organs. Among these are the ILO, the Food and Agriculture Organization (FAO), and UNESCO. Two of its organizations are directly concerned with health— WHO and UNICEF.

Other intergovernmental organizations concerned with health activities are the Pan American Health Organization (PAHO), the Caribbean Commission, the South Pacific Commission, and the Colombo Plan for Cooperative Economic Development in South and Southeast Asia.

Nurses have worked in these agencies. Some of the work they do will be described in this chapter.

The *bilateral* approach is a direct arrangement between 2 nations to improve health conditions in 1 of the 2 nations or its possessions.

Since World War II the USA has used the bilateral approach to develop programs through AID and the popular Peace Corps.

The World Health Organization

The World Health Organization (WHO), as pointed out previously, is one of the specialized agencies of the UN. It came into official existence as an intergovernmental agency of the UN on April 7, 1948, when the requisite 26th member of the UN ratified the WHO Constitution. As such, it has inherited the functions of antecedent organizations, such as the Office International d'Hygiène Publique, the Health Organization of the League of Nations, and the Health Division of the United Nations Relief and Rehabilitation Administration (UNRRA). Its principal aim is to bring all people to the highest possible level of health. As of November 1968, its membership included 131 countries. Its headquarters are in Geneva (Avenue Appia, 1211 Geneva, Switzerland). Regional offices are located in Alexandria, Brazzaville, Copenhagen, Manila, New Delhi, and Washington, D.C. (Pan American Sanitary Bureau).[11]

The scope of health interests and activities of WHO exceeds that of any previous international health organization. It acts as an international health coordinating authority. Its main activities include: assistance to countries for the improvement of health services, for education and training in the field of health, and for fighting communicable diseases; coordination and stimulation of medical research, exchange of information on public health and world-wide reporting on outbreaks of dangerous diseases; programs involving malaria and smallpox eradication, cancer and heart disease research, air and water pollution, dangerous drugs, and water supply.[12]

In recent years expanded research programs have been undertaken by WHO in collaboration with hundreds of national institutes and laboratories. In 1968, for example, a large number of research projects were underway in fields ranging from human genetics to insecticides, cancer and cardiovascular diseases. The World Health Assembly, the supreme governing body of WHO, meets annually, usually in Geneva but at times in other areas. In 1969, the Assembly met in Boston, Massachusetts.

More and more countries are requesting WHO's help in establishing or upgrading teaching and training facilities for all classes of medical personnel. WHO provides expert guidance and the services of highly qualified

[11] World Health Organization, *Facts in Brief,* Geneva, The Organization, no. 1, Nov. 1968.
[12] *Ibid.*

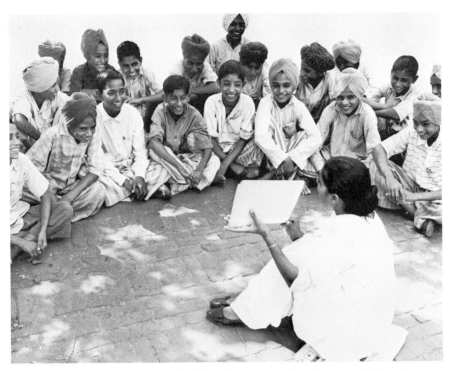

Fig. 25-5. An open-air class in health education conducted by a public health nurse in India. (WHO)

teaching personnel. It also gives fellowships and training grants each year — almost 30,000 fellowships have been given over the past 20 years.[13]

Nursing Activities. At the second World Health Assembly in 1949, it was recognized that every country has a shortage of nurses. Hence, the following types of questions were posed to be answered:

1. How can more and better qualified nurses be prepared?
2. Where can qualified teachers be found?
3. How can the less developed countries establish their programs quickly when they have practically no professional people and few, if any, training programs?
4. How can such programs be adapted to the countries where the bulk of the people are illiterate and the health problems tremendous?
5. How much can be done by a worker with very little preparation?
6. What kind of supervision will this worker need and by whom should it be given?

All these problems pointed to the need for surveying various countries before answers could be found.

[13] World Health Organization, *Twenty Years of Work,* Geneva, The Organization, Apr. 1968, p. 4.

In order to consider these problems and for other purposes, the Expert Committee on Nursing was formed. It held its first meeting in February 1950 in Geneva. Since then several meetings have been held to discuss problems in nursing. More recently, reports on *Public Health Nursing* (1959), *Post-Basic Education Programs for Foreign Students* (1959), *Aspects of Public Health Nursing* (1961), *The Nurse in Mental Health Practice* (1963), *World Directory of Post-Basic and Post-Graduate Schools of Nursing* (1965) and *The Midwife in Maternity Care* (1966) have been prepared for worldwide distribution.

Two nurses were appointed to the Geneva WHO office during 1949 — Olive Baggallay of Great Britain and Lyle Creelman of Canada. Others have been appointed to the Geneva office since then. At present (1970) Lily M. Turnbull is the chief nursing officer in the Geneva office. She was appointed in 1969, following Lyle Creelman's retirement in 1968. Nurse advisers also have been appointed on a regional basis. Agnes W. Chagas was the first nurse adviser for the Western Hemisphere in the regional office at Washington, D.C., in the Pan American Sanitary Bureau (PASB), the operating arm of the PAHO. She was succeeded by Kathleen Logan. The present (1970) chief officer is Margaret C. E. Cammaert. Helen K. Mus-

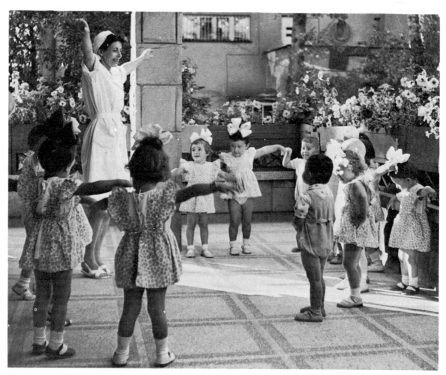

Fig. 25-6. Stoika Alexandrovna Balkanova, Bulgarian Nurse, conducts a child-education class. (WHO)

sallem, Executive Director of the Canadian Nurses' Association, was elected (1969) chairman of a newly-formed committee that advises the PAHO on ways and means of developing its nursing programs in Latin America.

Nursing has continued to be an essential part of all health and medical services of WHO. Almost every request for assistance has included the request for nursing support, either through treatment, surveillance, health education, or advice. In the 10-year period 1958 to 1967, nurses participated in approximately 160 country projects related directly to nursing and in over 230 other health field country projects. The latter included maternal and child health, tuberculosis, mental health, public health administration, health education and training, and communicable diseases. In addition to the country projects, during this same period nurses participated in 60 regional projects in nursing and about 30 regional projects in other health fields. The country projects dealt mostly with nursing education and provision of nursing advisory service to governments; the regional projects consisted mostly of educational meetings.[14]

Nursing activities in WHO include the following: (1) publication of reports of expert committees and of other advisory groups; (2) special studies; (3) organization of meetings, traveling seminars, workshops and training courses; (4) fellowships for study abroad, mainly post-basic or advanced; (5) provision of nurse advisers and short-term consultants who assist in assessing nursing and midwifery needs and resources, in training nursing and midwifery personnel, in strengthening educational institutions or establishing new ones and in demonstrating new methods and initiating research; and (6) supplying or arranging for provision of teaching equipment and nursing literature. The objective of all nursing activities is to provide quality care in the amount needed. Emphasis is placed not only on improving basic nursing education, but increasingly on comprehensive nursing education, post-basic and advanced education, and overall planning for nursing service at state or provincial and national levels.

Implied in this approach is the nurse's acceptance of a leadership role in nursing affairs. The approach also shows consideration of the cultural and social factors affecting the care of patients, the variety of clinical settings in which nurses serve, staffing patterns and facilities for basic nursing education.[15]

Special Activities of WHO in Relation to Nursing in the Western Hemisphere. The PASB functions as the regional office of WHO in this area, with headquarters in Washington, D.C. The fundamental purposes in this region, as elsewhere, are: (1) to give assistance on request through the ministries of health of each country, (2) to give such assistance in a realistic relation to the social and the economic development of the country, (3) to build up a na-

---

[14] *WHO Nursing Activities: A Review, 1958-1967.* Geneva, Switzerland, Nursing, World Health Organization, 1968, p. 2.
[15] *Ibid.,* pp. 2-4.

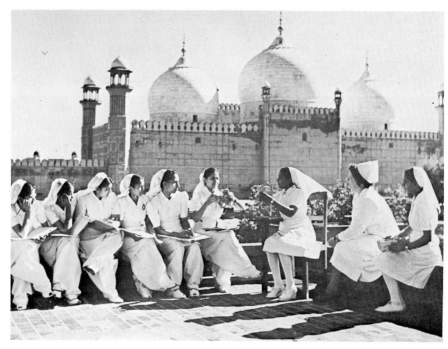

Fig. 25-7. Young Moslem girls who have thrown off their "burqua" (hood of purdah) to become health workers attend a midwifery class at a health center in Lahore, Pakistan. This is part of a course in Community Health Visiting organized by the Pakistan Government with the help of WHO and UNICEF. It is part of a scheme to increase Pakistan's women health workers from 1 to every 150,000 population, to 1 to every 10,000. (WHO)

tional group of nurses prepared to participate on the health teams and (4) to foster leadership in nursing within the country.

The emphasis, depending on the stage of development, has been on the following 4 elements in the various countries in the American region: (1) preservice education in nursing, (2) advanced education in nursing, (3) interchange of ideas on nursing and (4) assistance to national nursing associations.

In most of the activities of WHO in the Americas, other organizations have played an important part. The Rockefeller Foundation, the AID and its predecessors, and the W. K. Kellogg Foundation all have contributed numerous fellowships and grants for nursing service and nursing education projects.

In carrying out its nursing activities, WHO uses the standards of the ICN as a guide.

In 1948 there were 7 nurses on the WHO staff. By the end of 1967, there were 203 nurses working in 68 countries.[16] More are needed. Applications for positions may be made to: Personnel Unit, World Health Organization,

[16] *Ibid.,* p. 9.

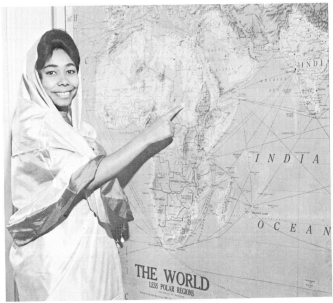

Fig. 25-8. Mrs. Awatif Ahmed Osman, Director, Khartoum Nursing College, Sudan—a fellowship student visiting the regional office of WHO in Washington, D.C., on her way to the School of Nursing of the University of California, San Francisco. Mrs. Osman is the first woman to hold a master's degree in nursing in the Sudan. (PAHO/WHO)

Palais des Nations, Geneva, Switzerland. A wide variety of nursing activities in WHO and AID are shown in Figures 25-5 through 25-13.

The Agency for International Development of the United States Department of State (AID)

Since the beginning of the foreign assistance program at the end of World War II, the USA has provided technical assistance in nursing to 47 countries on 5 continents, through programs of AID and its predecessor agencies—IIAA (Institute of Inter-American Affairs), TCA (Technical Cooperation Administration), MSA (Mutual Security Agency), ECA (Economic Cooperation Administration), FOA (Foreign Operations Administration) and ICA (International Cooperation Administration).[17] The goal of each of these agencies has been to help to create a community of free, independent and self-supporting nations. Our foreign aid program has shifted in scope and in emphasis to serve our national purposes and to deal effectively with the changing international situation, but it has always included a substantial

[17] Agency for International Development, *Taking a Look at Cooperation: An Assessment of 24 Years of AID Technical Assistance in Nursing,* Washington, D.C., U.S. Department of State, 1968, p. vi.

segment of technical assistance. Within recent years, increasing focus has been on long-term improvements in the social and economic structure of the recipient countries; a larger part of our foreign aid dollars is invested in economic development.

The locale of AID assistance has changed, too. Western Europe and Japan, who were helped early in the post-war years, are now themselves providers of aid. Some of the Latin American and Middle Eastern countries have achieved economic independence and no longer receive USA aid, while a number of new African nations have been added to the developing countries where AID programs are now active. Despite these changes, the fundamental objective of USA technical assistance has remained unchanged: to help other nations to help themselves.

Purposes of the Health Program. The broad health goal of the AID program is to bring the benefits of the medical and health sciences to people who, for centuries, have accepted disease and pain as an inevitable condition of life. More specifically, targets for the late 1960's and early 70's are to assist developing countries to eradicate or drastically reduce many preventable communicable diseases, to eliminate the severe nutritional disorders of infancy and childhood, to control rapid population growth and improve the health of families by making maternal and child health and family planning services widely available, to expand the health programs and services which contribute directly to the country's economic and social development, and to develop a broad range of health manpower needed to carry out these services.

Participation of Nurses. In the past 25 years, almost 500 USA nurses have worked in AID programs, either as direct employees of the Agency or as PHS officers detailed to AID. They have served as advisors to national ministries of health; participated in the establishment of schools of nursing and in the training of auxiliary health workers; given consultation and direct assistance in the organization of nursing services in hospitals and health centers; served as members of health teams with physicians, sanitary engineers, health educators and other health workers who have helped to carry out special programs in disease control, family planning and nutrition; and assisted in national planning and evaluation of health services. The largest number of AID nurses in 1969 were in Vietnam as part of a massive program to improve and expand the training of health personnel and to help to meet the needs of the civilian population for health and hospital services.

Effects of the Program. In cooperation with other agencies such as WHO and UNICEF and the bilateral aid programs of other countries, AID has assisted national health ministries in improving health institutions and the health of the people in more than 80 countries throughout the world.

Thousands of physicians, nurses, sanitary engineers and other health workers have been trained in schools and public health agencies in the USA. Health facilities have been established in scores of cities as well as in the most remote areas in countries where previously no health services existed. Schools of medicine, nursing and public health have been established;

Fig. 25-9. Kulwinder Kaur, a trained nurse in India, examining a pregnant woman. (WHO)

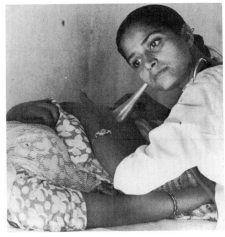

auxiliary health personnel have been trained; health departments have been improved; community water supplies have been developed; and sanitation procedures have been introduced. Infant death rates have declined, life spans have lengthened, and malaria has been eradicated or brought under control in a number of countries. In January 1968, a youngster in Ghana was

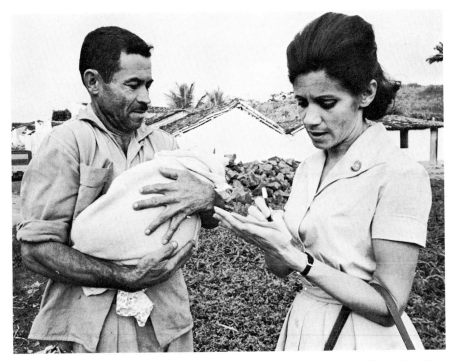

Fig. 25-10. Alvina Almeida, a registered nurse in public health practice in Brazil, is consulted by an anxious father. (WHO)

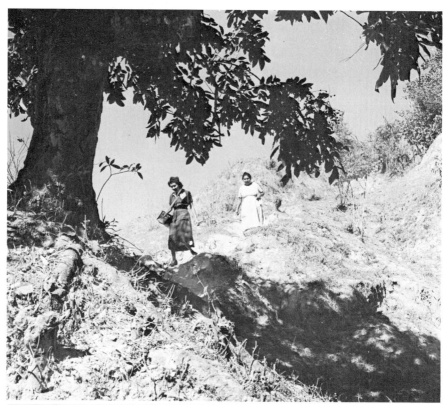

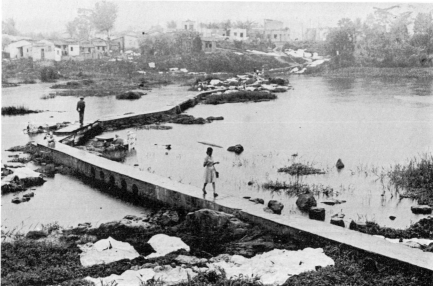

Fig. 25-11. Visiting nurses in good or bad weather are always on the job. *(Top)* Maria Marroquin, San Salvador. (UN). *(Bottom)* Alvina Almeida under an umbrella, Brazil. (WHO)

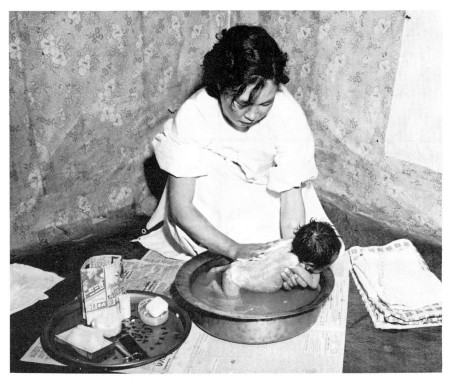

Fig. 25-12. Miss Kim Chung Bae, Assistant Nurse Advisor, UNC/OEC, tested the draft of a baby bath pamphlet by observing the return demonstration of a young Korean mother in her typical village home (AID)

the 25th millionth African to be vaccinated against smallpox in the current AID/PHS smallpox-measles program in 19 African countries.

New schools of nursing have been established in 19 countries — 42 countries have been assisted with subprofessional training of nurse and midwifery workers. Most of the approximately 800 nurses who have studied in the USA as AID participants have returned to positions of leadership in their countries' health services. National nursing associations have been created or strengthened in 35 of the countries where AID has been active, and 26 of these have met criteria for membership in the ICN.

Benefits from AID programs are not limited to the developing countries the Agency assists. Most of the approximately 500 USA nurses who have returned from AID assignments count their international experience as professionally rewarding as it was personally satisfying. The USA has a great deal to learn from these emerging countries about comprehensive national planning for health services and effective use of paramedical personnel.

For further information about AID, it is suggested that you read *Taking a Look at Cooperation: An Assessment of 24 Years of AID Technical Assistance in Nursing* published by AID in 1968 (see footnote number 17).

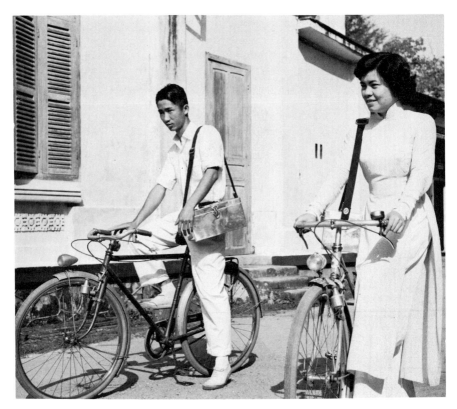

Fig. 25-13. Public health experience, AID. These second year students of the Health and Nursing Technician school in Hue, Vietnam, begin their city public health experience. This is the first class of students to have public health experience. (AID)

The Office of International Health of the Public Health Service

The Office of International Health (OIH), formerly a unit in the PHS, is now (1970) located in the Office of the Secretary of the U.S. Department of Health, Education, and Welfare (HEW). It serves as a center for the international health activities of the Federal Government's health services and its Director is the principal adviser to the Assistant Secretary for Health and Scientific Affairs regarding all international health concerns of HEW. It provides technical staff services to the Surgeon General of the PHS and other officials who represent the USA in the deliberations of the WHO, the PAHO and other international organizations.

The OIH maintains close contact with the U.S. State Department, AID and the Peace Corps in their concerns with health programs. The Director and personnel of the Office help to formulate USA policies in the field of international health. They participate in international negotiations on health; for example, on planning and operating the exchange scientific program. They serve as a technical resource staff to other agencies of the Federal government which have health programs overseas, assisting with program development, staff recruitment, project implementation and evaluation. They coordinate overseas health activities carried out by several operating units of the PHS and work closely with the PHS division that plans the USA programs for foreign health students and distinguished leaders in health and science from all over the world.

Nursing. The Nursing Unit of the OIH is part of its technical resources staff and is particularly concerned with the nursing and midwifery component of all international health programs. It recruits USA nurses for international agencies as well as for USA Government programs overseas. It serves as an information and counseling center for nurses who are interested in preparing themselves for careers in international health, and gives orientation and professional backstopping services to those nurses who are working overseas. One of its major functions is working with USA and international agencies in helping the governments of developing countries to plan for the nursing and midwifery services which will be needed to move their health plans and health goals from the drawing boards into the lives of their people.

The Peace Corps

The Peace Corps was established by Congress on September 22, 1961, as a semiautonomous unit within the U.S. Department of State. The primary purpose of the Corps is to promote world peace and friendship. The establishment of the Corps followed intensive study by a Presidential Task Force headed by Mr. R. Sargent Shriver. Important basic policies limited the work of the Peace Corps to countries to which it was invited, and stated that the Corps volunteers would be "doers," not "advisers." Volunteers would serve for 2 years, without salary, but would be provided a living allowance. A readjustment allowance of $75 was established, to be paid after return to the USA, for each month of satisfactory service. Within 18 months after the program was approved, nearly 5,000 volunteers, including nurses, were working in some 45 countries in Latin America, Africa, South Asia, the Far East and the Near East.[18] By June 1967, there were 11,912 Volunteers overseas in 50 nations, with another 3,056 in training — a total of 14,968 men and women.[19]

Participation of Nurses. In June 1967, 255 registered nurse volunteers were serving in 23 countries, and 100 more were selected to begin Peace Corps training during the next 3 months. Approximately 40 per cent of the nurse volunteers were graduates of baccalaureate programs in nursing, and the remainder were graduates of diploma programs.

The majority of Peace Corps nurses serve in a teaching capacity, in auxiliary nurse training programs, with inservice education of hospital or clinic nursing staffs, or in ward teaching and supervision of nursing students' practice. Their goal is to assist host-country nurses in developing and initiating better methods of nursing care and in preparing the various categories of

[18] Peace Corps, *Peace Corps Fact Book,* Washington, D.C., The Corps n.d., pp. 4-5.
[19] Peace Corps, *6th Annual Report,* Washington, D.C., The Corps, 1967, p. 35.

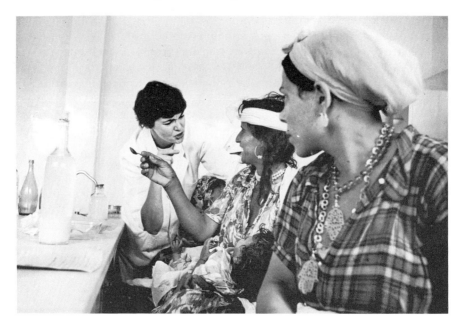

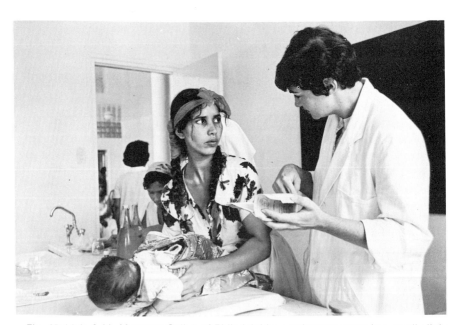

Fig. 25-14 (a & b). Margaret Gallen of Philadelphia, a volunteer nurse in a small clinic on the outskirts of Tunis, capital of Tunisia. She is shown here instructing mothers in the feeding of liquids to their infants. The major health problem with which she contends is infant dehydration. (Peace Corps)

nursing personnel to give safe, effective care to patients. Some nurse volunteers work on public health or community projects, assist host-country physicians with curative services, help with health education and take part in communicable disease control and family planning programs. Figure 25-14 shows nursing activities in the Peace Corps.

There is a continuing need for nurse volunteers. Qualifications considered desirable are good physical and mental health, adaptability and ability to relate well to people. A knowledge of another language in addition to English is not essential, but it is very helpful. Nursing students considering Peace Corps service after graduation might, if possible, plan to study a foreign language and perhaps select some courses in sociology or cultural anthropology, if time or electives permit. Participation in activities planned for students from other lands would also be helpful, if the opportunity is available. Training and experience in public health nursing or nursing education also provide valuable background.

Many Peace Corps nurses have found their overseas service not only personally rewarding, but also valuable in helping them decide on career plans when they return. Statistics are still sparse, but a large number have returned to school to get bachelor's or master's degrees, and even doctorates. These nurses have definite plans for acquiring the additional education and experience needed to enable them to serve effectively in their chosen specialty.[20]

Nurses on the Foreign Service Staff of the U.S. Department of State

The U.S. Department of State is the official channel through which the people of the USA conduct their relations with the other governments and peoples of the world. Within the Department of State, the Foreign Service Staff is a career corps of men and women serving in administrative, technical, stenographic and clerical positions. This group includes nurses.

The Foreign Service staffs the 290 embassies, legations and consulates maintained abroad. In the Department's effort to maintain and promote the health of its employees and their families and the personnel of other government agencies serving abroad, Foreign Service doctors and nurses serve at posts where medical facilities are substandard, and where health may be a problem.

The nurse may work alone or be under the direction of a Foreign Service physician. She is responsible for developing and administering a medical and health program for the embassy, and as required, for the consulates associated with the embassy. She serves as a health-room nurse to the employees of the USA government, their dependents and the local employees.

Because of the varied demands made on the nurse in Foreign Service, preference is given to nurses who have a baccalaureate degree in nursing and at least 3 years experience in nursing programs.

[20] Recently there has been some question about continuing the Corps. You may want to watch the newspapers for articles or announcements about this.

Private Foundations

The great Foundations, such as Rockefeller, W. K. Kellogg, Commonwealth Fund, Carnegie Corporation, and Russell Sage, have made significant contributions to nursing through sponsoring studies, granting scholarships and in many other ways. Two foundations that have made significant contributions to international nursing are described in this section.

International Health Activities of the Rockefeller Foundation. A few years after the Rockefeller Foundation was established in 1913 it began promoting interest in public health, the natural sciences, and the medical sciences in the Latin-American republics. This was done through the use of fellowships and grants-in-aid and the establishment of special health services within the host governments.

The Foundation placed particular stress on the training of the people in public health and allied fields within these countries. This provided a nucleus of trained personnel, many of whom later became leaders in their field.

The Rockefeller Foundation has not confined its activities to Latin America and public health. It has carried on many kinds of health projects all over the world, many of which relate to nursing. For example, in the early days the Foundation sent nurses to countries in Latin America and Europe to establish schools of nursing, courses in public health nursing, and public health nursing services.

From 1964 to 1968, the Rockefeller Foundation sponsored visiting professors at the University del Valle, Cali, Colombia.
These included:

Dorothy Brown — to develop and participate in the teaching of a Master's program in psychiatric nursing, 1964 to 1968
Carmela Cavero — to develop and participate in the teaching of a Master's program in maternal and infant care, 1966 to 1968
Lucille Mercadante — to work with the nursing service personnel, University Hospital, 1967 to 1968
Ruth A. Johnson — to assist with the integration of community health principles in all Masters' programs, 1968 to —
Esther Read — to develop and participate in the teaching of a Master's program in pediatric nursing, 1968 to —

Two nurses were serving (1969) as consultants in the field: Miss Thelma Ingles, Cali, Colombia, and Miss Ruby Wilson, Bangkok, Thailand.

International Program of the W. K. Kellogg Foundation. Although its assistance to international programs is independent of other similar programs, the W. K. Kellogg Foundation works with other agencies having like interests. For example, in Latin America it works with AID, PAHO/WHO, the PHS, and the Rockefeller Foundation.

The Foundation's professional education programs in Latin America are centered in leading universities. A major objective is to strengthen professional education in these universities. Fellowships are provided for selected members of faculties in these institutions, and library and other instructional materials, including laboratory equipment, are supplied also.

At present (1970), fellowships are provided in 4 areas — medicine, hospital administration, dentistry and nursing. These are given to strengthen and develop educational programs in selected professional schools. Therefore, fellowship students are selected with this in mind. All fellowship applicants from the various countries first must be screened and approved by a local selection committee in each country. They also must have studied English intensively for at least a year before coming to the USA. In addition, they are required to furnish evidence that they are being prepared for specific positions on their return to their own countries.

The scope of activities in nursing in Latin American countries has been enlarged. Currently included (1970) are such projects as advanced courses for graduate nurses, the improvement of new preservice nursing programs, the developing of a nursing care demonstration unit in a teaching hospital and assistance with new courses for auxiliary nursing personnel. A limited number of fellowships are provided to faculty in selected schools of nursing for graduate preparation in North American universities.

Barbara J. Lee is associate program director concerned with the nursing education interests of the W. K. Kellogg Foundation.

YOUR VISIT ABROAD

Are you thinking about studying or working in some foreign land after you become a nurse? If so, you will find that your membership in the ANA provides you with the privilege of international sponsorship and service. The ANA, along with other member associations of the ICN, is able to assist you in obtaining information about work experience abroad. Inquiries may be directed to the ANA Department of International Affairs. When feasible, it is desirable to plan for a personal interview with an ANA staff member regarding your special interests.

The requirements for assistance in obtaining work experience abroad include:

Membership in the ANA
At least 2 years of successful graduate experience in the USA
Compilation of a professional record with the ANA PC&PS

In addition, certain countries will require registration in their country and/or government working permits. Health and language certificates are also required.

All this is in the future, of course. But it is not too soon to start planning now. In most countries you need a working knowledge of the language in use, and languages, as you know, are not learned overnight. Also, there are the expenses to think about if your plan is for study or an observation visit. Even if you are looking forward to work experience, you will probably want extra money for a trip or two. Also, it is wise to have set aside the money for your return trip home. So start planning and saving now!

PROBLEMS

1. Watchwords of the ICN have been *work, courage, life, aspiration, peace, concordia, service, loyalty, faith, responsibility, wisdom, inquiry, tenacity* and *unity*. (a) Discuss the significance of these watchwords for an organization of international scope. (b) What future watchwords do you think would be suitable from the point of view of world affairs?

2. (a) Name the 3 USA nurses who have served as president of the ICN. (b) What other contributions have they made to nursing?

3. (a) Look at the most recent "Official Directory" of the *International Nursing Review*. (b) Then, make a list of the officers, the committee chairmen, and the staff personnel of the ICN. (c) How many of these are from the USA?

4. WHO works through governmental channels in relation to nursing problems. The ICN works through professional nursing organizations. What is the reason for this difference?

5. (a) What are the priority health problems in the Americas? (b) What is the effect of these problems on the economics of the countries involved?

6. In March 1961, the late President Kennedy proposed the "Alliance for Progress" program as a vast cooperative effort to satisfy the basic needs of the South American people for homes, work, land, health and schools. (a) How has the program operated? (b) What have been some major results? (c) What have been its failures?

7. In recent years, several voluntary health groups, such as Hope, have developed and maintained a variety of health programs in South America and throughout the world. (a) Make a survey to determine what groups have been organized. (b) Learn their specific objectives and programs.

8. What are the current purposes, programs and special features of the following associations? (a) United Nations (UN), (b) American Association for the United Nations (AAUN), (c) United Nations Children's Fund (UNICEF), (d) Pan American Health Organization (PAHO), (e) Organization of American States (OAS), (f) Inter-American Development Bank?

9. (a) Read *Nursing Legislation and Educations: A Study of the Role of National Governments and Voluntary Nursing Associations* (1963) by Eugenia K. Spalding published by the Catholic University of American Press, Washington, D.C. (b) Plan a group discussion to consider the importance of and the procedures for carrying out the recommendations listed in this report.

10. Select a country whose contemporary nursing program you would like to learn about. Prepare a report to be given before the entire school group. If each of you selects a different country on which to report, an international program can be planned. In making your reports, indicate the present concept of nursing held in the country studied, and present a review of contemporary nursing activities, achievements, leaders and professional organs for the dissemination of nursing information. Your bibliography could

be placed on cards and put in a cumulative file for the benefit of the school.

11. (a) Name several values that may be derived from a fuller understanding of nursing problems in other countries. (b) How would you interpret nursing in the USA – its aims, strengths, weaknesses and problems – to a nurse from, say, Peru, or Burma?

12. (a) What nursing magazines from Great Britain are available in your school of nursing library or other libraries that you use? (b) Consult a few recent numbers of those that are available, and compare the issues that are confronting British nurses, as reflected in these magazines, with those being discussed by nurses in the USA, as reflected in the professional journals described in Chapter 24. (c) Using *The Canadian Nurse,* make the same kind of comparison between our current issues and those in Canada.

13. Two-thirds of the world's people live in developing countries. Why and how do the conditions that exist in these lands cause barriers between peoples and nations?

14. (a) List the positions, the activities, or the outstanding achievements of each of the following, or give other interesting information about them: Dorothy Cornelius; Dr. Roger Egeberg; Alice Girard; Yvonne Hentsch; Abraham Horwitz; Thelma Ingles; Margrethe Kruse; Barbara J. Lee, Helen Mussallem, Sheila Quinn, Alice Thompson, Lily M. Turnbull, Doris de Vincenzo; (b) What other leaders in the field of international health would you add to this list?

SUGGESTED REFERENCES*

GENERAL

Boyle, R. E. "The First Three Years." *International Journal of Nursing Studies,* **4:**275-279, Dec. 1967.

Davidson, W. P. *International Political Communication.* New York, Frederick A. Praeger, 1965.

* Glaser, W. A. "American and Foreign Hospitals: Some Sociological Comparisons." *The Hospital in Modern Society.* New York, Free Press, 1963, pp. 37-62.

* Kona, W. "Foreign Journals in the Nursing School Library." *Nursing Outlook,* **10:**263-264, Apr. 1962.

* Matheu, R. "The Triple Role of International Organizations Today." *International Nursing Review,* **11:**8-12, July/Aug. 1964.

Nagano, S. "Nursing in Japan." *Canadian Nurse,* **65:**35-36, June 1969.

National Council of Women of the United States. *To Help to Unite Nations.* New York, The Council, n.d.

Restrepo, L. A. and de Garzon, E. C. "Nursing in Colombia." *Canadian Nurse,* **65:**37-39, June 1969.

The U.S. Department of State: What It Is . . . What It Does. Washington, D.C., Bureau of Public Affairs, The Department, Aug. 1963.

---

* In each chapter all citations are footnoted and are not included here. All starred references are recommended for additional reading.

INTERNATIONAL COUNCIL OF NURSES

American Nurses' Association. *Facts About Nursing: A Statistical Summary.* New York, The Association, 1968. pp. 237-238.

Breay, M. and Fenwick, E. G. *History of the International Council of Nurses, 1899-1925.* London, International Council of Nurses, 1931.

Bridges, D. C. "The Growth and Development of a Profession." *Canadian Nurse,* **65:**32-34, June 1969.

────. "International Nursing Review: Past, Present, and Progress." *International Nursing Review,* **15:**9-15, 1968.

Clamageran, A. "A Tribute to Helen Nussbaum." *International Nursing Review,* **14:**6-7, Aug. 1967.

* "1899-1959." *International Nursing Review,* **6:**3-101, July 1959.

"Frankfurt Congress ICN" *American Journal of Nursing,* **65:**88-97, Aug. 1965.

* Gage, N. D. "The International Council of Nurses." *American Journal of Nursing,* **29:**3-14, Jan. 1929.

"Guardian of World Health." *International Nursing Review,* **15:**101, Apr. 1968.

"International Congress of Nurses—Australia, April 17-22." *Nursing Outlook,* **9:**372-377, June 1961.

* International Council of Nurses. *Introducing the ICN.* Geneva, The Council, 1966.

* Nussbaum, H. "International Council of Nurses—Its Influence." *International Journal of Nursing Studies,* **1:**7-9, Dec. 1963.

* Quinn, S. "International Forum in Montreal." *Canadian Nurse,* **65:**31, June 1969.

* ────. "Issues Before the House." *American Journal of Nursing,* **69:**111-113, Jan. 1969.

────. "International Council of Nurses: Its Programmes and Activities." *Queensland Nurses Journal,* **9:**4-12, Nov. 1967.

* "With the ICN in Australia." *American Journal of Nursing,* **61:**60-71, July 1961.

"World Ethics Code Adopted by Nurses." *The New York Times,* July 19, 1953, sec. 1, p. 25.

* "The World of Nursing Meets in Montreal." *American Journal of Nursing,* **69:**1684-1699, Aug. 1969.

See routinely the *International Nursing Review* and *ICN Calling.*

Some ICN Publications

Henderson, V. *Basic Principles of Nursing Care.* Geneva, International Council of Nurses, 1960.

International Council of Nurses. *Salary and Employment Conditions in Nursing in Northern Countries of Europe.* Geneva, The Council, 1963.

PEACE CORPS

* Peace Corps. *Annual Report.* Washington, D.C., The Corps, Current issue.

* ────. *Fact Book and Directory.* Washington, D.C., The Corps, July 1968.

* ────. *Health Workers in the Peace Corps: The Pursuit of Life.* Washington, D.C., The Corps, n.d.

"Peace Corps Nurses." *Nursing Outlook,* **16:**40-41, Nov. 1968.

EXPERIENCES OF NURSES WORKING IN OTHER COUNTRIES

Campbell, T. "My World Health Organization Fellowship Experience." *Nursing Outlook,* **15:**40-42, Nov. 1967.

Erasmus, C. "Experiences of an Exchange-Visitor-Nurse." *International Nursing Review*, **14**:42-44, Aug. 1967.
Sister Genera. "Study Tour in Canada and the United States." *Irish Nurse*, **6**:267, Oct. 1967.
Kramer, M. "Comparative Study of Characteristics, Attitudes and Opinions of Neophyte British and American Nurses." *International Journal of Nursing Studies*, **4**:281-294, Dec. 1967.
Lund, J. "Public Health Nursing in the United States." *Tidsskrift for Sygeplejersker* (Denmark), **67**:529-530, Dec. 1967.

INTERNATIONAL COMMITTEE OF CATHOLIC NURSES

International Committee of Catholic Nurses. *C.I.C.I.A.M.S.* Brussels, Belgium, The Committee, n.d.
_____. *Statutes. C.I.C.I.A.M.S.,* Brussels, Belgium, The Committee, 1965.

WORLD HEALTH ORGANIZATION

* Creelman, L. "Quality Care in the Right Quantity: Two Decades of WHO Nursing Assistance." *International Nursing Review*, **15**:102-110, Apr. 1968.
* Taylor, J. "First Steps." *World Health: 20th Anniversary Issue*. Mar. 1968, pp. 3-5.
* "Twenty Years of Learning." *World Health: 20th Anniversary Issue*. Mar. 1968. pp. 6-10.
* World Health Organization. *Constitution of the World Health Organization.* Geneva, The Organization. Current edition.
_____. *The Work of WHO.* Geneva, The Organization. Published annually.
* _____. *The Second Ten Years of the World Health Organization, 1958-1967.* Geneva, The Organization, 1968.
_____. *Expert Committee on Nursing: Fifth Report.* Geneva, The Organization, 1966.
_____. *Report of the Travelling Seminar on Nursing in the USSR.* Geneva, The Organization, Oct. 1966.
* _____. *WHO – World Health Organization: What It Is . . . What It Does . . . How It Works.* Geneva, The Organization, 1963.
_____. Expert Committee on Nursing. *Expert Committee on Nursing: Second Report.* Geneva, The Organization, June 1952.
* _____. *Report on the First Session, Geneva, 20-26 February 1950.* Geneva, The Organization, 1950.
* "A Year's Work by WHO." *World Health,* Special issue. February 1964, pp. 2-30.

See *World Health,* a review published by the WHO since 1946. All publications of WHO can be secured from the Sales Section, Palais des Nations, Geneva, Switzerland, or from the International Documents Service, Columbia University Press, Columbia University, New York, New York, 10027.
See also *WHO Chronicle,* published monthly by WHO since 1947.

PAN AMERICAN HEALTH ORGANIZATION

* Pan American Health Organization. *Headquarters for Hemisphere Health.* Washington, D.C., The Organization, 1965.
_____. *PAHO/WHO, 1902-1967, 65 Years of Inter-American Health.* Washington, D.C., The Organization, 1968.
* Reno, N. "Sixty Years: The Story of the Pan American Health Organization." *Americas,* **14**:6-11, July 1962.

UNITED NATIONS

* American Association for the United Nations. *What It Is...What It Does... How It Works.* New York, The Association, Oct. 1968.
———. *Periodicals and Current Publications.* New York, United Nations. Issued periodically.
Straachan, M. "Nurse's Midwifery in UNICEF." *Bulletin of the American College of Nurse-Midwifery,* **8:**8-12, Spring 1963.
United Nations. *International Covenants on Human Rights.* New York, United Nations, Dec. 1967.
* United Nations Children's Fund. *UNICEF: What It Is...What It Does...How It Works.* New York, The Fund, 1963.

VOLUNTARY GROUPS IN INTERNATIONAL HEALTH PROGRAMS

* Fakkema, L. V. "Hope in Peru." *American Journal of Nursing,* **63:**114-115, Sept. 1963.
Fox, J. E. "Papal Volunteers in Peru." *American Journal of Nursing,* **67:**2565-2568, Dec. 1967.
Harris, F. M. and Campbell, T. M. "Hope Goes to Indonesia." *American Journal of Nursing.* **61:**79-81, July 1961.
* "The Kellogg Foundation: Helpful Endeavors on Four Continents." *Hospitals,* **38:**17-24, 128, Jan. 1, 1964.
The Rockefeller Foundation. *President's Review—1963.* New York, The Foundation, Dec. 1963. Published annually.

CHAPTER

26

American National
Red Cross

The American National Red Cross is a voluntary agency for the relief and the prevention of human suffering. Through its congressional charter it has certain responsibilities delegated to it by the USA Government. These are to furnish volunteer aid to the sick and the wounded of the armed forces in time of war; to act as a medium of voluntary relief and communication between the people of the USA and their armed forces; to provide a system of national and international disaster relief and to devise and carry on measures for preventing the sufferings caused by pestilence, famine, fire, floods and other great national calamities; and to assist the Government in carrying out the terms of the international treaties for the protection of war victims. With the consent of Congress, the charter has been broadly interpreted over the years to meet demonstrated needs in related fields of activity.

ORIGIN AND ORGANIZATION OF THE
AMERICAN RED CROSS

The American Red Cross is 1 of more than 100 national Red Cross, Red Crescent, and Red Lion and Sun Societies throughout the world.[1] All these

[1]The Red Cross movement in Moslem countries has adopted Islamic or national symbolism. Hence, the societies in most Moslem countries are known as the Red Crescent; Iran's society is called the Red Lion and Sun. See Chapter 1. p. 13.

societies have grown up as an intrinsic part of the international Red Cross movement, which had its formal beginning at Geneva in 1863 with the organization of the International Committee of the Red Cross. The founder of the Red Cross was Henri Dunant, a Swiss who, appalled by the suffering and neglect on the Italian battlefield of Solferino in 1859, organized a small band of local volunteers and worked with them to bind the injuries and bring food and water to the wounded of both sides. Haunted by the experience, Dunant wrote *Un Souvenir de Solferino,* a slim volume published in 1862, vividly picturing the suffering at Solferino and urging all countries to form committees of volunteers to care for war-wounded. In his effort to lighten suffering in war Dunant was influenced by the work of Florence Nightingale, who only a few years earlier, during the Crimean War, had taken a group of English nurses with her to Scutari and, in a short time, had greatly improved hospital conditions and the nursing care of the patients.

The next few years Dunant traveled throughout Europe, everywhere urging the need for organized groups in each country, trained to give medical and nursing services to armies. The first fruit of his work was the conference at Geneva, Switzerland, in 1863, at which the formation of volunteer aid societies was recommended for all countries. This conference also adopted a symbol, selecting, in honor of Dunant, a red cross on a white field – the colors of the Swiss flag reversed – as the emblem of the Societies. A year later a second conference – this one of government representatives with full power – drew up the first Geneva Convention, which provided that, during war, sick and wounded soldiers would be cared for irrespective of nationality and that hospitals, ambulances and people caring for patients would be safe from military attack.

Although 2 Americans, George G. Fogg and Charles Bowles, influenced the making of the first Geneva Treaty (their account of U.S. Sanitary Commission work during the Civil War stilled the objections in many quarters that nonmilitary workers in battle areas would act as spies), the USA in 1864 still viewed the signing of any treaty, however enlightened, as contrary to its policy of "no foreign entanglements." Ratification of the treaty by the U.S. Senate was not accomplished until 1882, after a long and almost single-handed campaign by Clara Barton. The American Association of the Red Cross (incorporated by act of Congress in 1900 as the American National Red Cross) had been founded in 1881, with Miss Barton as its first president.

The development of the concepts of disaster relief and general community-service work as the proper spheres of Red Cross activity is the unique contribution of the American society of the international Red Cross movement. Originally undertaken to assure the continuity of Red Cross preparedness between war emergencies, such services have become the foundation of the Red Cross in the USA today and have made the organization an integral part of the nation.

The American Red Cross operates through a national headquarters in

Washington, D.C., 4 area offices (Alexandria, Va.; Atlanta; St. Louis; and San Franciso), and 3,300 local chapters covering every county in the USA and the insular territories and possessions. Policies of the organization are determined by a board of governors, 30 of whose 50 members are elected by chapter delegates to the national convention. Of the remaining 20 members, 8 are appointed by the President of the USA, who is honorary chairman of the organization, and 12 are elected by the board itself.

THE INTERNATIONAL RED CROSS

The national Red Cross societies and 3 organized international groups form the International Red Cross, These 3 groups are:

1. *The International Committee of the Red Cross* is a group of no more than 25 Swiss citizens charged with maintaining Red Cross principles, recognizing newly established Red Cross societies, and acting as a neutral intermediary between belligerent governments.

2. *The League of Red Cross Societies,* a federation of some 100 national societies, was formed in 1919 to promote their activities and to facilitate cooperation among them. The League also acts as the representative of and spokesman for the Red Cross societies in relations with other international organizations. Among its many activities, the League maintains a nursing bureau that assists in the development of nursing services in national Red Cross societies, furnishes nursing information to the societies and encourages scholarships and study visits for nurses.

3. *The International Red Cross Conference* is composed of delegates from the national Red Cross societies, the International Committee, the League and the governments that have signed the Red Cross treaties. The highest deliberative body of the International Red Cross, the Conference meets regularly every 4 years to discuss such matters as Red Cross activities, the Geneva Conventions and humanitarian problems. Between meetings, a standing commission coordinates and harmonizes the work of the International Red Cross. The commission's membership includes 5 representatives from the national Red Cross societies, 2 from the League and 2 from the International Committee.

AMERICAN RED CROSS SERVICES

Briefly, the Red Cross provides welfare services and assistance programs to members of the armed forces, veterans and their families; conducts a nationwide disaster preparedness and relief program that includes emergency relief for disaster victims and needed assistance in restoring them to normal living; and carries on a year-round variety of health and safety programs in hometown communities. Included in such latter programs are home nursing, mother and baby care, mother's aide instruction, first aid and water safety education and a blood program that helps to meet the nation's need for blood and blood products. International services include emergency disaster relief and goodwill programs. Junior Red Cross and High School Red Cross members, enrolled in over 43,000 public, private and parochial schools and 1,300 colleges and universities, conduct community, national and international service programs and participate in volunteer work through local Red Cross chapters as well. During peace, the emphasis of Red Cross activity is on service that can be expanded as needed in a national emergency.

NURSING PROGRAMS

The Nursing Programs of the American Red Cross provides a reserve of professional nurses, both paid and volunteer, for Red Cross programs and for disaster relief work.

Following its reorganization in 1905, the Red Cross recognized that nurses would be needed in the programs developed to fulfill the terms of the organization's congressional charter. At first each state branch was given authority to enroll nurses, but the diversity of nursing standards from one state to another soon demonstrated the impracticality of this early method and the need for the establishment of nationwide qualifications for enrollment. This standardization of qualifications for Red Cross nurse enrollment was a forerunner of accreditation of schools of nursing as it is known today. Many schools of nursing improved their programs so that their graduates could be enrolled as Red Cross nurses.

With the assistance of the ANA, the nursing programs of the American National Red Cross were given official status when its organization was approved by the Executive Committee of the Red Cross in 1909. The first national director was Jane A. Delano, who resigned her position as superintendent of the Army Nurse Corps to become a full-time volunteer in the Red Cross so that she could help to develop a reserve nurse corps for military purposes and for disaster work.

Organization and Administration

The national headquarters Nursing Programs staff, composed of administrative and professional personnel, is responsible for the overall program-planning and for carrying out the specific nursing policies within the broad framework of policies established by the board of governors for approved nursing services. It provides technical and professional guidance and prepares instructional materials, courses, record forms, and the like. The national nursing staff also relates the Red Cross nursing program and its policies to the development of nursing as a whole and maintains relationships with other national health programs and organizations.

The National Nursing Advisory Committee, composed of leaders in the nursing profession, helps to standardize and guide the development of the various aspects of the Red Cross nursing programs and to appraise needs and progress. The Committee members are selected because of their interest in the Red Cross and in the national problem of providing good nursing care for the people who need it. The Committee, representing different parts of the country and different fields of nursing, assists those responsible for the nursing programs to maintain the high standards of Red Cross nursing in all its aspects and to modify programs to meet today's needs.

Recruitment for the Armed Forces

In 1911, President Taft designated the American Red Cross as the only volunteer relief agency officially authorized to give help to the Army and the Navy in wartime. This gave the stamp of approval to Miss Delano's plan for recruiting and maintaining a reserve of nurses for the Army and Navy Nurse Corps. In fulfilling this assignment, the Red Cross recruited most of the nurses who served with the armed forces during both World Wars (World War I – 24,000 of the 25,000 who served; World War II – almost all of the 77,800 who served). In World War II, the Red Cross actually certified 105,000 nurses for military service. This voluntary response was, in relation to resources, among the largest of the responses made by professional groups.

The need for the Red Cross to maintain a roster of reserve nurses ready for military duty ceased with the legislation in 1947 that established the status of the nurse corps for the armed forces, including the maintenance of their reserves. Since then the Red Cross chapters have enrolled nurses to serve only in their programs and to meet local and national emergencies.

Public Health Nursing

For many years after 1912, the Red Cross pioneered in rural public health nursing. Originally set up as a demonstration, the program contributed significantly to the development of the American public health facilities, which are among the most advanced in the world today. When the program was undertaken, only 8 nurses in the entire country were qualified to give instruction in public health nursing. By providing scholarships for nurses who wanted to enter the public health field, setting standards of organization and service, and conducting a community program of public health demonstrations that eventually reached over 1,800 counties, the Red Cross helped to make public health nursing the accepted community service it is today. By 1930, when most states had established departments of health and had written modern standards of public health practice into law, the job was largely done. However, it was not until 1950 that the Red Cross nursing in the public health program was terminated officially.

Instructional Programs

Other phases of the Red Cross nursing program have continued, or new ones have been developed. The home-nursing courses began as a primary method of ensuring the spread of good health practices throughout the communities. Today the need for instruction of families in caring for the sick at home is more important than ever, because of the increasing number of aging and chronically ill who can be cared for at home satisfactorily and economically. Early dismissal of patients from hospitals demands follow-up nursing care at home. The Office of Civil Defense, in planning for the care of the many who may be ill, injured, or displaced as a result of war, recognized the need for training thousands of homemakers to act as nursing assistants. In many places the home-nursing course is used as the basis for teaching nurse's aides in hospitals and auxiliary help in nursing homes. The home-nursing programmed instruction course is also taught in communities and schools. Thus the significance of teaching simple nursing skills through the Red Cross home-nursing program is increasing in today's society.

Red Cross nursing programs also include the preparation of Red Cross

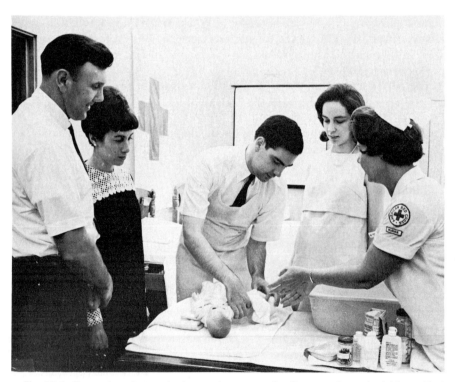

Fig. 26-1. Two pairs of expectant parents prepare for the experience by taking a Red Cross course in Mother and Baby Care. Under the supervision of a Red Cross Volunteer Nursing Instructor. An expectant father practices dressing the baby on a doll. His wife, second from right, and another expectant couple left, look on. (American National Red Cross)

volunteers who assist with nursing care in hospitals and nursing homes. These volunteers are given basic orientation to Red Cross and the specific preparation for hospital or agency requirements for the kind of personal-care services they will be administering to the patient. In each of the programs Red Cross is contributing to improving the quality of nursing care.

"Mother and Baby Care" (a 12-hour course) prepares parents for the

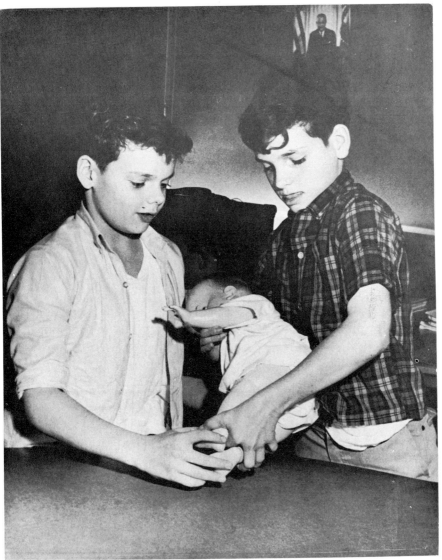

Fig. 26-2. Learning to Care . . . Many Red Cross chapters have special classes for young people in how to look after younger people. Running through a practice class exercise here are two students at the State Hospital for Crippled Children. (American National Red Cross)

arrival of the baby and helps parents in evaluating the growth, development and needs of the baby during his first year of life. The increasing number of births and the mobility of young parents have made this course very popular. Many hospitals and public health agencies also conduct maternity courses, but the assistance of the Red Cross, with its trained volunteer instructors, affords public health agencies opportunity to extend this instruction to all those who are interested. Fathers learning to give infant care are shown in Figure 26-1.

"Mother's Aide" (an 8-hour course) is designed to help upper elementary and junior high school students consider some important aspects of child care and learn some simple procedures they might be expected to use. This course, as are all Red Cross courses, is presented without charge to the community. Figure 26-2 shows young students learning child care.

"Fitness for the Future," a 4-session discussion course for people who are interested in preparing for their later years or for those who want to understand the older members of their families, stresses the importance of living healthfully, safely, wisely and leisurely. The group members have an opportunity to select subject matter within the framework of the above topics. These subjects might include the aging process, posture, medical supervision, nutrition, mental health and accident prevention, as well as financial planning for old age.

Geneva Conventions Orientation Lesson for Nurses is presented by Red Cross chapters to acquaint persons with the privileges provided and responsibilities delegated under the Geneva Conventions during war or internal strife.

Disaster Nursing

Disaster nursing is for many the most dramatic and satisfying experience of the Red Cross nurse. Nurses must be recruited and assigned quickly to care for the ill, the injured and the homeless. Since its early days, the Red Cross, from its roster of nurses, has been able to meet the nursing needs of communities hit by disaster. Red Cross disaster nurses may serve in shelters, man-aid stations during and after a disaster — many injuries occur to emergency workers clearing away debris in a disaster's aftermath — augment overworked hospital staffs and serve as members of volunteer Disaster Action Teams which respond around the clock to many of the 18,000 disasters that annually create a need for Red Cross service. In 1967, for example, a total of 1,200 nurses participated in Red Cross disaster operations. In the spring of that year, they were involved not only in helping victims of hundreds of fires, explosions and local disasters, but also in Red Cross efforts following floods and tornadoes in Arkansas, Kentucky, Ohio, Illinois, Iowa, Texas, Oklahoma and northern New Jersey. In Florida, they helped staff shelters open on a precautionary basis when Hurricane Abby threatened parts of Florida. The previous summer, hundreds of Red Cross

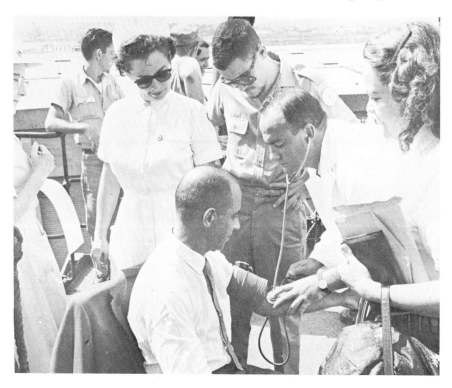

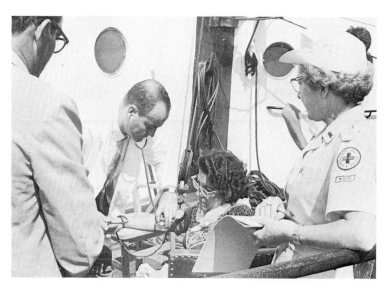

Fig. 26-3. Red Cross medical officer and Red Cross nurse examining Cuban refugees as they board the ship in Havana en route to the United States. (American National Red Cross)

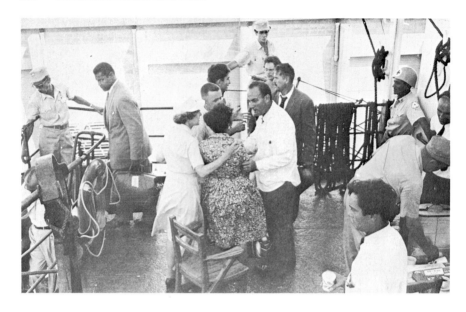

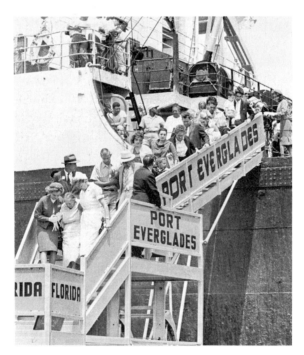

Fig. 26-3 *(Cont.)*. *(Top)* Red Cross personnel helping a sick refugee board the ship. *(Bottom)* Cuban refugees leaving the ship at Port Everglades, Florida. The Red Cross Nurse assists aged and ill down the ramp. (American National Red Cross)

nurses helped care for 30,000 people sheltered during and after the big
Fairbanks, Alaska floods, and during and after Hurricane Beulah and the
floods which followed in Texas. Work carried out with Cuban refugees is
shown in Figure 26-3. Figure 26-4 shows Red Cross personnel conferring
about care for flood refugees in Colorado. Disaster nursing training courses

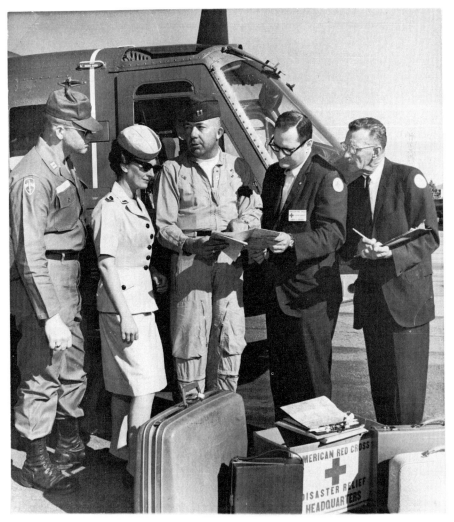

Fig. 26-4. Lowery Air Force Base, Colo. A Red Cross nurse and Red Cross disaster
officials receive pre-flight briefing from Capt. Harry V. Phillips, Jr., center, pilot of the
254th Medical Detachment Helicopter Ambulance Service, Ft. Carson, Colo. Subse-
quently, Mrs. Jean E. Lazar, R.N., of Falls Church, Va., took off for Lamar, Colo., to give
nursing care to 1,550 flood refugees there. Robert Freeman and J. White Gwyn, Red Cross
disaster officials, continued on the flight to survey flood damage. Capt. Kenneth Fitch,
left, was co-pilot of the craft. (American National Red Cross)

are conducted regularly by experienced Red Cross disaster nurses. Each year, tens of thousands of nurses attend such conferences.

It is suggested that you review Chapter 12, "Nurses in a National Disaster or Emergency," in connection with this section on "Disaster Nursing."

Nurse's Aides History

During World War II, 250,000 volunteer nurse's aides were trained as a supplementary nursing group in civilian and military hospitals. Their services in assisting with bedside care of patients, helping in clinics and in the Red Cross blood program are now extended to public health agencies for care of patients in homes. The work of well-trained volunteer nurse's aides has demonstrated the place of the volunteer auxiliary worker as a team member in patient care.

Blood Program

Professional nurses have played a major role in the Red Cross blood program from the time it was initiated in 1948. Assigned the important functions of donor screening and blood withdrawal, a highly skilled staff works closely with the physician-in-charge to assure the protection of both donors and recipients. In addition to assisting in the annual collection of over 3 million units of blood, this staff serves as a nucleus for training large numbers of both professional and lay volunteers in all phases of blood collection and, of perhaps even greater significance, stands ready as a reserve of trained personnel to render immeasurable help in a national emergency. Regularly, 72,800 professional nurses contribute their time and experience to assist in bringing Red Cross blood services to communities throughout the nation.

YOUR PLACE IN THE RED CROSS

Why Should You Enroll in Red Cross Nursing Programs?

Through its special nursing programs the Red Cross provides opportunity for instruction in group teaching for service in disasters or epidemics, for training and experience in blood collection procedures and for community service. Married and retired nurses have an unusual opportunity to contribute to community nursing programs and to keep up their professional skills through part-time work. Working in many capacities with members of other professions and with well-trained volunteers gives the nurse new experiences and interests that broaden her professional viewpoint and extend her social understanding.

The number of Red Cross programs that touch on nursing in one or more aspects makes it certain the nurse can find a place in Red Cross work that will allow her both to use her special skills and to gain new knowledge. Every eligible graduate of a nursing school should consider enrolling as a Red Cross nurse. The opportunities for service through the Red Cross challenge all nurses who wish to contribute to the betterment of the community, the nation and the world.

What Qualifications Must You Have?

An emergency call to the Red Cross to provide nurses leaves little time to investigate credentials and qualifications before making assignments. Enrolled Red Cross nurses have established their records at their local chapters and can be assigned promptly to the type of work for which they are best fitted.

Today (1970) the basic requirements for enrollment as a Red Cross nurse are:

1. State registration following graduation from a state-approved school of nursing.

2. Current registration, where required by law, for the type of work the nurse will do for the Red Cross.

3. Satisfactory personal, educational and professional qualifications and health for the work she will do as a Red Cross nurse.

4. Interest in Red Cross service and acceptance of Red Cross philosophy and purposes as evidenced by some pre-enrollment participation with the Red Cross.

How Will You Be Identified as a Red Cross Nurse?

Each enrolled nurse is given an appointment card and a badge with an identifying number as evidence of her enrollment as a Red Cross nurse. These serve as identification when the nurse is called for Red Cross service and indicate her willingness to use her specialized skills and experience for the relief and prevention of human suffering.

Use of the Red Cross emblem is protected by an act of Congress. The badge may be worn only by the nurse to whom it is issued and should be kept in her possession.

What Opportunities Are Open to Red Cross Nurses?

Nurses with the necessary requirements may be employed in several positions with the Red Cross. These are as follows: chapter director of nursing programs, instructor or instructor supervisor for Red Cross home nursing, chief or staff nurse in the blood program and member of the national staff in the field or in the office. Further information on these positions may be obtained from the National Director of Nursing Programs, American National Red Cross, Washington, D.C., 20006, or from the appropriate area office. (See ARC publication 1629-A, Nurses – A position for you with the American Red Cross as a nursing consultant.)

PROBLEMS

1. A tornado has struck your community, and you would like to make your services available to help the disaster victims. You have heard that there are about 200 people housed in the high school and that the hospital has just admitted 65 seriously injured people. There are also 2 first aid stations being set up to assist with the emergency treatment of the patients and the workers who are clearing up the debris. (a) How would you know where nurses were needed most urgently? (b) What would be your relationship with the American Red Cross on a disaster operation? (c) How could you prepare yourself for service in a disaster?

2. Riots across the USA have created emergency situations from time to time. If the Red Cross asked you to take charge of a first-aid station during such an event, how would you go about securing the required personnel, equipment and supplies?

3. An increasing older age group and the rising birth rate have posed problems to the health department in your community, as there is only 1 public health nurse in the entire county. (a) What kind of health education programs would help people meet these problems? (b) How could you, as a nurse, assist in such a community plan? (c) What kind of help could you expect from the Red Cross in your community?

SUGGESTED REFERENCES*

* American Natic a Red Cross. *Annual Report*. Washington, D.C., American National Red C oss. Current issue.

————. *Nurses – A Position for You With the ARC as a Nursing Consultant*. ARC 1629A. Washington, D.C., American National Red Cross, Jan. 1968.

————. *Nursing Services Instructional Program, A Guide for Chairmen*. ARC 1640D. Washington, D.C., American National Red Cross, Nov. 1967.

* ————. *American Red Cross Nursing Services*. ARC 1640A. Washington, D.C., American National Red Cross, July 1967.

* ————. *Home Nursing Programmed Instruction*. ARC 1671. Washington, D.C., American National Red Cross, Nov. 1966.

————. *The American Red Cross: A Brief Story*. ARC 626. Washington, D.C., American National Red Cross, July 1966.

————. *Blood . . . a Community Responsibility*. ARC 1735. Washington, D.C., American National Red Cross, June 1965.

* In each chapter all citations are footnoted and are not included here. All starred references are recommended for additional reading.

_____. *Nurses and the Geneva Conventions Orientation Lesson.* ARC 1669. Washington, D.C., American National Red Cross, Apr. 1965.

_____. *Student Nurse, See Yourself in the Red Cross.* ARC 1665. Washington, D.C., American National Red Cross, July 1963.

_____. *Wear It With Pride.* ARC 1638. Washington, D.C., American National Red Cross, Jan. 1956.

Dock, L. L., *et al. History of the American Red Cross Nursing.* New York, Macmillan, 1922.

* Jarvis, M. A., *et al.* "Health Larnin' in Appalachia." *American Journal of Nursing,* **67:**2345-2347, Nov. 1967.

* Lewis, E. P. "Night Boat from Havana." *American Journal of Nursing,* **63:**70-74, Apr. 1963.

* McGrath, M. E. "Teaching Students to Teach." *Nursing Outlook,* **15:**69-71, Sept. 1967.

"Red Cross in Disaster Relief." *British Medical Journal,* **2:**653-654, June 1967.

* "Red Cross Century Album." *World Health,* Special issue, Apr. 1963, pp. 4-46.

Steward, E. "Ready to Serve." *American Journal of Nursing,* **63:**85-87, Sept. 1963.

"A Thousand Plus Volunteers for Flood Emergency Duty." (news item) *American Journal of Nursing,* **67:**2246-2249, Nov. 1967.

CHAPTER

27

Legislation Affecting Nursing

What is law? What laws are of special concern to you? What legal requirements must you meet in order to practice nursing? What legislative responsibilities do nurses have?

President Nixon, just a few days before his election in the fall of 1968, wrote to the executive director of the ANA regarding his interest in nursing. He included in his remarks the statement that "few of our nation's professionals work as selflessly for human welfare as America's nurses. . . ."[1] As a student, as a graduate nurse and as a citizen you have a stake in promoting the best type of legislation for the public good as well as for the profession. And, as was indicated by President Nixon, nurses, through their professional association, have through the years had an enviable reputation for their wise and liberal stand on social welfare and health legislation.

This chapter reviews briefly the subject of legislation related to nursing. It is suggested that you read it in connection with Chapter 6, "Legal Issues in Nursing Practice," which deals with the nurse's legal responsibilities in practice and the issues and problems about which she must be knowledgeable.

[1] American Nurses' Association, "Nixon Favors Continued Federal Assistance to Nursing Education," *Capital Commentary*, p. 2, Nov.-Dec. 1968.

LAW IN GENERAL

What Is Law?

Blackstone defined municipal law as a "rule of civil conduct, prescribed by the supreme power in a state, commanding what is right, and prohibiting what is wrong."[2] Thomas Aquinas defined law as "Nothing other than an ordinance of reason for the common good, made by him who has care of the community, and promulgated."[3] Woodrow Wilson extended these definitions by considering law as "that portion of the established thought and habit which has gained distinct and formal recognition in the shape of uniform rules backed by the authority and power of government."[4] *Nursing law may be defined as that body of statutes, executive orders, regulations, rules and legal precedents which have for their objectives the promotion and the protection of individual and community health as it is affected by nursing and nursing services.*

Modern society has become very complex and interdependent. The only way order can be maintained is by the establishment and enforcement of laws. If there were no laws, chaos would result, similar to that which would exist if there were no rules to guide traffic or no controlling policies and regulations in a hospital.

The purpose of law is to promote the general good and welfare of the people by the regulation of human conduct in order to protect the individual from other individuals, groups, or the state, and vice versa. In a democracy, law represents community desires or commands; it is applicable to all in the community; it is backed by the power of the government; and it provides for all people the administration of justice under it.

Why Should You Be Concerned with Legislation?

There are several reasons for your being concerned with legislation. In a democracy like the USA, laws, in the last analysis, reflect the collective wishes of the people. As a citizen of a democracy, therefore, you have a responsibility to acquire a background about laws which will help you in evaluating them and in making known your wishes about legislation, as well as in abiding by the laws that have been established. Ignorance of the law is not taken as an excuse when an error is made.

Secondly, as a nurse you will have specific responsibilities and privileges assigned to you by law. Accordingly, you have the obligation of knowing what the laws which pertain to nursing mean to you, to the profession and to

[2] W. Blackstone, *Commentaries on the Laws of England; Book the Third of Private Wrongs,* Philadelphia, Childs, 1862, p. 1.

[3] Thomas Aquinas, *The Summa Theologica,* Vol. II, Chicago, Encyclopedia Britannica, 1952, Great Books of the Western World Series, p. 208. (Permission by Burns & Oates Ltd., London, and Benziger Brothers, Inc., New York, the original publishers.)

[4] W. Wilson, *The State: Elements of Historical and Practical Politics,* Boston, Heath, 1918, p. 69.

the public. You also need to be aware of your legal liability, for the purpose of knowing what protection to secure if you are sued for malpractice or negligence. You should have also some understanding of how well these laws accomplish what they are intended to accomplish and how, through changes in them, they might more effectively achieve their purposes.

Finally, you should be aware of new developments in legislation. The increased concern of the Government in health, welfare and education is broadening the scope of legislation that has a bearing on nursing and nurses. For example, the passage of *Public Law 89-239*, which established the Regional Medical Programs (1968), is of great interest to nursing and will probably have a significant effect on nursing practice and the provision of nursing services. It is important for you to acquire some background that will help you to decide whether the passage of new laws should be encouraged or discouraged.

Kinds of Laws

For you to exert your proper influence as a citizen and as a nurse on the improvement of existing laws and on the establishment of new ones, you need an understanding of the ways in which laws originate.

One way of thinking about the origin of a law is to consider the jurisdiction to which it pertains. As you know, the USA is a federation of 50 states, each with its history, economic and social problems, and interests. History reveals that the members of the Constitutional Convention turned over to the Federal Government the powers and the activities that were considered desirable and necessary for the common welfare and survival of all. Matters that could be handled adequately by the individual states were retained by the states.

Sometimes, however, this division is not clear-cut. Federal and state governments recognize some similar responsibilities, particularly in matters pertaining to social welfare. This has led to the passage of Federal and state laws that complement each other; for example, a Federal law may appropriate funds for programs that are administered by states under their own laws.

From the viewpoint of origin, laws may be classified also according to the kind of body that establishes them:

1. Constitutional law is developed by specially designated bodies or legislatures convened for the purpose of framing or amending a constitution.

2. Statutory law is enacted either by representative assemblies or by the process of initiative and referendum.

3. Administrative law includes rules, regulations, standards and orders issued by executives and administrative boards within the sphere of their legal competence and responsibility in order to carry out the intent of statutory laws.

4. Common law and equity consist of decisions made by courts in specific cases.

All laws, of course, can be changed, but it is harder to amend or repeal some than others. Generally speaking, administrative law is easier to change than statutory law, and statutory law is less difficult to amend than constitutional law.

In deciding how to proceed in getting changes made in an existing law, you will, of course, first want to find out what body in what jurisdiction is responsible for its establishment. In considering the passage of a new law, you will want to think about the geographic extent to which it should be applicable and whether it involves powers that belong to the states or to the Federal Government. You will want to consider also how enduring it should be and therefore whether it should be brought into existence as an amendment to the Federal or the state constitution, as a statute, or as an administrative regulation.

Legal Terminology

The following legal terms, often used in legislative activities, may serve you as a ready reference. Some of these are taken from a standard book of legal words and phrases.[5] Only a few important definitions are given here. A more comprehensive list may be found in law dictionaries. These dictionaries can be located usually in law libraries, court houses, state capitol buildings, or the private library of a lawyer.

Act (in legislation): A written law, formally ordained or passed by the legislative power of the state, called in England an "act of parliament" and in the USA an "act of congress" or of the "legislature"; a statute. (p. 42)
Affidavit: A written or printed declaration or statement of facts, made voluntarily, and confirmed by the oath or affirmation of the party making it, taken before an officer having authority to administer such oath. [Sometimes a small fee is charged for this service.] (p. 80)
Bill: A draft of an act presented to the legislature, but not [yet] enacted. (p. 209)
Certificate: An instrument accorded by a competent authority which confers the right to perform some act; also an instrument attesting a fact. The term *certificate* instead of *license* is used in some states.
Certified copy: A copy of a document or record, signed and certified as a true copy by the officer to whose custody the original is entrusted. (p. 287)
Diploma: An instrument given by schools and societies to an individual who has met certain qualifications.
Enact: To establish by law; to perform or effect; to decree. The usual introductory formula in making laws is, "Be it enacted." (p. 619)
License: A permission, [accorded] by a competent authority to do some act which without such authorization would be illegal, or would be a trespass or a tort. Also, the written evidence of such permission. [A trespass in its widest sense means any violation of a law. A tort is a civil wrong redressible in a civil proceeding.] (p. 1067)
Licensee: A person ... who holds a license. (p. 1070)
Licentiate: One who has license to practice any art or faculty. (p. 1071)
Mandatory nursing practice act: A law that gives to nursing personnel the legal right to practice nursing.

---

[5] H. C. Black, *Black's Law Dictionary,* St. Paul, West Publishing, 1951. The citations are from the pages of this book as indicated in parentheses.

Permissive nursing practice act: A law that gives to nursing personnel the legal right to use an approved legal title.
Permit: A written license or warrant, issued by a person in authority, empowering the grantee to do some act not forbidden by law, but not allowable without such authority. [A time limit usually is set.] (p. 1298)
Registered: Entered or recorded in some official register or record or list. (p. 1449)
Retroactive: Looking backward; contemplating what is past. [When a law is retroactive, it is effective as of a date prior to its passage.] (p. 1480)
Status: The legal relation of individual to the rest of the community. The rights, duties, capacities, and incapacities which determine a person to given class. (p. 1580)
Statute: An act of the legislature declaring, commanding, or prohibiting something; a particular law enacted and established by the will of the legislative department of government; the written will of the legislature, solemnly expressed according to the forms necessary to constitute it the law of the state. This word is used to designate the written law in contradistinction to the unwritten law. (p. 1581)
Waiver: In relation to a nursing practice act "waiver refers to definite or prudent time to permit nursing personnel, in practice at time of passage of the law, to attain legal recognition or work status as provided in the law."[6]

NURSING LEGISLATION IN GENERAL

Responsibility for Legislation

Legislation related to nurses and nursing, like all legislation in a democracy, is the responsibility of the citizens, and laws are established by them either directly or, as is more frequently the case, through their representatives. Often, however, citizens or their representatives need the advice of people or groups who have detailed knowledge about the subject with which the legislation is concerned. Therefore, for the development of sound legislation about nursing, the guidance of nurses is usually needed.

The American Nurses' Association (ANA) is the spokesman for the nursing profession on Federal legislative matters. The ANA encourages state nurses associations to take the leadership on state legislative matters. The ANA, in line with its legislative responsibility, not only makes known to lawmaking bodies the profession's position on pending legislation, but it also calls attention to the need for changing or repealing existing laws and for establishing new ones. Further, it develops materials which will help nurses and others keep informed on legislation about nursing and nurses and, through a council of state boards of nursing, studies problems involved in the licensing of nurses.

Objectives of Nursing Legislation

Laws which relate to nurses and nursing in the USA might be divided according to their major objectives into the 3 following groups:

[6] E. K. Spalding, *Nursing Legislation and Education: A Study of the Role of National Governments and Voluntary Nursing Associations,* Washington, D.C., The Catholic University of America, 1963, p. 48.

1. Laws designed to protect the public from unsafe nursing care. This is the primary purpose of laws which pertain to the registering and licensing of various kinds of nursing personnel. It is also an important objective of laws which establish merit systems for the selection of nurses in government agencies as well as for the selection of other health personnel employed by the government.

2. Laws directed toward providing the public with more and better nursing care and nursing services. This is the main objective of laws which provide funds for scholarships for the study of nursing, for the operation of educational programs in nursing, for construction of nursing education facilities and for research in nursing. Laws which provide for new positions for nurses in government agencies also might be included in this category.

3. Laws intended to promote the health, welfare and status of nurses. This legislative objective is not unique to nursing, of course, and many occupational groups are covered by most of the laws in this category, such as the *Social Security Act,* workmens' compensation and unemployment laws and Medicare and Medicaid acts. Some of these laws, however, are related to nurses only, such as those designed to secure appropriate status for nurses in the armed services.

Under this system of classification, you will note, laws are grouped according to their *primary* objective. It might be argued, however, that practically all nursing legislation is aimed at all 3 objectives. Laws which protect the public against unqualified practitioners also protect the qualified practitioner from unfair competition and are therefore of advantage to him. Laws which relate to nursing education redound to the benefit of those who receive scholarship help and to those whose educational preparation is of higher quality because of better prepared teachers and better financed schools. Laws which promote the welfare of nurses may well have the result of attracting more people into nursing and therefore bring about more nursing care for the public. Therefore, it might be said that no real distinction can be made between legislation pertaining to nursing and legislation pertaining to nurses. Laws which advance nursing are beneficial to nurses, and laws which promote the welfare of nurses result in more and better nursing. The public-at-large is the ultimate beneficiary of all such legislation.

NURSING PRACTICE ACTS

As has been stated, the main purpose of nursing practice legislation is to protect the public against unsafe nursing care. Such legislation is the prerogative and the responsibility of the individual states. As pointed out in Chapter 6, the right of the state to enact nursing practice laws derives from its police power and from its right to legislate for the health and the welfare of its citizens. Because of it, there is a basic agreement that there will be no laws for national licensing of nurses.

All states and territories of the USA and the District of Columbia provide for the licensing of professional and practical nurses (or vocational nurses as this category of nursing personnel is called in 2 states).

Historical Aspects of Nursing Practice Legislation

Legislation to give legal recognition to workers is not a modern movement in the world. In 1874 Dr. Acland, in England, wrote that the *Medical Act of 1858* provided for women to be legally registered as medical practitioners, but no provision was made for the legal recognition of nurses.

Although Great Britain was among the 1st countries to consider nursing practice legislation, a nurses' registration bill was not passed until 1919, after a 30-year bitter struggle.

The main arguments for nursing practice legislation in the early days were twofold. It was argued that:

1. Legal recognition of the people in any profession helped to promote its efficiency.

2. The community needed to be protected against ignorant and non-qualified workers.

The essential provisions of the early nursing practice legislation placed emphasis on:

1. The regulation of nurses' practice.

2. The licensing of those who were fully trained.

3. The prescription of a minimum program of training.

4. An examination of graduates of schools on the results of their training.

5. The legal inspection and approval of schools of nursing.

6. The ensuring of an adequate supply of nurses.

Cape Town, South Africa, had the 1st law in the entire world mentioning nursing. Legal registration of nurses was introduced there under the *Medical and Pharmacy Act of 1891* through the efforts of Sister Henrietta (Miss Stockdale), an English nurse of Kimberley. New Zealand, however, passed the 1st separate nursing practice law in 1901. This was brought about through the efforts of Mrs. Grace O'Neill, an English trained nurse, who was assistant inspector of hospitals and asylums under the direction of Dr. MacGregor, who helped her to bring into existence this 1st complete nursing practice act in history.

In the USA the first nursing practice act was passed in North Carolina in 1903. Three other states passed such laws in that same year – New Jersey, Virginia and New York.

The first public statement in the USA on the subject of nursing legislation was made by Sophia Palmer, head of the City Hospital in Rochester, in a paper read in 1898 before the New York State Federation of Women's

Clubs, a very influential body. She said, "It is of vital importance that examining boards shall be selected from among nurses."[7]

It was after this that state nurses associations were organized in the USA for the primary purpose of promoting legislation for the legal control of the practice of nursing. It was thought by the members of these associations that the legal control of nursing would protect the public by guaranteeing that those practicing nursing had met certain minimum educational requirements.

The first nurse licensing laws in the USA, in each jurisdiction, were permissive. From the beginning, however, the goal was to secure mandatory nursing practice acts. However, even in 1968, only 46 such laws were mandatory in character.[8]

The majority of countries (73), in which national nursing associations had full or associate membership in the ICN, as of 1962-1963, appeared to have some kind of nursing practice legislation. In each of these countries, except 5, these nursing practice laws were administered by the national government. The nursing practice laws are administered by states, provinces, or other types of local political jurisdictions in the following countries: Australia, Canada, German Federal Republic, India and the USA. In Switzerland the Swiss Red Cross, through a mandate from the Federal Government, registers nurses. Such a registered nurse is called a Swiss Red Cross registered nurse.[9]

To round out your knowledge of the historical aspects of nursing practice legislation we suggest that you review the references listed on this subject at the end of this Chapter.

Kinds of Nursing Licensing Laws

As said elsewhere, the basic nursing licensing law in a state of the USA is the nursing practice act, which is a statute. For a discussion of types of nursing practice acts refer to Chapter 6, "Legal Issues in Nursing Practice."

Qualifications for Licensure

The methods by which a person qualifies for a license, as defined in the nursing practice acts and the rules and regulations of the licensing authorities of the various states, are, broadly speaking, similar throughout the USA. In all jurisdictions the candidate for licensure as a registered nurse must have graduated from a school of nursing which meets specified stand-

---

[7] L. L. Dock, and I. M. Stewart, *A Short History of Nursing*, New York, Putnam, 1931, p. 169.

[8] American Nurses' Association, *Facts About Nursing: A Statistical Summary*, New York, The Association, 1968, p. 54.

[9] E. K. Spalding, *Nursing Legislation and Education: A Study of the Role of National Governments and Voluntary Nursing Associations*, Washington, D.C., Catholic University of America Press, 1963.

ards, as established through the law, and must pass a written examination. Similar requirements are in effect for the licensure of those who are beginning to practice practical nursing.

Although the statuatory requirements for licensure are essentially the same in most states, the educational standards and the passing scores required on the licensing examination may vary. Because nursing education programs have been improving and because states have moved toward more uniform passing scores on the State Board Test Pool licensing examination, nurses have little or no difficulty in securing a license to practice in another state.

The basic qualifications for licensure include high school graduation or the equivalent thereof, graduation from an approved school of nursing and good moral character. Some states require that the applicant be in good mental and physical health and some require the applicant to be a citizen of the USA.

Administration of Licensing Laws

Responsibility for the administration of licensing laws in the USA for professional nursing is vested in a body that is referred to as the *state board of nursing*, although it has different titles from state to state. The state board of nursing is considered an agent of the public rather than an agent of the nursing profession. The members of the board are usually appointed by the governor of the state and confirmed by the state senate. In some states the governor makes these appointments from a list submitted by the state nurses association. The ANA believes that this is the right procedure.

Laws governing the licensing of practical nurses are administered usually by the same board that administers professional nursing licensing laws. This is the plan that is supported by the ANA. In some instances, however, a separate board has been established for this purpose.

The main function of the state board of nursing is to license persons for nursing practice. Included in this function are the evaluation of the personal and educational qualifications of persons applying for licensure, the determination of the individual's competency to engage in nursing practice, and the prosecution of persons who misrepresent or violate the proper use of their skill or who are in other ways unfit to practice nursing.[10]

For examining candidates for licensure as registered nurses, the boards in all the states in this country and some of the provinces in Canada use the same written examination—the State Board Test Pool Examination. This examination is developed by boards of nursing that are in the State Board Test Pool. The examination is serviced by the NLN Measurement and Evaluation Services, which is also responsible for scoring the results. Through the ANA Council of State Boards of Nursing, members of the boards of

---

[10] ANA Council of State Boards of Nursing, *Manual for Members of State Boards of Nursing*, New York, The Association, 1959.

nursing participate in preparing the test plan and nominate expert nurse practitioners to write questions. The state boards also review the preliminary draft of the tests. Thus, the State Board Test Pool Examination is developed by many more experts than could probably be secured by a single state board if it were to construct its own examination. Moreover, the use of a single examination furthers the progress toward more uniform licensing standards which, as has been pointed out, is of benefit to both individual nurses and the public.

Members of state boards also participate in the construction of a licensing examination for practical nurses, which is developed, administered and scored by the NLN Measurement and Evaluation Services.

So that it may evaluate the educational preparation of candidates for licensure, the state board of nursing sets up minimum standards for an "approved school of professional nursing" and an "approved school of practical nursing," evaluates all the preservice educational programs in the state which prepare nursing practitioners, and sets up lists of approved schools for the state.

From this description of the functions of state boards of nursing, it is obvious that the members of these boards must be able to make sound judgments in a wide variety of matters concerning nursing practice and nursing education. It is important for board members to have an educational preparation that qualifies them to carry on these functions.

The ANA considers it desirable that all board members be professional registered nurses. In most states this is the case. In some states physicians serve on the board. In still others the membership of the board includes practical nurses, hospital administrators and lay persons. A few states have advisory committees composed of representatives of allied health and welfare groups and the public.

Importance of Nursing Practice Acts to Nursing

You can see that licensing laws and their administration have had and continue to have a considerable effect on the progress of nursing and nursing education. If there were no such laws, anyone could call himself a nurse. Or, licensing standards could vary so from state to state that the legal titles designating nursing personnel would not have any generally accepted meaning. Or again, minimum standards for approved schools could be so detailed and rigid as to prevent much-needed experimentation in nursing education.[11]

It is, therefore, fortunate that state boards of nursing have recognized the benefits that accrue to the public, whom they serve, from their working together and with the profession. And the profession should be congratulated for its readiness to cooperate with state boards in the solution of their problems.

---

[11] In Chapter 6 you will find illustrations of legal issues and implications that point up the significance of careful preparation of bills in securing sound nursing practice acts.

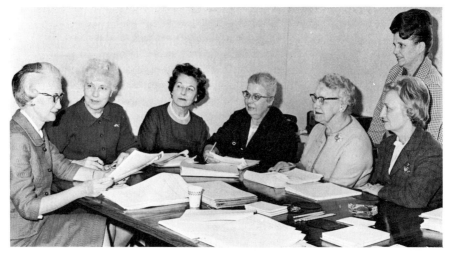

Fig. 27-1. ANA Subcommittee on Blueprint for Licensing Examinations confers on the preparation of the licensing test used in all states. (ANA)

Special mention might be made of the contribution of the ANA Council of State Boards of Nursing in furthering this cooperation. This Council is composed of professional nurse employees of boards of nursing, recommended by the respective boards and appointed by the ANA Board of Directors. This affords a means by which state board personnel from all over the country can work on common problems for the purpose of improving nursing education and practice and of contributing to the growth of the profession. The Council's functions include developing desirable and reasonable uniformity of standards, regulations, records and examinations; collecting of statistical data; recommending needed studies; promoting effective relationships with the association; and sponsoring an annual educational conference for State Boards of Nursing. A permanent subcommittee of the ANA Council on State Boards of Nursing is responsible for recommending educational standards for the use of state boards, and another committee is concerned with all aspects of the State Board Test Pool. Figure 27-1 shows an ANA subcommittee on licensing activities in action.

LICENSING AND THE INDIVIDUAL NURSE

What Do the Initials R.N. After Your Name Signify?

R.N. means *registered nurse*. It is not a degree but a legal title. These initials indicate that you have graduated from a state-approved nursing school and have met all other requirements of the nursing practice act within a state. They also mean that you are currently licensed, since they cannot be legally used by persons who have not renewed their licenses.

In some states your license must be duly registered in the county court-house office after you pass the examination. Some nurses fail to get their licenses recorded. In such instances the state boards cannot certify their licenses to other states until this is done. This creates problems, since all states do not require the recording of the license.

It is of importance to know that you are legally entitled to use the initials R.N. and to practice only within the boundaries of the state or the states in which you are registered. The initials R.N. not only denote that you have legal status, but they also signify that you can produce legal credentials. They are also an assurance to the public that you are qualified to practice as a registered nurse. Furthermore, state registration is an essential require-ment for all desirable positions in nursing, for membership in professional nursing organizations and for filing credentials with placement services for nurses.

How Do You Become Licensed?

Before you may use the letters R.N., or call yourself a registered nurse, you must pass the licensing examination, prior to which, with the coopera-tion of the director of your school of nursing, you must prepare the appli-cation to admit you to such an examination and make sure that the necessary credentials are sent in.

If you are an R.N. in one state and wish to practice nursing in another, it is necessary for you to apply for registration in that state. When requesting this application form, you might say that you wish to be "licensed by en-dorsement" or to be "licensed without examination."

You may wonder whether you can be licensed by reciprocity. Actually there is no such thing as reciprocity. Reciprocity, by definition, is a recipro-cal agreement whereby one state will do something if another state will do something in return. *Interstate licensure* is the correct term to use. Each in-dividual nurse must meet the requirements of the state to which she applies for licensure. Interstate licensure depends on the qualifications of the indi-vidual nurse, such as general education and professional education. Since you, as an individual nurse, must meet the requirements of the state to which you wish to go, you can see readily that states cannot make an agreement to exchange the courtesies of registration of all applicants without exception and irrespective of individual qualifications. For these reasons, and because the general requirements vary from state to state, it is necessary to write directly to the secretary of the state board of nursing in the state in which you desire to practice for information on the required procedure. It is im-portant that this be done prior to your arrival in the state, because some boards do not issue temporary permits, nor do they permit working until you are licensed.

The names and the addresses of the secretaries of state boards are listed in the "Official Directory" that appears in the January and July issues of the *American Journal of Nursing.*

Licensing of Nurses From Other Countries

The licensing of graduate nurses from outside our country differs in the various states. Some states give the same privileges as are given out-of-state nurses in the USA. Others think that it is too difficult to evaluate their education and insist on an examination. This does not always apply to Canada, where programs are comparable with our own. The fact that a nurse from another country becomes a citizen of the USA is, in itself, no criterion for measuring nursing competence.

FEDERAL LEGISLATION

Historical Background

The nursing profession in the USA has been active in the area of Federal legislation since about 1920. The first Federal legislation in which it became interested was the child-labor laws and the creation of the Childrens' Bureau.

The Women's Joint Congressional Committee, a clearing house for Federal legislation, composed of delegates and representatives of women's organizations such as the American Library Association and the ANA, was formed in 1920. The ANA had a representative then and has had delegates and representatives on this Committee ever since.

ANA representatives (volunteers) have appeared since 1920 as witnesses at Congressional hearings on all types of legislation that would affect health, welfare, education and nursing. However, it was not until 1951 that a full-time person, Julia C. Thompson, was stationed in Washington as a lobbyist for the ANA, which is the official spokesman for professional nurses on Federal legislation. The Washington office of the ANA continues to expand in activities and personnel. So does the New York office. Helen V. Connors presently is the director of the government relations department of the Association and is in the New York office.

Since 1951 the ANA has become increasingly active in Federal legislative matters, probably because 75 per cent, or more, of such legislation falls in categories that affect nursing and nurses.

Until 1954 ANA had 2 committees concerned with legislation, 1 with Federal and 1 with state. Since 1955 these 2 committees have been consolidated into 1 committee in order to:

1. Unify legislative efforts.

2. Get a better channel of communications to state nurses associations.

The ANA Committee on Legislation has as its functions:

1. Establishment of legislative priorities, which are reviewed each year.

2. Taking action on legislation in terms of policies and guides that have been approved by the ANA Board of Directors.

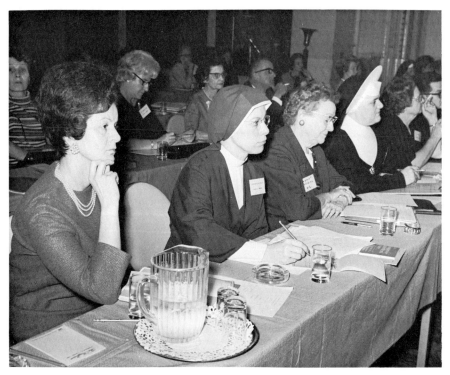

Fig. 27-2. Some Participants in ANA 1967 conference on legislation, Washington, D.C. One of the authors, Eugenia K. Spalding, is sitting 3rd from the left. (ANA)

You may wish to review some of the policies and guides which are listed at the end of this chapter under the various sections of the bibliography and suggested references.

Some direct Federal legislative concerns, among the many, of the ANA have been: Federal aid to education for nursing,[12] fair labor standards for hospital personnel, unemployment compensation, health and hospital insurance for the aged, social security, Medicare and Medicaid, community mental health centers and local teaching centers for the mentally retarded, hospital and medical facilities survey and construction, and the commissioning of men in the military nursing corps of the armed forces. Other kinds of legislation for which different groups have sought the support of the ANA are: migratory labor, child labor, food and drugs and other consumer protection, housing, accelerated public works and area redevelopment plans, school lunch programs, industrial safety, radiation safety, equal pay for equal work, adult literacy testing, retraining of youth, Peace Corps, human rights, War on Poverty, fair housing programs, manpower training and civil rights.

[12] A brief history of Federal financial aid to education for nursing appears in an unpublished master's dissertation (1961) by Sister Mary Jean Roth, which can be borrowed from the library of the Catholic University of America, Washington, D.C. The title of this report is *Federal Legislation Authorizing Financial Aid to Education for Nursing from 1935 to 1960: Purposes, Provisions, and Administration.*

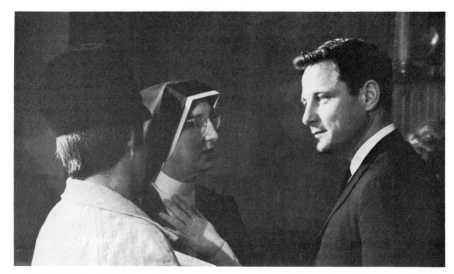

Fig. 27-3. Sister Delphine of Indianapolis discussing civil rights problems with Senator Birch Bayh of Indiana after presenting testimony on the *Civil Rights Bill* at a congressional hearing. (ANA)

The ANA has held 6 national conferences since 1950 to help nurses to develop skills and to increase their involvement in legislative matters, Federal and state (See Figure 27-2). The reports of these conferences (1954, 1958, 1961, 1963, 1965, 1967) are interesting and educational reading. These conferences will be held about every 2 years in the future. We suggest that you watch for the reports of them because a review of these is a good way to keep up-to-date. Reading of "At Press Time" in each issue of the *American Journal of Nursing* also would be very helpful in keeping you informed on current Federal legislation affecting nursing and nurses. *Capital Commentary,* distributed by the Government Relations Department of the ANA, also would be helpful.

The late Representative John Fogary said: "If every nurse in the country wrote to her Congressman on Federal legislation of concern to nurses they could have what they want."[13] However, it requires: (1) knowing the facts in the situation, (2) having an informed membership and (3) having a logical plan of action. Figures 27-3, 27-4, and 27-5 show various aspects of the ANA legislative program.

Federal Legislation Relating to Nursing Education

Unless we look up the statistics on financing of education, we tend to think that most young people or their families bear the costs of their edu-

[13] From notes taken by one of the authors on a lecture by Julia Thompson on "Legislation in Nursing" given to a class at the School of Nursing, The Catholic University of America, Washington, D.C., March 31, 1962.

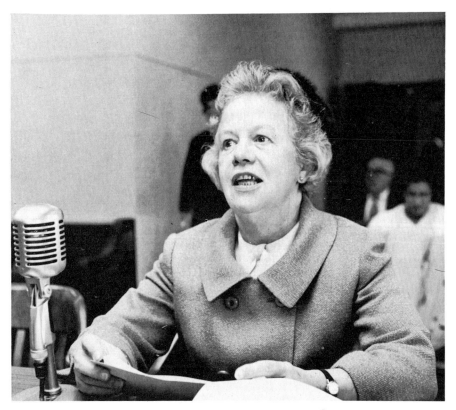

Fig. 27-4. Helen V. Connors, Director of Government Relations Department of the ANA, presenting testimony before a New York State committee in the legislature. (ANA)

Fig. 27-5. Testifying on behalf of ANA before U.S. Department of Health, Education, and Welfare officials in the Federal Court House, New York, Mrs. Eva Reese (right), a member of ANA's Commission on Nursing Services, protests Medicaid cutbacks. (ANA)

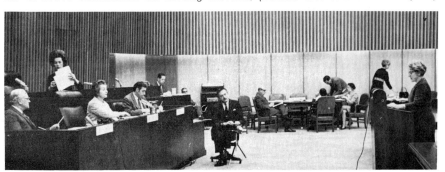

cation after high school. Actually, this is only partly true. Although they usually pay tuition fees, these fees, on the average, cover less than half the expense of their college education. The rest of the cost is covered by public funds, in the case of state, county, and municipal institutions, and, in private colleges and universities, by gifts from private individuals and groups and by income from endowments.

Nursing education is an exception to this general rule. The majority of educational programs in nursing are conducted by private rather than by public institutions and therefore are not supported by tax monies. Few of them have endowment funds. As long ago as 1950 it was estimated that only 7 per cent of the cost of nursing education was borne by the public through public funds or private donations.

This being the case, and because the public has such a great stake in the maintenance of an adequate supply of nursing personnel, it is appropriate that legislation be enacted for the financial assistance of educational programs in nursing and of students in these programs.

Both the state and the Federal governments have recognized the importance of such assistance. In some states the state government gives support to the schools of nursing in the state by paying them annually an amount for each student. Appropriations for scholarships have been voted by state legislatures for both preservice and graduate nurse students.

Except during World War II, when the U.S. Cadet Nurse program was in effect, Federal assistance for the development of preservice educational programs in nursing has been directed almost entirely toward educational programs to produce practical nurses. However, in 1963 the *Health Professions Educational Assistance Act (Public Law 88-129)* was passed. This law provided construction grants to schools of medicine, dentistry, public health, osteopathy, and to collegiate schools of nursing. Considerable recognition has been given to the need for helping graduate nurses to prepare for leadership positions in nursing. Through such legislation as the *Social Security Act (1935)* and the *Mental Health Act (1946)*, nurses as well as other health personnel have been given traineeships for preparing themselves in certain fields. Perhaps the greatest boost for graduate education for nurses to date was the passage, in 1956, of the *Health Amendments Act (Public Law 911)*. In 1959 the nurse traineeship section of *Public Law 911* was renewed as a separate law, *Public Law 105*. Under these 2 laws thousands of nurses have been enabled to prepare for administrative, supervisory, and teaching positions in nursing. In 1964 the ANA recommended that this legislation be expanded to include nursing specialists in clinical fields.

Public Law 88-581 or the *Nurse Training Act of 1964* was passed by the Congress on August 21, 1964, and was signed into Law by President Johnson on September 4, 1964. Some major provisions of the law are: supplying of funds for construction of teaching facilities for collegiate, associate degree and hospital schools of nursing; supplying of funds for a program of project grants for the improvement of nurse training in these schools; grants to hospital schools of nursing to defray a portion of the cost of training students of nursing; extension for 5 years of the professional nurse-traineeship program; loans to needy students of nursing in collegiate, associate degree and hospital schools of nursing; and an Advisory Council on Nurse Training to advise the Surgeon General of the Public Health Service on regulations and policies needed to administer the *Act* and to review applications for construction and for improvement of nurse training.

In 1968, the *Health Manpower Act of 1968* was signed into law *(Public Law 90-490)* by President Johnson. This Act continued and amended 4 major health programs, one of which was the *Nurse Training Act of 1964*. It extended Federal aid to nurse training through the fiscal years 1970 and 1971.[14] Later the same year, Congress appropriated $35,913,000 for 1969 for nursing education, which included $6.5 million in scholarships for needy students and more than $10 million for traineeships for professional nurses.[15] It will be helpful if you check each year to determine changes brought about through new Federal legislation on education for nursing.

This legislation relating to nursing education did not come about by chance. Behind its passage lies a vast amount work by the ANA, which has pressed continuously the needs of nursing education before legislative bodies, and by the NLN, which has amassed quantities of statistical data which give evidence of these needs. Because of the energy and the persistence of these organizations, you are probably receiving a better education from better prepared teachers than might otherwise have been available to you. In turn, you will be able to give your patients better care.

LEGISLATION AFFECTING THE WELFARE OF NURSES

To list and describe all the social welfare legislation that the Federal and state governments have enacted in recent years would require a number of books, particularly since legislation of this type varies considerably from state to state. Included in this category of legislation are social security laws (including Medicare), workmen's compensation laws, unemployment compensation laws, wage and hour laws, equal opportunity laws, labor-management relations laws and fair employment laws. Federal laws that now apply to most nurses include the *Equal Opportunity Law* (Title VII of the *Civil Rights Act of 1964)* and the *Wage and Hour Law (Fair Labor Standards*

[14] "President Signs Bill Aiding Nurse Education," *American Journal of Nursing,* **68:**2063, Oct. 1968.
[15] "Congress Votes $35,913,000 for Aid to Nurse Education," *American Journal of Nursing,* **68:**2503, Dec. 1968.

Act as amended in 1966). State laws in these same subject areas take precedence over Federal law when the state laws meet certain standards. For you to know just what rights you are entitled to under this type of legislation you should become acquainted with the provisions of these laws in your state.

A study of your state laws would probably reveal that nurses are not covered by some of them. Shorter working hours for nurses generally have been achieved through a program of education sponsored by the ANA rather than through legal compulsion. What may surprise you is that you will find yourself barred from some privileges to which other professional people and even other nurses are entitled because of the kind of organization for which you work.

In particular, you will probably find that the labor-management relations act in your state follows the Federal law in excluding employees of nonprofit hospitals from the benefits of its provisions. This law was designed primarily to protect employees in their right to organize, to choose their own representatives and to negotiate or bargain collectively. The exemption of nonprofit hospitals from its provisions takes from the majority of nurses the rights that are given to practically every other employee group. They are important rights, too. The ANA considers collective bargaining one of the tools for furthering the economic welfare of nurses. The right of nurses employed by nonprofit hospitals to bargain is now protected by the laws of 10 states (including Puerto Rico). In 6 states, nonprofit hospitals are not subject to the provisions of the state law. In the remaining states there is no applicable statute.

NARCOTIC LAWS

Illegal possession or use of narcotics is a crime of which a nurse may be guilty. It is very important that you know the provisions of the *Harrison Narcotic Law*. This act is set up to direct the manufacture and the distribution of narcotics through medical channels for medical purposes. According to the terms of this act, you may legally possess drugs only if you are so authorized by Federal license or if you are a patient or an agent of a licensed physician. As an agent, you may have only those drugs that are prescribed for your patient; and at the end of the case, or if you leave before the case is ended, you must give all the narcotics in your possession to the physician whose agent you are. Ignorance of the nature of the drugs you are handling or of the terms of the *Harrison Narcotic Law* will not be accepted as an excuse for violating this act.

In addition to the *Harrison Narcotic Law*, there are the following narcotic statutes: the *Narcotic Drugs Import and Export Act* and the *Uniform State Narcotics Act*. Information on Federal narcotic regulations may be secured from the district supervisor of the U.S. Bureau of Narcotics.

OBLIGATIONS OF THE INDIVIDUAL NURSE

From this it will be apparent that the ANA is always "on the job" protecting your legislative interests, whether they are at stake in a bill or law that applies to nursing only or in one that applies to a large group that does or should include nursing. Through this organization a single nurse or a small group of nurses can have the advantage of the combined strength of a large number of nurses. If you feel that you, as only one person, cannot make your voice heard in a legislative matter that concerns nursing or nurses, it might be well for you to participate in the legislative program of your professional organization.

The following is an excellent reference to review in connection with the nurse's responsibility as a citizen and her place in the political world: J. J. Albrect, "The Nurse as a Citizen or Politics is the Art of the Possible," *Maryland Nursing News*, **37**:6-21, Spring 1969.

This is one way you might begin to prepare yourself for such participation. Be sure to know the procedure of the legislature or Congress for the introduction of a bill and the steps leading to enactment. Keep informed on all nursing legislative problems and activities so that you can take part in group discussions for the purpose of arriving at worth-while solutions of the issues involved. You can do this by reading news on legislation in current issues of nursing, medical, and allied periodicals, by reading and analyzing bills, and by attending nursing meetings where such items are reviewed and considered. It is important for you and for every nurse to be able to interpret legislative issues to those from whom you wish support or defeat of bills. You also have an obligation to serve on legislative committees when asked to do so. You should be willing to do all in your power to advance sound and desirable legislation and to defeat undesirable and unfavorable legislation, for it is only through the combined efforts of all nurses that the true goals of nursing can be attained.

You may be asked to assist with the writing of testimony for use at Congressional or state legislative committee hearings. This requires the ability to analyze bills in the light of current principles and practices of nursing service and nursing education and to be able to write clearly and tersely in relation to the pros and cons of bills under consideration. If you are asked to present the testimony at legislative hearings, you will need to speak well and to answer questions relative to the proposed legislation spontaneously and to the point.

If you live in the vicinity of Washington, D.C., or if you plan to visit the capital city, it is suggested that you arrange for visits to the White House, some Congressional Committee hearings, the Senate, the House and the Supreme Court. You will find these rewarding experiences. It may be helpful to read Zinn's *How Our Laws are Made* (1969) in preparation for the proposed visits to Capitol Hill. Anyone who has ever worked in legislative programs can tell you, if you have not had this great opportunity and privilege, how exciting and worthwhile such an activity can be.

Chapter 17 discusses the leadership role of the professional nurse in some detail. You may wish to read it in connection with this Chapter.

PROBLEMS

1. (a) Read the article by Helen Creighton, entitled "Nursing Ethics and the Law" which begins on page 8 of the March 1960 issue of the *American Association of Industrial Nurses Journal.* (b) Create your own definitions showing the distinction between ethics and law.

2. (a) What are the provisions of the nursing practice act of your state, and when was it enacted? (b) What are the weaknesses of your present nursing practice act? (c) What are its good points? (d) Is the definition in your state law in accordance with that advocated by the ANA?

3. Suppose you live in Georgia and have just secured a position as an instructor in a nursing school in Colorado. What procedure should you follow to become a registered nurse in Colorado?

4. (a) If you were serving on a legislative committee in your state nurses association and were asked to assist in drafting a bill for introduction to the legislature, what steps would you take? (b) How does a bill become a law in your state?

5. (a) What is the difference between state accredited schools of nursing and those accredited by the NLN, a voluntary association? (b) Some nurses have proposed legislation that would require schools of nursing (professional, practical, or vocational) to be accredited by the NLN as a requirement for licensure of their graduates. This requirement would replace the present one, which requires surveying of these schools by the board of nursing employees as a basis of state board approval. What do you think of this idea?

6. Read the 1963 book by Eugenia K. Spalding, *Nursing Legislation and Education: A Study of the Role of National Governments and Voluntary Nursing Associations.* (a) Note how the role of government relative to nursing practice laws vary from country to country. (b) Compare the role of governments and national nursing associations in their legislative functions.

7. (a) What state in the USA passed the first law that specifically establishes the obligation of employers in nonprofit and proprietary hospitals and nursing homes to bargain with nurses? When did this occur? (b) What are the provisions of this *Act?* (c) What other states have similar legislation?

8. How have the following Federal acts and their revision influenced nursing? (a) *Mental Health Act (1946);* (b) *Hospital Construction Act (1946)* and its amendments; (c) *Health Amendments Act (1956);* (d) *Health Professions Educational Assistance Act (1963);* (e) *Mental Retardation Facilities Construction Act (1963);* (f) *Nurse Training Act (1964);* (g) *Fair Labor Standards Act (1966);* (h) *Regional Medical Programs Legislation (1968);* (i) *Health Manpower Act of 1966.*

9. (a) Under which occupational category do nurses come in the *Fair Labor Act?* (b) How did the *Taft-Hartley Act* affect nurses and other hospital personnel? (c) What is the present status of legislation relative to fair labor practices for hospital employees?

10. (a) What are the current provisions for Medicare and Medicaid? (b) Why is it important for nurses to be familiar with these provisions?

11. (a) What proposed legislation pertaining to health is now being considered by a Congressional committee or on the floor of the House of Representatives or the Senate? (b) Select 1 such piece of proposed legislation and write a letter to your Congressman or one of your state senators pointing out why its passage or defeat is in the best interest of the public.

12. How can voluntary professional and governmental health groups exercise control over standards for nursing care in nursing homes through systems of legal recognition of nursing personnel and accreditation programs?

13. The National Consumer's League led the successful effort to create the U.S. Children's Bureau over 50 years ago. (a) What are the League's current purposes? (b) Who are some nationally prominent members of the League?

14. On November 8, 1967, President Johnson signed into law a bill giving women in the armed forces equal opportunity with their male counterparts. For what does this law provide?

15. (a) What were the provisions of the Federal emergency assistance to states that caused widespread civil disorders in the Spring of 1968? (b) Why is it that the civil rights laws have not prevented such disorders and that civil disobedience has been on the increase in this country?

16. Discuss the contributions to nursing of the *Nurse Training Act of 1964* and the implications of the Act as extended and amended in the *Health Manpower Act of 1968 (Public Law 90-490)*.

17. The *Health Manpower Act of 1968* deleted the authority of the Commissioner of Education to accredit nursing education programs for purposes of receiving Federal funds (the Commissioner had previously delegated this authority to the NLN). Under the 1968 law an accredited program is defined as one accredited by an accrediting body of a state agency or a school of nursing, college, or university accredited by a recognized accrediting body. What are the disadvantages of this arrangement?

18. Among pertinent issues discussed by the Congress of the USA during the past several years have been the following: peace, disarmament, human rights (United Nations conventions), world trade, racism, anti-poverty programs, revised welfare system, education, treatment of crime, law enforcement, safety measures and national defense. (a) With which of these have nurses as health workers, been especially concerned? (b) What other issues (domestic and international) have been discussed recently by the Congress?

19. Which of the 2 national organizations (ANA and NLN) is tax exempt? (b) What is the significance of this status? (c) Who testifies for the nursing

profession on Federal legislative proposals for nursing? (d) What is the principal government agency that testifies at such hearings? (e) Who are the current ANA delegates and representatives on the Women's Joint Congressional Committee?

20. (a) Who have been the important leaders in nursing legislation in your state? (b) in the USA? (c) Discuss the legislative contribution or activities of the following: Bernice E. Anderson; Honorable Clinton P. Anderson; Wilbur J. Cohen; Helen V. Connors; Helen Creighton; Nathan Hershey; Honorable Lister Hill; Mrs. Virginia Knauer; Jean MacVicar; Honorable Wilber Mills; William C. Scott; Eleanor J. Smith; Eugenia K. Spalding; Honorable Harley Staggers; Julia C. Thompson; Sidney Willig.

SUGGESTED REFERENCES*

GENERAL

* American Nurses' Association. *Proceedings of the ANA Conference on Legislation, 1967*. New York, The Association, 1967.
_____. *Proceedings of ANA Conference on Legislation, 1965*. New York, The Association, 1965.
* _____. *Proceedings of the ANA Conference on Legislation, March 20-22, 1963, Washington, D.C.* New York, The Association, 1963.
_____. *Report of Conference on Legislation, March 22-24, 1961, Washington, D.C.* New York, The Association, 1961.
_____. *Report of Conference on Legislation, March 1958, Washington, D.C.* New York, The Association, 1958.
_____. *Report of Conference on Legislation, March 1954, Washington, D.C.* New York, The Association, 1954.
The Constitution of the United States of America. Washington, D.C., Government Printing Office, 1967.
The Constitution of the United States of America: Analysis and Interpretation. Washington, D.C., Government Printing Office, 1964.
Enactment of a Law: Procedural Steps in the Legislative Process. Washington, D.C., Government Printing Office, 1967.
*Inaugural Addresses of the Presidents of the United States of America. Washington, D.C., Government Printing Office, 1965.
*League of Women Voters of the United States. Choosing the President. Washington, D.C., The League, 1968.
Nomination and Election of the President and Vice President of the United States. Washington, D.C., Government Printing Office, 1968.
Our American Government: What is It? How Does It Function? Washington, D.C., Government Printing Office, 1967.
Samson, M. E. "From Bill to Law." *Nursing Outlook,* **16:**24-26, Dec. 1968.
United States Government Organization Manual, 1968-1969. Washington, D.C., Government Printing Office, 1968.
* Zinn, C. J. *How Our Laws are Made.* Washington, D.C., Government Printing Office, 1969.

---

* In each chapter all citations are footnoted and are not included here. All starred references are recommended for additional reading.

HISTORICAL BACKGROUND

Brown, E. L. *Nursing for the Future.* New York, Russell Sage Foundation, 1948. pp. 66-72.

Burgess, E. C. "What are Nurses Going to do About It?" *American Journal of Nursing,* **32:**553-556, May 1932.

Dock, L. L. "What We May Expect from the Law." *American Journal of Nursing,* **1:**8-12, Oct. 1900.

_____., and Stewart, I. M. *A Short History of Nursing.* New York, Putnam, 1931. pp. 168-170, 241-283.

Goldmark, J. *Nursing and Nursing Education in the United States.* New York, Macmillan, 1923. pp. 14-16, 26-28.

McManus, R. L. "The State Board Test Pool." *American Journal of Nursing,* **44:**380-384, Apr. 1964.

Nutting, M. A. and Dock, L. L. *A History of Nursing.* vol. III, New York, Putnam, 1912. pp. 30-61, 142-187.

Roberts, M. M. *American Nursing: History and Interpretation.* New York, Macmillan, 1954. pp. 72-75, 106-115, 127, 407.

Seymer, L. R. *A General History of Nursing.* New York, Macmillan, 1933. pp. 248-259.

Spalding, E. K. "Report of Committee to Prepare a Statement of Objectives Concerning Federal Aid for Nursing Education." *Annual Report and Record of Proceedings of Fifty-second Convention of National League of Nursing Education.* New York, The League, 1948. pp. 223-226.

Stewart, I. M. and Austin, A. *A History of Nursing.* New York, Putnam, 1962. pp. 167-169, 174-175, 223, 259-265, 269-271, 281, 290-294.

NURSING PRACTICE LEGISLATION

* American Nurses' Association. *Examination for State Licensure to Practice Nursing.* New York, The Association, n.d.

_____. *The Philosophy of Professional Licensure.* New York, The Association, n.d.

_____. "Nursing Concerns in the Home Health Services in Health Insurance for the Aged." *American Journal of Nursing,* **65:**72-73, Nov. 1965.

_____. *Nursing Practice Acts. Suggestions for Major Provisions to be Included.* New York, The Association, 1964.

_____. *Social Legislation and Nursing Practice.* New York, The Association, 1960.

* _____. *Principles of Legislation Relating to the Practice of Nursing. Ibid.,* Jan. 1958.

Kinney, L. B. "Professional Standards: Through Licensure or Certification?" *American Journal of Nursing,* **65:**118-121, Oct. 1965.

"Licensure of Nurses from Other Lands." *American Journal of Nursing,* **54:**1228-1231, Oct. 1954.

"Registered Nurses Responsibilities and Duties as Related to the Medical Practice Act." *Maryland Medical Journal,* **17:**80-82, Feb. 1968.

STATE BOARDS OF NURSING

American Nurses' Association. *Proceedings of Educational Conference for State Boards of Nursing, New York, 1967.* New York, The Association, 1967.

_____. *Proceedings of Educational Conference for State Boards of Nursing, San Francisco, 1966.* New York, The Association, 1966.

_____. *Proceedings of Educational Conference for State Boards of Nursing, San Francisco, 1965.* New York, The Association, 1965.

_____. *Proceedings of Work Conference on Survey Techniques for School Visitors.* New York, The Association, 1964.

_____. *Handbook on Policies, Functions and Activities of the ANA Council of State Boards of Nursing.* New York, The Association, 1963. (In process of revision.)

Baldwin, J. P., *et al.* "Factors Influencing Performance on State Board Test Pool Examinations." *Nursing Research,* **17**:170-172, Apr. 1968.

Barhan, V. Z. "State Board Examinations—Licensure and Yield." *National League for Nursing Conference Papers,* **27**:39, 1968.

Culver, V. M. "Flexible State Board Standards." *Nursing Outlook,* **12**:43-45, June 1964.

DeTornyay, R. "State Board Member." *American Journal of Nursing,* **69**:570-572, Mar. 1969.

"Directory of Practical Nursing State Associations and State Boards of Nursing." *Journal of Practical Nursing,* **18**:31-32, Feb. 1968.

Eskow, S. "State Board Examinations and Licensure and Yield." *National League for Nursing Conference Papers,* **24**-26, 1968.

"Let's Examine ... PNG, HSR and Licensure Results." *Nursing Outlook,* **15**:66, Nov. 1967.

FEDERAL LEGISLATION: GENERAL

* AFL-CIO. Department of Legislation. *Labor Looks at the 90th Congress: An AFL-CIO Legislative Report.* Washington, D.C., American Federation of Labor and Congress of Industrial Relations, Dec. 1968. Published annually.

* Albrect, J. J. "The Nurse as a Citizen or Politics is the Art of the Possible." *Maryland Nursing News,* **37**:9-21, Spring 1969.

Congressional Record: Proceedings and Debates of the Congress. Washington, D.C., Government Printing Office. Published daily while the Congress is in session.

Friend's Committee on National Legislation. *How to Visit Your Congressman.* Washington, D.C., The Committee, June 1962.

How to Find U.S. Statutes and U.S. Code Citations. Washington, D.C., Government Printing Office, 1965.

Library of Congress. *The Capitol.* 2 vols. Washington, D.C., Government Printing Office, 1964.

FEDERAL LEGISLATION: HEALTH AND NURSING

* American Nurses' Association. *Capital Commentary.* New York, The Association. Published monthly.

* At Press Time. *American Journal of Nursing.* Appears monthly.

"Federal Funds for Nursing Education." *American Journal of Nursing,* **68**:312-315, Feb. 1968.

* Gerds, G. *et al.* "Every Nurse a Lobbyist." *American Journal of Nursing,* **60**:1242-1245, Sept. 1960.

Hamilton, Dr. T. S. "Modern Medicine Requires Qualified Nurses." *Today's Health,* **41**:76, Aug. 1963.

U.S. Department of Health, Education, and Welfare. Public Health Service. *Nurse Training Act of 1964.* Washington, D.C., Government Printing Office, Dec. 1967.

_____. *Facts About the Hill-Burton Program.* Washington, D.C., The Service, 1964.

* _____. Surgeon General's Consultant Group. *Toward Quality Nursing.* Washington, D.C., Government Printing Office, 1963.

CHAPTER

28

Public Relations
in Nursing

What is the meaning of *public relations*? What is meant by *publicity*? What is *news*? What is the difference between these terms? These and similar questions arise when any nursing group plans a public information or, to use a better term, a public relations program. This chapter discusses some of the questions which arise and suggests their solution.

DEFINITIONS

Public Relations in Nursing

Public relations in nursing involves helping the members of the profession, members of groups associated with the profession, prospective students of nursing, and the public, or consumers of nursing, to understand the aims of nursing and the ways in which the members of these groups can assist in the achievement of these aims. It also involves securing reactions from these groups about the various phases of nursing with which they are concerned.

Distinctions Between *News, Publicity,* and *Public Relations*

News is a factual account of something new in the way of information touching on the general interests of those who learn about it. This means that it has to be prepared with the "learner" in mind. We who are not shoemakers are not interested in a new way to make shoes unless it means shoes will be cheaper, prettier, or more comfortable. If we accept this meaning of *news*, it must touch on our interests in beauty, economy and comfort.

If this is a correct belief about the meaning of *news*, then it follows that publicity must always be news. *Publicity* has a 3-fold meaning. It is the function of preparing news about an organization or an institution for publication. It is the act of placing this news before the public. It is the published result of news about an organization or an institution.

Public relations is interpreting the program of an organization to the public and educating the public about the aims and needs of the organization; it also is interpreting to the organization the needs of the public and its reactions to the organization's program. It is often an administrative function which: (1) evaluates the attitudes of the various publics with which the organization is concerned; (2) identifies the objectives, policies, and practices of the organization with the interests of the public; and (3) executes a program of action that will earn on its merits public understanding and public acceptance. On the other hand, it is also a function of every nurse in all of her contacts with the public.

Public relations is not "engineering the consent" of the public to accept an idea or to do something, as commonly is thought. It is not publicity. It is not lavish entertainment of people for the contribution they might make in return. It is not propaganda. Basically, it is the establishment of a climate of mutual understanding.

With this understanding of what public relations is and what it is not, you can see that everything an organization does in its public relations program must be in harmony with a basic purpose—improvement of its program.

Too often in our desires to impress an understanding of our organizational work or activities on the public, we assume that what is most important to us is equally as important to the public. An exaggeration of this attitude often results in bad public relations, even though excellent tools have been employed. There are occasions when those in charge of the public relations program, who must be objective all the time, need to be negative and say, "We don't want to emphasize this project or policy. . . . Yes, it is a big issue for us, but the public, lacking our specialized experience, will not understand or appreciate the finely drawn points we wish to make."

On the other hand, the ability of the public to understand technical advances should not be underestimated. This is particularly true in the health sciences. Since the promotion of health has become recognized as a national concern, and with the advent of newer methods of health education via radio and television, the public has developed a fairly sophisticated background of understanding about health practices on which new ideas can be built.

News and publicity are some of the tools by which a successful public relations program may be carried out by organizations, or other groups of nurses. Some hospitals today are using closed circuit TV within the hospital to interpret the hospital and the work of its personnel to patients and their families and friends.

The well-informed nurse is one of the most effective public relations tools we have in the profession. By her actions and her interpretation of nursing to others, she can do much to establish the image of nursing we wish the public to have. Her own pride in the profession and in herself as a nurse will be "caught" by others.

Nursing has several publics: the prospective student, the student of nursing, the nurse, the medical profession, other health professions and allied groups, and the public which constitutes the users of nursing service. This chapter deals primarily with public relations in regard to this last group.

PUBLIC RELATIONS PROGRAMS FOR NURSING

Why Should the Public Be Told About Nursing?

The right of the public to be told about nursing with its aims, needs and available services is based on several facts. The public is the purchaser of patient care and all types of nursing service. It helps to support nursing education, and from the public comes the supply of nurses. Furthermore, the public consists of potential patients, and it should know the types of nursing care available and how to get that care at the most reasonable cost. The public's stake in nursing cannot be overlooked, since its welfare is affected by the quality and the quantity of nursing service given. Therefore, the nurse has the responsibility of helping to educate the public with respect to its cooperation with the nurse in establishing or maintaining the quality of nursing required and in supplying nursing service to meet the public's nursing needs. It is a 2-way process.

The nursing profession needs the intelligent interest and cooperation of the public to promote adequate laws and to develop good educational facilities and nurse-placement agencies that will provide satisfactory distribution of nursing services. Therefore, the public must be told by those who are best qualified to speak — representatives of the nursing profession itself.

It is well to think of the public as a friend to whom you can tell the interesting news of the day's work. Of course, *news* and *publicity* might be put out on the basis that the public is a *supporter* or a *purchaser,* or "has the right to know." But the public is interested in people, and if the individual nurse is regarded as an interesting individual instead of as a cog in the machinery that goes into operation when accident or illness strikes, then nursing as a whole will benefit.

But it is wise to remember that regardless of how interesting nursing may be, the public is interested in it primarily as a service from which it can benefit, as its increasing interest in group hospitalization and in voluntary and compulsory health insurance, such as Medicare, has testified. It is through appealing to this interest that public relations for nursing will benefit. Participation by the public in activities of nursing organizations or institutions is an important mechanic in public relations. Actually, it is one of the most important means for maintaining sound public relations.

Who Is Responsible For Telling the Public About Nursing?

The responsibility for public relations programs that affect nursing as a whole must be assumed by the national nursing organizations. These organizations can provide a backdrop of information about broad national problems. They can, for example, help to bring about a better understanding of the relationship between the economic security of nurses or the better education of nurses and the quantity and quality of nursing care that is available to the public. They can arouse the interest of young people in selecting a career in nursing.

However, it is up to local groups and individual nurses to paint in the foreground of this picture. They can show the people in their communities how directly they are affected by the conditions in the nursing services and schools of nursing which serve them and how they can help to improve these conditions. They can help the young people whom they know personally to decide on a career and to choose a school in which to prepare for this career. They can help each member of the public, as he is confronted with information about the relation of the public to nursing, to think, "This means me."

It is well to remember, too, that nursing services are part of the broad welfare services which the community furnishes its members and that nursing education is a part of all higher education. Through participation in community health and welfare councils and groups concerned with post-high school education, nurses can help these groups to incorporate information about nursing in their public relations activities. Nursing's potential contribution to the rehabilitation of patients not only is a story in itself but is part of the bigger story of all the rehabilitative efforts made in hospitals, retraining centers, sheltered workshops and so on. The need for scholarships for students of nursing can be presented in pleas for scholarship help for various other groups of young people who are preparing to fill important roles in our society.

MEDIA FOR REACHING THE PUBLIC

If you were serving on a public relations committee, your first consideration would be to decide on the objectives of your particular public relations program. Included in these objectives would be the messages you wish to convey to the public. Then you would consider the means by which you could deliver these messages.

Newspapers

One way you can tell your story to the public is through the newspaper. News writing is an art in itself. Do not be misled by the simple arrangement of the completed stories you read in your daily paper. Only by long and laborious practice can you get all that you wish to say into the small space which newspapers can afford to give to their stories. Every word counts, and the editorial blue pencil eliminates all but the most essential.

The best way to acquire this art is to read the papers in your community and perhaps some outstanding newspapers from our largest cities. Clip news of the type you are interested in reproducing, and when the time comes to prepare an item concerning professional group and individual activities, follow the form acceptable to the paper to which it will be sent.

When newspaper reporters and publicity consultants write for the public, they assume that the reader never heard of the subject, knows nothing about it, and must be given full and complete information concerning it. They also know that the public does not understand technical terms, so they substitute more common words or define their terms. The first paragraph in a news-paper article is called the *lead*. It should tell *who, what, when, where* and *how,* and sometimes *why.* Nothing is taken for granted. As a result, each news story is complete in itself.

The news story form is the most natural form for telling about an occurrence. When you tell a friend of an event, you usually tell the most important or interesting thing first. Then you establish the time and the place and perhaps the persons concerned. When giving names, be sure to use full names and correct titles. Now you are ready to go into details. As you study news articles in newspapers, you will note that they do exactly that — only in a little more formal language than you use in conversation. In addition, a news story is constructed paragraph by paragraph in such a manner that the newspaper may cut the story without destroying its continuity. The first 2 paragraphs are the most important and should contain all of the pertinent facts. A study of what the paper prints and how it prints it is an excellent guide as to the way in which the story meets the requirements established by the individual paper.

Feature articles — either the short human-interest stories or the longer informational pieces that are not "spot" news but are mostly for background — may follow other patterns. They range from the story in a news pattern because it is tied to the news, through the chronological account, to the story with a surprise ending. Complete information on the source of the news is given, including the name of the person who is responsible for the release. In your own case, all that would probably be necessary would be the name of the organization you represent, the release date, your own name, and the telephone number in the upper left-hand corner.

After the first few releases, provided they are strictly factual and authoritative and are written without personal bias or opinion, your contacts should be well established. Type your stories on one side of the paper only. Begin your story, leaving the top one third of the paper blank for headlines. Do not write heads. Newspapers employ copy editors for this purpose. Use triple space. Write "more" at the lower right-hand corner of each sheet. Number each page and plainly indicate the end of the story. Each page ending should also be a paragraph ending. A *short* story always is preferred. Find out the *deadline* (the hour beyond which stories cannot be accepted). If possible, see that your copy to the paper is sent so as to arrive at least 24 hours before the deadline of a daily edition. Use mail or delivery service to the city room. Also, copy should be directed to city desks rather than to individuals (who may be sick or out-of-town). It is a good idea to send a copy of what is sent to the city editor, to the medical, or to other interested editors, if indicated. You can obtain their names by calling the newspaper. Remember that a story delivered soon after a meeting will get better space than one that is a day or two late. If the community has an evening paper, 12 hours is the life of a news story, such as reports of meetings, elections and similar events. Whenever a talk is to be delivered at a meeting, try to get an advance copy. If this is sent to the press with a statement as to when it will be given, a brief biographical sketch of the speaker, and a picture, if possible, the chances of coverage are increased considerably. In the case of Sunday editions, submit the copy from 3 to 5 days in advance, since most newspapers start setting up their Sunday editions by the middle of the week. If you are in an area where there are both morning and evening papers, try to give papers in each group a share of first releases. If you release a story to evening papers first, write a slightly different story for morning papers following.

Newspaper titles are not always fully descriptive, but usually your contact for ordinary news stories will be with the city editor. You should call or see him first. On some small newspapers the managing editor or the editor acts as the city editor. He may ask you to telephone or give your material regularly to a certain staff member, but he always will be willing to discuss special problems with you. Some of your strictly organizational material may be routed through the woman's editor or the society editor. Newspapers with Sunday editions frequently have a Sunday editor responsible for the feature or the magazine sections. Talk to him occasionally, especially about items that he may use for larger features on anniversaries or other important occasions. When you are engaged in a campaign, discuss your goals with the editor (editor-in-chief), for he has responsibility for editorial page expression. For example, if you are trying to recruit young men and women as nurses, it is the editor who can write an editorial appealing directly to the public to support you. He can express opinions that his news writers cannot.

If you are on a state or a district committee of a nursing organization, you may find that cooperation with the major press associations — AP (Associated Press), and UPI (United Press International), INS (International News Service) — will facilitate the distribution of legitimate news and features to newspapers in your area. Each service has one or more bureaus in each state, at the state capital and in the larger cities, presided over by a chief of bureau or a manager. He can help you. If you are an officer of an association, remember that an opinion from you, for example on legislation, often may be news.

If your newspaper carries a letter column, this often may be used to get across a message to the public directly. It also may be used to compliment those who help in public service or to complain when public officials or law-makers fail to give the cooperation deserved.

If a newspaper wants to do a story that you think may not be helpful to nursing, assist it in getting the facts needed to print an unbiased story. How-ever, it is wise not to make a nuisance of yourself or your cause. It needs to be remembered that the nursing group is one of many competing for space.

In local or area publicity efforts, do not overlook weekly newspapers, em-ployee publications in industrial plants, and publications of civic groups.

If you are nursing a patient, newspapers may call you for information regarding him, particularly if he is a prominent citizen or has figured in a news story, such as an accident. It is usually advisable to refer such inquiries to the attending physician and to the hospital administrator. In referring the inquiring reporter to the proper source of information, remember that he is doing his job, just as you are, and is not "snooping." By treating him cour-teously and helping him in whatever way you can, you are helping to create good will for the nursing profession and the hospital or agency with the working press.

It is well to remember also, when planning news releases or a publicity campaign, that stories and pictures of children and animals have a great appeal to the press and to the general reader. If you recall your current reading, you undoubtedly will remember that stories of children with rare ailments being rushed from the 4 corners of the world to clinics and spe-cialists for treatment have enlisted the aid of public and private agencies beyond all normal expectations, and the incidents have been covered in picture and paragraph in papers great and small in all parts of the country.

Stories about individual nurses are also interesting. What Jane Doe, R.N., does, or a problem faced by Mary Roe, R.N., may picture the services offered or the problems faced by the entire profession in an intimate and personal way. Often, a major point in a campaign or a story may be made when it is introduced by means of an attention-arresting, though basically minor, incident or event.

Localizing news is also important. For instance, when the chairman gets a statement from state or national organizations, if she puts in a local name and has the statement read at a local meeting, it will set the stage; then it will get better play. Local assets to spread news, such as civic club and women's club meetings, are always helpful.

Some papers may prefer to send their own reporters and photographers, especially for Sunday magazine type of features. This enlists personal inter-est of newspaper writers and photographers, which may be valuable on other occasions. It is advisable to learn the policy of the paper. Do not glut newspapers with materials they are unlikely to use or with too many stories alike in content. When talking to reporters, be prepared with the facts needed to provide background material regarding the story you want told. Avoid speaking "off the record;" if you do not want to say something in print simply say you have no comment. However, always be courteous. Be honest. If the reporter asks for facts you do not have, tell him you will get the facts for him later.

At convention luncheons and dinners, supply the photographers and the press with a list of people at the head table. At large gatherings the same may be done for the persons on the platform. Try to obtain advance copies of speeches and have them mimeographed for distribution to the press. When finances are at stake and banquet halls likely to be crowded, income-producing space may be sacrificed to press tables. The best plan under these circumstances is to arrange for the press to be fed beforehand. In the hall or the ballroom, they may be provided with a long, narrow table, depending on the number to be accommodated, directly in front of the platform. Here they may work uninterrupted and without in any way intruding on the smooth operation of the program.

These plans have been used with great success at meetings where thousands assemble for luncheon or dinner, or at meetings in some of the largest hotels in the country and where men of prominence, such as the President of the USA, may be present.

Papers in larger cities sometimes band together and formulate suggestions for hospitals on how to use the papers, when to call at night, and other items. It is suggested that you learn whether such rules have been prepared by papers in your community. The Cleveland Hospital Council, for example, worked out a set of rules and then submitted them to the newspapers, which accepted them.

Radio and Television

Radio and television have brought the whole world into the home. Each has had to develop a means of news coverage that is basically the same as that used in newspapers. However, the difference in the media has made it necessary for each to make its own rules to meet the particular physical, time and operational requirements. This extends beyond the news elements involved. It includes such matters as voice and, for the television screen, personal appearance. Tact and diplomacy will enter into this, for at times the expert or the celebrity may not find himself adaptable to the medium concerned. Each element requires its own careful study, and the one who adapts his program to the standards and the requirements of the medium concerned will meet the greatest success in the end. For example, note President Nixon's success on TV.

Among the developments in television that have attracted a great deal of interest and exceeded all expectations are the interview and the panel discussion. The general public likes such presentations and looks and listens in increasing numbers. A routine presentation often falls flat. What seems to attract most attention is when a celebrity can be put "on the spot." The naïve comments and questions of the novice to the television platform are remembered long after the celebrity is forgotten. In developing such a program it is customary for the panel to meet ahead of time for a discussion of the procedure. Often, questions or subject areas can be suggested to the interviewer. He usually welcomes ideas, and the suggestions help to ensure coverage of topics of primary interest to the interviewee. Spontaneous questions and replies are appreciated much more by the audience than are stereotyped or memorized performances. Most persons who appear on such programs understand they may be faced with the unexpected. It is part of the game. Skillfully handled, panel discussions and interviews can become most effective handmaidens in any publicity program.

Radio and television talks, interviews, and spot announcements are effective forms of local publicity and should be used frequently. Call or visit the program manager of each local radio or television station when planning your over-all publicity campaign. Provide him with a list of experienced speakers who are prepared to give talks or to be interviewed on the air. Submit spot announcements which are exactly timed — 20 seconds, 30 seconds, or 60 seconds. You can plan for a maximum of 50 words for a 30-second announcement. This kind of material is more likely to be used by stations than background material from which spot announcements have to be written. Send 4 to 5 copies of each spot announcement to make sure that it will be announced more than once, since a broadcaster may throw away copy after he reads it. For TV, if you can, send a picture that can be used with your announcement. Find out from the TV station how the picture should be prepared for their use. A note of appreciation to the program manager after the campaign is over will leave the door open for future contacts.

Speeches

In making a speech, tell the listeners what they are interested in hearing. If the material is reduced to one or two facts developed with good illustrations, it will be far more effective than a long-drawn-out, flowery oration. Make the talk very clear and simple and, by all means, keep to the point. Experienced speakers have a simple rule for keeping to the point: "Tell them what you're going to tell them; tell them; then tell them what you told them." Word your talk for the particular audience that you expect will hear it. For example, you would not handle a subject for a group of nursing students as you would for a medical society. On the other hand, if you were talking over the radio or making a television appearance, you would have to keep a great variety of people in mind. As one writer aptly says: "Word your talk and choose your stories so that they will be understood equally by the janitor's wife and the retired bank president."[1]

[1] V. McCormick, "The Nurse and the Public: Ways and Means in Public Information," *American Journal of Nursing,* **30:**444, Apr. 1930.

Bulletins and Form Letters

If your plan includes the use of bulletins, leaflets, or form letters, several of the directions already given can be observed. Be brief; select simple, vivid phrases; strive for uncluttered, easily read pages. Take advantage of type variations and use attractive forms. Use wide margins. Colored paper and line drawings add greatly to the effectiveness and make the material more interesting. Offset permits the use of pictures and designs without the cost for plates required in letter-press. Your printer or mimeographer can help you with type and arrangement. Too much dependence should not be placed on him, however, for he may be engaged in other projects in which he has a more personal interest. On the other hand, because he sees a number of different publications, he may have some excellent suggestions for your project. It is a good idea for you to lay aside for future reference letters, circulars, and folders that come through the mail which have in them an element of novelty or special appeal. Then, when occasion for your own publicity arises, go over them, selecting the ones most appropriate to the occasion, and make up your own, based on the best ideas that others have had to offer.

One important principle in writing form letters is to word them as if especially directed to the person addressed. When a relatively limited group or area is being addressed, a form letter (salutation and signature omitted) can be turned over to members of a committee who fill in the names of their friends or associates and sign their own names to the communication. If space also is left on the page, these people will add a personal message to supplement the letter, which will make a far greater impression than the impersonal form. This is a most effective device when applied to clubs or other organizations where the cooperating committee is known to the membership. In such cases, each person helping out should be given a list of the names and the addresses of the persons to whom he is to write. Better still, supply these correspondents with stamped, addressed envelopes, plus the form letters, and they also will take care of the mailing for you.

Photographs

If your picture is requested for publicity purposes, send a black and white glossy print. Do not write in pencil or ink on the backs of photographs you send to the press; such writing will show through. Write the name and other required information on back of the photo with wax crayon or attach the typed information to the back of the photograph with adhesive tape; for example, a caption for a photograph might be: MARY LISTON, DEAN, SCHOOL OF NURSING, THE CATHOLIC UNIVERSITY OF AMERICA, WASHINGTON, D.C., AT (place, date, name of group which is the audience), WHO WILL SPEAK ON "NURSING LOOKS TO THE FUTURE." This will prevent the caption from getting separated from the picture. Use picture credits whenever possible and win the good will of the photographer.

Even small papers use pictures. Tipping off city editors to picture possibilities, setting a definite time for picture-taking, and helping the photographer to take good pictures are important. This kind of cooperation with newspaper personnel avoids confusion.

At large meetings, to meet the needs of the photographers a special technique may be employed to reduce confusion and delays in carrying out the program. The chairman or the person in charge of publicity should decide beforehand what pictures are likely to be requested. A special room should be set aside in which the persons concerned and the photographers may be assembled. This may be done prior to the opening of the meeting, and the event may be "staged" for the press. Prepare a series of sheets of paper bearing the appropriate captions. Below, place squares in which the names of the persons are inserted. In proper sequence, bring the persons to a given spot, arrange them in proper order, and let the photographers do their work. Hand them the appropriate sheet and the job is done. This saves the photographers the job of rushing forward with notebooks and pencils to get the proper names, and it also enables the whole series to be taken with the least possible effort and delay.

Posters and Exhibits

Posters should be simple and striking. A single figure or group with only a few words addressed to the public is most effective. Let the newspaper article, leaflet, or radio talk tell the story, and use the poster only as a visual reminder. When planning the use of a poster, take into consideration first the size of the bulletin boards on which it is likely to be used. Many institutions and organizations overlook this elementary fact. If the poster conforms to the size normally displayed on public or institutional bulletin boards, it will be used; if you try to monopolize all the space with a large poster, you may find that it is tossed out as soon as it arrives, regardless of its importance or attractive appearance.

If you are planning a window display or exhibit, here are a few salient points to observe. Accuracy of detail is one of the most important considerations. But even to achieve accuracy, do not overcrowd. Bear in mind always the point of view of the public. Attempt to give local interest to the exhibit and make the necessary explanation as brief as possible.

PERSONAL INFLUENCE OF THE NURSE

The most important medium for reaching various groups or the public in general is the individual nurse through her professional, political and social contacts. Other people who are connected with nursing services—the telephone operator, the receptionist, the person who sends out bills—also have an effect on the relations which nursing has with the public. Perhaps the first phase of your public relations program, then, might be "internally directed" to yourself and those who are closely associated with you in your work.

Professional Attitudes

The best publicity that nursing can have comes from a satisfied patient who sings the praises of the nurse who helped him to recover and from the family of the patient who has been treated sympathetically by the nurse, even if the patient dies. Most harmful of all to nursing, however, is the nurse whose attitude and manner are unprofessional, curt or unfriendly in dealing with patients and their families and friends. Motion pictures and literature which depict nurses as persons with indifferent and unprofessional standards of conduct have an unfortunate influence on the public and prospective students.

The Nurse's Uniform

The ANA Committee on Ethical Standards has given careful consideration to the problem of the use of photographs of nurses in uniform or the appearance of nurses in uniform while engaged in nonprofessional activities. Statement 10 of the Code for Professional Nurses covers this area of conduct. The interpretation of statement 10 points out that the nurse may not allow her status or professional symbols, such as the uniform, to be used in promoting or advertising any commercial product or service.[2]

Telling Others About Nursing

A nurse's knowledge about the broad problems of nursing, as well as her behavior, can have a public relations impact for good or ill. It is not very fruitful, for example, to subject the public to a barrage of literature about the importance of providing nurses with good preparation if individual nurses are not convinced of the value of good nursing education or cannot explain how this education affects the kind of service they give. Therefore, it is important that you keep up to date by reading and through participating in the activities of nursing organizations, so that you can interpret the aims and problems of nursing to *your* public—your patients, associates and friends.

PROBLEMS

1. Suppose that you are the chairman of the committee on public relations of one of the societies in your school and you wish to write up a story of some school event for the newspaper. (a) With whom would you communicate to get the news into the paper? (b) Write up a story of some school event for publication in a newspaper. (c) Present your story in class for evaluation.

2. (a) Make a list of articles about nurses which have appeared in newspa-

[2] American Nurses' Association *Code for Nurses With Interpretative Statements*. New York, The Association, 1968.

pers and popular magazines during the last 6 months. (b) Using the guidelines for writing such stories, give a critique of 1 or more of these articles.

3. Begin to make a scrapbook of all news clippings about nursing and about yourself as an active participant in the profession. If you add to this scrapbook throughout your life you will have an invaluable historic record.

4. (a) If you were to appear on a television program, what preparation would you make? (b) When would you appear in uniform? Would you appear in uniform if you were on a recruitment program sponsored by a brewery or a tobacco company?

5. (a) Read the statements in the ANA publication, *Nursing and Commercial Advertising*. (b) Discuss the meaning of these statements, using examples of correct and incorrect usage. (c) Do you think the ANA should be concerned about "nursing and commercial advertising?" (d) Why do you feel this way?

6. (a) Discuss the current public information programs of the nursing organizations, including your student association, in your state. (b) Is there appropriate coordination of these programs? (c) How can you secure this information? (d) Evaluate these plans.

SUGGESTED REFERENCES*

* American Hospital Association. *People Caring for People*. Chicago, The Association, 1968.
Dale, E. *You Give the Public What It Wants*. New York, Cowles, 1967.
Fillmore, G. "When You Are Asking About Nursing." *American Journal of Nursing*, **63:**74-76, Aug. 1963.
* Geister, J. M. "Public Relations Begins at the Bedside." *American Journal of Nursing*, **50:**463-464, Aug. 1950.
Goddard, H. A. "The Art of Interviewing." *Nursing Mirror*, **126:**39, Feb. 23, 1968.
Goldsborough, J. "Involvement." *American Journal of Nursing*, **69:**66-68, Jan. 1969.
* Lippitt, G. L. "An Analysis of Factors Affecting the Public's Perception of National Organizations." *International Nursing Review*, **9:**34-37, Jan./Feb. 1962.
* Rockefeller, M. C. "The Why of Citizen Involvement in Patient Care." *Nursing Outlook*, **12:**580-581, Aug. 1963.
* Schorr, T. "Nursing's TV Image." *American Journal of Nursing*, **63:**119-121, Oct. 1963.
"21 Ways to Improve Your Conversation." *Christopher News Notes*, New York, May 1964.
Weiner, H. N. "Making Your Public Relations Program Work." *Nursing Outlook*, **11:**654-655, Sept. 1963.

* In each chapter all citations are footnoted and are not included here. All starred references are recommended for additional reading.

CHAPTER

29

Skills and Practices Which Aid in Professional Activities

More and more we need to recognize the vital role that we play in our civic as well as in our professional organizations. Organization work can be exciting and interesting, depending on the interest and commitment of the members and the vitality of the program. Much of the success of any organization depends on its officers and committees, and upon their ability to define goals, to plan and organize activities and to motivate participation through effective communication. They cannot carry on the work alone, however. All members must be interested and prepared to participate.

Some procedures that need to be understood by officers, committee members, and all of us as individual members, if we are to participate effectively, are:

How to formulate and revise constitutions and bylaws.
How to be good committee members.
How to plan, carry out and follow up programs.
How to develop and participate in meetings.
How to prepare agenda for meetings.
How to preside.
How to record minutes.
How to expedite business through the use of parliamentary procedure.

How to participate effectively as a leader or a member of a group when parliamentary procedure is not required.

How to formulate and give reports and to do professional writing.

How to speak in public and to participate in general discussion and debate.

How to secure information through interviews, questionnaires, books, pamphlets, magazines and other sources.

How to make use of this information to develop informed opinion.

These are some of the major skills and procedures with which organization members need to be familiar. Some of them will be discussed briefly in this chapter. It is not intended to tell you exactly how you can master these skills, but rather to emphasize their importance and to suggest sources of information. Probably you have been introduced to most of these by participation in school organizations, in the National Student Nurses' Association and in other group activities. You will need to master them if you expect to get maximum benefit from your organization activities or any group learning.

ORGANIZATIONAL STRUCTURE

Every member of an organization, if he is to participate effectively and help shape opinion or develop activities, should be acquainted with the way in which it is governed. He should know how it is organized and his place, as a member, in its organizational structure. Does he hold direct membership with the right to an individual vote on all matters that come before the membership? Or is he a member by virtue of belonging to an association or agency that is a voting member? Or is he both an individual member and a member of a constituent agency?

Again, he should know what person, group, or groups can take action in the name of the organization. How are they selected? What is the extent of their responsibility and authority? What are the channels through which desirable change is introduced?

Bylaws

The regulations by which an organization is governed are found in the bylaws, which incorporate the certificate of incorporation, or the constitution, and the bylaws. These enunciate the purpose of the organization and spell out the operating rules or standards designed to facilitate smooth functioning. The bylaws should be consistent throughout with the purpose and functions of the association.

It is important to remember that bylaws are not "written in stone." Changes may be required from time to time. Many organizations have a committee that periodically reviews the bylaws and proposes revisions that will keep them up to date. It is through this committee that you, as a member, can suggest changes that you think should be made.

Officers

The provisions of the bylaws should be familiar to all the members of an organization — but especially to those elected to office. Besides knowing the regulations of the organization and having a real understanding of its purposes, an officer should possess certain qualifications: tact, sense of humor, enthusiasm, dignity, fairness, initiative, integrity, and executive ability. It is understood that anyone who is even considered for an office has a sincere interest in the organization and is willing to work hard to accomplish its ends. Only those who are sensitive to the needs of the groups to be served and who really can promote the best interests of these groups should be considered. Another consideration in nominating and electing officers is their ability to work together as a group. No matter how well qualified an individual may be otherwise, he will not be a good officer unless he is congenial and co-operative.

Faulty selection of officers and committee members is a frequent cause of failure in organization work. Obviously, officers or committee chairmen who wish to hold office merely for personal prestige or to attain their own objectives should not be selected because they usually will not serve the best interests of the organization. Sometimes an officer or a committee member is selected just because he is "nice," or because he is willing to serve, not because he has the knowledge and the experience that fit him for the function he is expected to perform. Such a procedure may be fatal to success.

The competence of potential officers is determined on the basis of their past performance. As a rule, the important offices are held by those who have secured their preparation by working in less important positions first.

If you are assisting in the selection of officers or committee members, or if you are asked to serve in such capacity, you cannot be too careful in considering the qualifications that are essential for the performance of the duties involved.

The officers of an organization usually consist of a president, one or more vice-presidents, a secretary and a treasurer.

The president has certain functions defined by the bylaws of the particular association. The usual functions are:

1. To guide and direct the organization and to promote its program.
2. To protect the members in their rights.
3. To carry out the will of the members, expressed by a majority vote.
4. To act as the representative and spokesman of the society.
5. To preside at meetings of the board of directors, the executive committee and house of delegates or general membership meetings.
6. To call special meetings.
7. To sign orders to the treasurer for the payment of bills.
8. To serve ex officio on all committees except the nominating committee.
9. To appoint committees not otherwise provided for in the bylaws.

This list does not describe the full extent of the president's obligation to keep constantly in touch with the organization's activities and to exert the type of leadership that will keep it moving toward its goals.

The secretary's functions are also prescribed by the bylaws of an organization. In addition to possessing the other qualifications of every efficient officer, he must be systematic and responsible. The usual duties are:

1. To be present at all meetings, both regular and special, of the board of directors, the executive committee, the house of delegates and general membership meetings.

2. To keep an accurate, complete record of the proceedings of each meeting.

3. To read the minutes of the previous meeting.

4. To maintain a file of all correspondence and official documents so that they are available to other officers and members.

5. To prepare, with the president, an agenda of the business to be attended to before the meeting; during the meeting he should assist the chairman and the group to focus on the purposes of the meeting.

The recording secretary also sends out notices of meetings, prepares publicity items for the press unless there is a special committee or a public relations consultant for this, and handles the correspondence. If there is a corresponding secretary, however, he performs these duties. When there is more than one secretary, the title *secretary* refers to the recording officer.

The keeping of minutes and the handling and filing of correspondence for a large and active organization can total up to a staggering load for an elected officer who cannot devote full time to secretarial responsibilities. Moreover, some of the secretary's functions mesh closely with those of employed staff members when these exist. For these reasons, the chief administrator of the staff sometimes serves also as secretary of the organization.

The responsibilities of the other officers of an organization may vary. In general, the vice-president carries out the functions of the president in his absence or disability. If the president should die or resign, the vice-president automatically assumes the presidency unless there are other provisions in the bylaws of the association.

The treasurer is responsible for seeing that adequate records are maintained to record the receipts of all monies and authorized disbursements, and that complete reports can be prepared from the records maintained. Usually there is an auditor or an auditing committee appointed to examine the treasurer's books at regular intervals. If this is done, the treasurer's yearly report need not include details, but only the amount of money on hand at the beginning of the year, the total receipts and expenditures, and the balance at the end of the year. If there is no auditor, an itemized report must be given; but, for his own protection, the treasurer always should request an audit. It is a safe measure, also, to follow the policy of bonding the treasurer and the officers who handle funds of the organization.

Board of Directors

Unless the members of an organization can meet frequently as a total group, it is usually impossible for them to make all the decisions necessary for the organization to move ahead. Instead, through the bylaws, they delegate many powers to a group which usually is called the board of directors.

The board of directors includes the officers of the organization and other members as indicated in the bylaws. Sometimes, to assure a cross section of viewpoint on the board, the bylaws stipulate a number of interests that must be represented on it.

The responsibilities of the board are great, and board members should be selected for their judgment, their breadth of viewpoint and their vision. It is particularly important that those who represent a particular group should not wear "special interest blinders" but should be able to see matters relating to their own fields in the context of the organization's total program.

Committees

A committee is a small group elected or selected to perform a task that can be done more effectively by a small than by a large group or that requires special knowledge and skills. Its functions are fixed by the vote creating it or by the bylaws. Sometimes the committee's task involves guidance in one of the organization's major programs, and its functions are broadly enough stated to permit it to engage in a number of activities as the need arises. At other times, it is assigned to one specific task.

The chairman is the leader for the committee. He is chosen for his ability to administer the details of the assignment. He must be generally intelligent, have a sense of humor, and have the respect of the other members of the committee. He may be selected by appointment by the president of the organization or a presiding officer at a particular meeting, by election by the organization or parent body, or by election by members of the committee.

Committee members are appointed or elected by the organization or the parent body. They should be people who are willing and capable of carrying out the task assigned. The number of people selected and their specific background of knowledge depend on the assignment.

The chairman has the responsibility for making plans and arrangements for meetings. He also is responsible for calling the meeting at the scheduled time; introducing the problem or the topic of discussion; conducting the discussion of the problem; summarizing the discussion; and preparing the report for submission to the appropriate group. The recorder is responsible for keeping the record and assisting the chairman in any way possible.

All members are responsible for analyzing the problem; doing the study needed to arrive at the solution; suggesting a plan of action; and acting, if acting is the stated responsibility of the committee.

It is important that a committee keep fairly well to its assignment and not wander down all the bypaths that may turn up during its deliberations. It is only human to prefer giving advice to rolling up one's sleeves and working, and it is not unheard of for a committee that has been assigned a particular piece of work to end its meeting with a recommendation that a committee be appointed to undertake that selfsame work assignment. The parent group, of course, welcomes any recommendations that are by-products of the committee's work, but it also counts on the committee to complete the job for which it was created.

If you serve on a committee, and particularly if you are its chairman, you might keep asking yourself: What precisely is this committee's assignment? Was it asked to formulate recommendations about policy or about how a task should be done, or is it a production committee with instructions to do a piece of work? Was it appointed "with power" to follow through on some of its decisions, or must it secure the approval of the parent body before it can take further steps?

Committee work trains potential leaders, gets work done that could not be done efficiently in a large group, and gives better opportunity for exploring a problem, doing the necessary research, and arriving at a solution that can be considered by the parent body.

Some limitations are encountered if the members have been chosen poorly, if the committee members live too far apart to meet and the job has to be done by correspondence, if the members are biased, or if 1 or 2 members dominate the group and its activities.

Members

If you decide to become a member of any organization, make up your mind to be an effective member, one who is able to take an intelligent part in discussions and to expedite the business of its meetings.

Not only the officers and directors of an organization, but the members as well, have certain responsibilities. All members, whether officers or committee members or not, need to be loyal to the organization. It is not sufficient to be present and on time at meetings; in addition, you should prepare yourself to be an active member. You can do this by studying the bylaws of the organization and by finding out what its general policy has been in the past. Acquaint yourself with the issues that the group expects to discuss, and study both sides of the questions. Read about them and talk them over with your friends before the meeting, so that during the meeting you will be able to discuss them intelligently and to offer some suggestions.

To be an effective member you must also know and apply parliamentary procedure. The best and the only way to acquire this knowledge is to learn the rules and then to practice them. If you have a working knowledge of parliamentary procedure, you will be able to protect and further those movements in which you are interested. By offering certain motions and applying particular rules, you may secure immediate action on a motion or delay it as long as possible. You will find that parliamentary procedure enhances discussion and provides an orderly way of resolving differences.

You may be called on to serve on a committee or to act as chairman of one. Anyone has the right to refuse, but unless you have a good reason for declining, you should welcome the opportunity. Once you have agreed to serve, do not withdraw at the last minute. There is hard work connected with any active organization, and it is unfair to expect the same few people to do all of it. Anyone who promises his assistance and then withholds it causes much confusion and extra work for someone else. In case something unforeseen arises that makes it impossible for you to fulfill your promise to help, explain the difficulty to the person in charge, ask to be excused, and express your regret and your desire to serve another time. If it is possible, you might also offer to find someone to take your place.

At times you may not think you are sufficiently prepared for the office you are called on to take. However, if the group with whom you are asked to cooperate is prepared to do the work, it may be wise for you to accept, as you will be sure to learn a great deal about essential organization principles and practices.

If the organization has a staff of employed workers, you must be careful not to put on their shoulders the responsibilities that belong to the total membership or to a group of members. Some of these employees may be experts in fields connected with the organization's activities. Most of them will have the detailed knowledge of the organization's program that can only be acquired through day-in, day-out association with it. It is therefore tempting for a group that has been assigned a task to say, "The staff members know more about this than we do. Let them decide." Later, it is just as tempting to remark on "those bureaucrats." The solution is, of course, to call on the employed staff for the facts in their possession and even for their opinions. But the final decision should be made by the group charged with that responsibility. Sometimes staff members of an organization may be inclined to make decisions and to assume activities that are the responsibilities of officers, sections, committees, or membership. It is your responsibility, as a member of the organization, to see that this does not happen.

In addition to knowing the obligations of the members and the officers of an organization, you also should know how a meeting is conducted. You will find the rules for the conducting of business in the constitution and the by-laws and in the book on parliamentary usage that has been selected for guidance of the organization.

KINDS OF MEETINGS

Even if you are not a member of a board of directors or of a committee, you will doubtless participate in a considerable number of meetings if you are an active member of an organization. Nursing organizations operate on the belief that the best way to reach down-to-earth, acceptable solutions to problems is to arrange for all those concerned with these problems to work on them together. For this reason, they make provision for meetings at which the total membership or groups of constituents can explore problems and thrash out issues before action is taken on these problems and issues. The type of meeting held depends upon the nature of the problem to be dealt with or upon the purpose of the meeting.

Business Meetings

The business meeting provides an opportunity for the entire membership of an organization to keep abreast of the organization's activities and to take action on matters or issues that are the prerogative of the membership or that the board of directors thinks the membership should consider. It is at this meeting that the officers and the committees give their reports. The president's report is particularly important. He is obligated to report to the membership what he has done in its behalf as spokesman and representative of the organization, what he conceives the state of the organization to be, and what new developments, if any, he believes affect the organization and its program.

Usually the bylaws of an organization indicate how frequently such a meeting must be held and make provision for the calling of other special business meetings if the need for them arises. The bylaws also spell out certain details about the business meeting, such as how it is called and what constitutes a quorum.

Institutes

An institute is a series of sessions that may be held on 1 day or may continue for several days or weeks, arranged for a group of people who come together to learn about a specific field. Its several purposes are to present information, to identify and explore a problem or a group of related problems in a specific field, to solve a problem and to stimulate the members to do further exploration of the field on their own.

It provides a method of presenting new ideas and practices. It allows those attending to ask questions, express their views and to discuss their problems and views with others who are equally interested in the subject of the institute. It furnishes a method for presenting material in a unified way. Its success depends upon having lecturers and leaders with the necessary training and experience, and upon participants who prepare adequately for the discussions.

Workshops

A workshop is a short or long course in which the participants focus on the solution of a problem of concern to all or in which each participant works on a problem of particular concern to him. The characteristics of the workshop include the following: (1) participants assist in the planning sessions so that all members of the group are involved from the beginning; (2) considerable time is allotted to small group work sessions, and there is time for feed-back from each small group to the whole group; (3) resources are available, such as pertinent literature, visual aides and consultants; (4) there is time for individual conferences with consultants and those responsible for the workshop; (5) time is allowed for oral summarizing and evaluating from time to time and at the end of the workshop; (6) there is no formal final examination, although group evaluation of the workshop is usually made; and (7) a written report may be prepared for the participants and for publication.

Conferences

A conference is a discussion group working together for a common purpose on a problem or problems where group agreement on a reasonable solution grows from pooling the results of each participant's best thinking. The participants usually are selected because of the contributions they can make to the solution of the problem. Provision is made for all the available facts connected with the problem to be put at the disposal of the conferees, and the conference is so planned that each participant can make his maximum contribution to it.

Agreements on how the problem might be solved result sometimes in a recommendation or a series of recommendations to the conferees themselves or to the body that called the conference. At other times, the conference results in a report of the facts that have a bearing on the problem and suggestions about ways in which the problem might best be approached. At times a conference may result in both a majority and a minority report.

Seminars

A seminar is a group of persons who come together for the purpose of studying a problem or a variety of problems under the leadership of an expert. It is used to identify, explore and solve problems. It involves the consideration of how to plan the method of approach involved in the research and the appropriate sources to use. It provides an opportunity for members of the group to share learnings and findings and to gain experience in reporting and recording.

Each seminar member identifies and selects a problem to study; prepares a method of attack; uses appropriate sources, such as reading, interviews, or case studies; prepares a report; shares his findings with the group; and participates in all discussion periods at all stages of the problem-solving process being used by each member of the group.

The seminar enables the members to study under a learned person. It stimulates active participation. It helps members to gain new information, and the learning situation is a vital one. However, if the leader is not an expert and will not permit new and opposing points of view to be expressed, a seminar experience may be deadening. If members are reluctant to participate, it is not an effective educational method, or if time allotted is inadequate for a complete exploration of the individual problems, it is frustrating.

PLANNING FOR MEETINGS

From the description of the various kinds of meetings, you can see that the type of meeting that is planned usually is determined by its purpose. If, for example, the meeting is aimed toward helping a group of people to gain an understanding of how a nursing team operates, an institute might be held. A workshop might be chosen for helping team leaders to find methods of working with specific problems that they have encountered in their work. If there is need to develop plans for the preparation of team leaders, arrangements might be made for a conference of people with various types of expert knowledge — knowledge about nursing education, about how people are trained on the job for leadership responsibilities, about how people learn and about the qualities and abilities needed by team leaders. Again, a comparatively small number of people who have studied various aspects of team leadership might come together in a seminar.

A good meeting doesn't just happen; it is usually the result of considerable planning and real work by those who are responsible for it. Decisions must be made about the short-term and long-range objectives. The ways in which information is to be presented and discussions and work are to be carried on must be determined. Participants must be invited, and arrangements must be made for registering and housing them. Meeting rooms must be obtained and equipped. Speakers, chairmen and consultants must be secured, and source materials must be accumulated. Arrangements must be made for briefing leadership teams, panel discussants and others with important roles and for intergroup communications. Plans are drafted for evaluating the meeting and for the preparation and the publication of written materials that emanate from it. Attention must be paid to the public relations and publicity aspects. Very often there is a whole network of committees to handle this work — an overall planning committee and committees on program, arrangements, evaluation, public relations, reports and so on.

Whole books have been written on the subject of how to plan and hold meetings. One that, although not new, might be useful to you if you are on a committee with responsibilities for a meeting is:

Beckhard, Richard. *How to Plan and Conduct Workshops and Conferences.* New York, Association Press, 1956.

Even if you are not concerned with arrangements for a meeting, you, as a participant have certain responsibilities to prepare for the meeting, to contribute to it, to help in evaluating it and to follow through on it. It is these participant responsibilities that we perhaps should talk about here.

PARTICIPATION IN MEETINGS

Responsibilities of Participants

All participants should come to a meeting ready to contribute their share. Thoughtful preparation in advance is necessary to accomplish this.

Sometimes those who have planned a conference or workshop send a questionnaire to the participants in advance, asking them to indicate specific problems that they think might be discussed and to make other suggestions about the program and arrangements. By providing thoughtful and prompt answers to such a questionnaire, you can do your bit toward planning a meeting that will have real meaning to you and others like you. Also, you should go over carefully any study materials that are sent you before the meeting. You might even pay a visit to your library and look up articles or books about the subject of the meeting. If you are attending the meeting as a representative of a group, you should enlist the help of its members in answering the questionnaire and in studying the materials that have been sent you.

When you participate in a meeting, you need to keep in mind that the discussion is a quest for the right answer and should not be argumentative. There should be a centering on real differences. Arguments over technicalities should be avoided, and no one should take a point of view merely for the sake of an argument. Avoid tangles over words and definitions. When there are such conflicts get some good illustrations and then go ahead. Brief statements are much more to the point than long speeches. What is wanted is a give-and-take to mold ideas that lead to a solution.

It is important in a group discussion that the members trust each other. There is usually no one in it who is not superior to the rest in at least one respect, but the experience of all is more valuable than the experience of any 1 person. In other words, the group as a whole can probably see farther and better than its 1 best member.

Some members in a group actually prevent any real accomplishments. They do this by:

Failing to come to the meeting with an open mind.
Failing to participate but taking away all that they can.
Talking too much.
Being irrelevant in making points.
Letting their pet points of view interfere with the discussion.
Refusing to drop a subject when the others wish to do so.
Showing lack of interest.
Being late or irregular in attendance.

For you to participate effectively in a meeting, you should have an understanding of your role and the roles of the other participants. This involves, in turn, a knowledge of the ways in which information is collected or given, experiences are shared and decisions are arrived at. A description of some of the ways in which you may participate in a meeting therefore may be of help.

Parliamentary Procedure

Parliamentary law is the accepted system of rules for conducting business, preserving order and governing debate in legislative or other bodies meeting for deliberative purposes.

It is based on the regulations used in the British Parliament, but several changes have been introduced into the procedure used in the USA.

Common sense is the basis of all parliamentary law. Its 4 fundamental principles are: (1) equality and fairness, (2) orderly transaction of business, (3) majority rule and (4) protection of the rights of the minority.

These rules effectively cover any problem or situation that arises in the course of a business meeting, and adherence to them will assure order, clarity and economy of time. Parliamentary procedure is a method to expedite the work of the group. However, the procedure should never become so rigid that this purpose is lost. There may be times when, by general concensus, the procedure is dispensed with temporarily in order to enable the group to move forward.

Although all parliamentary procedure is based on the same general principles, various systems differ slightly in details. Therefore, an organization should select and follow one particular system. Some of the authoritative sources are listed at the end of this chapter.

Parliamentary procedure often is thought of in connection with a business meeting, but it is useful in many other types of meetings, particularly when the number of participants is large. At a large conference, for example, the participants may wish to make recommendations to the parent body, and it is important to be sure that such recommendations express the beliefs of the majority of the participants. This frequently requires the use of parliamentary procedure.

It is generally thought that to have a satisfactory business meeting only the chairman and perhaps one or two others need to be familiar with parliamentary law. This is not enough. The cooperation of all present is a prime requisite for the success of a meeting; if everyone knows the rules of parliamentary procedure, the greatest cooperation can be secured. Moreover, no matter how well versed the chairman may be in correct technique, this knowledge is of little avail in an assembly where the members speak from the floor without first addressing the chair, or do not know the correct way to offer a motion.

The Motion. A motion is a proposal that the group take certain action or express itself as holding certain views. To make a motion, a member obtains the floor and says, "I move that such and such be done." Before making a motion it is a good idea to write it out and read it over to yourself. This will help you to make sure that you are saying what you mean to say. It will also assist you if you are called on to repeat the motion. In fact, the chairman has the right to require that any main motion be put in writing.

With certain exceptions, every motion should be seconded. This is to prevent consideration of a question that only one person is concerned with.

When a motion is offered, the chairman states it by saying: "It has been moved and seconded that we do so and so." If the motion is debatable, the chairman says, "Are there any remarks?" When debate lags, he says, "Are you ready for the question?"

The chairman puts the question to vote by "All in favor say *aye*," a pause, and then "Those opposed *no*," or, often preferably, by asking for a show of hands. The chairman thereupon declares the motion carried or not carried.

The Chairman. As the presiding officer at a meeting, the function of the chairman is to preserve order, state each motion offered, put it to a vote at the proper time, and announce the result. The chairman himself may not offer, second, or discuss a motion while he occupies the chair. If the need should arise for him to take part in the debate, he must leave the chair and speak from the floor as a member. When this happens, the vice-chairman presides and continues to act as chairman until the question has been settled. Although provision is made for such a situation, it is not good policy for the chairman to take part in debate, for he is supposed to be an impartial executive who carries out the wishes of the members.

The chairman does not forfeit his right to vote, but exercises it only when the vote is taken by ballot or by roll call. In the latter case, his name is called last of all. If he wishes, he may vote if there is a tie or if his vote will make it a tie. If the vote has been taken by ballot, he may not cast the deciding vote, for the secrecy of the ballot must be preserved.

At the opening of a business meeting the chairman says, "This meeting will now come to order; the secretary will call the roll," and, at the conclusion of the roll call and if a quorum is present, "The secretary will read the minutes." At the close of the reading of the minutes, the chairman says, "You have heard the minutes of the last meeting; if there are no corrections or amendments, the minutes stand approved." He pauses a moment; then if there are no corrections, he says, "They are approved."

The chairman calls for reports of officers and committees and then for unfinished and new business. It is the responsibility of the chairman to see that all recommendations are given consideration by being included either in the acceptance of reports or in new business.

When the chairman is corrected, he says: "The chair stands corrected."

After the vote for adjournment, the motion for which frequently specifies the time of the next meeting, the chairman formally announces that the meeting is adjourned.

Further suggestions for the chairman and the secretary will be found in Part Two of the Appendix, where there is a sample form that may be used as a guide in recording minutes.

FACE-TO-FACE GROUPS

In a small meeting, such as a board or committee meeting, there is an opportunity for members to "bat a question back and forth," without the use of parliamentary procedure, before they come to a decision about it. In a large meeting, however, there is often not time or opportunity for all members to engage in such an interchange of opinion. Moreover, some people who have real contributions to make may hesitate to "speak up" before a large audience.

To bring the advantages of a small meeting to the large meeting, conference, workshop, or institute, arrangements frequently are made for the total group to be subdivided, from time to time, into smaller groups of not more than 10 to 20 members. This can be done even in the face of limited facilities: it is not always necessary for subgroups to meet in different rooms; they may be divided into small groups in the main meeting room. The facts found, problems identified, or conclusions reached in these subgroups are "fed back" to the total group at intervals so that all participants can consider the findings of all subgroups as they proceed with their assignments.

Sometimes all subgroups are assigned the same problems to work on. In such instances, an effort is usually made to have all the interests represented at the conference represented on each subgroup as well. At other times, the participants are subdivided according to areas of special knowledge or interest, and each subgroup studies the aspects of the problem that are of most concern to its members.

Roles

Beginning in your student experience and continuing throughout most of your adult life, you no doubt will be involved in small group meetings. Much of the business of organizations, as well as committee activities in your own place of work, and in the many other groups of which you will be a part, will be carried out in small group meetings. It is very important, therefore, that you have a working knowledge of how these groups function. When you find yourself in a subgroup, you will discover that certain people in it have been asked to assume certain roles, such as leader, recorder, content resource person, and observer (if appropriate).

You may have been asked to assume one of these roles. If so, you probably will be told about your responsibilities in a "leadership briefing session" before the meeting begins. During the course of the conference or workshop, other meetings of all the leadership teams are likely to be called at which the progress of the various subgroups can be discussed and their findings to date can be coordinated. However, it might be well for you to have some idea about the general type of responsibilities that are assigned to each member of the leadership team.

The Leader. It is the leader's responsibility to make it possible for members of the group to think creatively together. His main functions are to help the group to define the problem that it wishes to discuss, to see that all points of view are given a chance to contribute to the group thinking, to keep the discussion of the group on the subject, to clarify and summarize the progress of the group from time to time and to try to maintain an atmosphere in which the greatest cooperation and production can be achieved.

One important function of the discussion leader is to secure participation from all. He should attempt to draw out the shy people with friendly encouragement and, if necessary, subdue the more aggressive to give the quiet ones an opportunity to comment. Unlike the presiding officer at a large meeting, the leader should feel at liberty to participate in the discussion and express his opinions. In small groups it is possible, and even desirable at times, for different people to emerge as leaders at different stages of discussion.

The Recorder. The main responsibilities of the content recorder are to get down the chief points of content that the group thinking produces. This includes the major issues discussed by the group, with the pros and cons indicated; the major agreements reached by the group; the decisions made; and the recommendations agreed on. The recorder also has the job of seeing that his group's thinking is shared by other groups of his conference, if a large one, in general sessions and by a wider public through the reports which the conference prepares.

Recording conference discussions requires a keen and alert mind and the ability to pick out essentials quickly and accurately and express them in good clear English, to get on well with others, to lessen friction when necessary, and to summarize discussion when called on.

The Content Resource Person. The resource person has expert knowledge of the subject under discussion. However, he tries not to act like an expert or to give lectures on the subject unless he is called on by the group to give technical or background information. Instead, he asks the group leading questions that will stimulate the members to think or calls attention to factual information that is available in the source materials or elsewhere.

One or more content resource persons may be assigned to each subgroup. Or there may be a group of such people who serve, on call, all the subgroups of the meeting.

The Observer. An observer may or may not be provided for each subgroup. The observer's task is to help the group over the hurdles that may be blocking the discussion. For example, 2 participants may believe that they are arguing about the same matter from 2 points of view, whereas in reality they may be talking about 2 entirely different things. The observer could help the leader in letting the group see that this misunderstanding is holding up their progress. However, it is not his function to try to analyze the group or its members.

In order to perform his function, the observer is a nonparticipating member of the group—that is, he does not take part in the discussions.

The above discussion of the roles and functions of members of small groups is brief, and we suggest that you familiarize yourself with the references on group work such as those issued periodically by the Adult Education Association of the USA, 1225 Nineteenth Street, N.W., Washington, D.C. 20036, and the National Education Association, 1201 Sixteenth Street, N.W., Washington, D.C. 20036.

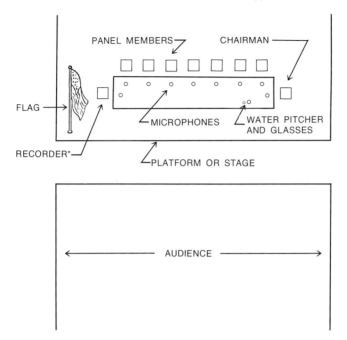

Fig. 29-1. Suggested arrangement for a panel discussion.

* A tape recorder may be used to record the discussion at meetings of this kind. If a stenotypist is used he would probably be placed in front of and below the platform.

TYPES OF PRESENTATIONS

As has been noted, all of you will very likely have many opportunities for participation in meetings—as participant, as leader or chairman, as resource person, as recorder, or as observer. The type and the extent of your participation will depend on the responsibility that you are assigned or have accepted, and on the kind of meeting that is involved. Thus far our discussion has been related mainly to participation in business meetings, conventions, conferences, or small group meetings (for example, committee meetings). You also will be participating, as a member of the audience or as a speaker, in other types of meetings such as those discussed next. Again, the type of meeting selected will depend upon the nature of the subject to be discussed.

The Panel Discussion

In the panel method, several people (4 to 6) with special knowledge on a topic carry on an informal discussion before an audience. It is sometimes referred to as a panel forum. It is not a debate. It is a socialized conversation in which different points of view are expressed. As a rule, a panel discussion is best used to consider a controversial issue by attempting to view all sides of the question. Other purposes of the panel discussion are to secure audience participation, to obtain the attitude and the general opinion of the group, to offer information in an informal manner and to establish informal contact with the audience. It does not always attempt to reach a final solution; its aim is better understanding of the issue. The panel discussion is used frequently on TV.

Together with the discussion leader the panel members are seated at a table on a platform, and all face the audience. See Figure 29-1 for a suggested arrangement. For about one half the time allotted, the topic is discussed from every angle by those on the platform, and then the leader invites the listeners to join in. The entire proceeding is informal. There are no written or rehearsed speeches. The speakers do not rise, and the atmosphere is that of an animated conversation among friends.

The nature of the topic under discussion, the capability of the leader, the suitability of the members on the panel, and careful preliminary planning determine the ultimate success or failure of the panel discussion.

The topic should be one in which people are vitally interested and which they are eager to discuss. It must necessarily be one that admits of discussion and that must be viewed from several angles before a satisfactory decision can be reached. It is also important that the subject be clearly worded in exact language, so that there may be no misconception of terms and so that everyone may have the same understanding of the question.

Planning. Preliminary planning for panel discussions is extremely important. The planning committee or the leader must select the members known to have knowledge of the subject and reasonable skill in conversing in public. If the subject is a controversial one, all points of view should be represented by the panel members. It is important for the panel members to meet once or twice before the discussion to get used to each other and to clarify their thinking and positions on the issue. This getting together of the panel members should never be used for rehearsal because that destroys spontaneity. If a report of the meeting is planned, a recorder should be present. Frequently a tape recording is made of the meeting and later transcribed; or a stenotypist may be used.

The Leader. An able leader of a panel discussion is one who is conversant with every phase of the question. He does not take part in the discussion, but guides it so that it remains relevant and balanced.

The duties of a leader are similar to those he has in a group discussion. He introduces the panel members to the audience, explains the procedure to be followed, gives a brief explanation of the question and presents it to the panel. During the discussion he must see that a free give-and-take is maintained, with no one talking too much and everyone taking part, and with all sides of the question presented fairly. When the leader thinks that the problem has been sufficiently clarified, he throws the discussion open to the audience. The panel members also join in this general discussion.

Intelligence, tact, and a sense of humor are necessary qualifications of a leader, so that spontaneity, tolerance, and good-natured exchange may characterize the conference. If the people taking part really are interested, they may become so earnest that the discussion will become tense unless the leader can enliven it with humor.

Advantages. The value of the panel method is the stimulus that it gives to thinking about important issues. No one in the audience can listen to an enthusiastic, controversial discussion on some vital topic without formulating ideas of his own and becoming eager to impart these to his neighbors, only to find that his neighbors also have ideas on the subject, some of them conflicting with his. Another friendly argument begins, and in this way the topic of the panel is carried home, thought about and discussed. The very fact that the discussion may end without having reached any definite conclusion is not a disadvantage in itself, for undoubtedly people have begun to think about the problem and the way is paved for further consideration of the issue with the aim of resolving it.

The Symposium

A symposium frequently is confused with the panel discussion. A symposium is a series of speeches on various phases of a topic by individual speakers, which may or may not be followed by open discussion. The several speakers and the leader sit on a platform facing the audience, but the similarity goes no farther. The job of the leader is more like that of a chairman of a public meeting.

The symposium is used to accomplish one or more of the following purposes: to present impartial and objective points of view on the various phases of the subject under consideration; to present an analysis of several sides of a controversial subject; to present information; to provide opportunity for audience participation, if the symposium is the forum type; to assist people to clarify parts of a problem and to see the unity of their relationship; to identify or explore a problem; or to direct the audience to subsequent inquiry and reading.

Planning. Before speakers are selected, a topic must be decided on and analyzed, so that it can be broken into several subtopics. Then the very best speaker obtainable must be selected to present each subtopic. He should be able to discuss it in terms of the purpose of the whole subject and of those who are expected to attend.

The next step consists of organizing the program and briefing the speakers. Those planning for the symposium must be sure that each speaker understands the purpose of the discussion, the general plan of procedure to be followed in the meeting, the exact time limit for each speaker, and the equipment to be used, such as blackboard or other visual aids. It is a good idea to ask the speakers to submit their papers in advance of the meeting. These papers may be used in preparing the final report.

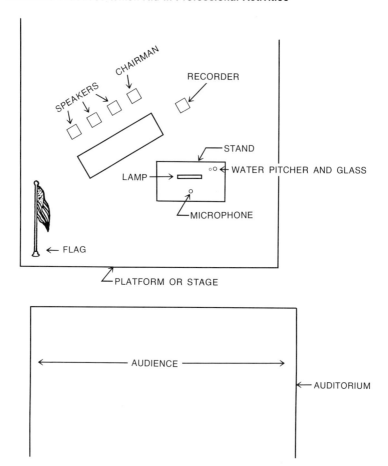

Fig. 29-2. Suggested arrangement for a symposium.

The Chairman. There are several main functions of the chairman in the actual conducting of a symposium: (1) starting the meeting promptly at the time scheduled, (2) welcoming the group, (3) introducing speakers and subject, (4) presiding over the discussion, (5) summarizing the symposium and (6) closing the meeting. All questions and comments from the audience, if it is the forum type of symposium, are held until the last speaker has concluded. In summarizing, the chairman tries to indicate points of agreement or disagreement, if any, before opening the discussion to the listeners. Sometimes the chairman appoints another person to give the summary. In either case, the resumé should be accurate and objective.

Advantages. One of the advantages of a symposium is that it provides a coordinated consideration of a question. This is especially true if the summary is well done. A disadvantage in the forum type is encountered if the symposium is permitted to continue without allowing time for discussion and a summary.

Figure 29-2 shows a suggested arrangement for a symposium.

The Debate

A debate may be planned to deal with an issue about which there are 2 commonly accepted but different points of view, or on which 2 positions have been taken. Speakers are selected to present the 2 or more opposing viewpoints. Their presentation is followed by general discussion. The purpose of a debate is to bring forth the various aspects of the differing positions and to discuss these objectively in order to: (1) arrive at a better understanding of the issue, or issues involved and (2) develop informed opinion. For this purpose, well-informed speakers should be selected who understand the point of view they espouse and who can defend their stand by a logical and objective presentation.

Dramatic Presentations

We have all experienced the feeling, while watching a good play, that the story is a real one. Sometimes we even identify with one of the characters and have the same emotional reactions as he or she does. Because of the power of dramatic presentations to give a situation a real-life quality, such devices as motion pictures, skits and role-playing sessions frequently are employed in meetings. Other devices also in use include tape recordings, television, and video-tape recordings. Dramatic presentations are best used when you wish to present several dimensions of the subject at once — factual content plus human relations and interaction.

What you may not realize is the amount of thought that has gone into the teacher's preparation for the showing. She has selected the film or video-tape with a view to its appropriateness for you at the present stage of your educational development. She has probably viewed it several times, noting down questions that might be raised in the discussion that follows its presentation. And she has not allowed its real-life quality to lure her into blind acceptance of all its details. Undoubtedly, she challenges you to spot such flaws as errors in nursing procedures. Even the best films can incorporate inaccuracies.

Practice in the use of films or video-tape in your class is the best way to prepare yourself for leading or participating in a discussion of a film at a meeting. It is very important to plan carefully for the discussion that is to follow the film or video-tape showing. Usually it is necessary to prepare your audience for the showing and to preplan the discussion. Sometimes it is useful to present, before the showing, the questions to be discussed so that thinking will be focused on the material that you wish to highlight by using the film, or the video-tape.

Here are a few suggestions regarding film or video-tape showings:

1. Use a film or video-tape only if it will help the meeting to move toward its goal; otherwise it may be a waste of time.

2. Select a film or video-tape that is not likely to have been seen by most of the audience.

3. Do not attempt to lead the discussion of a film or video-tape that you have not had opportunity to study carefully.

4. A film or video-tape cannot be expected to accomplish too much in 1 showing. Films which teach complex procedures should be reserved for small groups. Inspirational films, or films that make people aware of a problem, are more suitable for large audiences.

Skits. It would be presumptuous for anyone to tell students of nursing what a skit is or how to put one on. The students' skits are among the high points of our national conventions.

However, you may not be aware of the ways in which a skit may be used to help people to study a situation. For an example of how a skit was used in conferences of nurse educators, you might refer to the skit about a student-instructor conference in:

Elliott, F. *Viewpoints on Curriculum Development Expressed at the 1957 Curriculum Conferences of the National League for Nursing.* New York, The League, 1957. pp. 16-21.

Although this is an old skit, it exemplifies a good one. You will note that the teachers who saw this skit talk about it as if it had really happened. They discuss the ways in which the teacher was helpful to the student and how she might have been more helpful. You, as students, probably could give them the real "low-down." Do you agree with their evaluation of the teacher's behavior?

You will also note that during the first 2 conferences at which this skit was presented, no time was allotted for discussion of it. The participants did not like this. They wanted a chance to analyze and discuss it. You might read also about the provisions that were made for discussion at subsequent conferences. Which do you think helped the participants most—discussion in a general session or in small groups?

Role Playing. Role playing is another device for getting an audience to see a situation as it might occur in real life. Unlike a skit, it is not structured —that is, every detail of the actors' behavior has not been planned beforehand, and they have not been rehearsed for their parts. Instead, they are told the situation in which they are being placed and are given a thumbnail sketch about the roles and personal characteristics of the people whom they are portraying. They are urged to enter into their roles and to behave as they would if they were placed in the situation in real life.

The spontaneity of the performance makes role players feel as though they are really living through the situation. The audience, too, can be drawn into it. Sometimes the group watching the performance is divided into subgroups, each one of which is told to identify with one or more role players. In this way, each member of the audience can experience, at least vicariously, what the role player is going through, how he is feeling, what his "inside" reactions are.

Role playing can be a very effective device for bringing about an awareness that, in turn, can help people change their attitudes, emotions, and behavior. But, without expert help, this awareness may be only a vague feeling that "I've done something irritating," or "I sure have muffed this situation somehow." It can be shattering, too, to see ourselves as others see us. Many people believe that role playing should not be undertaken without the help of a person who has had experience in its use.

The Speech

We have purposely placed speech making last in the list of ways in which you may participate in a meeting, because public speaking is an art which is useful on many occasions. A knowledge of its principles will be helpful not only when you give a formal talk, but also when you give an oral report as a chairman of a committee or speak impromptu at a meeting in favor of or in opposition to some proposed measure. The essentials of effective speaking are always the same, though the technique must be adapted to the occasion. There naturally would be more preparation for a talk that you are to give as a guest speaker than is required for a committee report, while for an impromptu discussion there would be none at all.

Fundamentally, there is little difference between addressing an audience and talking with a group of friends. Public speaking is merely an enlarged conversation. The most effective speaker is not one who delivers an eloquent discourse, but rather one who talks to his audience in a natural conversational manner. He convinces them of the sincerity of his purpose and inspires them with new ideas and incentives for further thought. When you speak in public, your aim need not be to secure the complete agreement of the audience. You may intend to convince them of the wisdom of some line of thought or action, but you may be most successful if your remarks produce some dissension. Any opposition based on honest opinion should be welcomed and encouraged, since a discussion will arouse the interest of the audience and will enable you to bring out or stress points that might be overlooked otherwise. The ability to view things from more than one aspect is a rare gift and usually impresses an audience.

Preparation. Discussing points of your talk with the audience means that you must be well prepared and thoroughly acquainted with your subject. You should have an awareness of the occasion, the composition of the audience, the events immediately preceding the particular meeting, and the events to follow. Ignorance and unpreparedness are an insult to your audience and are detected easily.[1]

---

[1] This is an age when ghost-writers are sometimes used. Should you make use of a ghost-writer, you will still need to carefully plan what you want to say and talk this over with him.

Whether you are asked to speak in public often or seldom, 4 factors will determine the impression you make: appropriate material, adequate preparation, use of good illustrations and effective delivery.

One of the worst ways in the world to prepare a talk is to provide yourself with paper and pencil and sit down with the fixed intention of writing the speech in an hour or so and "getting it over with." Possibly you may write as though you were inspired, but it is more likely that your mind will remain void of suggestions. Instead, think over your subject for several days before attempting to write anything. Let your "subconscious" mind do some work too. It will if you give it time. Read what others have to say about it and decide whether you agree with them. Do not place complete confidence in what has been written already, but adopt a critical attitude toward it. Examine this material for helpfulness and integrity, and regard it as a source of new ideas and new points of view. It may be helpful to jot down some of the thoughts you have while you are reading these articles or considering your talk. A record of such observations will be useful when you begin to organize your material.

After you have spent some time in reflection and study, you are ready to begin the actual preparation. In most cases it is better to outline tentatively what you intend to say. A carefully made outline, even though tentative, helps sound, logical thinking. It also ensures those 3 fundamentals of good composition, both written and spoken — unity, coherence and emphasis — and is thus a safeguard against aimlessness.

When you have revamped the outline and are sure that it contains all your main points, practice talking the speech, using the outline as a guide. Practice in an empty room before a mirror, if possible. If you have an obliging friend ask him to listen to you and then criticize. Do this several times, with different people if possible, trying to use different wording and phrasing each time. This method of talking over the subject before an imaginary audience makes it easier for you to face the real audience and find words readily. You may find it helpful to have a few notes on cards which you can hold in your hand. These notes may include a brief outline of your topic, dates or figures that you are likely to forget, or important points that you want to be sure to include. It is frequently helpful to think through or write out the exact wording of the introduction and the conclusion ahead of time, particularly if you feel a need for developing security.

Objection may be raised that a speech prepared in this way will be rather extemporaneous and, as a result, less polished and more rambling than one that is written out entirely and memorized. However, careful planning will eliminate most of the unfavorable aspects of extemporaneous speaking, leaving unaltered the genuineness and the spontaneity in which lies its attractiveness. This is one of the best methods of preparing a talk. It is almost always fatal to memorize a speech, for it will probably appear stilted and will lack that touch of lightness and informality which attracts the audience. The danger of becoming confused and excited if you should forget a phrase or two is another drawback to this practice.

Unless you are the first speaker on a program, you often can refer to or make use in some way of something that has been mentioned by someone else. You can do this especially in your opening sentence, which plays so important a role in securing the listeners' attention.

Often a speaker is asked to submit his speech in advance of the meeting so that it can be used for publicity purposes and for publication in the proceedings of the meeting or in a journal. He should not ignore this request. Many people, including those who could not get to the meeting, may want to read about his experiences and ideas and refer to them. The fact that he has prepared a speech in writing, however, does not mean that he should read it at the meeting. He can use the outline of his written speech as the outline for his talk.

Some speakers advocate the practice of writing out the speech in full, then talking it, using the written manuscript as a guide. This method is very effective when used by accomplished speakers. It requires the knack of reading aloud in a pleasant, conversational tone, with the proper emphasis and expression, while at the same time you are looking ahead at the next few lines, and also looking at the audience. Practice is necessary to perfect this method. Also, the speech should be written for talking purposes, not for publication. We tend to use shorter words and sentences and to repeat our thoughts more often when we tell something to someone than we do when we write it. An interesting article may prove very dull and boring when it is delivered as a speech. For this reason audiences seem to have a horror of manuscripts, and the minute they see one they groan in spirit and adopt an attitude of resignation which can seriously affect your chance of success before you have said one word.

Delivery. No matter how well prepared your talk may be, no audience will remain attentive unless you are relevant and interesting. Therefore, keep in mind the interests and the attitude of the group whom you are addressing, their reasons for attending, and also your reasons for speaking.

Usually your purpose is to communicate your ideas to others, inspiring them to a certain line of thought or action. An audience rarely takes away from a speech more than 1 or 2 ideas. Therefore, it is well to let all your remarks tend to bring into focus the thoughts you want to leave. With this end in view express yourself in vivid, forceful language and concrete, familiar terms. It is a well-known fact that our interest in a subject is proportional to our knowledge of it. You can create interest in something new by associating it with something already familiar and interesting to your listeners.

If you wish to impress your audience with a particular idea, it is not enough to say it once or twice. Refer to it throughout your talk, present the thought in varying aspects, and approach it from different angles. Finally, summarize what you have said. Repetition can be overdone, of course, and care must be taken that your talk does not become a monotonous repetition of one idea. Give each repetition a new styling, creating variety of presentation.

An excellent way to hold the attention of others and to make an impression is to bring in one or two pertinent illustrations, for long after the speaker's words have slipped from the mind a graphic example, illustration, or parable recalls his message. Finding a telling illustration is well worth the time and the effort spent, because it is so useful. Another way to sustain interest and pinpoint issues is to use carefully selected visual aids in connection with your talk.

The effectiveness of your talk depends finally on the way that you give it. Courtesy demands that you talk so that you may be heard and understood without effort. Therefore, it is best to speak in a natural, conversational style, free from mannerisms. Gestures that are entirely natural and not too frequent often help to convey your meaning.

As in any conversation, try to be pleasant, alert and sincere; make your words clear-cut and distinct; look at your audience. Let your opening sentence arouse immediate interest and attention. Avoid saying, "I have come here tonight to speak to you on —"; instead, start out with some interesting or striking phase of your topic, one that will provoke instant curiosity and interest which you should try to sustain. Let your listeners feel that you actually are talking to them by frequently using the pronoun "you"; rhetorical questions beginning with "Wouldn't you —" and "Don't you think that —" are a great help in creating a personal bond between the speaker and the audience.

Do not be afraid to talk the American language; this does not mean slang, but it does include certain expressions peculiarly American and exceptionally expressive. Some people seem to think that whenever they speak they should impress the audience with their wonderful range of vocabulary, so they fill their talk with words that they would never use in ordinary conversation. Remember that your purpose in speaking is to inspire, persuade, or instruct others, not to bore them with big words. Avoid the use of superlatives and trite expressions, as well as vague, meaningless terms. Use plain talk — it is an art.

A great deal can be done to maintain interest through the proper variance of pitch, volume and speed. An effective sedative is a voice that goes on and on, pitched always the same. A change in volume is useful to express emphasis, but it should be saved for the really important points. Speaking more slowly is also a means of stressing certain ideas. Some experts say that your speed should vary from about 120 to 140 words a minute. A pause properly placed can be as effective as words. You might watch how expert speakers on TV gain attention.

There are several stratagems to overcome any feeling of fright which you may experience as an amateur. Several long, deep breaths just before you begin to speak usually quiet nervousness. You may try concentrating on someone who appears to be very bored, and forget yourself in an effort to elicit a response. Remember that most of the people in front of you are there because they are interested in the topic you are going to discuss and are eager to hear your viewpoint. See that you are well groomed and present an attractive appearance, but don't let your costume be so striking that what you wear gets more attention than what you say.

Length. It is unnecessary to mention the importance of promptness both in beginning and in concluding your talk. If you are one of several speakers, ascertain from the chairman how long you are expected to talk, and plan your material with the time in view. Some say, "Never speak beyond 45 minutes." In any kind of speech or report, brevity is always welcome and increases your popularity as a speaker. Never pad a speech. Someone has said that most people stop listening to a speaker after 15 minutes. When you have covered the points you wished to make, stop.

FOLLOW-UP OF MEETINGS

The speeches, panel discussions, group sessions and business meetings are over. In a sense, however, the meeting is still going on. You feel "filled to the brim" with it and are anxious to try out all your new ideas with your colleagues. The small group meeting or committee meeting is over, but now come the steps of interpretation and application, of action recommended, or if you represented a group, the report to them. In many instances, also, when the meeting is away from the place where you work, you know the back-homers will be expecting a report from you. No, the meeting is definitely not over yet. But the nature of your action back home will depend upon how deeply involved you became with the issue and upon how you interpret your commitment to bring your new ideas back to your colleagues at home.

Reports

Attendance at meetings may be looked upon as a real privilege, for usually you will find that you gain much more than you give. If you have been selected to represent a group, you have the responsibility: (1) to participate to the extent you can and (2) to bring back as faithful a report as you can, together with your own reactions to the meeting. Your interest and involvement in the meeting and your enthusiasm will also affect your report to your coworkers.

Kinds of Reports. The written materials that emanate from a meeting will help you to refresh your memory about it and to carry your message back home. While most of this section, and the one following, is geared to reports following attendance at conventions, conferences, or workshops, the points made are also applicable, in part, to reports following small group or committee meetings at home. These written materials might include:

    1. Committee minutes, or summaries of action taken in small group sessions.

    2. Minutes of business sessions to which are sometimes appended full reports of the officers and committees. Sometimes the reports are given to

you in a take-home packet, but the minutes probably will not be available for some time.

3. Abstracts of speeches. These may or may not be available in take-home packets.

4. Full speeches. Some of these may be available at the meeting. Others may appear later in the official journal of the organization under whose auspices the meeting was held. For others you may have to await the report of the meeting if one is issued.

5. Daily reports from small group sessions that are sometimes distributed during a meeting to further the internal communications.

6. News sheets such as *Convention Journal* and *Convention Outlook,* which the AJN Co. publishes at the biennial conventions of the ANA and the NLN.

7. Report of the meeting. This may be of several varieties, such as: the full proceedings of the meeting; a report of the recommendations made and a summary of all discussions plus those speeches which will not be published elsewhere; an account of what took place at the meeting with an interpretation of its effect on the participants as judged by their performance during the meeting and their answers to evaluation questionnaires.

The decision about what kinds of written materials will be made available is made often by the group or, if the meeting is a large important one, by a committee. If you ever serve on such a committee, you will find that the following points must be considered:

1. The usefulness of the materials for achieving the objectives of the meeting. If the main objectives of a meeting are to bring about changes in attitudes, it may be decided that written materials will contribute little to their achievement.

2. The historic importance of the meeting or some speech or session.

3. The expense of reproduction: (a) immediately and (b) after the meeting.

4. The availability of the speeches and discussions in writing or on tape recordings.

Your Responsibility for Reports. After you have wrestled with the problems involved in reports of meetings, you will understand why an organization or group sometimes cannot furnish participants with all the materials that they think they need the moment they want them. You also will be careful to do your share toward lessening the work of those who issue the reports. In particular, you will:

1. Put any records or minutes that you take in good form, and submit them promptly.

2. Write out legibly and hand to the secretary any motions that you make.

3. Send in your speech in advance of the meeting if you have been asked to do so; otherwise have a copy available to give to the secretary or recorder at the meeting. (A written speech is far less expensive to repro-

duce than is one that has to be transcribed from a tape recorder. And the good, but unwritten, unrecorded speech has caused many a reports committee to wring its collective hands.)

4. Hand in any outline or rough notes that you have made in preparation for your participation in a panel discussion.

5. Make any reports that you prepare as a recorder meaningful and legible.

Back Home Reporting. Loaded down with materials though you may be, you still have the problem of how you will make your report and get your ideas accepted by your colleagues. In some meetings there is a session at which the participants can discuss plans for reporting the meeting to those whom they represent. You may leave such a meeting eager and "raring to go." However, if you are wise, you will leaven your enthusiasm with realistic foresight. The written materials that you have will not of themselves change the attitudes of others who have not had your recent experiences. Here is some advice for you to refer to if you feel yourself becoming too starry-eyed.

1. Make haste slowly. People find it hard to change ideas, habits and procedures; be aware of this and move gently.

2. The back-home group must understand and want to change their procedures or habits before the change will really work.

3. As a participant, be prepared for some difficulties back home. You have been to a strange land, even if it was only a staff committee meeting, and the stay-at-homes are bound to be a little suspicious — perhaps envious — and they will be more so if you attended outside meetings.

4. Be careful about using the "strange language" you may have picked up at a conference — technical terms or jargon when misapplied can hurt the reception of your ideas by your colleagues.[2]

Evaluation of Meetings: Questions. Your reactions to the meeting and the reception of your ideas by your colleagues back home are, of course, of great interest to those who conducted the meeting. They will want to know, first of all, the degree to which the meeting accomplished its objectives. Did the participants arrive at reasonable, workable solutions to the problems which gave rise to the meeting? Does their apparent agreement on these solutions mean real acceptance — that is, will they try to adapt them to their problems at home? Will they be able to "sell" these solutions to the back-home group? The success of the meeting hinges on the answers to these questions. These answers also will indicate what further efforts should be made by the sponsoring organization to achieve the objectives of the meeting.

Secondly, those responsible for the meeting will want to know how it could have been improved. Was the program as a whole well planned? What sessions were most helpful to the participants? Which were least helpful? Were the physical arrangements conducive to work and study? In the

---

[2] Adapted from R. Beckhard, *How to Plan and Conduct Workshops and Conferences*, New York, Association Press, 1956, p. 62.

case of long meetings, daily evaluations of this kind may help the steering committee to make adjustments in the program and the physical environment. After the meeting, such appraisals are guides for the planning of future meetings.

Lastly, those who planned the meeting will want to know about any by-product values that were derived from it. You came to the meeting with some objectives of your own in addition to those that you shared with the other participants. Were your expectations met? Was the meeting fruitful in ways that you did not expect? The unanticipated results of a meeting sometimes can be as important as the hoped-for outcomes.

Evaluation of Meetings: Your Answers. There are several ways in which you can cooperate with the meeting planners in their search for answers to these questions. You may be asked to answer a daily reaction form and a questionnaire at the close of the meeting. Or you may be chosen for a sample 5-minute interview at which you are questioned about your satisfactions.

Give thought before answering these questions. Your first reaction may be that the most entertaining presentation was the best one; on second thought you may decide that you derived the most benefit from a less dramatic but meaty speech. You may have gained little information from the content presented in a panel discussion, but your participation has taught you something about the technique of this form that will be useful to you at home. Although you would have liked tea instead of the coffee that was served, the lack of a cup of tea did not really interfere with your work at the meeting. On the other hand, the poor ventilation in one of the rooms contributed considerably to your fatigue, and you think that planners of future meetings may want to know what a difference an air-conditioned meeting room would have made.

Then, several months after the conference another questionnaire may arrive, asking you what effects, if any, the meeting has had on your work. Again, think carefully before you answer. The purpose of the meeting may have been to show you how to train nurse aides to do simple procedures. The training methods you learned have been adopted in your hospital, and you have noticed that the patients are getting better care as a result of the improved on-the-job training program. But is this all? You seem to be getting along better with your supervisor. Could this have anything to do with that role playing session at the meeting? The supervisor in it, with whom your subgroup was asked to identify, was subjected to such terrific pressures. Maybe. . . .

Of course, there are other ways by which meetings are evaluated. Sometimes a consultant from the sponsoring organization pays a postmeeting visit to help the participant to apply her new skills. Visitors and consultants who come to your institution for other reasons are alert to signs of improvement that may have resulted from the meeting.

Regardless of the valuation devices that are used by the meeting planners, however, it is important that you reflect from time to time on what the meeting meant to you. Whenever you feel that glow of satisfaction that comes from a situation well handled, stop and say to yourself, "What has made me so smart all of a sudden? Could it have been that meeting?"

Surely, your answer will sometimes be "Yes." As the "yeses" pile up, you will begin to see how much participation in organizational work really contributes to your development as a nurse and as a person.

WRITING

One way to participate in organizational activities is through the written word. You may, of course, desire to write because you like to put your ideas on paper. However, even if you do not particularly care for writing, you will find it a useful skill, and, as you develop this skill through practice, you may "catch the writing bug." You may even choose writing as a career and eventually may earn a livelihood in that way. Nurses today are writing books on professional subjects, articles for their professional journals, and even fiction and poetry for the general public.

Opportunities

You may find it necessary to make written reports. Whenever you act as a committee chairman, you probably will have to submit a written account of the proceedings and the recommendations of the committee of which you are head. The ability to convey your ideas in clear, brief terms with vivid illustrations is important. Too many committee reports are tedious to read.

Preparing articles for newspapers and magazines affords you an excellent opportunity to show your skills as a writer. Be sure that you write about a subject with which you are quite familiar. The official professional magazines, the *American Journal of Nursing, Nursing Outlook,* and the *International Nursing Review,* the periodicals published by state nurses associations, and the independent nonofficial magazines, encourage their readers to submit articles and opinions drawn from their own experience. Also, if you have participated in any project or activity that you think would be useful to people in nursing services or schools of nursing, you might write it up and submit it to the NLN for publication in the *League Exchange.* Even though you may not be gifted with literary ability, editors of the nursing profession's magazines may be able to use your articles, especially if they are a genuine contribution to patient care and/or to the nursing profession generally.

A well-prepared nurse should be equipped to write effective content. Your training prepares you to observe thoughtfully and to record accurately, while your professional background supplies you with abundant interesting material. A frequent complaint of magazine editors is that the articles sent them by would-be authors have nothing in them worth telling. Nursing enables you to meet and study people and to encounter interesting situations, so that you have a story to tell.

To furnish you with ideas and material, if the occasion arises, it is sometimes helpful to keep a record of new activities in which you are engaged, or of out-of-the-ordinary happenings. Simple recordings of the way that certain patients respond to particular nursing activities may give you the basis of a very practical article. The practice of recording what you observe in brief, concise terms teaches precision and accuracy — qualities ranking with brilliance in their importance for good writing. It is necessary, of course, to adopt a natural, readable style for this type of writing, but this will come with practice.

Preparing a Manuscript

The following suggestions might serve you as a guide in preparing an article for a periodical. If a magazine follows any special rules, however, it is best to secure such rules from the editor. Many magazines furnish guides to the preparation of articles.

1. Use plain white paper of good quality, $8\frac{1}{2} \times 11$ inches, and number each page, preferably in the center at the top of the page.

2. Type on one side of paper only; double space; leave a wide margin on all sides.

3. Type your name and address on each sheet in the left-hand upper corner. (Some editors prefer this information in the right-hand upper corner, because this information is obscured sometimes by the paper clip and the manuscript comment clip which is attached when the manuscript is circulated for review.) On the first page in the right-hand corner, note the estimated number of words.

4. Halfway down the first page, type the title of your article and under it your name as you wish it to appear in the published article.

5. Send 2 copies of the manuscript to the editor with an appropriate letter of transmittal.

6. As a rule, a pseudonym is not desirable.

7. Make a carbon copy of your manuscript for yourself, and keep a record of the date that it was sent out and where, so that after a reasonable time you can check on it.

8. Do not fold or roll the paper; send it flat. It is important to send a clean original manuscript.

9. Use a large envelope and enclose a stamped self-addressed envelope.

10. Do not get discouraged at rejection slips. Try again! As you have seen in Chapter 24, there are a variety of nursing magazines from which to select.

Submitting a Manuscript

Knowing where to send a manuscript is as important as familiarity with the method of preparing it. Use foresight in selecting the magazines in the first place. It frequently happens that articles are never published, simply because they were sent to the wrong magazines. Familiarize yourself with the nursing periodicals, their purpose, content and style before deciding on the one to which you will submit your manuscript. Before submitting any article to a magazine, analyze it to see that there is no conflict in tone, arrangement, or material. This same approach should be used if you are considering submitting an article to a popular magazine.

Breaking into Print

If possible, question editors to find out just what kind of articles they want. This query can be in the form of a short letter with an outline of the proposed article, or just a presentation of the article idea and a request that the editor, if interested, indicate the treatment that he would like. While such a query to the editor will not guarantee that an article will be acceptable, it does save both the author's and the editor's time by giving the editor a chance to reject immediately any article suggestion which is obviously unsuitable or which simply duplicates an article the magazine, or another magazine in the same field, has printed recently.

If you are new at writing, an excellent way to start is to write your first article about something you know well. If you have been working with cardiac patients, you will know from your experience many of the important phases in nursing of such patients and certainly enough to make a tentative outline.

To broaden the content of the article, you will want to see what else has been written on the subject and what authorities in the field say about it. Some of your review of the subject can be done by talking to the doctors with whom you work. Other information can be gleaned from your co-workers and from the patients you observe and care for. Although this would be done informally, it would be interviewing. Taking notes either on the spot or recording results right after such interviewing is extremely important.

The writing itself requires that you get away by yourself and use your pencil and paper to advantage. Many suggestions have been given in this chapter about it.

How an Article Is Evaluated

No matter what kind of article you submit, or to what type of periodical you submit it, it will be examined according to form and content. Both are important. Simplicity is the keynote of form, and interest the keynote of content. Observance of the rules of grammar and punctuation and the principles of structure, together with ease and clarity of expression, will do much toward making an article acceptable.

There are few rules to follow to become a good writer. Read widely and reflect on what you read. It is impossible to read a great deal without absorbing part of what you have read. In your own writing you will reproduce unconsciously the styles of various authors, and the addition of your personal touch to this potpourri probably will result in an individual style of your own. The more you read, the better able you will be to evaluate your own work. Adopt a critical attitude toward whatever you write. Strive especially for spontaneity. Sincerity and naturalness are fundamental, and their absence is detected readily.

Try not to think of rules while you are actually writing the article, but keep them in mind while you are planning what to write and apply them as a test to the completed composition. You are more likely to write naturally and simply if you forget rules while writing.

Use the waste basket copiously until you get the content and the style you want. While a fine flow of creation is appealing and exciting, the majority of successful article writers do not submit a manuscript until they have revised it, rewritten it, and polished it to the best of their ability. Many times an editor rejects an article because, among other reasons, the thought is so disconnected and the logic so obscure that it would necessitate a complete rewriting before it could be printed. The more nurses can become aware that a term paper, be it ever so neatly footnoted, is not going to be acceptable to a magazine unless it is rewritten for magazine readers, the easier it will be to find publishers for their articles.

When you use footnotes and references, if possible follow the style of the magazine, or other acceptable style. In any case, check your footnotes and references, and any quotations you use, for accuracy.

Finally, do not hesitate to go to others for assistance. The staffs of medical centers frequently include editorial personnel and research librarians who are willing to help people like you to tell their stories in writing. Again, the editor of the professional magazine to which you submit your article may make a few changes in it. Do not resent this; be grateful for the help and try to figure out why the change was made. This will assist you to improve your style and to move further along the path of becoming a forceful and interesting writer.

PROBLEMS

1. (a) Consider some speakers whom you have heard recently and decide whether they were successful. (b) Think over their talks and list the reasons for their success or failure. (c) From these lists set up criteria by which the effectiveness of any speaker can be determined.

2. Select a topic of current interest and write an article which you hope to send to some magazine for publication. If there is a school paper, it could be given to the editor for possible publication therein.

3. (a) Determine the characteristics of a committee report. (b) Secure

copies of some reports of committees in nursing organizations, and evaluate them.

4. Find 3 reports of recent nursing conferences or workshops in your library, and evaluate them from the following standpoints: (a) their effectiveness in stimulating you, a nonparticipant, to want to do something about the problems discussed at the meeting; (b) their usefulness as source materials on the content of the meeting; (c) their helpfulness to one who is participating in making plans for a similar meeting.

5. Suppose that you have been selected by your school to be a delegate to a meeting of the National Student Nurses' Association. What should you do to fulfill your functions effectively?

6. (a) Consult some pertinent references and learn what some of the authorities say about the general characteristics of the following devices used for meetings and group work: sensitivity training, colloquy, convention, plenary session, round table, clinic, convocation, town meeting and congress. (b) If each of you selects a different device to study, you could report your findings to your class group.

7. Listen to some television interview shows such as "Meet the Press," "Face the Nation," or "Issues and Answers." Evaluate the procedure and performance of the leader and participants. What was the purpose of the interview and how well did it accomplish this purpose?

8. Make an annotated list of the latest and best resources you can locate on communications and its importance as an effective and essential aid in professional activities.

9. In what way do you think the public relations of the nursing profession could be affected if nurses wrote articles for popular magazines?

SUGGESTED REFERENCES*

GROUP WORK

* *Adult Leadership: A Periodical.* Adult Education Association of the USA, 1225 Nineteenth Street N.W., Washington, D.C.
* *Assessment of Leader Behaviors: First Regional Conference, Sigma Theta Tau, held October 17-18, 1968 in Cleveland, Ohio.* 20 Hillside Circle, Storrs, Connecticut, Sigma Theta Tau, 1969.
Beebe, J. E., *et al.* "Bench Conference in a Large Obstetric Clinic." *American Journal of Nursing,* **68**:85-87, Jan. 1968.
* Bennis, E. G., *et al. The Planning of Change.* New York, Holt, Rinehart and Winston, 1969.
* Bergevin, P. E. *Adult Education Procedures.* New York, Seabury, 1963.
Blake, R. R. and Mouton, J. S. *Group Dynamics — Key to Decision Making.* Houston, Texas. Gulf Publishing, 1961.
Bradford, L. P., *et al. T-Group Theory and Laboratory Method. Innovation on Reeducation.* New York, Wiley, 1964.

* In each chapter all citations are footnoted and are not included here. All starred references are recommended for additional reading.

Brown, B. S., *et al.* "The Role of the Leader in Formal Staff Process." *Comprenensive Psychiatry,* **8:**217-223, Aug. 1967.

Burnside, I. M. "Group Work Among the Aged." *Nursing Outlook,* **17:**68-71, June 1969.

Cartwright, D. and Zander, A. *Group Dynamics.* Evanston, Illinois, Row-Peterson, 1960.

Chase, S. *Guides to Straight Thinking.* New York, Harper, 1956.

Dabis, A. J. "Skills of Communications." *American Journal of Nursing,* **63:**66-70, Jan. 1963.

Hall, B. L. and Little, D. E. "Group Project and Learning Outcomes." *Nursing Outlook,* **17:**82-83, June 1969.

Homans, G. *Human Group.* New York, Harcourt, 1950.

"How to Succeed as a Conventioneer." *American Journal of Nursing,* **64:**116-118, June 1964.

Kron, T. *Communication in Nursing.* Philadelphia, Saunders, 1967.

Leadership in Nursing Series, Washington, D.C. Leadership Resources, 1966.

Lippitt, R., *et al. The Dynamics of Planned Change.* New York, Harcourt, Brace, 1958.

Merton, R. K. "Dilemmas of Democracy in the Voluntary Association." *American Journal of Nursing,* **66:**1055-1061, May 1966.

Miles, M. B. *Learning to Work in Groups.* New York, Bureau of Publications, Teachers College, Columbia University, 1959.

* Seashore, C. "What Is Sensitivity Training?" *NTL Institute: News and Reports,* **2(2):** Apr. 1968. Reprint can be secured from NTL Institute for Applied Behavioral Science associated with the National Education Association, 1201 Sixteenth Street, N.W., Washington, D.C. 20036.

PARLIAMENTARY LAW

Fauber, J. C. "Keeping Minutes." *American Journal of Nursing,* **55:**934-935, Aug. 1955.

"On Conducting A Meeting." *American Association of Industrial Nurses Journal,* **10:**26-29, Feb. 1962.

Roberts, H. *Roberts Rules of Order.* Old Tappan, N.J., Revell, 1967.

Scrimshaw, F. "The Parliamentarian—What She Is and What She Does." *American Journal of Nursing,* **59:**373-374, Mar. 1959.

THE WORKSHOP

Cheavens, F. *Developing Discussion Leaders in Brief Workshops.* Austin, Texas, University of Texas Printing Division, 1963.

* Creighton H. and Armington, Sister Catherine. "Workshops." *International Journal of Nursing Studies,* **5:**293-301, Dec. 1968.

* Diers, D. and Johnson, J. E. "How Workshops Prepare Nurses for the Therapeutic Role." *Nursing Outlook,* **17:**30-31, June 1969.

Fancovic, G. B. "For the Doldrums: A Workshop." *American Journal of Nursing,* **62:**100-102, Jan. 1962.

Linsky, A. S. "Why Evaluate Work Conferences?" *Nursing Outlook,* **11:**656-659, Sept. 1963.

THE SEMINAR

Bergevin, P. and Morris, D. *Group Processes for Adult Education.* 1804 East 10th St., Bloomington, Ind., Community Services in Adult Education, 1951. pp. 65-66.

Buxton, C. E. *College Teaching.* New York, Harcourt, Brace, 1956. pp. 189-193.

PANEL DISCUSSION

Auer, J. J. and Ewbank, H. L. *Handbook for Discussion Leaders.* New York, Harper, 1947. pp. 71-77.
* Bergevin, P. and Morris, D. *Group Processes for Adult Education.* 1804 East 10th St., Bloomington, Ind., Community Services in Adult Education, 1951. pp. 21-28, 40-43.
* Peplau, H. E. "Panel Discussion: A Democratic Participation Technic." *American Journal of Nursing,* **47:**334, May 1947.

THE SYMPOSIUM

* Auer, J. J. and Ewbank, H. L. *Handbook for Discussion Leaders.* New York, Harper, 1947. pp. 78-81.
Bergevin, P. and Morris, D. *Group Processes for Adult Education.* 1804 East 10th St., Bloomington, Ind., Community Services in Adult Education, 1951. pp. 29-39.

THE DEBATE

Cobb, M., *et al.* "The Pros and Cons of Formal Evaluation Conferences: A Faculty Debate." *Nursing Forum,* **4(4):**57-75, 1965.
Pender, N. J. "The Debate as a Teaching and Learning Tool." *Nursing Outlook,* **15:**42-43, Dec. 1967.

PUBLIC SPEAKING

* Anderson, V. A. *Training the Speaking Voice.* New York, Oxford University Press, 1961.
* Babcock, C. M. *The Harper Handbook of Communication Skills.* New York, Harper, 1957.
* Flesch, R. *How to Make Sense.* New York, Harper, 1954.
* Reed, E. "Don't Read Your Speech!" *American Journal of Nursing,* **55:**1212-1213, Oct. 1955.

WRITING

Benner, J. N. "Planning to Write a Manual." *Nursing Outlook,* **11:**118-120, Feb. 1963.
* Dickson, F. A. (ed.) *Handbook of Article Writing.* New York, Holt, Rinehart and Winston, 1968.
* Freeman, R. B. "The Nurse as a Writer." *Nursing Science,* **1:**156-161, Aug.-Sept., 1963.
Gilzean, E. "My Nursing Has Paid Me Twice." *Nursing Times,* **63:**1723, Dec. 22, 1967.
Gould, J. R. "Communication Through Professional Writing." *Journal of the American Dietetic Association,* **41:**315-318, Oct. 1962.
Gunning, R. *How To Take The Fog Out of Writing.* Chicago, Dartnell Corporation, 1964.
Ju.ian, F. "The Annual Report." *Nursing Outlook,* **8:**141, Mar. 1960.
A Manual of Style. Chicago, Chicago University Press, 1969.
Shannon, J. R. "Art in Writing for Educational Periodicals." *Journal of Educational Research,* **44:**599-610, Apr. 1951; **46:**333-345, Jan. 1953.
Skillin, M. and Gay, R. *Words Into Type.* New York, Appleton-Century-Crofts, 1964.
Taylor, S. D. "How to Prepare an Abstract." *Nursing Outlook,* **15:**61-63. Sept. 1967.

Turabian, K. L. *Manual for Writers of Term Papers, Theses and Dissertations.* Chicago, University of Chicago Press, 1963.
"Will Nursing Outlook Print It?" New York, *Nursing Outlook,* n.d.
"Will The Journal Print It?" New York, *American Journal of Nursing,* n.d.

DRAMATIC PRESENTATIONS

Harty, M. B. "Role-playing as a Teaching Technique." *Nursing Outlook,* **9:**563-564, Sept. 1961.
* Keaney, M. C. "Staging a Nursing Production." *Nursing Outlook,* **11:**444-446, June 1963.
Lippitt, R. "Role Playing." *American Journal of Nursing,* **53:**693-696, June 1953.
* Speroff, B. J. "Role Playing Versus Acting With Scripts." *Nursing Outlook,* **3:**377-379, July 1955.
* Williams, M. M. "Role Playing: A Teaching Method for Increasing Professional Skills." *Nursing Times,* **64:** Supplement: 32, Feb. 23, 1968.

VISUAL AIDS*

* American Nurses' Association. *Continuing Education for Nursing. Tools and Techniques.* New York, The Association, 1968.
Deegan, M., *et al.* "An Audiotutorial Approach to Learning." *Nursing Outlook,* **16:**46-48, Mar. 1968.
Griffin, G. J., *et al.* "Clinical Nursing Instruction and Closed Circuit TV." *Nursing Research,* **13:**196-204, Summer 1964.
Hornbeck, M. S. and Hornbeck, H. L. "Party Line for Nurses." *Nursing Outlook,* **16:**30-31, May 1968.
Hutchins, N. "Mediated Self-Instruction in Nursing Education." *Journal of Nursing Education,* **7:**3-8, 24-26, Apr. 1968.
Koch, H. B. "Television in Nursing Education." *Journal of Nursing Education,* **7:**37-43, Apr. 1968.
Narrow, B. W. "8mm Film Loops: An Exciting New Media for Nursing Education." *Journal of Nursing Education,* **7:**15-21, Apr. 1968.
National League for Nursing. *Audio-Visual Resources for Teaching and Learning.* New York, The League, 1965.
Reed, E. "Exhibits for Meetings: The Whats, Whys, and Hows of Successful Displays." *American Journal of Nursing,* **50:**468-469, Aug. 1950.
Reed, S. D. "The Overhead Projector and Transparencies." *Journal of Nursing Education,* **7:**9-14, Apr. 1968.
Remillet, J. G. "The 8mm Film in Student and Patient Education." *Journal of Nursing Education,* **7:**27-35, Apr. 1968.
Westley, B. H. and Hornback, M. "An Experimental Study of the Use of Television in Teaching Basic Nursing Skills." *Nursing Research,* **13:**205-209, Summer 1964.
Wilcox, J. "Adventuring with Television." *Nursing Outlook,* **10:**527-529, Aug. 1962.

---

* For information and film library list of nursing films write the Education Services Division, American Journal of Nursing Co., 10 Columbus Circle, New York, New York 10019.

APPENDIX

PART I

Reference Materials for Nurses[1]

Reference tools may serve you in 2 ways. They may supply direct information, or they may indicate the place where information is found. Encyclopedias, dictionaries, directories, almanacs and similar works are examples of the first way; bibliographies and indexes are examples of the second way.

The following is a list of a few of the most frequently used general reference tools and of some that are related particularly to nursing. No attempt is made to do more than to introduce you to these printed materials. If you desire to pursue this subject further, it is suggested that you consult the following:

Barton, Mary N. *Reference Books: A Brief Guide for Students and Other Users of the Library.* Baltimore, Enoch Pratt Free Library, 1962.
The Booklist and Subscription Books Bulletin, 1930-. Chicago, American Library Association, 1930-.
Gates, Jean K. *Guide to the Use of Books and Libraries.* New York, McGraw-Hill, 1962.
Wilson Library Bulletin. "Current Reference Books." Ed. by Frances N. Cheney. New York, Wilson. Issued monthly.
Winchell, Constance M. *Guide to Reference Books.* Chicago, American Library Association, 1967.

The following list of reference books and other reference materials is designed for the nurse, to suggest to her sources of information necessary or helpful in the effective performance of her work. Whether she gives direct care to patients, teaches students of nursing or is herself a student, administers a preservice or a graduate program of nursing education, directs the nursing service of a hospital or public health or other community agency, serves as an officer of a nursing organization, or pursues her professional functions in some other capacity, she will find useful some or all of the sources listed here.

With few exceptions, "basic" nursing, medical and related texts do not appear as individual entries; however, several bibliographies listing such

[1] Much of the material in this section is adapted from *Reference Tools For Nursing,* revised April 1968 and prepared by a Committee of the Interagency Council on Library Tools for Nursing. Revised periodically.

texts, as well as other materials, are included. Effort has been made to check the most recent sources or to consult the publishers as to editions, year and other items; however, editions are subject to change.

The selection of sources is not geared to the needs of any one type of user, either librarian or nurse. A nursing school library, the library in a university offering graduate programs in nursing, the medical library, the nursing organization headquarters office, the public library—any of these may be called on for information contained in some or all of the references on this list.

Nursing Reference Tools

"*Abstracts of Hospital Management Studies.* Ann Arbor, Michigan, University of Michigan. Published quarterly, with annual cumulations.

"Abstracts of Reports of Studies in Nursing." In *Nursing Research,* beginning in vol. 9, no. 2, 1960. Abstracts in vol. 9, no. 2 through vol. 11, no. 2, were prepared under the direction of the Institute of Research and Service in Nursing Education, Teachers College, Columbia University; beginning with vol. 11, no. 3, 1962, under the direction of the American Nurses' Foundation. Indexed by author and subjects in *Cumulative Index to Nursing Research,* vols. 1 to 12, 1952-1963. (See also *Nursing Research* annual Indexes.)

"Abstracts of Studies in Public Health Nursing, 1924-1957." In Nursing Research, 8:45-115, Spring 1959. Prepared under the direction of the Institute of Research and Service in Nursing Education, Teachers College, Columbia University. Indexed by author and subject in *Cumulative Index to Nursing Research,* vols. 1 to 12, 1952-1963. (See also *Nursing Research* annual Indexes.)

American Journal of Nursing Indexes: Annual index is published separately and available on request; sent routinely to schools of nursing. Cumulative Indexes—latest cumulation, vols. 61 to 65, 1961-1965. Earlier cumulative indexes, now out of print but available in many libraries: vols. 1 to 10, Oct. 1900-Sept. 1910; vols. 11 to 20, Oct. 1910-Sept. 1920; vols. 21 to 30, Oct. 1920-Dec. 1930; vols. 31 to 40, 1931-1940; vols. 41 to 45, 1941-1945; vols. 46 to 50, 1946-1950; vols. 51 to 55, 1951-1955; vols. 56-60, 1956-1960.

Austin, A. L., ed. *History of Nursing Source Book.* New York, Putnam, 1957.

Concordia, Sister M. *Basic Book and Periodical List for Nursing School and Small Medical Library.* LaSalle, Illinois, St. Mary's Hospital, 1967.

Cumulative Index to Nursing Literature. Glendale, Cal., Glendale Sanitarium and Hospital Publications Service, Box 871. Quarterly index to periodical literature in nursing and related fields by subject and author. Published bimonthly, with annual cumulations.

Educational Programs in Nursing. Lists published by the National League for Nursing, 10 Columbus Circle, New York, N.Y.

> *Baccalaureate and Masters Degree Programs in Nursing Accredited by the National League for Nursing.* Published annually in *Nursing Outlook.*
>
> *College-Controlled Programs in Nurse Education leading to an Associate Degree,* 1964.
>
> Collete Education: Key to a Professional Career in Nursing. Published annually.
>
> *Educational Programs Accredited for Public Health Nursing Preparation by the National League for Nursing.* 1968.
>
> *Educational Programs in Nursing Accredited by the National League for Nursing, Department of Associate Degree Programs.* Published annually in *Nursing Outlook.*
>
> *Educational Programs in Nursing Accredited by the National League for Nursing, Department of Diploma Programs.* Published annually in *Nursing Outlook.*
>
> *Let's Be Practical About a Nursing Career.* With a List of State-Approved Schools of Practical Nursing. Published annually.
>
> *Masters Education. Route to Opportunities In Modern Nursing.* Published annually.
>
> *State-Approved Schools of Nursing, L.P.N./L.V.N.* Published annually.
>
> *State-Approved Schools of Nursing, R.N.* Published annually.

Facts About Nursing. New York, American Nurses' Association. Published annually, except 1962. A statistical review.

Guide for the Development of Libraries in Schools of Nursing. New York, National League for Nursing, 1964.

Hayt, E., *et al. Law of Hospital and Nurse.* New York, Hospital Textbook Co., 1958.

International Nursing Index. New York, American Journal of Nursing Co., 10 Columbus Circle. Beginning in 1966. A cumulative quarterly index to nursing literature by subject and author. The annual cumulation also lists all nursing books published during the year and all doctoral dissertations by nurses for the year.

Lesnik, M. and Anderson, B. E. *Nursing Practice and the Law.* Philadelphia, Lippincott, 1962.

Library Handbook for Schools of Nursing. New York, National League for Nursing, 1953. Classification schedule designed for nursing and related literature; subject heading list; library organization and administration.

Medical Care Review. Succeeded *Public Health Economics and Medical Care Abstracts.* Ann Arbor, Michigan, Bureau of Public Health Economics, School of Public Health, University of Michigan. Published monthly, except September.

Nursing Outlook Indexes:

   Annual Index. Published in Dec. issue from 1957 to 1967. Available upon request beginning in 1968 and sent routinely to school of nursing libraries.

   Cumulative Indexes. vols. 1 to 5, 1953-1957, vols. 6 to 10, 1958-1962.

Nursing Research Indexes:

   Annual Index. Published in final issue of each volume.

   Cumulative Index. vols. 1 to 12, 1952-1963. In 3 parts. *Part 1.* Index to Articles, Briefs, Research Reporter and Researcher's Bookshelf; *Part 2.* Index to Abstracts, 1959-1963; *Part 3.* Alphabetical subject list of Studies in Nursing (summaries), 1954-1959. New York, American Journal of Nursing Co., 1964. (The studies indexed in Part 3 consist mainly of those carried out by nurses at colleges and universities in the USA in partial fulfillment of the requirements for Master's and Doctoral degrees.)

Nursing Studies Index. By V. Henderson, *et al.* vol. 3, 1950-1956; vol. 4, 1957-1959. Philadelphia, Lippincott, 1963. A retrospective annotated guide to reported studies, research in progress, research methods and historical materials. Prepared by the Yale University School of Nursing index staff under direction of Miss Henderson. Four volumes are planned, covering the period 1900-1959.

Nursing Thesaurus. Issued annually as Part 2 of the No. 1 issue of the *International Nursing Index.* New York, American Journal of Nursing Co.

Nutting, M. A. and Dock, L. L. *History of Nursing.* New York, Putnam, 1907-1912. 4 vols. (vols. 3 and 4 were edited and in part written by Miss Dock.) Out of print, but available in many libraries. Especially valuable for earlier history and the comprehensive bibliography.

Official Directories. The *American Journal of Nursing* and *Nursing Outlook* each carry an Official Directory twice a year (of nursing and related organizations, including Federal and state governmental bureaus, departments—their officers and personnel, and other information). Consult the table of contents of any issue of these periodicals to discover which issues contain the directory. See also entries under *Hospital Progress* and *Hospitals:* "Guide Issue."

Lists of educational programs for nurses are found in the annual indexes of the *American Journal of Nursing* and *Nursing Outlook* and also in the *Catholic Hospital Association Directory,* the *Education Index* and the "Guide Issue" of *Hospitals.*

Reports and proceedings of conventions: Among the best ways to keep up to date on recent and authoritative materials is to review reports and proceedings of conventions. It is suggested that you note the nursing and allied associations that issue volumes of annual proceedings. These annual or biennial publications include reports and papers on problems and trends discussed at the yearly or periodical conventions of the organizations concerned. There follows a list of 5 important publications of this nature and the addresses of the organizations from which they can be secured:

Annual Reports of the National League of Nursing Education. Volumes 1 to 56 (1897-1952) are available in many nursing libraries. They were discontinued in 1952 when the NLNE became part of the NLN.

Biennial Reports of the National League for Nursing. 10 Columbus Circle, New York, National League for Nursing. Issued biennially.

National Reports of Member Associations. 37, rue de Vermont, 1202 Geneva, Switzerland, The International Council of Nurses. Issued quadrennially.

Proceedings of the American Hospital Association. 18 East Division St., Chicago, American Hospital Association. Issued annually.

Proceedings of Biennial Convention of the American Nurses' Association. 10 Columbus Circle, New York, American Nurses' Association. Issued biennially.

Roberts, M. M. *American Nursing:* History and Interpretation. New York, Macmillan, 1954.

Sarner, H. *Nurse and the Law.* Philadelphia, Saunders, 1968.

Studies in Nursing (Clearing House List). New York, American Nurses' Association, 1950-1955. Supplements: 1955-1956; 1957-1958; 1959-1961.

The Yearbook of Modern Nursing. Ed. by M. Cordelia Cowan. New York, Putnam, 1956; 1957-1958 (out of print but available in some libraries); 1959.

General Reference Works

American Catholic Who's Who. Detroit, Walter Romig, 1934/35. Biennial.

Bartlett, John. *Familiar Quotations.* 13th ed. Boston, Little, Brown, 1955.

The Bible. King James, Douay, or Modern Version and the Confraternity-Douay version of the Old Testament and the New Testament, Confraternity Edition, and *The Jerusalem Bible,* published by Doubleday in 1968.

Biography Index: A Cumulative Index to Biographical Material in Books and Magazines, 1946-. New York, Wilson, September 1946-.

Catholic Periodical Index, 1930-. New York, The Catholic Library Association, 1939-.

Cumulative Book Index. New York, Wilson, 1933-. Published monthly, except July and August.

Dictionary of Education. Ed. by Carter V. Good. New York, McGraw-Hill, 1959.

Doris, L. and Miller, B. M. *Complete Secretary's Handbook.* Englewood Cliffs, New Jersey, Prentice-Hall, 1960.

Education Index. New York, Wilson, monthly, except July and August. A cumulated index to materials in the fields of curriculum, educational administration, adult education, guidance and other areas.

Encyclopaedia Britannica. Chicago, Encyclopaedia Britannica, Inc. 24 vols. Continuous revision.

Encyclopedia Americana. New York, Americana Corp. Continuous revision.

Encyclopedia of Associations. Detroit, Gale Research Co., 2200 Book Tower, 1968. vol. 1, National Associations of the U.S. Revised periodically.

Foundation Library Center, *Foundation Directory.* New York, Russell Sage, 1967.

Home Book of Quotations, Classical and Modern, Ed. by B. E. Stevenson. New York, Dodd-Mead, 1967.

Hutchinson, L. I. *Standard Handbook for Secretaries.* New York, McGraw-Hill, 1956.

Kane, J. N. *Famous First Facts.* New York, Wilson, 1964.

Lincoln Library of Essential Information. Buffalo, N.Y., Frontier Press, 1963.

Rand McNally New Cosmopolitan Atlas. Chicago, Rand McNally, 1968.

Readers' Guide to Periodical Literature. New York, Wilson, semi-monthly, September-June; monthly, July and August.

Robert, H. M. *Robert's Rules of Order.* Old Tappan, N.J.,, Revell, 1967.

Roget, P. M. *Roget's International Thesaurus.* New York, Crowell, 1962.

Scientific and Technical Societies of the U.S. and Canada. Washington, D.C., National Academy of Sciences—National Research Council, 1968.

Social Sciences and Humanities Index. New York, Wilson. Quarterly guide to periodical literature in the social sciences and humanities, formerly the *International Index.*

Turabian, K. L. *Manual for Writers of Term Papers, Theses and Dissertations.* Chicago, University of Chicago Press, 1967.

Ulrich's Periodical Directory, 2 vols. New York, Bowker, 1967-1968.

United States Catalogue, New York, Wilson, 1928.

U.S. Census Bureau. *Historical Statistics of the United States, Colonial Times to 1957.* A Statistical Abstract supplement. Washington, D.C., U.S. Government Printing Office, 1960. A statistical summary of American social and economic development. Includes, among other data, figures for births and deaths, housing, education, immi-

gration, population, prices, wages and hours, wealth and income.
———. *Statistical Abstract of the United States*. Washington, D.C., U.S. Government Printing Office. Published annually.

U.S. Government Organization Manual. Washington, D.C., U.S. Government Printing Office. Published annually.

US. Interdepartmental Committee on the Status of Women. *American Women 1963-1968*. Washington, D.C. U.S. Government Printing Office, 1968.

U.S. Office of Education. *Education Directory*. Washington, D.C., U.S. Government Printing Office. Published annually. In 4 parts. Part 3, *Higher Education,* lists all institutions of higher learning in the USA that meet certain requirements as to accreditation; names officers, department heads and accrediting bodies; and specifies types of programs offered, including nursing.

U.S. President's Commission on the Status of Women. *American Women*. Washington, D.C., U.S. Government Printing Office, 1963. Data on life span of American women, employment, education, marriage and other information.

Vanderbilt, A. *Amy Vanderbilt's New Complete Book of Etiquette*. New York, Doubleday, 1963.

Webster's New Dictionary of Synonyms. Springfield, Mass., Merriam, 1968.

Webster's Seventh New Collegiate Dictionary. Springfield, Mass., Merriam, 1967.

Webster's Third New International Dictionary. Springfield, Mass., Merriam, 1961.

Who's Who in America. Chicago, Marquis, revised and reissued biennially.

Who's Who in American Education, Ed. by R. C. Cook, Nashville, Tenn., Who's Who in American Education, 1928-, biennial.

Who's Who in the East. (Middle Atlantic and Northeastern States and Eastern Canada.) Chicago, Marquis, 1943-, biennial.

Who's Who of American Women. Chicago, Marquis, revised biennially.

World Almanac. New York, World-Telegram and Sun. Published annually.

Yearbook of International Organizations. Brussels, Union of International Associations, revised annually.

Reference Tools in Medical, Paramedical and Basic Sciences

Abstract Journals. Many journals limit their content to abstracts of the literature in the fields of medicine and the related sciences. The most comprehensive of these is *Excerpta Medica*. Others are *Biological Abstracts, Chemical Abstracts, Nutrition Abstracts* and *Psychological Abstracts,* to name but a few. For a more complete listing and the sources, see "Basic Reference Aids For Small Medical Libraries," *Bulletin of the Medical Library Association,* **55:**160-175, Apr. 1967. See also *Hospital Abstracts.* Abstracts also appear in many health science journals.

American Medical Association. *Current Medical Terminology.* Chicago, The Association, 1966.

———. *Standard Nomenclature of Disease and Operations.* Ed. by E. Thompson and A. C. Hayden. New York, Blakiston, McGraw-Hill, 1961.

———. Council on Drugs. *New and Non-Official Drugs.* Philadelphia, Lippincott. Published annually.

American Medical Directory. Chicago, American Medical Association. Published biennially.

American Men of Science. 5 vols. Physiologic and biologic sciences: vols. A to E and F to K, 1960; vols. L to R and S to Z, 1961. Sociologic and behavioral sciences, 1962. Tempe, Arizona, Jaques Cattell Press.

"Basic Reference Aids For Small Medical Libraries." Rev. by E. D. Blair. *Bulletin of the Medical Library Association,* **55:**160-175, Apr. 1967.

Catholic Hospital Association Directory. 1438 So. Grand Blvd., St. Louis, Catholic Hospital Association. Published annually.

Cumulated Index Medicus. Chicago, American Medical Association, vols. 1, 2 and 3, 1960, 1961 and 1962, out of print but available in many libraries. vol. 4, 1963. Annual cumulation of *Index Medicus,* new series, published by the National Library of Medicine, Bethesda, Md. Author and subject volumes.

Cumulative Index of Hospital Literature. Chicago, American Hospital Association, 1945-1949, 1950-1954 (out of print but available in many libraries), 1955-1959, 1960-1965.

Current List of Medical Literature. Bethesda, Md., National Library of Medicine, vols. 1 to 36, 1941-1959. No longer published but available in many libraries; replaced by *Index Medicus,* new series.

Directory of Medical Specialists, Chicago, Marquis, vol. 11, 1963-1964.

U.S. Dispensatory and Physician's Pharmacology. Ed. by A. Osol, *et al.* Philadelphia, Lippincott, 1967.

Drugs of Choice, 1968-1969. Ed. by Walter Modell, St. Louis, Mosby, 1968.

Facts on the Major Killing and Crippling Diseases in the U.S. Today. 135 E. 42nd St., New York, National Health Education Committee. Published annually.

Federal Advisory Council on Medical Training Aids. *Film Reference Guide for Medicine and Allied Sciences.* Washington, D.C., U.S. Government Printing Office. Revised annually. Comprehensive list of films on medical, surgical, nursing and related subjects; well indexed.

Garrison, F. H. *History of Medicine.* Philadelphia, Saunders, 1929. Reprinted 1960.

Goodale, R. E. *Clinical Interpretation of Laboratory Tests.* Philadelphia, Davis, 1964.

Health Economics Studies Information Exchange. Loose-leaf, 1965-. Medical Care Administration. U.S. Public Health Service. Succeeds *Inventory of Social and Economic Research in Health* which ceased publication in 1965.

Health Organizations of the United States and Canada: National, Regional and State. Ithaca, N.Y. Cornell University, Graduate School of Business and Public Administration, 1961-.

Hospital Abstracts. H. M. Stationery Office, P. O. Box 569, London, S.E.1, England. Published monthly, from 1961. Survey of world hospital literature, prepared by the Ministry of Health and covering whole field of hospitals and their administration, with special section for nursing staff.

Hospital Literature Index. Chicago, American Hospital Association, quarterly. Annual cumulation with the fourth issue.

Hospital Purchasing File. 1050 Merchandise Mart, Chicago, Hospital Purchasing Files, Inc. Published annually. (Controlled distribution.)

Hospitals. "Guide Issue." Part 2 of Aug. 1 issue of *Hospitals,* Journal of the American Hospital Association, Chicago, American Hospital Association, annually.

Medical Dictionaries and Word Books:

American Psychiatric Association. Committee on Public Information. *Psychiatric Glossary.* 1700 18th St., N.W., Washington, D.C., The Association, 1964.

Blakiston's New Gould Medical Dictionary. Ed. by N. L. Hoerr and A. Osol. New York, Blakiston, McGraw-Hill, 1956.

Current Medical Terminology. Ed. by B. L. Gordon. Chicago, American Medical Association. Published annually.

Dorland's Illustrated Medical Dictionary. Ed. by L. B. Arey, *et al.* Philadelphia, Saunders, 1965.

English, H. B. and English, A. C. *Comprehensive Dictionary of Psychological and Psychoanalytical Terms.* New York, McKay, 1958.

Frenay, Sister M. Agnes Clare. *Understanding Medical Terminology.* 1438 So. Grand, St. Louis, Catholic Hospital Association, 1969.

Hinsie, L. E. and Campbell, R. J. *Psychiatric Dictionary.* New York, Oxford, 1960.

Pepper, O. H. P. *Medical Etymology.* Philadelphia, Saunders, 1949. (The history and derivation of medical terms.)

Skinner, H. A. L. *Origin of Medical Terms.* Baltimore, Williams & Wilkins, 1961.

Stedman, T. L. *Medical Dictionary.* Baltimore, Williams & Wilkins, 1966.

Medical Library Association. *Handbook of Medical Library Practice.* Third edition by Gertrude L. Annan and Jacqueline W. Felter. 919 N. Michigan Ave., Chicago, Medical Library Association, 1970.

Merck Index of Chemicals and Drugs. Rahway, N.J., Merck & Co. 1968.

Merck Manual of Diagnosis and Therapy. Rahway, N.J. Merck & Co. 1966.

Modern Drug Encyclopedia and Therapeutic Index. New York. Reuben Donnelley Corp., 1970. Quarterly supplements for two years.

National Library of Medicine. *Bibliography of Medical Reviews.* Bethesda, Md., The Library. Published annually.

_____. *Biomedical Serials, 1950-1960.* Washington, D.C., U.S. Government Printing Office, 1962.

_____. *Index Medicus.* Washington, D.C., U.S. Government Printing Office. Published monthly from 1960. Subject and author index to articles selected from more than 2,300 medical and related journals, including some nursing periodicals.

_____. "Medical Subject Headings." Part 2, Jan. issue of *Index Medicus.* Washington, D.C., U.S. Government Printing Office.

Pearsall, M. *Medical Behavioral Science: A Selected Bibliography of Cultural Anthropology, Social Psychology, and Sociology in Medicine.* Lexington, Ky., University of Kentucky Press, 1963.

Physicians' Desk Reference to Pharmaceutical Specialties and Biologicals. Oradell, N.J., Medical Economics. Published annually.

Quarterly Cumulative Index Medicus. Old series, vols. 1 to 12, 1916-1926, new series, vols. 1 to 60, 1927-1956. Chicago, American Medical Association. Out of print but available in many libraries.

U.S. Department of Health, Education, and Welfare. *Health, Education, and Welfare Trends.* Washington, D.C., U.S. Government Printing Office. Published annually.

_____. *Medical and Health Related Thesaurus.* Washington, D.C., U.S. Government Printing Office, 1963.

_____. National Vital Statistics Division. *Vital Statistics of the United States.* Washington, D.C., U.S. Government Printing Office. Published annually. Official data on births, deaths, marriages and divorces. Current bound volumes cover the year 1961 as follows: vol. I. Natality; vol. II. Mortality—part A and part B: vol. III. Marriage and Divorce.

World Health Organization. *Catalog of Publications.* 2960 Broadway, New York, New York, International Documents Service, Columbia University Press. Published periodically.

_____. *International Classification of Diseases.* 1965 revision. Geneva, W.H.O. 1967.

PART 2

A Suggested Form for Minutes

The following outline of "A Suggested Form for Minutes of an Alumni Association" has been adapted from Ada K. Gannon's *Thumb Prints of Parliamentary Points*.[1] Although this form has been designed for an alumni association, it will be useful as a guide to secretaries of any type of organization. The annual meeting has been selected for the sample because it includes election of officers and other additional procedures not usually included in the ordinary meeting.

It is suggested that the secretary keep the minutes on the right-hand page of the minute book. The left-hand page is reserved for corrections, insertions, amendments to minutes, or any other important notations. A wide margin for reference and index is suggested for the inside of the right-hand page.

It is customary for every society having a permanent existence to adopt an order of business or agenda for its meetings. When no rule has been adopted, the order suggested by the parliamentary authority which is recognized by the association as its guide is followed.

*Margin for Reference
and Index*

PLACE AND TIME

The . . . School Alumni Association, Columbus, Ohio, met in regular session in the School of Nursing Auditorium, Tuesday, January, 2, 19 — — , at 2:30 P.M.

PRESIDING

Miss Ruth Allen, President, in the Chair.

SECRETARY

Miss Mary Hamilton, Secretary.

ROLL CALL
(See A.R.C. Page 3
Col. 5)[2]

Roll Call, 102 present, 30 absent.

[1] A. K. Gannon, *Thumb Prints of Parliamentary Points,* 518 Victoria Building, St. Louis, Mo., 1934, pp. 27-28. Out of print.
[2] A.R.C. means — Attendance Roll Call.

*Margin for Reference
and Index*

MINUTES OF PREVIOUS MEETING	Minutes of previous meeting, held on November 4, 19— —, were read, corrected and approved.
MINUTES OF BOARD OF DIRECTORS	Minutes of the meeting of the Board of Directors, held immediately preceding this meeting, were read.[3]

REPORTS OF OFFICERS

ANNUAL REPORT OF SECRETARY	The Secretary presented the following annual report. (Insert report.)
Filed: Officer's Reports	Moved by Miss B., and seconded, that the annual report of the Secretary be accepted.[4]
ANNUAL REPORT OF TREASURER	The Treasurer presented the following annual report. (Insert Treasurer's audited report.)
Filed: Officer's Reports	Moved by Miss C., and seconded, that the annual report of the Treasurer, as audited, be accepted.[5] Motion carried.[6]

REPORTS OF STANDING
COMMITTEES

MEMBERSHIP AND CREDENTIALS	ˌThe Chairman of the Committee on Membership and Credentials presented the following annual report. (Insert report.)
Filed: Committee Reports	Moved by Miss S., and seconded, that the annual report of the Committee on Membership and Credentials be accepted and the recommendations adopted.[7]

[3] Board minutes are approved in Board meetings.

[4] The name of seconder is not entered in the minutes and he may talk against the motion he seconded and vote against it. The one who offers the motion may not talk against his own motion, though he may vote against it.

[5] The treasurer does not move that his own report be accepted; also a treasurer's report is never accepted until it has been audited.

[6] Reports of other officers may be included here. If so, they should be given in order of rank.

[7] Move to accept a report. Move to adopt recommendations. If recommendations are other than pertinent to "credentials"—i.e., embodying new business—recommendations should be referred to "new business" in agenda for adoption.

Margin for Reference
and Index

PROGRAM AND
ARRANGEMENTS

Filed: Committee
Reports

PUBLIC RELATIONS

Filed: Committee
Reports

REVISION OF BYLAWS

Filed: Committee
Reports

The Chairman of the Committee on Program and Arrangements presented the following annual report.
(Insert report.)

Moved by Miss R., and seconded, that the annual report of the Committee on Program and Arrangements be accepted.
Motion carried.

The Chairman of the Committee on Public Relations presented the following annual report.
(Insert report.)

Moved by Miss D., and seconded, that the annual report of the Committee on Public Relations be accepted. Recommendations referred to new business on agenda.
Motion carried.

The Chairman of the Committee on Revision of Bylaws presented the following report.
(Insert report, which includes statement that proposed revisions have been prepared by the Committee and copies of same sent to each member of the association. Include revisions proposed, also.)

Miss D., Chairman of the Committee on the Revision of Bylaws, read the report of the Committee on Revision of Bylaws.[8]

Moved by Miss K., and seconded, that Article I of the Bylaws be amended by striking out the words " . . . " and inserting the words " . . . "
Motion carried.

Moved by Miss R., and seconded, that Article III, Section 2, of the Bylaws, be amended by substituting the words " . . . " in lieu of the words " . . . "
Motion carried.

[8] The Chair presents each article to be revised.

*Margin for Reference
and Index*

Moved by Miss D. that the proposed revision of the Bylaws be adopted as amended.[9]
Motion carried.

LEGISLATION

The Chairman of the Committee on Legislation presented the following report.
(Insert report.)

Filed: Committee
Reports

Moved by Miss G., and seconded, that the annual report of the Committee on Legislation be accepted.
Motion carried.

NOMINATIONS

The Chairman of the Committee on Nominations presented the following report.
(Insert the report, including the proposed ticket.)

Filed: Committee
Reports

Moved by Miss E., and seconded, that the report of the Committee on Nominations be accepted.
Motion carried.
The Chair called for nominations from floor.[10]
Miss J. nominated Miss O. for president.
Miss T. nominated Miss N. for treasurer.
The Chair instructed the Secretary to see that the names of the nominees were placed on the ballots in their respective places.
Moved by Miss R., and seconded, that nominations be closed.[11]
Motion carried.

COMMUNICATIONS

The Secretary presented communications from the following.

Filed and referred to
Committee on Legislation and Books.

Letter from the Honorable Mr. James Brown, *re* current legislation on funds for nursing education.

Filed and referred to
Committee on
Scholarships.

Miss Emily Robertson, Director of . . . School of Nursing, *re* scholarships.
Correspondence referred to proper committees.

[9] When all articles have been considered, the main motion on the adoption of the total Bylaws is considered and acted upon. Therefore, action on the main motion is recorded at the end.
[10] The Chairman must always call for other nominations from the floor.
[11] If other nominations are made from the floor, the names are included in the proper place on the ballot.

*Margin for Reference
and Index*

MEMBERSHIP CARDS

Moved by Miss A., and seconded, that each member be requested to present her membership card at each meeting.

Moved by Miss L., and seconded, to table.

Motion carried.

SCHOLARSHIP
CONTRIBUTION

Moved by Miss C., and seconded, that we give $200 to the Nurses' Educational Funds, Inc., as a contribution for scholarships.

Moved by Miss F., and seconded, to amend by striking out $200 and inserting $250.

Amendment carried.

Motion as amended carried.[12]

ORIENTAL TEA

Moved by Miss Z., and seconded, that we have an Oriental Tea for the special book fund.

Moved by Miss R., and seconded, to amend by adding the words "on Easter Monday."

Amendment carried.

Moved by Miss L., and seconded, to amend by striking out the words "Oriental Tea" and inserting the words "card party."

Amendment not carried.[13]

Motion as amended, that we have an Oriental Tea on Easter Monday, carried.

Chair appointed a committee of three to complete arrangements for the tea: Miss Z., Miss R., and Miss C.

SAMUEL E. BROWN

Moved by Miss C., and seconded, that we endorse Samuel E. Brown for mayor of...

Objection raised by Chair to consideration of question.

Objection sustained by two-thirds *no* vote.

Chair ruled "Politics" a forbidden question.

Appeal from decision of the Chair offered by Miss X.

Chair sustained.

[12] There are five methods of amending: (1) by striking out a certain word or words, (2) by inserting or adding certain word or words, (3) by striking out and inserting certain word or words, (4) by substituting and (5) by dividing the question.

[13] Motions not carried are just as important as those which are carried and must always be recorded in the minutes.

Secret ballot method of voting was used for the election of officers and directors.

The Chair appointed as Committee on Elections: Miss D., Mrs. A., Miss J.[14]

Miss D., the Chairman of the Committee on Elections, read the following report.

REPORT OF COMMITTEE ON ELECTIONS[15]

Total number of ballots cast 102
Number required to elect 53
Illegal ballots 2
Legal ballots 100
Required to elect 51
President — Miss C. received 52
              Miss E. received 40
              Miss O. received 8
First Vice-President
              Miss X. received 60
              Miss L. received 40
Second Vice-President
              Miss G. received 25
              Miss F. received 75
Secretary
              Miss R. received 30
              Miss T. received 70
Treasurer
              Miss Z. received 80
              Miss H. received 4
              Miss N. received 16
Directors
              Miss A. received 20
              Miss I. received 80

Moved by Miss D., and seconded, that the report of the Committee on Elections be accepted.

Motion carried.

---

[14] The Committee on Elections is sometimes referred to as tellers. Candidates may not be tellers.

[15] Tellers should count every ballot and report every vote.

*Margin for Reference
and Index*

NEW OFFICERS

The Chair declared the following elected.[16]
(Include names of those elected to the various offices.)

DESTROYING OF
BALLOTS

Moved by Mrs. A., a member of Committee on Elections, and seconded, that the ballots be destroyed.
Motion carried.

ADJOURNMENT

Moved by Miss D., and seconded, that we adjourn.
Motion carried.
Meeting adjourned at 4:30 P.M.

Ruth Allen, R.N.
(Miss) Ruth Allen, R.N.
President

Mary Hamilton, R.N.
(Miss) Mary Hamilton, R.N.
Secretary

PROGRAM

An address on " . . . ," was given by Mrs. R. T. C. . . . of . . . .
Vocal solos were given by Miss E. L. and Miss A. D.

---

[16] The chairman does not declare her own election. This may be done by the vice-president or secretary.

Index

Page numbers in *italics* indicate illustrations. Page numbers followed by the letter "t" indicate tabular material, and page numbers followed by the letter "n" indicate material in footnotes.